EDUCATIONAL AUDIOLOGY HANDBOOK

A Singular Audiology Text
Jeffrey L. Danhauer, Ph.D.
Audiology Editor

EDUCATIONAL AUDIOLOGY HANDBOOK

Cheryl DeConde Johnson, Ed.D.
Colorado Department of Education and Greeley-Evans School District 6
Greeley, Colorado

Peggy V. Benson, Ed.S.
Educational Audiology Consultant
Manassas, Virginia

Jane B. Seaton, M.S.
Seaton Consultants
Athens, Georgia

SINGULAR
™
THOMSON LEARNING

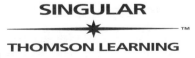

Africa • Australia • Canada • Denmark • Japan • Mexico • New Zealand • Philippines
Puerto Rico • Singapore • Spain • United Kingdom • United States

NOTICE TO THE READER

COPYRIGHT © 1997 Delmar. Singular Publishing Group is an imprint of Delmar, a division of Thomson Learning. Thomson Learning™ is a trademark used herein under license.

Printed in the United States of America
3 4 5 6 7 8 XXX 03 02 01 00

For more information, contact Singular Publishing Group, 401 West "A" Street, Suite 325 San Diego, CA 92101-7904; or find us on the World Wide Web at http://www.singpub.com

For permission to use material from this text or product contact us by
Tel (800) 730-2214; Fax (800) 730-2215; www.thomsonrights.com

Library of Congress Cataloging-in-Publication Data

Johnson, Cheryl DeConde.
    Educational audiology handbook / Cheryl Deconde Johnson, Peggy
V. Benson, Jane B. Seaton.
       p.   cm.
    Includes bibliographical references and index.
    ISBN 1-56593-8232
    1. Audiology. 2. Hearing impaired children—Services for
I. Benson, Peggy V. II. Seaton, Jane B. III. Title.
RF291.5 C45J64 1997
618.92' 0978—dc21   97-11045
                               CIP

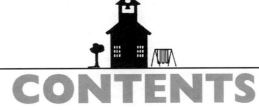

CONTENTS

References   513

Index   519

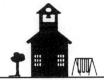

PREFACE

This handbook represents the culmination of our experiences as educational audiologists—a combination of more than seventy years. We have collected and consolidated the best of the information we have learned in a format we hope is practical and easy to use. This handbook is not meant to provide comprehensive information in the traditional areas of audiology because volumes have already been written elsewhere. However, we have included several topics which are unique to our school environments and not found in other audiology texts. Our goal is to provide the reader with information that is essential to the practice of audiology in the school setting.

How to Use This Handbook

The main text of this handbook is divided into sections which reflect basic practice areas, relations with others, and program effectiveness. Educational audiologists often find that in the school environment, they need to focus more on the application of audiology practices than on the audiology skills themselves. Therefore, this text emphasizes areas and material which should be helpful in achieving more effective practices.

Since the responsibilities of educational audiologists and formats of programs vary, we have chosen to introduce topic areas by chapters organized into subcategories. Chapters usually begin with a list of questions that can assist in the development and implementation of the task under consideration. Although we offer our suggestions as "best practice" solutions to many of those questions, educational audiologists should seek input from others as well as derive answers from their own experiences.

The Appendixes are a significant portion of this handbook. They are divided into sections that correspond with the chapter numbers and correlating content. Each Appendix section begins with a Contents page, which also indicates materials that are available on computer disk which is available for separate purchase.

The computer disk contains forms and handouts that the user can download and add local identifying information, such as school name, if desired. Material created by the authors is identified with the handbook, title, authors, and publishers, which should remain at the bottom of the page to retain the original identification. Further computer disk instructions are included on the computer disk contents.

Terminology

For ease in flow of reading we have used the following terms interchangeably: children/students, hearing impairments/deaf and hard-of-hearing, case manager/service coordinator, and educational audiologist/school-based audiologist. In addition, the term aural (re)habilitation was used to include both habilitation and rehabilitation.

Photography (by Cheryl DeConde Johnson)

Capturing the individual chapter concepts in a photograph would be difficult. Instead we focused on the people—the children, the parents, the teachers, and the other professionals—we touch through our work as educational audiologists. Although the impact of our involvement with these individuals may not always be readily apparent or acknowledged, we should never underestimate the influence that we can have in the lives of the children, and those associated with the children, with whom we work. We hope that these photographs will be a reminder to you of the children and other individuals we meet and assist every day.

Acknowledgments

We would like to recognize all educational audiologists. Without your dedication to provide the highest quality audiology services in schools many children would be unable to realize their full potential for hearing and learning in school. Our future is not only in the identification and treatment of children with hearing problems but also in supporting a quality listening and learning environment for all children.

To all of our educational audiology colleagues who have shared their insights, expertise, and materials with us, we thank you. We could not imagine a more satisfactory setting to practice audiology than the schools, and there could not be a greater group of professionals and friends with whom to work.

Finally, we would like to acknowledge our families, especially our husbands, Roger Johnson, Serge Benson, and Hal Seaton, who provided endless support and encouragement as well as back rubs, pizza, and M & Ms during the course of this project.

C.D.J., P.B., & J.S.

OPTIONAL COMPUTER DISK

As an optional feature of this Handbook, computer disks may be purchased which contain forms and handouts from the text appendixes. These documents are contained in two disks representing Macintosh (MAC) and PC-Windows formats. The disk feature provides the user the advantage of printing original copywork as well as the flexibility to adapt the documents with program or school names. Users are asked to retain the book title, authors, and publisher printed at the bottom to maintain the original identity with the Handbook.

Materials which are authored by others should not be adapted unless permission of the original authors is obtained.

Prior to using the disks, copy the contents to a separate disk to use as the working file. The contents of the disks are listed below. All documents were originally developed in MAC format. Due to difficulties translating to PC-Windows, some documents are not available in the PC format.

CONTENTS

APPENDIX TITLE

EDUCATIONAL AUDIOLOGY PRACTICES

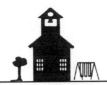

CHAPTER I

EDUCATIONAL AUDIOLOGY

How Did We Get Here?

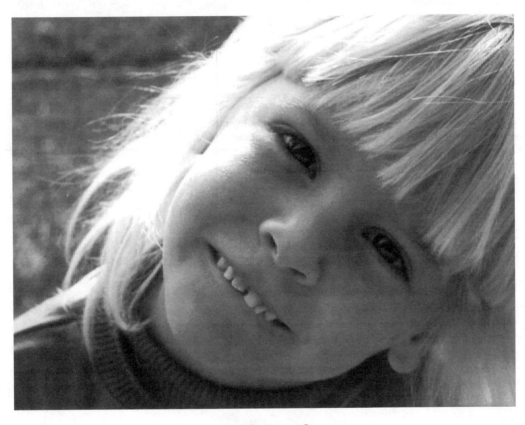

Jennifer at age 5

CONTENTS

Educational audiology continues to represent one of the most challenging and rewarding practice areas of our profession. The challenge is in reconciling the sheer numbers of children and their diverse needs with insufficient support, equipment, money, and staff to meet those needs. The reward is the opportunity to make a difference in a child's life every day.

What are some of the challenges facing audiologists in educational settings?

➤ A large in-school population—about 42,933,325 children ages 6–17 years in the United States based on the July 1993 census (U.S. Department of Education, 1994b).
➤ A large out-of-school population—about 11,921,381 children who are in the birth—2 age group, 11,312,565

children ages 3–5, and 14,609,114 individuals who are 18–21 years of age (U.S. Department of Education, 1994b). From these populations, children with hearing impairments must be identified, and appropriate services must be provided to all but the birth to 2-year-old children in most states.
➤ A consistently growing percentage of children and youth served by special education and related serves (4.5% reported in 1976–77 to 6.4% reported in 1992–93 according to the U.S. Department of Education, 1994b).
➤ An alarming shortage of audiologists to provide audiological services to these children. As shown in Table 1–1, 997 audiologists were reported to be employed in school settings in the United States during the 1991–92 school year, representing an

Table 1–1. Estimated number of children 3–21 years of age, number of audiologists employed by and needed by states, and audiologists to child ratio during the 1991–1992 school year.[1]

State	Number of Estimated 3–21	Number of Audiologists Employed	Number of Audiologists Needed[2]	Full-TIme Equivalent Ratio
Alabama	1,159.000	8	0	1:144,875
Alaska	178,000	4	0	1:44,500
Arizona	1,042,000	16	1	1:65,125
Arkansas	669,000	4	0	1:167,250
California	8,325,000	51	3	1:163,235
Colorado	924,000	31	1	1:29,032
Connecticut	803,000	15	0	1:53,533
Delaware	178,000	2	1	1:89,000
District of Columbia	134,000	4	0	1:33,500
Florida	3,126,000	47	3	1:66,510
Georgia	1,882,000	39	3	1:48,256
Hawaii	299,000	3	0	1:99,666
Idaho	333,000	10	2	1:33,300
Illinois	3,142,000	48	0	1:65,458
Indiana	1,580,000	14	3	1:112,857
Iowa	778,000	58	0	1:13,413
Kansas	706,000	19	0	1:37,157
Kentucky	1,042,000	4	3	1:260,500
Louisiana	1,302,000	15	6	1:86,800
Maine	333,000	11	0	1:33,454
Maryland	1,241,000	25	1	1:49,640
Massachusetts	1,479,000			no data avail
Michigan	2,630,000	20	1	1:131,500
Minnesota	1,237,000	26	3	1:53,576
Mississippi	812,000	9	0	1:90,222
Missouri	1,415,000	13	0	1:108,846
Montana	233,000	4	2	1:58,250
Nebraska	457,000	3	0	1:152,333
Nevada	325,000	3	2	1:108,333
New Hampshire	293,000	1	0	1:293,000
New Jersey	1,916,000	44	0	1:43,545
New Mexico	472,000	21	2	1:22,476

(continued)

State	Number of Estimated 3–21	Number of Audiologists Employed	Number of Audiologists Needed[2]	Full-Time Equivalent Ratio
New York	4,601,000	21	0	1:219,095
North Carolina	1,794,000	32	24	1: 56,062
North Dakota	187,000	3		1: 62,333
Ohio	3,000,000	26	0	1:115,384
Oklahoma	902,000	4	1	1:225,500
Oregon	782,000	64	3	1: 12,218
Pennsylvania	3,041,000	25	3	1:121,640
Rhode Island	254,000	2	0	1:127,000
South Carolina	1,016,000	17	6	1: 59,764
South Dakota	209,000	3	3	1: 69,666
Tennessee	1,330,000	32	2	1: 41,562
Texas	5,181,000	21	0	1:246,714
Utah	661,000	22	2	1: 30,045
Vermont	157,000	2	0	1: 78,500
Virginia	1,658,000	127	1	1: 13,055
Washington	1,362,000	0	2	0:1,362,000
West Virginia	489,000	5	0	1: 97,800
Wisconsin	1,387,000	12	0	1:115,583
Wyoming	142,000	8	0	1: 17,750
Bureau of Indian Affairs		(1)	(15)	
TOTALS	**68,598,000**	**997**	**82**	**1: 68,804**

[1]U.S. Department of Education (1994b). *Sixteenth Annual Report to Congress on the Implementation of The Individuals with Disabilities Education Act,* p. A–212.

[2]Represents the number of vacant positions.

average ratio of one audiologist for every 68,804 children. An analysis of the data reported for the 1992–93 school year identified a decrease to 883 audiologists, yielding an average of 1:78,628 (U.S. Department of Education, 1995).

➤ Working with regular and special education administrators who often have limited, if any, knowledge about audiological and hearing needs of children.

➤ Limited financial resources to provide the necessary amplification equipment and services for each child.

➤ Limited time to conduct the audiological services as stipulated in state and federal regulations (i.e., The Individuals with Disabilities Education Act, IDEA, formerly PL 94-142).

➤ A federal law that is interpreted differently by each state, resulting in services that vary significantly among states. These services also may vary within states, depending on the individual school district's understanding, commitment, and willingness to provide audiology services.

➤ Adaptation of a traditionally medical model of audiology into an educational one and the development of a service that is functional, meaningful, and responsive within the educational context.

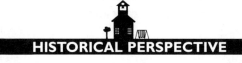

HISTORICAL PERSPECTIVE

The Sixties

Most practices and specialties develop to meet specific services required for a particular population. Educational audiology, the practice of audiology in educational or school settings, has developed as a specialty within audiology for that exact purpose. Although the majority of growth in educational audiology has arisen from federal legislation mandating specific services for children with disabilities, the provision of audiology services for educational purposes actually began in the 1960s. Figure 1–1 summarizes the historical progression of important activities and legislation related to the development of educational audiology.

Joint Committee on Audiology and Education of the Deaf

The first major step toward the use and role of audiologists in school environments was taken at the National Conference on Audiology and Education of

Joint Committee on Audiology & Education of the Deaf	1963–1966	
	1965	The Babbidge Report
Fletcher/Berg definition of Educational Audiology	1970	
	1973	Section 504, Rehabilitation Act
PL 33-380: Education of the Handicapped Amendments	1974	
	1975	PL 94-142: Education for all Handicapped Children Act
PL 99-457: Education of the Handicapped Act Amendments	1986	
	1988	Commission on the Education of the Deaf
PL 101-336: Americans with Disabilities Act	1990	PL 101-476: Individuals with Disabilities Act
Davilla: U.S. Department of Policy & Guidance Statement	1992	
	1994	GOALS 2000
IDEA Re-authorization	1997?	

Figure 1–1. Educational audiology: Summary of key events.

the Deaf held in Tucson, Arizona in 1964. The proceedings from that conference, along with summaries of the other meetings and activities of a 2-year (1963–65) federally funded project of the Vocational Rehabilitation Administration at the U.S. Department of Health, Education, and Welfare, were published in a report, *Audiology and Education of the Deaf: a Research Project and Training Manual* sponsored by the Joint Committee on Audiology and Education of the Deaf (Ventry, 1965). The Joint Committee was made up of members of the American Speech and Hearing Association and the Conference of Executives of American Schools for the Deaf

Many significant recommendations regarding audiology services for children in schools resulted from this project. The role of the audiologist in educational programs and the qualifications and competencies needed to provide audiologic services to children in educational settings were the two major areas of discussion. The report discussed the importance of the knowledge about education of the deaf and the "validation" of this knowledge through experiences with children with hearing impairments as key to audiologists' ability to influence educational programs for children. In an attempt to define and clarify the role of the audiologist, the participants passed the following resolutions:

> RESOLVED that it be recognized that audiologists should participate in the habilitation and rehabilitation, as well as the identification, evaluation, and assessment of hearing handicapped individuals. WHEREAS clinical audiology encompasses many aspects of hearing and deafness, and WHEREAS recent emphases have conveyed an impression that hearing testing and audiologic evaluations are the sole functions of the clinical audiologists, RESOLVED that among the contributions of a clinical audiologists are the following:
>
> (1) Assessment of hearing function and communication skills.
> (2) Interpretation of the results of the assessment.
> (3) Application of psychoacoustic and auditory information to all aspects of aural rehabilitation (p. 89)

Another resolution was passed recommending that the audiologist be a "full-time participating member of the instructional staff of each education program for deaf children" (p. 101). For audiologists to "make meaningful rehabilitative and educational recommendations to educators, parents, and deaf individuals" (p. 90), specific recommendations for their academic preparation were also made. Suggested coursework included "language development and language disorders caused by deafness, history of education of

the deaf, educational philosophies and controversies, and psychological and social aspects of deafness" (p. 90).

The National Conference recommended specific audiologic services for children in the educational setting. One area particularly emphasized was the need for audiologists to provide interpretive information regarding (a) specific implications of children's hearing losses relative to the use of audition for learning, (b) a suitable physical environment, and (c) equipment involved in testing and (re)habilitation. Research activities were also singled out as a special need for school audiologists, particularly by administrators of deaf education programs who gave highest priority to collaborative audiology research projects between schools and college or university programs. They also noted that research might provide inducements for audiologists to work in school programs. The following list is not exhaustive, but represents the most important of the audiology services recommended by the national conference:

> ➤ Complete audiological evaluation of children related to their admission to the educational program,
> ➤ Annual assessment of children's hearing, including an interpretation of the results to the teacher,
> ➤ Hearing aid selection, orientation, and maintenance,
> ➤ Application of knowledge about speech perception and speech pathology to the speech problems of deaf children,
> ➤ Inservice training to help keep teachers abreast of new techniques and new information,
> ➤ Parent counseling,
> ➤ Evaluation, application, and selection of the amplifying systems and equipment used in the school,
> ➤ Liaison between the school and the college or university training program and/or community speech and hearing center, and
> ➤ Research. (pp. 99–100)

The Babbidge Report

Another impetus to improving services to children with hearing impairments was the Babbidge Report, published in 1965, by the U.S. Department of Health, Education, and Welfare (Babbidge, 1965). An 11-member advisory committee, headed by Homer D. Babbidge, was appointed by the federal government to assess the status and needs of the education of deaf individuals from preschool through adulthood. The report was based on a study of 920 students who left residential schools during the 1963–64 school year and cited the limited academic success of these children. The report also supported the need for children to have services that facilitated language and speech preparation and that stressed the maximum use of residual hearing.

The federal government's involvement in the specialization of audiology services to school children continued in 1966 through a training grant awarded by the U.S. Office of Education to Utah State University. Spurred by the 1965 Commission and Babbidge reports, the Utah State University curriculum was designated as educational audiology and considered a specialty within audiology due to its greater emphasis on educational management. The curriculum was designed to:

➤ Encompass the total characteristics and needs of children who were hard-of-hearing
➤ Isolate the parameters of hearing impairment, identify the deficiencies rising from hearing disability, relate these to the unique characteristics of individuals, and develop educational programs designed for children who were hard-of-hearing
➤ Acknowledge that a coordination of skills of varied professionals and adjustment of various laymen are needed to help children to the utmost
➤ Recognize that the newer developments in education–increasing reliance on behavioral engineering, sensory aids, and instructional technology–are critically relevant to the educational management of persons who are hard-of-hearing
➤ Design a program to prepare specialists to meet the certification and coming licensing requirements in both audiology and education of the hearing impaired with a focus on children who are hard-of-hearing in regular school settings. (Berg, 1976, p. 31)

Soon after initiating this specialization, Fletcher and Berg proposed the following definition of educational audiology:

Educational audiology seeks to isolate the parameters of hearing impairment, to identify the deficiencies rising from hearing disabilities, to relate these to the unique characteristics of individuals, and to develop educational programs specifically for hard-of-hearing children. (Berg, 1970, p. 275)

The Seventies

The federal legislation of the 1970s was most active regarding provisions for children with disabilities. The first federal legislation (Public Law 19-8) affecting individuals with disabilities was passed in 1827 establishing an asylum for the deaf in Kentucky. Between that law and the passage of Public Law 94-142 in 1975, 195 federal laws were enacted specific to persons with disabilities (Weintraub, Abeson, Ballard, & La Vor, 1976). In the period between March 1970 and November 1975, 61 of these laws were passed. The civil rights activities of the 1960s and 1970s had a significant impact on legislation for individuals with disabilities. Increase in social awareness and responsiveness were important for these individuals, as well as for other minority populations.

Laws passed by the federal government usually result in state legislation to ensure that state statutes are in compliance with the federal laws. Although legislation should define public policy, assuring that individual rights are protected, services are provided, and a level of quality is maintained (Meyen, 1978), it does not ensure that sufficient funds are provided or that compliance is adequately enforced. Advocacy groups have played a major role in the interpretation and monitoring of legislative actions. The area of special education, having some of the most active, productive, and influential public and professional advocacy groups in the United States, is an excellent example of how public policy can be influenced by groups heralding a common cause.

Important Legislation of the Seventies

Among the various laws passed affecting education during the 1970s, three are most significant:

➤ Section 504 of the Rehabilitation Act of 1973
➤ PL 93-380, the Education of the Handicapped Amendments of 1974
➤ PL 94-142, Education for all Handicapped Children Act, passed in 1975.

SECTION 504 OF THE REHABILITATION ACT OF 1973. This act is commonly referred to as the civil rights legislation for the handicapped because it was the first law that specifically protected the rights of handicapped persons by prohibiting recipients of federal funds from discriminating against "otherwise qualified individuals" (34 CFR Part 104). The provisions of this law are almost identical to the nondiscriminatory provisions related to race in Title VI of the Civil Rights Act of 1964 and to gender in Title IX of the Education Amendments of 1972. This Act defined a "handicapped" individual as:

any person who (A) has a physical or mental impairment which substantially limits one or more of such person's major life activities, (B) has a record of such an impairment, or (C) is regarded as having such an impairment.

Initially this law was restricted to employment of the handicapped, but through amendments passed in 1974, Section 504 was applied to a wider array of services including education (academic, nonacademic, and extracurricular services and activities). There are six subparts of the Act either administered by the U.S. Department of Health and Human Services or the U.S. Department of Education, depending on where funds originate. The Federal Regulations for Section 504: Subpart D–Preschool, Elementary, and Secondary Education are reprinted in Appendix 1–A.

Section 504-Subpart D and IDEA-B (the current version of PL 94-142) have many similarities that together provide comprehensive protection to all children whether or not they are identified as disabled under the special education statues. Key components that differentiate these laws include:

➤ "Eligibility" for services under IDEA compared to "protected" under Section 504: While IDEA-B requires the existence of a handicapping condition (as identified in the IDEA-B regulations, 34 CFR Part 300, Section 300.5) that adversely affects educational performance necessitating special education services, Section 504's broader definition includes persons with handicaps not mentioned in IDEA or state education policies. Therefore, the obligation to provide appropriate education may extend beyond the traditionally operated special education programs.

➤ Because a school district is obligated to provide services (evaluations, regular education, reasonable accommodations, related services, and related aids) regardless of eligibility for special education under IDEA-B, the school district may be obligated to use regular education funds to provide related services and/or aids for a handicapped child.

➤ Simply because a child receives a free and appropriate education (FAPE) through a school district's special education program does not necessarily mean that the situation is in compliance with Section 504 (example: a child receiving special education services in a building or classroom segregated from the other regular students). (National Association of State Directors of Special Education [NASDSE], 1991, p. 6)

We are just beginning to realize the tremendous impact of Section 504 for children having milder, yet still significant, disabilities who may not meet special education "eligibility" requirements. Two groups for which this law has significant implications are children with milder hearing impairments and children having central auditory processing difficulties. For both of these groups, acoustic accessibility is an invisible barrier to their hearing and/or understanding

of auditory information. This area is typically overlooked unless knowledgeable audiologists, teachers, or other individuals are representing the needs of these children in schools. Amplification systems and classroom and communication accommodations are critical regular education adaptations that can be implemented for students to provide accessibility without special education eligibility (see Chapter 11, Individual Planning, for more information on Section 504, and Chapter 7, Case Management and Aural (Re)habilitation, for additional information about management needs and services).

PL 93-380, THE EDUCATION OF THE HANDICAPPED AMENDMENTS OF 1974. This law was an extension and amendment to the Elementary and Secondary Education Act of 1965, which included provisions for handicapped children that were to become the basis for many of the specific aspects of PL 94-142. PL 93-380 established the right to equal educational opportunity (Title VIII, Section 901), including a specific goal for handicapped children that also identified, as a priority, the use of funds for handicapped children who were not receiving an education. The law also included provisions for procedural safeguards and due process (Section 613 [A]).

PL 94-142, THE EDUCATION FOR ALL HANDICAPPED CHILDREN ACT. The most notable of legislation for children with disabilities, PL 94-142, was passed in 1975. This law states:

> *All children who are handicapped and in need of special education and related services must be identified, evaluated, and assured a free appropriate public education in the least restrictive environment.*

Although the provisions of this law are now generally known, Table 1–2 summarizes its major principles.

The Rules and Regulations for PL 94-142 (U.S. Department of Health, Education, and Welfare, August 23, 1977) in addition to articulating the specific rights of handicapped children identified previously, provided definitions for handicapped, special education, and related services, as well as specified the federal government's fiscal responsibility for excess cost in order to assist states in assuring these children a free and appropriate education, and specified a timeline by which states and local education agencies or school districts must comply with the regulations. This first reference to audiology, as a special education related service, is described as follows in the regulations:

Audiology includes:

(i) *Identification of children with hearing loss;*

Table 1–2. Major principles of PL 94-142.

Zero Reject/Child	➤ Requires that all children with handicaps be provided with a free, appropriate education (FAPE).
Identification	➤ Requires a child find program to locate, identify, and evaluate all children who are handicapped who live in the jurisdiction of each public agency.
Multidisciplinary Evaluation	➤ Requires a full individual comprehensive evaluation prior to placement in a special education program.
	➤ Evaluation must be multidisciplinary, meet specified standards, and interpretation must consider information from a variety of sources.
Individualized Education	➤ Development and implementation of the IEP ensures that educational programs are determined on an individual basis to meet the needs of students with handicaps.
Program IEP	➤ IEP requirements specify content, scope, timeliness for writing IEPs, participants in the IEP meeting, parent participation, private school placements, and accountability.
Least Restrictive Environment (LRE)	➤ Placement of children occurs so that, to the maximum possible, children with handicaps are educated with children who are not handicapped.
	➤ Removal to special classes occurs only when the nature or severity of the handicap prevents successful education in regular classes, even with the use of supplementary aids and services.
	➤ A continuum of alternative educational services from more restrictive to less restrictive is provided by the public agency.
	➤ Placement decisions are determined by the goals and objectives of the student's IEP and are reviewed annually.
Due Process	➤ Establishes and implements regulations, standards, and procedures for compliance with all procedural safeguards, including written notice to parents of referral, confidentiality of information, right to independent educational evaluation, parental consent for placement, due process hearings, and appointment of surrogate parents when needed
	➤ Ensures fairness of educational decisions and the accountability for making decisions for both professionals and parents.

(ii) *Determination of the range, nature, and degree of hearing loss, including referral for medical or other professional attention for the habilitation of hearing;*

(iii) *Provision of habilitation activities, such as language habilitation, auditory training, speech reading, (lipreading), hearing evaluation, and speech conservation;*

(iv) *Creation and administration of programs for prevention of hearing loss;*

(v) *Counseling and guidance of pupils, parents, and teachers regarding hearing loss;*

(vi) *Determination of the child's need for group and individual amplification, selecting and fitting an appropriate aid, and evaluating the effectiveness of amplification.* (34 CFR 300.12[b])

The authors of these rules and regulations, generally personnel from the U.S. Office of Education's Bureau of Education for the Handicapped (now the Office of Special Education Programs), must be commended for their understanding and knowledge of the concerns and needs of children with hearing impairments. The definition of audiology continues to stand today as representative of the scope of services necessary for children with hearing impairments in the schools. An additional regulation recognized the concern regarding the condition of hearing

aids worn by children in public schools. This provision was based on the results of a Bureau of Education of the Handicapped study, conducted at the request of the 1976 House of Representatives Appropriations Committee, which found up to one-third of the hearing aids worn by children in schools were malfunctioning. This regulation is identified as:

> *Proper function of hearing aids.*
> *Each public agency shall ensure that the hearing aids worn by children with hearing impairment including deafness in school are functioning properly.* (34 CFR 300.303)

Appendix 1–B includes definitions for special education, deafness, deaf-blindness, hearing impairment, related services, and assistive technology, as well as other pertinent portions of the most recent Rules and Regulations for PL 94-142, now IDEA-B, from the *Federal Register* (U.S. Department of Education, September 29,1992) that pertain to audiology and education of children with hearing impairments.

Major limitations of this legislation, as indicated earlier, are that individual states have a great deal of latitude in their interpretation of the provisions and that the federal government lacks significant consequences in its compliance monitoring system. These problems result in substantial variability in services among states. A review of litigation related to special education law, however, shows that it is the court system that provides the greatest control over compliance. Coincidentally, the first case decided by the U.S. Supreme Court involving PL 94-142 was Hendrick Hudson School District Board of Education v. Rowley in 1982, regarding the use of a sign language interpreter for a mainstreamed elementary school child. Following a general societal pattern, the reliance on the court system to define these rights for children continues to escalate. Unfortunately, litigation requires parents who have the time, money, and perseverance to take on their local school programs. Such litigation may not be in the best interest of the involved children because their parents are often pitted against their school systems in bitter disputes rather than working together for the children.

The IEP (individual education plan) is the legal document that defines the program and services for each student. For students to receive related services (such as audiology), they must meet the eligibility requirements for special education according to the criteria used to determine that students cannot receive reasonable educational benefit from regular education. In other words, students could have a physical impairment, such as a hearing loss, that does not result in significant educational problems and would then not meet the special education eligibility requirements. These students should then be considered for 504 services because they may have a documented condition (disability) by virtue of their hearing impairment which requires certain accommodations as part of regular education (504 plans are discussed more in Chapter 11).

Because the IEP is the key to ensuring that appropriate services are provided for students with hearing impairments, it is imperative that their IEPs be developed by individuals knowledgeable about the peculiar needs of students with hearing impairment. All students with hearing impairments must therefore have their needs represented on the IEP team by a specialist in the area of hearing ("specialist" may be defined by each state plan, but usually is an audiologist, a teacher of the deaf or hard-of-hearing, or sometimes a speech-language pathologist who can interpret test results and make appropriate recommendations). The PL 94-142 requirements that must be included on each IEP are:

1. A statement of annual goals, including short-term objectives.
2. A statement of the specific special education and related services to be provided.
3. The extent to which the child will be able to participate in regular education programs.
4. A statement of the child's present levels of educational performance.
5. The projected dates for initiation of services and the anticipated duration of the services.
6. Appropriate objective criteria and evaluation procedures and schedules for determining whether the objectives are achieved.

A major need for school-based audiologists is to understand their role in the IEP planning meeting. This role will be discussed in more detail in Chapter 11, Individual Planning.

The Eighties

A major focus of the 1980s was directed at refining the legislation of the previous decade. Although court decisions provided further clarification of PL 94-142 and upheld its provisions, professional groups and individual state and local education agencies struggled with interpretative, logistic, and financial impacts of the law. Parental and advocacy groups became increasingly more powerful and sophisticated in bringing about the changes they supported.

Important Legislation of the Eighties: PL 99-457

The major legislative accomplishment of the 1980s was the passage of PL 99-457, the Education of the Handicapped Act Amendments (EHA) of 1986. In response to the growing evidence attributing to the benefits of early intervention, the re-authorization of PL 94-142 included two significant new programs. First, the service provisions of PL 94-142 were extended to all handicapped children aged 3 to 5 years (provisions for children aged 3 to 21 years were identified as Part B of the EHA), and second, the legislation authorized early intervention services to handicapped infants and toddlers and their families birth to age 2, inclusive (Part H of the EHA). In addition, Part H mandated statewide and community coordination efforts to serve special-needs and at-risk children and emphasized the important role of the family in these services. Although the Part H portion of the law was permissive, states choosing not to participate stood to lose all preschool federal grant moneys. In this law, the term "handicapped infants and toddlers" was defined to include those *experiencing developmental delays*, those having *a diagnosed physical or mental condition which has a high probability of resulting in developmental delay*, and, at an individual state's discretion, those *who are at risk of having substantial developmental delays if early intervention services are not provided*.

Important provisions of this law included financial assistance to each state to assist in the development of *a statewide, comprehensive, coordinated, multidisciplinary, interagency system to provide early intervention services for handicapped infants and toddlers and their families* (Sec. 673), *establishment of a State Interagency Coordinating Council* (Sec. 674), and implementation of the *Individual Family Service Plan* (Sec. 677). Audiologists are included as one of the "qualified personnel" for providing early intervention services. The definition of audiology here contains some subtle differences (bolded) from that used in PL 94-142:

(i) *Identification of children with impairments,* **using at risk criteria and appropriate audiological screening techniques;**

(ii) *Determination of the range, nature, and degree of hearing loss and* **communication functions***, by use of audiologic evaluation procedures;*

(iii) *Referral for medical and other services necessary for the habilitation or rehabilitation of children with auditory impairment;*

(iv) *Provision of auditory training, aural rehabilitation, speech reading and* **listening device orientation and training***, and other services;*

(v) *Provision of services for the prevention of hearing loss; and*

(vi) *Determination of the child's need for individual amplification, including selecting, fitting, and* **dispensing** *of appropriate listening and vibrotactile devices, and evaluating the effectiveness of those devices.* (34 CFR 303.12[d])

A controversial audiology service under Part H is the **dispensing** of amplification devices. It must be remembered that Part H is not a school responsibility, but rather a community one. Therefore, if hearing aids or other amplification devices are necessary for a child, it is a community responsibility to determine how they are provided to the family. Part H stipulates that services are provided at no cost unless the state has a federal or state system of payments by families, including a schedule of sliding fees (Sec. 672 [2] [B]). Although several state and community resources exist to pay for hearing aids, this provision appears to be poorly understood and under-utilized. Pertinent sections of the most recent rules and regulations (1993) of PL 99-457, now IDEA, are reprinted in Appendix 1–C.

Commission on Education of the Deaf

In 1988, the Commission on Education of the Deaf published its report *Toward Equality: Education of the Deaf*, which was submitted to the President and the Congress of the United States. The report focused on the unsatisfactory educational performance of deaf students and in particular the problems associated with inappropriate mainstreamed placements (least restrictive environment [LRE] interpretation issues). In all, 52 recommendations were made regarding prevention and early identification, language acquisition, appropriate education, least restrictive environment, parents' rights, evaluation and assessment, program standards, quality education, American Sign Language, federal postsecondary education systems, research, evaluation, outreach, professional standards and training, technology, clearinghouses, and committees on deaf/blindness. Many of these recommendations were addressed in a U.S. Department of Education Notice of Policy Guidance statement by the Director of the Office of Special Education and Rehabilitative Services, Robert Davila, and the Secretary of Education, Lamar Alexander (U.S. Department of Education, October 30, 1992) (Reprinted in Appendix 1-G). The establishment of the National Institute on Deafness and Other Communication Disorders within the National Institutes of Health was another outcome of the Commission Report. Recognizing that the problems identified in the Commission Report exist for many deaf and hard-of-hearing students, it should be noted that the report did not differentiate degree of hearing loss, using the term deaf to refer to all persons with hearing impairment, including those who are hard-of-hearing and those deafened later in life.

GUIDING POLICIES FOR THE NINETIES

The inclusion movement had the greatest impact in special education services for children with disabilities in the 1990s. No longer are children mainstreamed only for classes where it is thought they could benefit from the regular curriculum with minor adaptations. Rather, children with disabilities are considered to be equal members of the regular education classroom every day and are separated only when specific instruction or therapy cannot occur within the child's classroom. Inclusion has had the most profound effect on children with severe disabilities who previously were educated or maintained in separate rooms. In fact, it is the advocates for these children who are responsible for the inclusion movement (Fuchs & Fuchs, 1994). Although the benefit actually derived by some of these children from the regular classroom setting is controversial, they can be found, with the support of aides, in regular classrooms across the country.

Audiology has been significantly impacted by the increased inclusion of children with auditory, language, and learning problems in regular classrooms. With fewer children educated in small groups in resource rooms that can be controlled for noise and distance from the speaker, auditory learning problems have escalated. In addition to children with hearing impairments, audiologists are now fitting assistive listening systems on children with normal hearing who have other language and/or learning problems in order to counteract the effects of the noise and distance listening problems. These issues will be discussed further in Chapter 6, Amplification and Classroom Hearing Technology, Chapter 11, Individual Planning, and Chapter 13, Marketing.

Important Legislation of the Nineties

Two major pieces of legislation were passed in 1990: The Americans with Disabilities Act , (PL 101-336) and the Individuals with Disabilities Education Act (PL 101-476).

The Americans with Disabilities Act (ADA)

The ADA was enacted to provide protection from discrimination based on disability, just as the 1964 Civil Rights Act prohibited discrimination based on race, sex, creed, and national origin. Modeled after the Rehabilitation Act of 1973, the ADA replaces the word "handicap" with "disability" and pertains to all employers, not just those receiving federal funds. The Act includes five sections (called Titles) covering employment, public services and transportation, public accommodations and commercial facilities, telecommunications, and miscellaneous provisions. *Communication and the ADA*, a document prepared by the American Speech-Language-Hearing Association (ASHA), explains many of the pertinent aspects of the law relating to speech, language, and hearing disabilities. It is reprinted in Appendix 2–A.

Individuals with Disabilities Education Act (IDEA)

This most recent law pertaining to children with disabilities combines all of the amendments to PL 94-142 and PL 99-457. Part H of IDEA, the Early Intervention Program for Infants and Toddlers with Disabilities, contains the most recent 1991 amendments and "promotes a seamless system of services for children with disabilities from birth through five years of age and their families" (34 CFR Part 303, U.S. Department of Education, July 30, 1993). Part B of IDEA, the Education of Children with Disabilities program, pertains

to preschool (Part 301) and school-age children (Part 300). The final regulations (U.S. Department of Education, September 29, 1992) incorporated changes made by the Handicapped Programs Technical Amendments Act of 1988, the 1990 Amendments (PL 101-476), the National Literacy Act of 1991 (PL 102-73), and the 1991 Amendments. (PL 102-119). In addition to changing the terminology ("handicap" to "disability"), the disabilities and definitions for autism and traumatic brain injury were added, as well as definitions for rehabilitation counseling services and transitions services. More important for audiology, statutory definitions of "assistive technology device" and "assistive technology service" were made (reprinted in Appendix 1-F), including *a requirement that if a child with a disability requires a device and services in order to receive a free and appropriate education (FAPE), the public agency must ensure that they are made available.* The definitions of "device" and "service" are important:

> 300.5 *"Assistive technology device" means any item, piece of equipment, or product system, whether acquired commercially off the shelf, modified, or customized, that is used to increase, maintain, or improve the functional capabilities of children with disabilities.*
> 300.6 *"Assistive technology service" means any service that directly assists a child with a disability in the selection, acquisition, or use of an assistive technology device. The term includes*
> *(a) The evaluation of the needs of a child with a disability, including a functional evaluation of the child in the child's customary environment;*
> *(b) Purchasing, leasing, or otherwise providing for the acquisition of assistive technology devices by children with disabilities;*
> *(c) Selecting, designing, fitting, customizing, adapting, applying, retaining, repairing, or replacing assistive technology devices;*
> *(d) Coordinating and using other therapies, interventions, or services with assistive technology devices, such as those associated with existing education and rehabilitation plans and programs;*
> *(e) Training or technical assistance for a child with a disability or, if appropriate, that child's family; and*
> *(f) Training or technical assistance for professionals (including individuals providing education or rehabilitation services), employers, or other individuals who provide services to, employ, or are otherwise substantially involved in the major life functions of children with disabilities.*

Interpretation of this rule should be in the context of what a child needs to "receive reasonable benefit" from the educational program. For example, if a parent requested a certain brand of FM system, the school would not be obligated to supply that brand as long as the FM system they did provide met the needs of the student. Considering individual needs, however, is important. For example, arguments for a BTE (behind-the-ear) FM system could potentially be justified if the student refused to wear a body-worn system for cosmetic reasons, but would use a BTE model. Pertinent sections of the most recent rules and regulations for IDEA, Part B, are reprinted in Appendix 1–B and for IDEA, Part H, in Appendix 1–C. A comparison of Section 504, IDEA, and ADA can be found in Appendix 1–E.

The Regular Education Initiative

This initiative seeks to establish the regular classroom as the appropriate environment for all children with disabilities. Like inclusion, this movement has been driven by parents of children with severe disabilities who have typically been educated in more segregated facilities or classrooms. Paramount to the success of such programs is the provision of adequate support personnel and services to assist with the regular classroom placements. Another unresolved issue is the argument concerning the cost effectiveness of such inclusion practices versus the benefit derived by the student. Inclusion is discussed in more detail under IEP planning and least restrictive environment (LRE) in Chapter 7, Case Management and Aural (Re)habilitation.

Goals 2000

These goals were the focus of the Educate America Act of the U.S. Department of Education (PL 103-227, 1994a). This school reform effort was in response to "A Nation at Risk," a report by the National Commission on Excellence in Education (1983) and subsequent studies that continue to focus on the achievement problems of students in public schools in the United States. Goals 2000 include the following objectives:

1. All Children will start school ready to learn.
2. The high school graduation rate will be 90%.
3. Students will demonstrate competencies in core subjects in 4th, 8th, and 12th grades.
4. The United States will be first in the world in the fields of science and math.
5. Every adult will be literate and able to compete in the marketplace.
6. Every school will be safe, disciplined, and free of drugs.

The Goals 2000 initiative and other reform efforts have led to a movement in many school districts toward outcome-based or standards-based education. These

standards or outcomes raise questions of relevance for many students with special needs. Alternative graduation requirements, usually based on each student's IEP goals, rather than the school's assessment standards, are typically used. However, the issues around differentiated diplomas and certificates of attendance as alternatives to actual diplomas are still being resolved. It is hoped that students with special needs will be recognized in the educational reform movement and that the results will be greater opportunities to learn and improved performance.

Re-authorization of IDEA

At the time of this writing, re-authorization of IDEA is involved in re-election politics. Re-authorization has been controversial due to changes certain legislators hope to make based on constituency, special interest, and political party concerns. A trend to de-emphasize the federal government's role in education and special education clouds the entire process, leaving many of the provisions of IDEA vulnerable. Legislators are also concerned about the continuing problem created by unfunded federal mandates. The state block grant concept and health care reform are two issues that could impact the future of how children access and receive services. Shortages in some related service areas, the use of aides and support personnel, qualified provider issues, and the cost to provide some of the services (especially those involving technology) will be some of the key discussions in ongoing re-authorization considerations. However, professional and advocacy groups for the various disabilities are strong, and it is hoped that major changes in disability legislation will not occur. What is critical, though, is that parent and professional groups put aside their differences and unite to fight to maintain the rights and services that have taken so much time, pain, and hard work to obtain.

SUMMARY

With time, federal laws may define parameters of service, but the guarantees are still dependent on the interpretation and will of local administrative agencies and the motivation of parents or advocacy groups who support individual services for children. Judicial decisions have continued to further define the specific provisions of disability legislation and we hope will remain perceptive to the services the education system can reasonably provide. Cases impacting services to children with hearing impairments are summarized in Appendix 1–D. As practicing school-based audiologists, we know that our time, finances, and administrative support have a significant impact on the services we can deliver. Another major factor is the intensity of demands that children's parents make; schools often succumb to vocal parents' wishes rather than risk a lawsuit. The result, unfortunately, is that children of vocal parents often get more services than those of quiet, compliant families, even though their children may be just as needy.

The pendulum of the education clock continues to swing back and forth. Finding a comfortable balance between what should and what should not be, and what schools can and cannot afford, is not easy. Reform often seems more like new names for old practices, rather than a systemic difference in how education works. Efforts to change are often driven by small vocal groups rather than by a consensus process. Of utmost importance is that *each* child is an individual with unique characteristics and needs; a particular method or system that may work well for one does not necessarily work well or may not be appropriate for another.

Although most school-based audiologists have much to be proud of, as a profession we are still wrestling with many of the same issues raised in the 1965 Joint Committee Report (Ventry, 1965), "Audiology and Education of the Deaf." That project was identified as a beginning to resolve the issues experienced at the time. Read the summary statements from that project below and compare them to the list of challenges identified at the opening of this chapter. Expanding "deaf" to "deaf and hard-of-hearing," do you think we are there yet?

1. There is an undeniable need for increased emphasis to be placed on education of the deaf in audiology training programs. There is also a need, perhaps to a somewhat lesser extent, for increased emphasis on audiology in teacher of the deaf training programs.
2. There is a need for clarification of the roles and responsibilities of both audiologists and teachers of the deaf.
3. Interprofessional relationships need to be improved. One major method of accomplishing this is to increase contact and communication between the practicing teacher of the deaf and the clinical audiologist.
4. The audiologist needs greater exposure, probably by means of direct contact, to the educational and language problems imposed by deafness. Teachers need to be better able to utilize audiologic information in planning an educational program.
5. The audiologists can play an important and significant role in an educational program for deaf children. There needs, however, to be greater utilization of audiologic personnel in such programs.
6. If services are to be offered to deaf clients, they must be offered by individuals who are knowledgeable about problems related to deafness and who have had experience with deaf people.
7. Audiologic research has much to contribute to deaf education, but there needs to be more cooperative research efforts, and these efforts need to be designed to solve, in part, some of the problems facing educators of the deaf.
8. Deaf education programs need to take greater advantage of the audiologic services available at speech and hearing centers. This is particularly true if the centers can offer a wide variety of services, especially diagnostic services.
9. The role of the speech pathologist in dealing with the speech and language problems associated with deafness needs to be re-evaluated.
10. Greater understanding, appreciation, and respect for the contributions made by each professional group need to be fostered and enhanced.
11. The final conclusion is that maximum audiologic services are not currently being provided to, or utilized by, deaf children and adults. As a result, many deaf individuals fail to achieve their maximum potential. (p. 116)

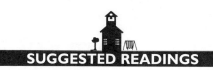

SUGGESTED READINGS

National Association of State Directors of Special Education. (1994). *Deaf & hard-of-hearing students, educational services guidelines*. Alexandria, VA: Author.

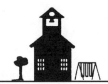

CHAPTER 2

ROLES AND RESPONSIBILITIES OF THE EDUCATIONAL AUDIOLOGIST

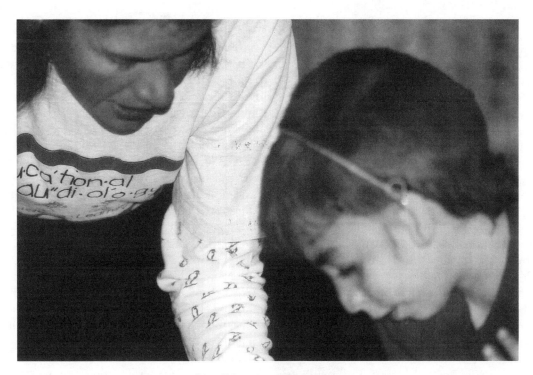

Lisa, Educational Audiologist

CONTENTS

To those of us who have worked in the schools, the importance of having audiologists in that environment is obvious. School-based audiologists are in a unique position to facilitate and support the educational management of students with hearing losses. Unfortunately, the need for comprehensive audiological services in the schools is less obvious to school administrators, teachers, and parents. These individuals may be aware of the legal mandate to provide services for students with hearing losses, but they may seek to do so using a clinical model of audiological services. The clinical model focuses on diagnosis of the child's hearing loss, and remediation is typically limited to medical management and/or the provision of amplification. These services are important, but the educational impact of the hearing loss must be determined and managed so that the needs of the student are fully addressed.

To create an educational audiology position in a school district or to expand existing services, it is important that educational audiologists understand their role in the educational system. Educational audiologists must work with the school administration to define their positions and to develop a comprehensive system of delivering audiological services to all students, both those with hearing and listening disorders and those with normal hearing. Once audiology services are in place in a school system, it is important that educational audiologists continue to advocate for their services. Without continued awareness of the importance of educational audiology services, these services may not be used effectively and may eventually be reduced or eliminated.

This chapter addresses the following questions:

➤ What are the roles of educational audiologists?
➤ What responsibilities do educational audiologists have in the school district?
➤ What training is necessary for educational audiologists?
➤ What are the various delivery systems that can be used for educational audiology services?

➤ What can educational audiologists do to improve audiological services in the schools?

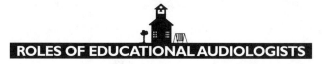

ROLES OF EDUCATIONAL AUDIOLOGISTS

The roles of educational audiologists will vary depending on the other services and personnel available to help children within the school system. Educational audiologists are members of the educational team, and, in addition to performing audiological activities, may serve at various times in any or all of the following capacities:

➤ Service coordinator
➤ Instructional team member
➤ Consultant

Educational Audiologists as Service Coordinators

In situations where a student with a hearing loss is not receiving any direct special education services, the educational audiologist often functions as the student's service coordinator, and, as a result, is the individual responsible for monitoring and coordinating the educational program for the student. The educational audiologist may also be designated by the educational team as the service coordinator for a student with a hearing loss who is receiving multiple special education services. In either of these situations, the educational audiologist provides routine diagnostic audiology services, but also works with the regular and special education teachers, the student, the parents, and others involved with the student to see that appropriate services and classroom modifications are provided. As the service coordinator, the educational audiologist is responsible for monitoring the student's educational progress and plays a key role in recommending changes in educational placement when necessary. English (1995) provided the following list of responsibilities for service coordinators:

➤ Maintain complete and updated information regarding the placement options available within the district for students with hearing losses
➤ Prepare teachers and other service providers for working with students having hearing losses
➤ Ensure that all appropriate services (e.g., speech-language pathology, occupational therapy) are coordinated and implemented in a timely fashion
➤ Maintain contact with teachers and provide technical support as necessary
➤ Monitor the student's placement and progress

➤ Support transitions to other grades, schools, and programs

➤ Evaluate each student's placement and make recommendations for changes as needed. (p. 58)

A more detailed discussion on the implementation of these responsibilities is provided in Chapter 7, Case Management and Aural (Re)habilitation.

Educational Audiologists as Instructional Team Members

There are many circumstances in which an educational audiologist functions as a member of the instructional team, providing support to teachers and other staff. When a student is enrolled in a special education program, whether a program for children who are deaf and hard-of-hearing or a program for students with other disabilities, the audiologist typically provides support to the special education teacher, the regular education teacher, the student, and the parents. This support is focused most often on assessment of the hearing loss and on management of amplification, but may include direct (re)habilitation services or other activities when needed. When the teachers are not familiar with hearing loss and its effects, the support provided by the educational audiologist is typically expanded and may include the provision of inservice and/or consultation with other members of the educational team. Expanded discussions of the educational audiologist's activities as a member of the instructional team can be found in Chapter 7, Case Management and Aural (Re)habilitation, and Chapter 12, Inservice.

Educational Audiologists as Consultants

It is becoming increasingly more common for educational audiologists to provide consultation to all teachers, including those who may not have children with identified hearing losses in their classrooms. Teachers may request any of the following:

➤ Information on a specific child's hearing sensitivity or auditory processing ability

➤ Suggested activities for improving their students' listening skills

➤ Classroom presentations related to the function of the ear, hearing loss, or hearing conservation

➤ Information on classroom acoustics

➤ Assistance with the use of classroom amplification systems

➤ Information about how to integrate auditory skills into the school curricula

These consultative services are often focused on children with normal-hearing sensitivity, but the teachers'

concerns are ones that educational audiologists are uniquely qualified to address.

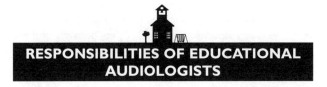

RESPONSIBILITIES OF EDUCATIONAL AUDIOLOGISTS

Regardless of the roles assumed by educational audiologists, there are many responsibilities they must address. Suggested responsibilities for audiologists who are employed in the schools, as described in the American Speech-Language-Hearing Association's *Guidelines for Audiology Services in the Schools* (1993), are listed in Table 2–1. The complete guidelines are reproduced in Appendix 2–B. The responsibilities of educational audiologists can be grouped into the following areas:

➤ Hearing conservation

➤ Identification of hearing loss

➤ Assessment of hearing loss and other abilities

➤ Amplification and other assistive technology

➤ Educational planning and support

➤ Direct (re)habilitation services

➤ Family support

At times the responsibilities of educational audiologists may overlap with those of other school staff, particularly nurses and teachers of the deaf and hard-of-hearing. When this occurs, it is important to delineate which individual is primarily responsible for each activity. Table 2–2 provides an example of how identification, referral, evaluation, and monitoring can be assigned to the various members of the hearing team.

Hearing Conservation

One of the responsibilities often assumed by educational audiologists is educating parents, teachers, and students about hearing loss and ways to prevent hearing loss. This education may be accomplished through inservice programs for teachers, direct instruction to students, or monitoring of noise levels during various school activities. Hearing conservation activities often have a lower priority than our other responsibilities, but they are important and can be a means of increasing the awareness of teachers about educational audiology services. More information on hearing conservation activities is contained in Chapter 8, Hearing Conservation.

Identification of Hearing Loss

Identification of hearing loss is one responsibility that is almost always a part of the educational audiolo-

Table 2–1. Suggested responsibilities of audiologists who are employed in the schools.

➤ Provide community leadership to ensure that all infants, toddlers, and youth with impaired hearing are promptly identified, evaluated, and provided with appropriate intervention services

➤ Collaborate with community resources to develop a high-risk registry and follow-up

➤ Develop and supervise a hearing screening program for preschool and school-age children

➤ Train audiometric technicians or other appropriate personnel to screen for hearing loss

➤ Perform follow-up comprehensive audiological evaluations

➤ Assess central auditory function

➤ Make appropriate referrals for further audiological, communication, educational, psychosocial, or medical assessment

➤ Interpret audiological assessment results to other school personnel

➤ Serve as a member of the educational team in the evaluation, planning, and placement process. Make recommendations regarding placement, related service needs, communication needs, and modification of classroom environments for students with hearing impairments and other auditory problems

➤ Provide in-service training on hearing and hearing impairments and their implications to school personnel, children, and parents

➤ Educate parents, children, and school personnel about hearing loss prevention

➤ Make recommendations about use of hearing aids, cochlear implants, group and classroom amplification, and assistive listening devices

➤ Ensure the proper fit and functioning of hearing aids, cochlear implants, group and classroom amplification, and assistive listening devices

➤ Analyze classroom noise and acoustics and make recommendations for improving the listening environment

➤ Manage the use and calibration of audiometric equipment

➤ Collaborate with the school, parents, teachers, special support personnel, and relevant community agencies and professionals to ensure delivery of appropriate services

➤ Make recommendations for assistive devices (radio/television, telephone, alerting, convenience) for students with hearing impairments

➤ Provide services, including home programming if appropriate, in the areas of speechreading, listening, communication strategies, use and care of amplification, including cochlear implants, and self-management of hearing needs

Source: From "Guidelines for audiology services in the schools" by the American Speech-Language-Hearing Association, 1995, *Asha Desk Reference for Audiology and Speech-Language Pathology, II,* p. 71. Available for sale from ASHA Fullfillment Operations (301-897-5700 x218). Reprinted with permission.

gist's role. Educational audiologists generally do not provide direct screening services, but they may be responsible for the administration and supervision of the school hearing screening program. They may also collaborate with community audiologists and agencies to facilitate the identification of infants, toddlers, and preschoolers with hearing losses. A full discussion of hearing identification programs is provided in Chapter 3, Identification Practices, and Chapter 9, Community Collaboration, includes more information about community collaboration.

Assessment of Hearing Loss and Other Abilities

Another responsibility routinely assumed by educational audiologists is that of providing comprehensive audiological evaluations, including the assessment of central auditory functioning. Although audiological assessment is a primary activity, we believe that the responsibility of educational audiologists must go beyond that. Awareness of the effects of hearing losses and listening disorders, as well as the ability to recognize other problems a student may have, is critical. Additionally, school-based audiologists must make appropriate referrals and be able to discuss the relationship of a hearing loss or a central auditory processing disorder to the student's overall functioning. Issues related to assessment of hearing losses are ad-

dressed more completely in Chapter 4, Assessment Practices, and information on central auditory processing disorders is contained in Chapter 5, Central Auditory Processing Disorders.

Amplification and Other Assistive Technology

Working with amplification and other assistive technology is an area of major responsibility for most educational audiologists. Although either clinical audiologists or educational audiologists may make recommendations about a child's use of hearing aids, cochlear implants, tactile devices, or other amplification systems, the educational audiologist is the individual responsible for ensuring that these devices are functioning and are being used correctly and appropriately in the classroom. The educational audiologist is also the person who most often makes recommendations for the use of group or classroom amplification systems and other assistive listening devices and monitors their function in the learning environment. This topic is covered in more detail in Chapter 6, Amplification and Classroom Hearing Technology.

Educational Planning and Support

Another responsibility unique to educational audiologists is their role in collaboration with parents, teach-

Table 2–2. Suggested responsibilities for nurses, audiologists, and teachers of deaf and hard-of-hearing students.

Nurses
➤ Conduct screening (preschool and school-age) using referral criteria determined by audiologist
➤ Cooperate with other agencies to ensure hearing loss identification and appropriate referrals
➤ Conduct follow-up to ensure those referred have received appropriate care

Audiologists
➤ Work with nurses, hearing team, and community resources to develop hearing loss identification, assessment, and referral process
➤ Manage hearing screening program, including training of support personnel; participate in screening when necessary
➤ Conduct comprehensive hearing evaluations for all students with identified hearing losses who have not had complete evaluations (annually for those who meet educationally significant criteria)
➤ Provide assessment to determine the range and nature of hearing loss and to evaluate the effectiveness of hearing aids and FM amplification when prescribed
➤ Interpret educational implications of assessments
➤ Monitor hearing of those with hearing losses which are educationally nonsignificant
➤ Make recommendations for amplification and assistive listening devices
➤ Attend IEP meetings for children with educationally significant hearing loss (ESHL) to provide input regarding the associated educational implications of the loss
➤ Monitor functioning of hearing aids and FM systems
➤ Provide teacher inservice regarding hearing aids, amplification, and classroom and instructional modifications
➤ Refer all those with ESHL to the teacher of the deaf and hard-of-hearing for consideration of needs and services
➤ Provide education to students about hearing loss prevention

Teachers of the Deaf and Hard-of-Hearing
➤ Annually conduct SIFTERs to monitor educational performance on all those with known ESHL who are not staffed
➤ Conduct SIFTERs on those referred by audiologist with newly identified ESHL
➤ Schedule pre-conferences on all those referred with ESHL to discuss hearing impairment, associated educational concerns, and appropriate instructional modifications and adaptations
➤ Schedule pre-assessment conferences and staffings for those with associated educational concerns who need to be considered for hearing disability and services
➤ Act as case manager for students with ESHL
➤ Provide direct services to students who are deaf or hard-of-hearing

All
➤ Attend periodic hearing team meetings for communication, case review, and update of status of hearing services

ers, and school administrators to ensure that appropriate educational services are delivered to each student with a hearing loss. The educational audiologist is a member of the educational team that evaluates each student and subsequently makes appropriate educational placements. In addition to documenting the hearing loss, describing the student's use of audition, defining the implications of the hearing loss, and making recommendations regarding amplification, the educational audiologist is often responsible for analyzing classroom acoustics and improving the listening environment for the child. The educational audiologist may also provide support to the classroom teacher and other professionals who work with the student with a hearing loss. These issues are addressed more completely in Chapter 7, Case Management and Aural (Re)habilitation, and Chapter 11, Individual Planning.

Direct (Re)habilitation Services

Although not all educational audiologists assume responsibility for providing direct treatment services for students, school-based audiologists have an ongoing role in (re)habilitation. If educational audiologists do not provide comprehensive (re)habilitation services, they should work with the educational team to determine what services are needed and to ensure that all services are provided. Frequently, educational audiologists will consult with other professionals who are providing direct services to make these services more appropriate for students. Direct services may focus on any or all of the following:

➤ Speechreading
➤ Listening
➤ Communication strategies

➤ Hearing aid orientation
➤ Use and care of amplification
➤ Self-management of hearing needs
➤ Self-esteem building

More information on implementing aural (re)habilitation services is provided in Chapter 7, Case Management and Aural (Re)habilitation.

Family Support

To be effective, we believe it is important for educational audiologists to work closely with the families of children with hearing losses. Family-centered interventon is mandated with infants and toddlers, but as the child gets older, families are often less involved in their child's education. This lack of parent involvement is unfortunate, because parents usually know their child best and often can provide information that can result in more productive management of the child. Additionally, parents are primary case managers during periods when school personnel are not available, such as during the summer months and holiday vacations. Educational audiologists should work with families to empower them in their child's education and to utilize their resources to assist the child.

When working with families, educational audiologists must be sensitive to diversity. Families may include only a single parent, or there may be a large extended family actively involved with the child. There is also a multitude of socioeconomic and cultural differences with which educational audiologists must work. Additionally, educational audiologists should be aware of the Deaf Culture, both when working with Deaf parents and with students who view themselves as Deaf. Educational audiologists must be aware of various parent options regarding educational placements, communication systems, amplification, and other issues. They must be able to provide unbiased information about these options to the parents and then support the parents' decisions. Working with families is discussed in more detail in Chapter 10, Relationships with Families.

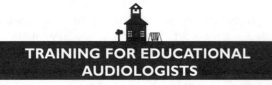

TRAINING FOR EDUCATIONAL AUDIOLOGISTS

To be qualified for all of the responsibilities described previously, it is obvious that educational audiologists must have training beyond that provided to most clinical audiologists. Surveys have routinely indicated that practicing educational audiologists do not believe they were adequately prepared to meet the responsibilities they have in the schools (Blair, Wilson-Vlotman, & Von Almen, 1989; Seaton, Von Almen, & Blair, 1994; Wilson-Vlotman & Blair, 1986). Areas of training that were reported as inadequate in these surveys include:

➤ Amplification
➤ Educational management of children with hearing losses
➤ Mainstreaming
➤ Auditory (re)habilitation
➤ Working with special populations
➤ Sign language
➤ Counseling

Additionally, two-thirds of the respondents to the survey conducted by Seaton, Von Almen, and Blair (1994) stated that an externship in an educational setting would have been helpful.

In recognition of the deficiencies currently existing in the training of educational audiologists, the Educational Audiology Association approved *Minimum Competencies for Educational Audiologists* in 1994 (see Appendix 2–M). These competencies focus on the knowledge, skills, and abilities necessary to provide effective, comprehensive audiology services in the schools. Although many of the competencies are also necessary for clinical audiologists, competency in the areas listed below are unique to the educational setting:

➤ Educational referral, follow-up procedures, and special education eligibility requirements
➤ Evaluation of the need for, selection, and maintenance of personal and classroom FM systems and other hearing assistance technology used in educational environments
➤ The structure of the learning environment, including classroom acoustics and implications for learning
➤ IFSP/IEP planning process and procedures, including interpretation of auditory assessment results and their implications, educational options, and legal issues and procedures
➤ Consultation and collaboration with classroom teachers and other professionals regarding the relationship of hearing and hearing loss to the development of academic and psychosocial skills
➤ Participation in team management of communication treatment
➤ Knowledge of communication systems and language used by individuals who are deaf and hard-of-hearing
➤ Implementation of inservice training for educational staff and support personnel
➤ Knowledge of school systems, multidisciplinary

teams, and community and professional resources The Educational Audiology Association also recommended that all audiologists employed in the schools complete an internship in a school setting under the supervision of an educational audiologist, preferably a full-time experience lasting at least 6 weeks. These recommendations have been used to encourage university training programs to upgrade their curricula for educational audiologists and can be a means of informing school administrators about the special knowledge, skills, and abilities of educational audiologists.

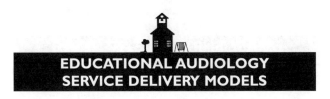

EDUCATIONAL AUDIOLOGY SERVICE DELIVERY MODELS

There are several different ways that educational audiology services can be delivered within a school district. Although at least five different models have been discussed in the literature (Blair, 1991), most are merely modifications of two basic models:

➤ School-based
➤ Contractual agreement

Both models can be used to provide effective educational audiology services in schools, and it may be possible that a district will find it beneficial to provide services using a combination of the two models. Neither of these models is superior to the other, but they each have specific advantages and disadvantages (see Table 2–3 for a comparison of the two models).

School-Based

In a school-based model of services, the educational audiologist is a direct employee of the school district or education agency. Most school-based audiologists are relatively autonomous in defining their positions in the schools and are, therefore, able to include comprehensive educational audiology services in their job description. Because school-based audiologists are employees of the system, they are peers of teachers and other school personnel and are perceived as providing services within the system, rather than as an outsider. Scheduling flexibility for consultation and follow-up can also be an advantage of this model. A major disadvantage is that many districts assume that the school-based audiologist can provide services to an infinite number of students. This model is effective only if the audiologist's caseload is reasonable. The ASHA *Guidelines for Audiology Services in the Schools* (1993) suggest that there should be a minimum of one educational audiologist to every 12,000 students in a school district.

Contractual Agreement

A school district may choose to provide educational audiology services using a contractual agreement. In this instance, the district contracts with the audiologist to perform specified services for students in the district. This model can be cost-effective and may be the only means of obtaining audiological services in some rural districts. If the contract is comprehensive, the services provided to the students may not differ from those provided by school-based audiologists.

Table 2–3. Comparison of school-based and contractual agreement service delivery models.

School-Based Audiology Services	Contracted Audiology Services
➤ Direct employee	➤ Contracted employee
➤ Relatively autonomous	➤ Completely autonomous
➤ Services typically comprehensive, based on job description	➤ Services may be limited by scope of contract
➤ Peer of other school employees; perceived as "insider"	➤ Considered an "outside expert"; collaboration with teachers may be difficult
➤ Caseload often very large	➤ Caseload can be specified in contract
➤ District often purchases and maintains audiological equipment	➤ District usually not responsible for diagnostic audiological equipment
➤ Cost to district may be greater	➤ Cost-effective
➤ Often less efficient in small, rural systems due to small caseload	➤ Appropriate for small, rural systems

However, many districts limit services in their contracts so that the majority of the services related to the educational support for students with hearing losses are addressed only minimally, if at all. Also, with this model educational audiologists often are viewed as "outside experts," and their effectiveness in collaboration with teachers may be limited.

Audiologists providing contracted audiology services should emphasize to administrators that a full range of audiology services must be provided. Differences between educational and clinical audiology services may need to be clarified as the contract is being developed. Table 2–4 describes the different functions of educational and clinical audiologists. In addition to hearing assessments, activities such as classroom observations, teacher collaboration, attendance at IEP meetings, equipment maintenance and repair, and inservice should be specified in the contract.

Combined School-Based and Contractual Agreement

At times it may be advantageous for a school district or educational agency to use a combination of both school-based and contractual agreement services. This model can be particularly useful when the school-based audiologist is not able to provide service to all the students within the district or when an audiologist with

specialized skills is needed. The contracted audiologist may provide comprehensive services to specified students within the district, such as those who live in a specific geographical area or those with specific disabilities. Optionally, the contracted audiologist may provide specified services (e.g., central auditory processing assessments) to all students within the district. For this model to work effectively, both the school-based and the contractual audiologist must have well-articulated responsibilities, a clear understanding of what the other is doing, and an ability to collaborate so that comprehensive services are provided.

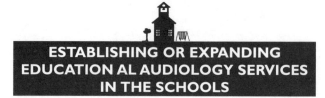

ESTABLISHING OR EXPANDING EDUCATIONAL AUDIOLOGY SERVICES IN THE SCHOOLS

Although educational audiologists have been employed in some school systems for many years, there are still many areas in which educational audiology services are minimal or nonexistent. Only a few states have guidelines which ensure that there is at least one educational audiologist for every 12,000 students in a school system, as recommended by ASHA's *Guidelines for Audiology Services in the Schools* (1993).

Table 2–4. Educational versus clinical audiology.

Educational Audiology	Clinical Audiology
➤ Identify hearing loss at earliest age	➤ Identify hearing loss at earliest age
➤ Diagnose hearing impairment	➤ Diagnose hearing impairment to
➤ Make appropriate referrals for	—Assist with medical management
—Medical attention and management	—Assist with (re)habilitative needs
—Personal amplification	➤ Communicate with physicians and
➤ Evaluate hearing abilities to establish	referral source
auditory skill development and to	➤ Dispense and monitor appropriate
determine hearing function in various	amplification
communication and learning settings	
➤ Select and fit appropriate assistive	
amplification devices	
➤ Interpret audiological information for	
educational implications	
➤ Determine appropriate instructional	
modifications and accomodations	
➤ Consult with student, teachers, parents,	
and other necessary staff regarding	
hearing and amplification needs	
➤ Ensure that amplification is working	
properly	
➤ Provide and/or assist with	
(re)habilitative needs within	
learning environment	

To create new educational audiology positions or to expand existing services, the educational audiologist must have a clear idea of what changes should be made and how these changes can be accomplished. Change is often difficult, but a systematic approach will help educational audiologists stay focused on the goals they set. A process described by Blair (1991) that can facilitate the improvement of audiology services in the schools is as follows:

➤ Develop a written proposal for the educational audiology program

➤ Review the current program and services to determine what changes should be made

➤ Prioritize long-term and short-term goals for the program

➤ Identify and obtain support from key decision makers at the district and state levels

➤ Implement new services according to the approved plans

➤ Evaluate the changes in the program at least annually to determine program's progress and any additional needs

➤ Keep key decision makers aware of progress

Chapter 13, Marketing, contains more information on marketing educational audiology, and program development, planning, and evaluation are specifically dealt with in Chapter 14, Program Development, Evaluation, and Mangement.

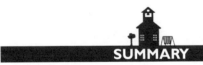

SUMMARY

The roles and responsibilities of educational audiologists in the total management of students with hearing losses are quite comprehensive. Unfortunately, administrators and others in the schools are often not aware of the broad scope of practice for educational audiologists, and educational audiology services are frequently not available or are under-utilized. There are many ways that educational audiology services can be delivered in a school system, but it is important for us to recognize what we can do to market our services. It is possible to enhance audiology services in the schools, but it takes a planned, consistent effort on the part of educational audiologists. The changes required are not easy to accomplish, but they are necessary to ensure comprehensive services to students with hearing losses.

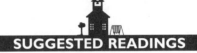

SUGGESTED READINGS

Berg, F., Blair, J., Viehweg, S., & Wilson-Vlotman, A. (1986). *Educational audiology for the hard of hearing child*. Orlando, FL: Grune & Stratton, Inc.

English, K. M. (1995). *Educational audiology across the lifespan*. Baltimore, MD: Paul H. Brookes Publishing Co.

Hull, R., & Dilka, K. (Eds.). (1984). *The hearing-impaired child in school*. Orlando, FL: Grune & Stratton, Inc.

Maxon, A., & Brackett, D. (1992). *The hearing-impaired child: Infancy through high school years*. Boston, MA: Andover Medical Publishers.

Roeser, R. J., & Downs, M. P. (1988). *Auditory disorders in school children* (2nd ed.). New York: Thieme Medical Publishers, Inc.

Ross, M., Brackett, D., & Maxon, A. (1991). *Assessment and management of mainstreamed hearing-impaired children: Principles and practices*. Austin, TX: Pro-Ed, Inc.

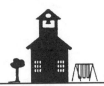

CHAPTER 3

IDENTIFICATION PRACTICES

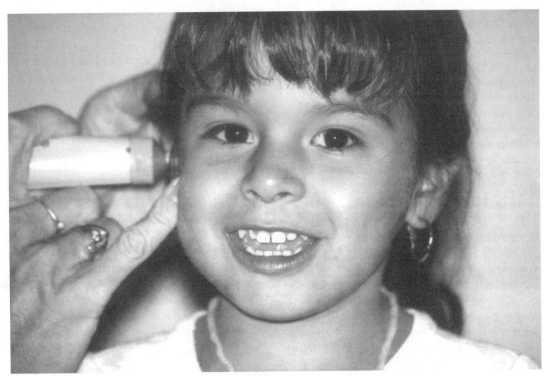

Olivia, age 4

CONTENTS

The initial step in any school-based audiology program is to establish some method of identifying those children who have hearing losses or auditory problems. This is typically done, at least in part, through a hearing screening or identification program. A hearing screening program's purpose is to identify those children who *might* have a hearing loss, whereas a hearing loss identification program should identify those who *definitely* have a hearing loss. A hearing screening program should separate a large population of children into two groups—those who have normal results (pass) and those who have abnormal results who need further testing (rescreen or refer). Because a hearing loss identification program is designed to determine the presence or absence of hearing loss, diagnostic testing beyond the hearing screening must be included. This chapter deals with issues specific to hearing screening, and Chapter 4, Assessment Practices, addresses diagnostic testing.

Questions to be addressed when developing and implementing a hearing screening program include the following:

➤ What are the existing state mandates for hearing screening?
➤ What are the purposes of the hearing screening program?
➤ What resources are available to the program?
➤ What children will be screened and how will they be referred for screening?
➤ What tests will be used for screening?
➤ How will children who cannot respond to traditional techniques be screened?
➤ What personnel will be necessary for the screening program?
➤ What pass/fail criteria will be used for screening?
➤ What equipment will be necessary, and how will it be maintained?
➤ What environment will be used for the screening?
➤ How will the screening program be organized?
➤ What follow-up procedures will be used for screening failures and absentees?
➤ What recordkeeping and reporting will be used in the screening program?
➤ What will be done to determine the effectiveness of the screening program?

It is impossible to provide specific answers for each of these questions because the needs of each screening program will vary. This chapter addresses each of these questions, providing options that the educational audiologist can consider when implementing a hearing screening program. Issues related to screening for central auditory processing disorders are not specifically addressed in this chapter, but are discussed in Chapter 5, Central Auditory Processing Disorders.

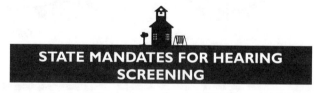

STATE MANDATES FOR HEARING SCREENING

The state laws that govern hearing screening vary a great deal and may be nonexistent for certain populations in some states. Blake and Hall (1990) found that only 14 states had a legislative mandate for neonatal hearing screening using a high-risk register, but that 12 additional states had addressed neonatal screening in some manner. There rarely are state mandates for screening the hearing of toddlers and preschoolers, but implementation of PL 99-457 often provides a vehicle through which these services can be provided. Most states require hearing screening for school-age children, but there is a great deal of variability in the specificity of the laws. The laws may indicate who should be screened and the screening criteria, or they may be more general, only providing for the screening in general terms. It is critical that all educational audiologists know the mandates regarding hearing screening in their states.

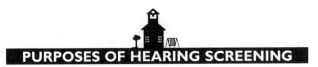

PURPOSES OF HEARING SCREENING

Before beginning a hearing screening program, the educational audiologist must have the specific outcomes of the program clearly in mind. These purposes may differ depending on the ages of the children to be screened and the philosophy of the program.

Age Considerations

A major concern for infants, toddlers, and preschoolers is the development of speech, language, and cognitive skills. As a result, most hearing screening programs for this age group will have as their goal the detection of hearing losses that may affect the development of these skills. School-age children also may develop or are at risk for delays in speech, language, and cognitive development when a hearing loss is present. These delays are often manifested by poor academic performance. As a result many screening programs for school-age children will have the identification of educationally significant auditory disorders (i.e., those disorders that potentially affect a child's communication and learning skills) as their goal.

Programmatic Considerations

The efficacy and criteria for failure for hearing screening programs, especially for immittance and central auditory processing screening, are not well specified in the literature. The philosophy of the program and of the audiologist will therefore play an important role in determining what will be included in the program, the specific criteria for failure, and the protocol for follow-up. For example, the audiologist's belief about the educational impact of minimal and fluctuating conductive hearing losses may affect the screening level used for pure-tone screening and the inclusion of immittance screening in the program. Likewise, the belief about the efficacy of the evaluation and treatment of central auditory processing disorders will dictate what attempts will be made to identify these disorders.

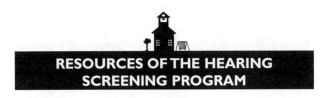

RESOURCES OF THE HEARING SCREENING PROGRAM

Personnel and Time

Resources available for screening and follow-up will impact the development of a hearing screening program. Personnel and time are critical factors to be considered in determining the scope and protocol of the screening program. Regardless of the desire of an audiologist to identify all educationally significant auditory disorders, it is frustrating to screen for these disorders when resources for follow-up are not available. In fact, screening without adequate follow-up can potentially cause more harm than if the screening was not done. If follow-up testing is significantly delayed or is not done at all, teachers and parents may believe that a child, who actually has an auditory problem, has normal hearing abilities. Likewise, if teachers and parents are aware that a child has failed a hearing screening test, they may blame hearing loss for all difficulties the child is having when, in fact, other reasons for academic failure may exist.

Working with Staff and Schedules

The audiologist must work closely with the schools and with others involved in the screening program and be sensitive to their needs. Even the best hearing screening program will experience failure if the screening or follow-up is scheduled on the same day as an assembly or other school activity. Teachers who do not understand the importance of the hearing screening program or the protocol that will be used may object to having their classes participate in the screening. Also, because of the fluctuating nature of some hearing losses and the conditions under which screening programs are conducted, no program will identify all of the children who have auditory problems. It is, therefore, critical that the audiologist maintain contact with teachers and parents to encourage questions about specific children and referrals for additional testing.

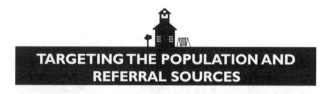

TARGETING THE POPULATION AND REFERRAL SOURCES

Screening and Referrals for Infants, Toddlers, and Preschoolers

Screening programs to detect hearing losses among school-age children have existed in most school systems in the United States for many years. It is also advantageous for educational audiologists to be involved in the screening of infants, toddlers, and preschoolers in order to facilitate early identification and intervention for children with hearing losses. In states where the health department is responsible for services to infants and toddlers under Public Law 99-457, educational audiologists may serve as consultants to the program or may function as advocates for the program. However, when the education agency is responsible for these services, it is imperative that educational audiologists be directly involved in developing, implementing, and monitoring the hearing screening program for infants and toddlers. Regardless of the role played by educational audiologists in such programs, they should be aware of the screening protocols appropriate for infants, toddlers, and preschoolers.

The American Speech-Language-Hearing Association (ASHA) guidelines, *Audiologic Screening of Newborn Infants Who Are At Risk for Hearing Impairment* (see Appendix 2–C), were published in 1989. The guidelines are valuable to the educational audiologist, but they are somewhat dated because the high-risk criteria provided by the Joint Committee on Infant Hearing (1994) have been updated and because technological advances have made universal neonatal screening a possibility. Currently hearing screening for infants, toddlers, and preschoolers may be promoted by a variety of activities, including:

➤ High-risk registers
➤ Universal hearing screening of infants

➤ Developmental checklists
➤ Education of other professionals

High-Risk Registers

Until recently, the accepted protocol for screening for hearing loss in infants was the use of a high-risk register. In 1994 the Joint Committee on Infant Hearing provided an updated list of criteria that put a neonate at risk for hearing impairment (see Table 3–1). Recognizing that not all hearing losses will be present at birth, the Joint Committee on Infant Hearing also provided high-risk criteria for infants from 29 days through 2 years of age (see Table 3–2).

Universal Hearing Screening

Unfortunately, only about 50% of infants with hearing losses will be identified through a high-risk register. Because of this fact and the improved technology available for infant hearing screening, the National Institutes of Health (NIH) Consensus Development Conference on Early Identification of Hearing Impairment in Infants and Young Children (1993) recommended universal hearing screening of all infants within the first 3 months of life. Not all professionals have accepted the NIH Conference recommendation, but there is considerable effort currently being made to establish universal hearing screening programs.

Developmental Checklists and Professional Education

With universal neonatal hearing screening, early identification of hearing losses will be greatly enhanced. However, late-onset and progressive hearing losses will not be identified by this method, and conductive hearing losses may or may not be present at birth. Ideally all children, birth to age 7, should receive annual hearing screenings. Ensuring these annual screenings is currently impossible because there is no established environment to conduct such a mass screening in the preschool years. Educational audiologists should educate physicians, health departments, and early childhood care agencies regarding the importance and necessity of annual screenings in order to establish community, statewide, and national support for such a standard of care. This education will have the added advantage of encouraging hearing screenings during routine, well-baby checks.

It is necessary for educational audiologists to continue to be alert to the concerns that parents and other caregivers have about the status of a child's hearing. Developmental checklists produced by several orga-

Table 3–1. Risk criteria for neonates (birth–28 days) when universal screening is not available.

1. Family history of hereditary childhood sensorineural hearing loss.
2. In utero infection, such as cytomegalovirus, rubella, syphilis, herpes, and toxoplasmosis.
3. Craniofacial anomalies, including those with morphologic abnormalities of the pinna and ear canal.
4. Birth weight less than 1500 grams (3.3 lbs.).
5. Hyperbilirubinemia at a serum level requiring exchange transfusion.
6. Ototoxic medications, including but not limited to the aminoglycosides, used in multiple courses or in combination with loop diuretics.
7. Bacterial meningitis.
8. Apgar scores of 0–4 at 1 minute or 0–6 at 5 minutes.
9. Mechanical ventilation lasting 5 days or longer.
10. Stigmata or other findings associated with a syndrome known to include a sensorineural and/or conductive hearing loss.

Source: From "Joint Committee on Infant Hearing position statement" by the Joint Committee on Infant Hearing, 1994.

Table 3–2. Risk criteria for infants (29 days–2 years).

Infants with Certain Health Conditions that Require Screening

1. Parent/caregiver concern regarding hearing, speech, language and/or developmental delay.
2. Bacterial meningitis and other infections associated with sensorineural hearing loss.
3. Head trauma associated with loss of consciousness or skull fracture.
4. Stigmata or other findings associated with a syndrome known to include a sensorineural and/or conductive hearing loss.
5. Ototoxic medications, including but not limited to chemotherapeutic agents or aminoglycosides, used in multiple courses or in combination with loop diuretics.
6. Recurrent or persistent otitis media with effusion for at least 3 months.

Infants Who Require Periodic Monitoring of Hearing

Some newborns and infants may pass initial hearing screening but require periodic monitoring of hearing to detect delayed-onset sensorineural and/or conductive hearing loss. Infants with these indicators require hearing evaluation at least every 6 months until age 3 years and at appropriate intervals thereafter. Indicators associated with delayed onset sensorineural hearing loss include:
1. Family history of hereditary childhood hearing loss.
2. In utero infection, such as cytomegalovirus, rubella, syphilis, herpes, or toxoplasmosis.
3. Neurofibromatosis Type II and neurodegenerative disorders.

Indicators Associated with Conductive Hearing Loss include:

1. Recurrent or persistent otitis media with effusion.
2. Anatomic deformities and other disorders that affect eustachian tube function.
3. Neurodegenerative disorders.

Source: From "Joint Committee on Infant Hearing position statement" by the Joint Committee on Infant Hearing, 1994.

nizations and agencies (see Appendix 16–B for a list of available checklists) are useful in educating parents about the expected auditory and communication behaviors of their children at specific ages.

Screening and Referrals for School-Age Children

School-age children will typically be referred for hearing screening through one of the following protocols:

➤ Mass hearing screening
➤ Special education hearing screening
➤ Teacher, parent, or physician referrals
➤ Teacher or parent checklists

Mass Hearing Screening

The concept of mass hearing screening for school-age children is fairly universal, but the specific grades screened vary a great deal from state to state, as well as from program to program. Most of the programs in a recent survey (Roush & Davidson, as cited in Roush, 1992) provided pure-tone screening for all kindergarten and first-grade students. Beyond the first grade, the survey revealed that mass screening tends to occur every other year, with fewer students being screened at the secondary level. The inclusion of immittance screening as part of the mass screening program is much less common at all grades, but is more frequently included in the lower elementary grades.

Special Education Hearing Screening

In many states it is required that all students referred for special education programs have a vision and hearing screening prior to their educational evaluation. This is a useful practice because the screenings can detect sensory deficits that might interfere with testing or relate to the identified problem, ultimately affecting the child's placement. It is also advantageous to screen the hearing of all special education students periodically so that there is not an unidentified hearing loss that could interfere with their educational progress.

Teacher, Parent, or Physician Referrals

Referrals from teachers, parents, or physicians are critical in seeking to identify children with educationally significant auditory disorders. Traditional mass hearing screening programs will not identify the hearing losses of students who are absent when the screening occurs or those not in the grades routinely screened. Also missed will be students who have fluctuating hearing losses but who had normal hearing during the mass screening and those with central auditory processing disorders. Mass screening programs may also mistakenly pass some children who actually have hearing losses (false negative responses). It is important to encourage, both formally and informally, referrals from teachers, parents, and physicians. Because many referrals are obtained informally as the educational audiologist has contact with teachers, parents, or physicians, it is critical that information about behaviors that may indicate that a child has a hearing loss be provided to potential referral sources. A sample list of these behaviors, which can be given to teachers, parents, and physicians and/or be used as the basis for inservice training sessions, is provided in Appendix 3–A.

Teacher or Parent Checklists

To supplement the informal referrals for hearing screenings, some school districts use formalized checklists to encourage referrals from parents, teachers, or other school personnel. To identify children with chronic middle ear problems or known sensorineural hearing losses, it has been suggested that all parents be required to complete a hearing history form (see Appendix 3–B) when they enroll their child in school each year. The Colorado Front Range Educational Audiology Group designed a Hearing Questionnaire (see Appendix 3–C) that can be completed by teachers, parents, or other persons familiar with the child to document his or her responses to sound. Although specifically designed to screen children for central audi-

tory processing disorders, the Fisher's Auditory Problems Checklist (Fisher, 1985) could be adapted to obtain referrals from teachers for children suspected of having hearing problems. A copy of this checklist is in Appendix 3–D.

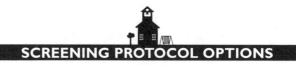

SCREENING PROTOCOL OPTIONS

Infants, Toddlers, and Preschoolers

Procedures used in a hearing screening program for infants, toddlers, and preschoolers vary depending on the age of the child and the resources available to the program. These procedures, summarized in Table 3–3, include:

➤ High-risk register
➤ Electrophysiologic screening
    Auditory brainstem response (ABR)
    Transiently evoked otoacoustic emissions (TEOAEs)
    Distortion product otoacoustic emissions (DPOAEs)
➤ Behavioral screening
    Visual reinforcement audiometry (VRA)
    Conditioned play audiometry (CPA)
➤ Immittance screening

For infants, electrophysiologic screening tests have become the preferred method of screening, whereas behavioral tests are most often used for screening the hearing of toddlers and preschoolers. For all age groups, immittance screening is invaluable in determining the status of the middle ear system.

High-Risk Register

As stated previously, one of the accepted protocols for screening the hearing of infants and toddlers is the high-risk register, using a list of criteria similar to the ones published in 1994 by the Joint Committee on Infant Hearing (see Tables 3–1 and 3–2). With this method, children are screened, using either birth certificates or information provided in the child's medical chart, to determine if the factors on the high-risk register are present. If any of the factors are present, the child is referred for additional electrophysiologic or behavioral testing. Although high-risk registers are relatively easy to administer and volunteers can be used to review the birth certificates or charts, less than 50% of the children who have sensorineural hearing losses are identified by a high-risk register (Mauk, White, Mortensen, & Behrens, 1991).

Table 3–3. Summary of pediatric hearing screening procedures.

Procedure	Developmental Age of Target Population	Advantages	Limitations
High-risk register (HRR)	Birth–2 years; Possible for all ages	Easy to administer Volunteers easily trained	Only 50% of hearing losses identified May require time-consuming chart review Follow-up difficult
Auditory brainstem response (ABR)	All ages	Effective for losses greater than 30 dB HL Ear-specific Minimal cooperation required	Expensive equipment Interpretation complex Not frequency-specific Difficult to interpret if CNS pathology present Measures only to brainstem
Otoacoustic emissions: Transient evoked (TEOAE) or DIstortion product (DPOAE)	All ages	Effective for losses greater than 30 dB HL Noninvasive, simple procedure Quick, easy to administer Useful with neurologically compromised Frequency-specific Ear-specific Minimal cooperation required	Expensive equipment Valid screening difficult prior to 24 hours of age Measures only to cochlea Compromised by middle or outer ear involvement
Visual reinforcement audiometry (VRA)	6 months–2.5 years	Valid responses to low-level stimuli Inexpensive equipment Sound-field or ear-specific Frequency-specific	2-year-olds frequently habituate rapidly Requires trained administrator(s)
Conditioned play audiometry (CPA)	2.5–5 years	Valid responses to low-level stimuli Inexpensive equipment Sound-field or ear-specific Frequency-specific Variety of play tasks	Requires trained administrator Requires child cooperation
Immittance	6 months and older	Valid indicator of middle ear function Quick, easy to administer Inexpensive equipment	Does not assess hearing sensitivity Questionable follow-up protocol

Electrophysiologic Screening

The two electrophysiologic tests that are most often used for hearing screening are the auditory brainstem response (ABR) test and, more recently, otoacoustic emissions using transient evoked (TEOAE) and/or distortion product (DPOAE) stimuli. Traditional ABR screening has been shown to be an effective technique for detecting hearing losses that are greater than 30 dB HL. Some limitations in the use of this technique are that the equipment is relatively expensive and the technique requires the use of highly trained personnel for both administration and interpretation of the tests. These disadvantages have been solved to some extent by automated ABR screeners, but the automated screen-er has stringent requirements for electrode imped-ance, ambient noise level, and muscle artifact that pro-hibit its use in some environments. Even though the automated screener has overcome some of the disad-vantages of the traditional ABR unit and has become a viable means of screening the hearing of infants, it should be remembered that ABR using click stimuli is not effective in the identification of children who have low-frequency hearing losses. Additionally, ABR tests measure responses of the neural system only as far as the brainstem; purely cortical auditory disorders will not be detected by this screening.

TEOAE and DPOAE tests have been shown to sepa-rate ears with normal cochlear functioning from those with a hearing loss greater than approximately 30 dB

HL. These tests are quickly and easily administered and can provide frequency-specific information across a relatively wide range of frequencies. Although the equipment is expensive at this time, it is easy to use and volunteers or medical personnel can be trained to administer the tests effectively. Because infants are often discharged from the hospital quickly, the high failure rate for OAE screenings during the first 24 hours of life often makes it difficult to get a valid screening before the baby leaves the hospital. Additionally, the results of OAE screenings may be compromised if the child has outer or middle ear problems. A final disadvantage of OAE screening is that it only measures cochlear functioning and does not give an indication of the child's auditory status at levels higher than the cochlea.

Behavioral Screening

Behavioral screening tests have been used with neonates in the past, but they are typically more effective for children who are 6 months of age or older. For infants older than 6 months of age, toddlers, and preschoolers, the two most common behavioral tests are visual reinforcement audiometry (VRA) and conditioned play audiometry (CPA). VRA is very successful with children who are developmentally from 6 months through 2½ years of age. With it valid responses to very low-level sounds can be obtained either in sound-field or under earphones. VRA does require a specialized reinforcement design, but portable units are now available. This equipment is not very expensive and is useful to educational audiologists in a variety of screening situations. Although a major drawback to the use of VRA is that 2-year-old children can quickly habituate to this technique, it can be quite helpful when screening children who have developmental disabilities.

Conditioned play audiometry (CPA) is a very effective technique with most preschoolers above the age of 2½ years. It requires very little specialized equipment, and because of the variety of play tasks that can be used, children rarely habituate to the task. With either VRA or CPA, children may object to wearing standard earphones. The availability of insert earphones has alleviated this concern in many instances.

Immittance Screening

Although the need for monitoring the middle ear status of preschool children is well recognized, the protocol to be used has been fairly controversial. Historically, immittance screening protocols have used both tympanometry and acoustic reflex screening, but the most recent guidelines published by the American Speech-Language-Hearing Association (1990b) have suggested the use of only tympanometry to reduce the high number of false positive results.

The scheduling and follow-up protocols for immittance screenings is another area of controversy. It is difficult to know when and how often to perform immittance screening. If the screening is scheduled during the winter months when the incidence of middle ear problems is greatest, the failure rate will be higher than if the screening is done at another time of the year. Likewise, because middle ear problems are transitory in nature, the fact that children pass a screening does not mean they are clear of middle ear diseases at another point in time. It may be necessary to use repeated screenings to identify all children with chronic middle ear disorders. It is difficult to determine the most effective immittance screening protocol, but the potential deleterious effects of chronic middle ear disease on learning make it critical that immittance screening be routinely provided for infants, toddlers, and preschoolers.

School-Age Children

Screening tests for school-age children routinely include one or more of the following tests:

➤ Pure-tone screening
➤ Immittance screening
➤ OAE screening

Pure-tone screening is the most frequently used technique for this population, but the inclusion of immittance and OAE screenings is becoming more common, especially for kindergarten and first-grade children.

Pure-Tone Screening

Pure-tone screening is a quick procedure, the screening can be easily done by a trained volunteer or paraprofessional, and the test can be completed by most school-age children with relative ease. Assuming that the number of frequencies screened, typically three or four, is sufficient, pure-tone screening is effective in identifying students who might have a peripheral hearing loss in one or both ears. It is not, however, possible to identify hearing losses that are milder than the screening level used. Because of the limitations imposed by noise levels in the environment in which screenings often occur, pure-tone screenings frequently use screening levels that are higher than would be ideal for the identification of mild hearing losses.

Immittance Screening

Middle ear disorders are common in school-age children in the lower elementary grades, and immittance screening has been shown to be an effective way to detect these problems. It should be emphasized that immittance testing is not effective in determining a child's hearing sensitivity. Pure-tone or other screening tests are necessary to determine the presence of a hearing loss because immittance screening primarily measures middle ear functioning. As was noted in the previous discussion of immittance screening, the immittance screening protocols and the most effective follow-up strategies are still subject to much debate. When immittance screening is used as part of a mass screening program, it is typically used in lower elementary grades (kindergarten, first grade) due to the higher incidence of middle ear problems in younger children. Another alternative, supported by Bluestone et al. (1986), is to provide immittance screening only for high-risk "special populations." Examples of these high-risk populations are children who are Native Americans (Indians or Eskimos), children with cleft palates or other craniofacial anomalies, and children with Down syndrome.

Otoacoustic Emissions Screening

The use of otoacoustic emissions as part of school hearing screening programs is a relatively new occurrence. Although OAE equipment is somewhat expensive at this time, some school districts have purchased equipment and are using it to provide either TEOAE or DPOAE screenings for school-age children. OAE screenings provide frequency-specific, objective data. They can be quickly and easily administered, and volunteers can be trained to perform the screenings. Despite these advantages, it must be remembered that OAEs will detect only those cochlear hearing losses greater than 30 dB HL. It is not, therefore, effective in screening for very mild hearing losses that may have academic significance.

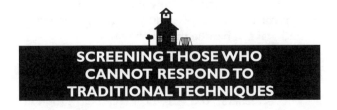

SCREENING THOSE WHO CANNOT RESPOND TO TRADITIONAL TECHNIQUES

Although pure-tone and immittance screening will be appropriate for most school-age children, some children have mental, physical, or emotional disabilities that make it impossible for them to respond to traditional screening techniques. Screening tests appropriate for younger children, including both behavioral and electrophysiologic techniques, may have to be used to determine the status of their auditory systems. Screening utilizing otoacoustic emissions promises to be an effective technique for use with this population. It should be emphasized that the hearing status of every child must be determined as part of initial placement in special education, either through screening or further evaluation. With the technology and resources currently available, DNT (did not test) or CNT (cannot test) should never be accepted as the final screening result for any child.

Because of limited resources for equipment in the schools, it may be necessary for some children to be tested by a clinical audiologist apart from the school system. Although this may be relatively expensive, all children, regardless of functioning level, should have their hearing screened at least once to determine if they have a hearing loss. Once it has been determined that a child has normal hearing sensitivity, outside referrals to monitor the child's hearing may not be necessary on an annual basis. Instead, a teacher checklist, perhaps based on the Functional Communication Measures developed in 1994 by the ASHA Task Force on Treatment Outcomes and Cost Effectiveness (see Appendix 2–D) or the Hearing Questionnaire developed by the Colorado Front Range Educational Audiology Group (see Appendix 3–C), can be used to monitor the child's responses to auditory stimuli. Additionally, all of these children should be tested at least annually using immittance and, if available, OAE measures. If changes in the teacher's observations or the immittance and OAE results are observed, the child should be immediately referred for another hearing screening or for a diagnostic evaluation.

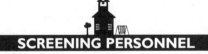

SCREENING PERSONNEL

Numerous persons, including audiologists, speech-language pathologists, school nurses, paraprofessionals, and parent volunteers, have traditionally been involved in hearing screening programs in the schools. In determining the personnel for a specific program, it is important to look at the cost effectiveness of using various personnel, while ensuring there is adequate expertise and supervision for the program.

Audiologists

Audiologists play a key role in hearing screening programs. However, it is generally not cost effective for the audiologist to be involved in the actual administration of the screening tests. Technicians, paid or volunteer, can be adequately trained to perform routine screenings, thus saving the district the higher salary of the audiologist for this task. The exception to using audiologists to perform actual screening tests is in the screening of infants, toddlers, and other students who cannot respond to standard techniques. Even though technicians can sometimes be trained to screen this population, the complexity of screening these students requires that the audiologist be actively involved in the administration and interpretation of the tests.

Activities related to hearing screening typically performed by the audiologist include the following:

➤ Planning and administering the hearing screening program
➤ Coordinating with other community agencies for infant/toddler early identification programs
➤ Training and supervising screening personnel
➤ Performing follow-up services, including rescreening, diagnostic evaluation, referral to other agencies, and educational management

Speech-Language Pathologists

Quite often speech-language pathologists perform puretone hearing screenings in the schools. They are often given this task because they are in every school on a regular basis and because they have received training to conduct screenings. It is not, however, cost effective to have speech-language pathologists conduct the initial screenings. Individuals with less training can adequately provide the screenings at a lower cost, without interfering with the regular workload of the speech-language pathologist. An American Speech-Language-Hearing Association Issues in Ethics statement (ASHA, 1994a) indicated that speech-language pathologists could conduct pure-tone air-conduction hearing screening independently, but that they could not perform immittance screening unless they were functioning as support personnel under the supervision of an audiologist. It would therefore be necessary to have the speech-language pathologists supervised by an audiologist if they were going to conduct immittance screening. Although not specifically addressed by ASHA at this time, similar comments could probably be made regarding OAE testing. Regardless of the speech-language pathologist's role, the entire screening program needs to be planned and supervised by an audiologist.

Parent Volunteers, School Nurses, and Paraprofessionals

As stated previously, it is more cost-effective to have someone other than the audiologist or speech-language pathologist actually administer the screening tests. When adequately trained and provided with supervised practice, parent volunteers, school nurses, and paraprofessionals can do routine screening quite effectively. The use of volunteers in a screening program is attractive because they cost the school district nothing. However, because they are not paid, they may not always show up at the scheduled time, and their abilities and motivation can vary widely. Procedural consistency may also cause problems when the volunteers change frequently. For these reasons, the use of school nurses or paraprofessionals may be more effective. It is also likely that school nurses or paraprofessionals who would be with the screening program over a period of several years would have better screening skills, thus making their screening results more reliable.

Training of Support Personnel

Some states have licensure laws that regulate the training and use of technicians who perform hearing screening. It is critical that educational audiologists be aware of such regulations in their states and follow them as a minimum standard for working with technicians. Recently, the Consensus Panel on Support Personnel in Audiology (1996), consisting of representatives of most audiology organizations, developed a draft position statement and guidelines for the utilization of support personnel in audiology. These guidelines address qualifications, training, role, and supervision for support personnel. They are reproduced in Appendix 2–O.

To be adequately trained to perform hearing screenings, the people doing the screening need to learn more than how to perform the actual screening test. Some topics that should be presented to potential screeners include:

➤ The purpose of hearing screening
➤ The screening equipment, including how to set it up, how to check its functioning, how to identify possible malfunctions in the equipment, and how to do basic troubleshooting if a problem occurs
➤ Typical behaviors of children during screenings and ways to handle these behaviors
➤ How the screening program will operate and how the results of the program will be reported to parents and teachers
➤ The screeners' role in the screening program, including an understanding that they cannot diagnose hearing loss nor report results independently
➤ Supervised practice under the direction of an audiologist, including screening of peers and of children who are the same ages as those who will be screened

Training sessions for routine pure-tone screening can usually be accomplished in a half-day. Additional training time may be needed depending on the background knowledge of the screeners, the population being screened, and the procedures used. Review sessions should be provided each year for those who have satisfactorily completed the initial training session.

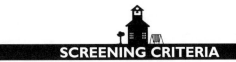

SCREENING CRITERIA

There are several sets of published guidelines that specify the criteria for various hearing screening procedures. It should be recognized that these guidelines contain only the recommendations of a group of experts, not specific criteria that *must* be followed in every situation. The actual criteria used by a district or agency may vary depending on the goals of the program and the state laws that must be followed. For example, if a school district has as its goal the identification of every hearing loss that *might* be educationally significant, including minimal hearing losses, a screening level of 15 dB HL may be selected by the district. On the other hand, if the district wants to identify only those losses that have a high likelihood of being educationally significant, a higher screening level, such as 25 dB HL, may be chosen.

Electrophysiologic Screening Tests

There are no universally recognized guidelines specifying the criteria for either auditory brainstem response (ABR) or otoacoustic emissions (OAE) screening, but large-scale research and clinical programs have recommended criteria that are generally well accepted. For ABR screening, the criteria for passing is the presence of an electrophysiologic response to the click stimuli in each ear at a specified intensity level, usually 30 or 40 dB nHL. A definite response in each of the frequency bands from 1000 through 5000 Hz in each ear is usually required to pass the OAE screening. Those wishing to use an electrophysiologic screening procedure should do additional research prior to beginning their screening program in order to determine the specific test parameters that should be used. As the parameters of the tests are varied, the criteria for the screening tests may differ from those given in this section.

Pure-Tone Screening Tests

For pure-tone screening, the most commonly used set of criteria is contained in the American Speech-Language-Hearing Association *Guidelines for Identification Audiometry* (ASHA, 1985). A summary of the screening criteria is provided in Table 3–4, and the complete guidelines are reproduced in Appendix 2–E. These guidelines recommend screening the frequencies of 1000, 2000, and 4000 Hz at a level of 20 dB. If immittance screening is not used in conjunction with the pure-tone screening, the guidelines further suggest the screening of 500 Hz, also at a 20 dB level. It should be noted that when 500 Hz is included, there is an increased likelihood of obtaining false positive results because environmental noise often makes it difficult for children to detect the 500-Hz tone. The criterion for passing the pure-tone screening is a response to each tone as it is presented to each ear individually. It is recommended that children who do not pass the screening be rescreened on the day of the screening or within 2 weeks of the initial screening. Children who fail the rescreening should be referred for audiological evaluation.

Some school screening programs modify the ASHA guidelines to include the frequency of 6000 Hz in order to obtain information relative to high-frequency hearing ability. Others screen the various frequencies at a level other than 20 dB. It is the responsibility of the educational audiologist to ensure that modifications to the criteria recommended by ASHA are appropriate for the purposes of the screening program.

Immittance Screening Tests

The criteria used for immittance screening are less defined than those for pure-tone screening. In an attempt to reduce the high number of false positive results from its earlier immittance screening protocol, the American Speech-Language-Hearing Association published *Guidelines for Screening for Hearing Impairment and Middle-Ear Disorders* (ASHA, 1990b). Table 3–4 summarizes these screening criteria, and Appendix 2–F contains the complete guidelines. These guidelines are comprehensive, suggesting that screening include four aspects: history, visual inspection, pure-tone screening, and immittance screening. The immittance screening protocol considers static acoustic immittance, equivalent ear canal volume, and tympanometric width or gradient. The specific criteria for each of these factors are not included in the guidelines, but some interim criteria are provided in an appendix to the guidelines. The criteria provided in the appendix recommend that a static acoustic immittance value greater than .2 cm^3 and a tympanometric width (a measure of gradient) less than 150 daPa be required for passing the screening. We have found the gradient value of 150 daPa to over-refer for middle ear conditions and recommend use of a value in the 180–200 daPa range, depending on local findings. Ear canal volume measurements are considered only if a child has a low static acoustic admittance

Table 3–4. Summary of Guidelines for Identification Audiometry (ASHA, 1985) and Guidelines for Screening for Hearing Impairments and Middle Ear Disorders (ASHA, 1990).

Screening Test	Screening Protocol	Criteria for Failure
History	History of ear pain (otalgia)	Recent positive history
	History of ear drainage (otorrhea)	Recent positive history
Visual Inspection	External ear, head, and neck	Structural defect
	Ear canal	Abnormality (blood, effusion, inflammation, excessive cerumen, tumor, foreign material)
	Eardrum	Abnormality (abnormal color, bulging eardrum, fluid line or bubbles, perforation, retraction)
Pure-tone	Response to 1000, 2000, and 4000 Hz at 20 dB level in each ear;	Lack of response to one tone in either ear
	Response to 500 Hz at 20 dB level if immittance not included	
Immittance	Measurement of static acoustic immitance	Less than .2 cm³*
	Measurement of tympanometric width or gradient	Greater than 150 daPa*
	Measurement of equivalent ear canal volume	Greater than 1.0 cm³ if static acoustic immitance is less than .2 cm³*

*Interim values

value. If the admittance is low in the presence of a volume measurement greater than 1.0 cm³, it is recommended that the child be immediately referred for medical evaluation. The guidelines further recommend that children with low static acoustic admittance values in the absence of a large volume measurement and children with large tympanometric widths be rescreened in 4 to 6 weeks. If they fail the rescreening, they should be referred for an audiological evaluation.

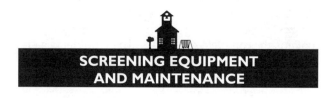

SCREENING EQUIPMENT AND MAINTENANCE

Screening Equipment

Electrophysiologic Screening

The types of equipment used for electrophysiologic screening will vary depending on the resources available to the program, the environment in which the screening will occur, and the expertise of the screeners. Auditory brainstem response (ABR) screening can be done with a variety of equipment, but the use of automated screeners has become more common in recent years. These screeners are less expensive than

diagnostic ABR equipment, and they are typically easier to use, an important consideration if volunteers or technicians will be used for the screenings. Equipment for OAE screening is increasing in availability, options, portability, and pricing, making it more and more attractive as a screening and diagnostic tool.

In addition to the actual equipment used, there are supplies that must be available for electrophysiologic screenings. Auditory brainstem response screenings require the use of electrodes that may or may not be reusable. Otoacoustic emissions screening utilizes a probe tip for each child who is screened. These tips are reusable, but care must be taken to ensure they are properly sanitized before they are used again (see section on infection control).

Pure-Tone Screening

Pure-tone screening requires the use of a pure-tone audiometer. Although there are screening audiometers with limited frequencies and intensity levels available, it is typically more cost effective to use a single-channel audiometer that uses two earphones and produces at least octave frequencies between 250 and 8000 Hz at levels ranging from 0 to at least 90 dB. The money that will be saved when purchasing a screening audiometer is not worth the flexibility that is lost with its limitations. With a standard pure-tone audiometer, the audiologist can determine the screening level and the frequencies to be screened, rather than using the predetermined levels and frequencies set by a screening audiometer. Additionally, the standard pure-tone audiometer can be used for both screening and diagnostic purposes, whereas the screening audiometer can be used only for screening.

The pure-tone audiometer that will be used for screening should be lightweight and durable. Most audiometers require the use of an electrical plug for power, but some audiometers are designed to be powered by a battery. This may be an advantage in some situations, as long as there is a warning light to signal when the battery is low. Some screening environments with older electrical wiring may have outlets that are not compatible with the three-pronged plugs on newer audiometers. The use of adapters may not meet electrical and/or fire code requirements, so screening audiometers with three-pronged plugs may have limited use in older school facilities. Educational audiologists should consult with school safety directors to determine if any special electrical requirements must be met before purchasing any audiometric equipment.

Immittance Screening

There are several tympanometers and portable immittance bridges that are available and can be used for immittance screening. Tympanometers typically are more automated and often provide quicker results than portable bridges. They are therefore better suited for the immittance screenings that will be performed by technicians or volunteers. Portable bridges, however, offer more flexibility and can be used by the audiologist to do diagnostic testing. Regardless of the type of equipment used, the audiologist should be certain that the equipment can quickly and easily provide measurements of the components that will be considered in the screening. For example, several tympanometers do not provide a direct measure of gradient, making it difficult to determine if a child has passed or failed if gradient is one of the screening criteria. As with the pure-tone audiometers, an immittance screener that is lightweight and durable is advantageous.

If immittance screening is done, it is advantageous to use an otoscope for a visual inspection of the ear canal and tympanic membrane prior to inserting the probe tip. In fact, many professionals agree that otoscopic examination should be completed on every ear before any audiologic testing is done. Although the many different otoscopes available offer a variety of features that may be convenient, such as the use of rechargeable batteries, the main requirement is that there be sufficient light to view the ear canal adequately.

For each child who participates in the immittance screening, a reusable immittance probe tip and either a disposable or reusable specula for the otoscope are used. As was noted when otoacoustic emissions screenings were discussed, the educational audiologist must ensure that the tips and specula are properly sanitized before they are used again (see section on infection control).

Equipment Maintenance

Regardless of the type of equipment used in a screening program, it is critical that it be working properly on the day of the screening. Unless the equipment is performing as it is supposed to be, the screening will not be accurate, resulting either in passing some children who have a hearing problem or in excessive failures. A back-up plan with loaner equipment should be developed for emergencies. All equipment should be calibrated at least annually, and screeners should be trained to perform a daily calibration check prior to the use of the equipment. Additionally, screeners should be alert to excessive failures during the screening, and they should check the equipment any time it seems to be functioning improperly.

Infection Control

Infection control has recently become a critical concern for audiologists (Kemp, Roeser, Pearson, & Ballachanda, 1995) and is particularly important in screening programs. The screeners see many different children in one day, thus increasing the chance of getting an infection from a child or passing an infection from one child to another. The best way for screeners to avoid the spread of disease is to wash their hands thoroughly with disinfectant soap as often as possible (ideally between each child tested) and to avoid putting their hands near their faces, eyes, and mouths. When it is impractical to stop and wash their hands, screeners can use a product such as Audiologist's Choice disinfectant hand lotion (see Appendix 16–C for ordering information) to clean their hands. Additionally, screeners should periodically wipe table surfaces and toys used for play audiometry with a disinfectant, because they are potential vehicles for infectious diseases.

Typically earphones are not a major source of infection. However, if they are put on a child who has excessive cerumen, drainage from the ears, open sores near the ears, or head lice, the earphone cushions should be wiped with a disinfectant before they are placed on another child. Ideally, disposable earphone covers should be changed between each test. The probe tips used for otoacoustic emissions or immittance screening and the specula on otoscopes are a much greater potential source of infection because they are actually inserted into the ear canal. When possible, disposable probe tips and specula should be used. If reusable tips or specula are used during screening, it is important that they be thoroughly disinfected (most of the germs killed) or sterilized (all of the germs killed) before they are used again. Merely washing them in soapy water or cleaning them with an alcohol wipe will not provide the necessary protection. Oaktree Products (see Appendix 16–C for address) and other companies offer a variety of disinfectants and sterilants that can be used to clean the probe tips and specula effectively.

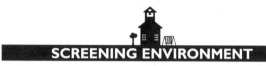

SCREENING ENVIRONMENT

Electrophysiologic Screening

Typically, electrophysiologic screenings are conducted in a hospital or clinic environment. Although the noise levels of the room are not as critical as with pure-tone screening, it is usually best to perform electrophysiologic screenings in a relatively quiet location. Both auditory brainstem response and otoacoustic emissions screening use a computer-averaging technique that will not measure a response if the ambient noise level is too high. The screening procedure will take longer than usual, or may not be completed, if the noise level in the test room, or that produced by the child, exceeds the ambient noise limit.

Pure-Tone Screening

When selecting the location for pure-tone screening, the following variables must be considered:

➤ Location of the screening room
➤ Noise levels
➤ Electrical outlets
➤ Size of the screening room

Location of the Screening Room

Typically, the audiologist wants to find a location for screening that is as quiet as possible and is away from the main traffic flow of the building. In the absence of a sound-treated room or a mobile screening vehicle that can be brought to the school, possible locations for hearing screening include vacant classrooms, the clinic, and the media center. Even though storage closets are considered a bad joke, they often provide suit-

able acoustics for screening. At times, administrators may suggest screening in the children's classroom, but this is usually not an efficient procedure because it necessitates moving the equipment from one classroom to the next.

Noise Levels

The place in which hearing screenings occur is a critical concern for audiologists working in the schools because it is difficult to find an ideal environment for pure-tone screening. The maximum allowable ambient noise levels for octave bands, when screening at a 20 dB level, are provided in Table 3–5. It is obvious that the frequency that will be the most difficult to screen in a less-than-ideal environment is 500 Hz.

If forced to screen in an environment that is too noisy, there will be an excessive number of failures on the screening test, and the actual screening will take longer than when done in a quiet environment. This means there are longer interruptions in the school's schedule on the day of the screening and also during follow-up testing. Typical screening data, including the number of children screened per hour and the number of failures, can be compared to similar data obtained when screening in a poor acoustic environment in order to educate administrators as to the importance and cost effectiveness of a good environment for the screening.

It is *never* acceptable to raise the intensity of the signal to compensate for a noisy environment. If the noise problems in the test room cannot be resolved, it may be necessary to terminate the screening. Audiologists are often too accommodating to school administrators, and, in the process, lead them to believe that these poor environments are acceptable.

Other Factors

Although noise is the primary environmental concern for pure-tone screening, there are some other factors that must be considered. A sufficient number of electrical outlets should be available. It is possible to run extension cords to outlets in another location, but this may create a safety problem if the cords are not taped securely to the floor and fire codes considered. The room must also be large enough to accommodate the screeners and the children comfortably. Depending on the organization used during the screening, the room may need to be only large enough to hold two people, or it may need to accommodate an entire classroom of children and several screening stations. This latter design is less desirable due to added noise.

Table 3–5. Approximate allowable ambient noise levels for octave bands for screening at 20 db HL.

Center Frequency for Octave Band	Maximum Allowable Level
500 Hz	41.5 dB SPL
1000 Hz	49.5 dB SPL
2000 Hz	54.5 dB SPL
4000 Hz	62 dB SPL

Source: From "Guidelines for identification audiometry" by American Speech-Language-Hearing Association, 1995, *Asha Desk Reference for Audiology and Speech-Language Pathology, II,* p. 12. Available for sale from ASHA Fullfillment Operations (301-897-5700, ext. 218). Adapted by permission.

Immittance Screening

The environment for immittance screening is much less critical. Immittance testing is not affected by noise, so it may be performed in less acoustically controlled situations. It is still important to have sufficient electrical outlets of the appropriate design and enough space in the screening location. Seating location and height can also facilitate both otoscopic and immittance screening.

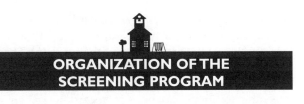

ORGANIZATION OF THE SCREENING PROGRAM

When developing the screening program, it is important to consider how it will be organized. A well-organized program will run more efficiently, and those involved in the program will be more aware of what to expect. Important items to consider include:

➤ Scheduling of the screening
   Consulting the principal or school nurse to determine dates
➤ Activities prior to the screening
   Notifying parents
   Educating teachers and administrators
   Completing necessary forms
   Determining the school's daily schedule
   Training technicians/volunteers/assistants
➤ Activities during the screening
   Providing advance notification to classes
   Getting classes to the screening location
   Completing necessary forms and paperwork

Scheduling of the Screening

When setting up a mass screening program, it is critical to consider when the screenings will occur. For newborn screenings, it is obvious that the screenings will be ongoing. In school systems, screenings of special education and other referrals will also be ongoing, but the mass hearing screening will likely occur only once during the school year. Screening in the fall is advantageous because there is maximum time for follow-up during the remainder of the school year. In addition, the failure rate will typically be lower in the fall than in the winter months when children are more prone to have ear infections. However, when scheduling mass screenings, the resources of the program must be considered. If personnel and time are not available to rescreen the students who fail shortly after the initial screening, it may be better to postpone the initial screening of some schools or grades until later in the school year.

It is also necessary to determine if the mass hearing screening for each school will be completed in one day or over a period of several days. It is usually easier to limit the initial screening to one day if volunteers are used. If there is only one screener in the school district, it may take several days to screen all of the children in each school. Typically, this does not present a problem in elementary schools because each class is interrupted only once during the initial screening. There may, however, be a problem at the secondary level because screening over several days could be very disruptive to the school's schedule. The principal, school nurse, or other representative must be contacted to determine the actual screening dates to avoid conflicts with other school activities.

Activities Prior to the Screening

Parent Notification

Although parent permission is not required for mass hearing screenings in most schools because the screening is a routine part of the district's program, some parents may prefer that their child not participate. It is, therefore, wise to let parents know through a note, a newsletter, or a meeting that the screening will occur and that they will be notified if their child has a possible problem. It is also helpful to ask parents to let the screening program know of any past or present hearing loss or middle ear problems their child has experienced. If history of recent ear problems is part of the screening protocol, a form to obtain this information can be included with the parental notification (see Appendix 3–E).

Education of School Personnel

Teachers and administrators need to be aware of the purpose of the hearing screening program and how the program will be implemented in the school. This information may be provided in written form, but it is usually more effective to have a brief inservice to let the school staff know about the program. It may be possible to provide this information to teachers with other general health services information in order to limit the amount of time required by the teachers. Information that should be provided includes:

➤ The purpose and importance of the hearing screening program
➤ Where and when the screening will take place
➤ How classes will be notified when it is time for them to be screened
➤ How the school will be notified of the screening results
➤ How follow-up will occur

If teachers are aware of the procedure, they can answer their students' questions about the screening and help them know what to do. Likewise, school nurses and administrators who understand the screening program can help facilitate it.

Other Considerations

If class lists or individual screening forms will be used, they should be prepared in advance and ready for use on the day of the screening. Notes to be sent to the students' parents to notify them of the screening results should also be ready if they will be used. It is helpful to know the school's schedule for lunch, recess, and exploratory classes prior to the day of screening so that classes can be screened at convenient times. It is usually best to screen younger students earlier in the day when they are more alert, but the arrangement of the school's schedule may dictate that a different order be used for screening. A final consideration prior to screening is to provide local physicians and pediatricians with information concerning the hearing screening and follow-up procedures.

Activities During the Screening

Organization

For a mass hearing screening program in a school system to be efficient, it is important that the organization on the day or days of the screening be carefully planned. Depending on the number of screeners, it typically works best to bring a small group or an entire class to the screening location at one time. Because some children may be out of the classroom for special education classes or other activities, the teacher should be notified approximately 10 minutes prior to the screening so that the children can all be in a single location prior to their screening time. Instructions for the screening can be given to the children as a group, or they can be given to each child individually. Younger children may benefit from both. Once children have been screened, it is advantageous to send them back to the classroom immediately in order to reduce the noise from children who have completed the screening and to reduce missed class time.

Use of Assistants

For the screening to run efficiently, it is helpful to have the assistance of one or two paraprofessionals or parent volunteers who are familiar with the school. These assistants can alert classes approximately 10 minutes before they will be screened, can bring classes to the screening location, can help in recording screening results, can handle necessary screening forms, and can keep quiet and order in the screening room.

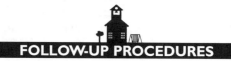

FOLLOW-UP PROCEDURES

The most critical part of any hearing screening program is the follow-up. Without appropriate follow-up, all of the effort invested in the screenings will be in vain. More importantly, the presence of a screening program without appropriate follow-up may be misleading and even harmful to the children. Parents or teachers may know that the screening was done and may assume that a child's hearing is normal when, in fact, there is a hearing loss present. The parents or teachers will therefore not attend to the auditory needs of the child and will look for other reasons to explain the difficulties the child is having. The opposite can also occur. Children who have normal hearing, but fail a screening, may have academic problems incorrectly attributed to hearing loss. Follow-up for screening programs should always include:

➤ Rescreening of failures and absentees from the initial screening
➤ Referrals for further evaluations for all rescreening failures
  Audiological
  Medical
  Educational screenings/evaluations

Rescreening

The first step in any follow-up program is the rescreening of all children who failed or who were absent for the initial screening. The rescreenings should be scheduled within a reasonable length of time, but the length of time between the initial screening and the rescreening will vary depending on the screening tests that were used. The ASHA guidelines recommend that pure-tone failures be rescreened as soon as possible after the initial screening, preferably on the same day of the screening (ASHA, 1985) and that immittance failures be rescreened in 4 to 6 weeks (ASHA, 1990b). Currently, there are no guidelines recommending when OAE failures should be rescreened, but these failures should also be rescreened as soon as possible after the initial screening. Rescreening at these time intervals will not present difficulty if a school district uses only pure-tone, immittance, or OAE screening. However, if immittance screening is performed in combination with either pure-tone or OAE screening, it may be awkward and disruptive to the school to come back on one day to rescreen the pure-tone or OAE failures and on a second day to rescreen the immittance failures. The recommended schedule will work if it is possible to rescreen the pure-tone or OAE failures on the same day as the initial screening. Otherwise, the audiologist may want to schedule the rescreening of all failures at the same time, perhaps 3 to 4 weeks after the initial screening. If a student does not pass the rescreening, it is very helpful to establish pure-tone threshold estimates at the time of rescreening. Threshold information helps prioritize students for audiological assessment referrals, as well as provides physicians valuable information on the hearing implications of middle ear problems.

Referrals for Diagnostic Evaluations

Students who fail the rescreening should be referred for a more thorough evaluation. Typically, referrals will be made either to an audiologist or, after review of rescreening results by the audiologist, immediately to a physician. As with other facets of the screening program, the resources of the program may dictate to

whom the referrals are initially made. Ideally all referrals should be made to an audiologist who can determine the nature and degree of the hearing loss and then refer the child to a physician when necessary. However, if it will be several weeks before a child can be seen by an audiologist, it may be beneficial to set criteria for referring some children to the physician as the first step in the follow-up process. For example, children who fail the immittance rescreening likely have some middle ear problem and could be initially referred to a physician.

It is important that all children who fail the rescreening be seen by an audiologist at some point in the follow-up process to determine if there is any significant hearing loss that may affect academic performance. In addition to the necessity of a medical referral, the audiologist should be aware of the need to refer to other professionals when appropriate. Educational audiologists may be able to determine the need for further evaluation by informally discussing children's performance with their parents or teachers. Another alternative for determining educational implications is to use a form, such as the Screening Instrument for Targeting Educational Risk (S.I.F.T.E.R.) (Anderson, 1989) or the Preschool S.I.F.T.E.R. (Anderson & Matkin, 1996) (see Appendixes 3–F and 3–G), that can be completed by the children's teacher. The audiologist who evaluates any child who fails the screening should communicate directly with the school system to ensure that all of the child's needs, not just the medical or audiological ones, are addressed as a result of the hearing screening.

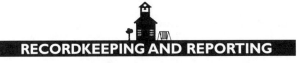

RECORDKEEPING AND REPORTING

It is important for the screening program to keep accurate records of the students who are screened and of the results of the screening. In addition to deciding what forms will be used to document the screening results, it is important to consider:

➤ Reporting to the school
➤ Reporting to parents
➤ Receiving information regarding follow-up

Screening Record Forms
Screening Forms

Many ways have been used to maintain screening records, including the use of both individual and class reporting forms. Individual forms have an advantage because they can be placed in each child's permanent file, thus documenting the hearing screening date and result. A disadvantage in using individual forms is the large volume of paper that will be used during the screening. To cut down on the amount of paper required, some school districts use class forms on which all the students in one class are listed and where the results of the screening are recorded. If the school maintains individual health cumulative files, results could be transferred to a chart in that folder. With the wider use of computers in the schools, some districts have opted to record screening results in a database. The specific form used may be determined by the method the school uses for maintaining results on health records, as well as how the screening is set up. There may also be legal requirements regarding information necessary to be maintained. Examples of both individual and class forms are provided in Appendix 3–H.

Rescreening Forms

In addition to the use of some type of form for recording the results of the initial screening, it is important to keep a record of those students who need to be rescreened and the results of the rescreening. If a class form is used, this information can be provided on the same form as the original screening results. Another alternative is to use a separate form listing those students who were absent on the day of the screening and those needing to be rescreened. An example of such a form is provided in Appendix 3–I.

Reporting to the School

Screening Results

In addition to the recordkeeping that the screening program does for its own use, it is important to communicate the results of the screening to principals, special education coordinators, teachers, and school nurses. The administrators will be interested in the total number screened and the number who passed and failed. Teachers will want to know the specific results for each child in their classroom. This can be accomplished by giving the teacher a copy of the class record form or by returning the individual record forms to the teacher once those needing to be rescreened are recorded. This information, along with a written or verbal explanation of what follow-up is recommended, should be provided to the teacher as soon as possible after the screening. If other school personnel, such as speech-language pathologists, special education teachers, or social workers, are involved

with these students, a system to facilitate providing the screening results to them should be in place.

Rescreening Results

The results of the rescreening should also be provided to school personnel. Although administrators may want to know the number of students who were rescreened and the number referred for further evaluation, they should also be alerted to any students who are of concern because of suspected hearing problems that may be affecting classroom performance. This will allow the administrators to work with the teachers and parents to ensure that follow-up is done in a timely manner. School nurses should also receive information on individual students who failed the screening so they can maintain accurate health records and assist with follow-up. Because the number of students to be rescreened is relatively small, it is often possible to provide the teachers with information about their students on an individual basis (see Appendix 3–J for sample form). This helps the teachers become aware of potential hearing problems and allows them an opportunity to let the screening program know their observations about the child in question. This information exchange can often prove helpful in the final management of the child.

Reporting to Parents

Screening Results

Parents should also be notified in a timely manner about the results of the hearing screening. Some districts notify the parents immediately by sending a note home with the child on the day of the initial screening. Samples of parental notification letters for children who passed the hearing screening and for children who will be rescreened can be found in Appendix 3–K. Other school districts notify parents only if the child is referred from the rescreening and needs to receive medical or audiological attention. There are advantages and disadvantages to each method for notifying parents. The first method requires that a note be available for each child to take home, but it does provide the parent with immediate information about the results of the screening. When parents are only notified if the child is referred from the screening, parents whose children passed the screening may not be aware that their child was screened. Another alternative for parental notification is to let parents know the screening date and advise them to contact the child's teacher or the school nurse shortly after the screening if they want to know the results for their child. This would cut down on the amount of paperwork for the screening program, but still allow parents to have access to the information.

Rescreening Results

Regardless of if and how parents are notified of the hearing screening results, it is critical that they receive timely notification if their child needs to be referred for follow-up. Parents may be referred to their physician or health provider, to the school district's audiologist, or to a private audiologist for follow-up evaluation. The parent notification letter should emphasize that only a hearing screening was done and that more testing is necessary to determine if there is a hearing loss and, if so, the type and severity of the loss. If parent permission is required for follow-up services within the school system, an appropriate form should be enclosed for parents to sign and return. The information sent to the parent should motivate them to follow-up and should also provide the referral agency with the reason for referral and an easy way to return information to the schools. It may also be helpful to provide the parents with a list of practitioners within the community who are available to provide the recommended follow-up services. Examples of parent notification letters are provided in Appendix 3–L.

Receiving Information Regarding Follow-Up

To have complete information, the screening program will ideally receive a report on each child who was referred for medical or audiological evaluation. This can be facilitated by having a report form similar to the one included in Appendix 3–M for the referring agency to compete and return to the screening program. It is often difficult to obtain this information from referral agencies, and documentation of follow-up can become very time-consuming. Forms should be brief and clear and require minimal time to complete by the referral agency or individual. These forms can be included with the screening results sent to parents to hand-carry to the audiologist or physician or can be sent directly to the professional who has seen the child. In either case, written permission will need to be given by the parent for the school to receive a report from an outside agency. Alternatives to this procedure are to contact the parents to determine what action was taken or to have the individual school responsible for ensuring that appropriate follow-up is completed. A database, similar to the one described in Appendix 3–N, may be helpful in monitoring the status of follow-up for each child referred for audiological, medical, or educational evaluation.

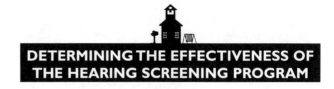

DETERMINING THE EFFECTIVENESS OF THE HEARING SCREENING PROGRAM

The final aspect of a good hearing screening program is an evaluation to determine its effectiveness. This is important for at least two reasons. First, it is critical to monitor the program to ensure that it is running efficiently. A review of data from the program may reveal a need to modify the screening protocol to make it more effective. Second, information about the effectiveness of the hearing screening program is useful in convincing administrators, teachers, and parents of the importance of the program. As people see the number of children screened, identified, and treated as a result of the hearing screening program, support for the program will increase.

Data from Screening Program

Types of information that will help determine the program's effectiveness are:

➤ Total number of children screened
➤ Number and percentage of children who failed the initial screening
➤ Number and percentage who failed the rescreening
➤ Number and percentage who were seen for follow-up evaluations (audiological, medical, and/or educational)
➤ Number and percentage who had problems on final evaluation and the type of problems found
➤ Actual numbers and percentage who passed the hearing screening but were later found to have a hearing loss

The audiologist can use these data to monitor the efficiency and success of the program. For example, if the number failing the initial screening seems too high, the initial screening procedure can be examined to determine if the screeners were not testing properly, if the noise level in the environment was too high, or if the equipment was not functioning properly. Based on this information, steps can be taken to alleviate problems identified. Likewise, the number of children actually seen for follow-up and the results of the follow-up evaluation are critical. If most of the children are not seen for follow-up, the efforts of the screening program are wasted. Additionally, if many of the children seen for follow-up evaluation are found to have normal hearing, additional contact with the referral agencies may be necessary to clarify the findings, or it may be necessary to modify the screening protocol to provide more efficient referrals.

Sensitivity and Specificity

Although the screening tests used by most educational audiologists have been shown to be effective, it may be useful for educational audiologists to determine the sensitivity and specificity of the screening test for the specific population they are testing. Sensitivity is a measure of how well the screening test detects those people who actually have a hearing loss, whereas specificity measures how well the screening test determines those people who do not have a hearing loss. Sensitivity can be thought of as the true positive rate, and specificity is the true negative rate. A chart showing how to determine sensitivity and specificity for a specific test is provided in Figure 3–1.

Cost Effectiveness

Another factor that should be considered in the evaluation of a screening program is the cost effectiveness of the program. The total cost of personnel, equipment,

equipment maintenance, and forms for each year can be compared to the number of children screened to determine the cost of screening each child. Additionally, the number of children identified as having a hearing loss can be compared to the total cost of the program to determine the cost of identifying each child with a hearing loss. The benefits of the screening program, including the number of children seen for medical treatment, the number fit with hearing aids or assistive technology, and the number provided educational consultation and assistance, can also be considered in terms of the total cost of the program.

SUMMARY

The hearing screening program is the basis for most of the other services that we provide as educational audiologists. It is critical that it be effective and well-supported. It is, therefore, important to plan and administer the program effectively, and then to share data and information from the program with administrators, teachers, parents, and the public. As others see the effectiveness of the program, particularly the benefits to the children who are identified as having hearing losses, the programs will gain the support necessary for its continuation and growth.

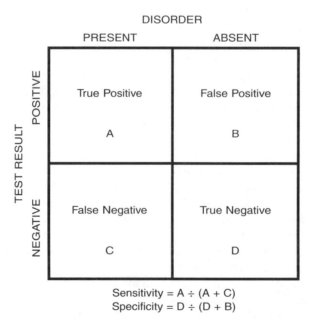

Figure 3–1. Determining sensitivity and specificity of screening tests.

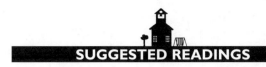

SUGGESTED READINGS

American Speech-Language-Hearing Association Committee on Quality Assurance. (1991). Chronic communicable diseases and risk management in the schools. *Language, Speech, and Hearing Services in Schools, 22,* 345–352.

Anderson, K. L. (1991). Hearing conservation in the public schools revisited. *Seminars in Hearing, 12*(4), 340–364.

Barrett, K. A. (1994). Hearing and middle-ear screening of school-age children. In J. Katz (Ed.), *Handbook of clinical audiology* (pp. 476–489). Baltimore, MD: Williams and Wilkins.

Bess, F. H., & Hall, J. W. (1992). *Screening children for auditory function.* Nashville, TN: Bill Wilkerson Center Press.

Kemp, R. J., Roeser, R. J., Pearson, D., & Ballachanda, B. (1995). *Infection control for the professions of audiology and speech-language pathology.* San Diego, CA: Singular Publishing Group, Inc.

Kenworthy, O. T. (1987). Identification of hearing loss in infancy and early childhood. In J. G. Alpiner & P. McCarthy (Eds.), *Rehabilitative audiology: Children and adults* (pp. 18–43). Baltimore, MD: Williams and Wilkins.

Roush, J. (1990). Identification of hearing loss and middle ear disease in preschool and school-age children. *Seminars in Hearing, 11*(4), 357–371.

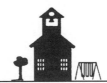

CHAPTER 4

ASSESSMENT PRACTICES

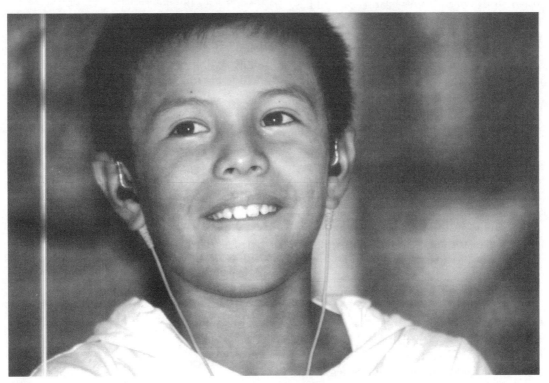

Sammy, age 10

CONTENTS

Assessment of the Educational Effects of Hearing Loss

One of the major activities of educational audiologists is the assessment of children's hearing capabilities. Although the administration of audiologic tests to determine the nature and degree of hearing losses is of primary importance, the area of educationally related auditory assessment includes much more. As educational audiologists, we need to focus on the educational implications of the hearing or listening disorder and on the benefits, if any, that can be received from personal or classroom amplification. For educational audiologists, the purposes of assessment include the following:

➤ Determination of the presence of a hearing loss or central auditory processing disorder
➤ Monitoring of changes in hearing sensitivity
➤ Determination of the educational effects of a hearing loss or central auditory processing disorder
➤ Determination of the need for personal and classroom amplification
➤ Monitoring the benefit from personal and classroom amplification

Although all educational audiologists may not perform every one of these assessment activities, instead referring to other audiologists and/or related professionals for specific services, they are responsible for seeing that all aspects of a comprehensive assessment are provided for the children in their target student population.

This chapter discusses most of the purposes of assessment in the schools, but issues related to central auditory processing disorders are in Chapter 5, Central Auditory Processing Disorders, and amplification issues are in Chapter 6, Amplification and Classroom Hearing Technology. Specifically, this chapter addresses the following questions:

➤ What is included in a basic assessment of hearing loss?
➤ What modifications in the assessment protocol are useful with special populations?
➤ What special audiometric tests might be needed?

➤ What is involved in monitoring hearing sensitivity?
➤ What additional audiologic information should be obtained to determine the effects of a hearing loss?
➤ How can the educational effects of hearing losses be assessed?
➤ How should results of assessments be communicated to parents, teachers, other school personnel, and other professionals?

BASIC ASSESSMENT OF HEARING LOSS

The basic audiologic assessment for a child is required to identify the presence of a hearing loss and to determine the nature and degree of the hearing loss. Additionally, it will provide information about the child's ability to understand speech. Basic assessment should include the following:

➤ Case history
➤ Pure-tone air- and bone-conduction thresholds
➤ Speech thresholds
➤ Word recognition ability
➤ Otoscopy
➤ Immittance testing

Before discussing each of these topics, it is important to remember that during all assessment procedures, audiologists must be aware of the need for infection control and must take necessary precautions to protect themselves and their clients. More specific information on infection control procedures can be found in Chapter 3, Identification Practices.

Case History

The case history is a critical part of every audiologic assessment. It not only provides information that may assist in the diagnosis of a hearing loss, but also can help in determining the effects of the hearing loss and planning for management. Knowledge of the occurrence and success or failure of prior medical treatment and/or educational intervention is often valuable when planning future management. Another example of how history information may be useful is when a family history of hearing loss is identified. Subsequent referral of the familiy for genetic counseling may not only help the parents with future family planning, but may also identify a syndrome with associated characteristics that could have an impact on educational performance. A list of information typically included in an initial case history is included in Table 4–1.

Table 4–1. Information to be obtained from case history.

➤ Major concern(s) about child

➤ Pregnancy and birth information

➤ Medical history
  General
  Ear

➤ Developmental history
  Auditory
  Speech and language
  Motor
  Cognitive
  Social and emotional

➤ Family history
  History of hearing loss or deafness
  History of ear disease
  Educational difficulty
  Speech-language difficulty

➤ Educational experiences
  Regular education
  Special education

Usually one or both of the parents will be the primary source for the case history information. The case history interview can be a useful mechanism for evaluating the parents' perception of the child's current and prior auditory function. However, the value of input from teachers and others involved with the child should not be overlooked. It takes additional time for the educational audiologist to contact other professionals working with the child, but this effort can be beneficial in providing more complete information about the child's background and day-to-day performance.

Case history information can be obtained through the use of a form and/or an interview. The logistics of sending and obtaining a case history form may be difficult in a school system. However, if used, it can be completed by the parent or teacher prior to the diagnostic evaluation and will be especially useful if the parent or teacher is not present for the assessment. It is helpful for the audiologist to review the information on the form with the parent or teacher in a personal or telephone interview whenever possible. Sometimes the informants may have misunderstood a question on the case history form, or they may have provided incomplete information. The interview will also be helpful in providing the educational audiologist with a sense of how the informant views the child and in establishing trust between the audiologist and the informant.

Pure-Tone Air- and Bone-Conduction Thresholds

Pure-tone air-conduction thresholds determine if a hearing loss is present and provide a direct indication of the amount of hearing loss at each frequency. A comparison of the air and bone thresholds will indicate if the loss is conductive, sensorineural, or mixed in nature, and a comparison of the thresholds obtained from the two ears will determine if there is a loss in one or both ears and which ear is better.

By recording the child's thresholds on audiograms with familiar sounds or other speech information plotted on them, we can predict the effects of the child's hearing loss on the perception of speech while graphically helping the parents and teachers begin to understand the impact of the hearing loss. Examples of audiograms that may be useful include one with the "speech banana" (Watkins, 1993), one with pictures of familiar sounds on it (American Academy of Audiology, 1993), one with percentages of normal conversational speech heard at various levels (Pascoe, 1980, as cited in Olsen, Hawkins, & Van Tasell, 1987), and the "Count-the-Dot" audiogram (Mueller & Killion, 1990). For the first three audiograms, the area above the child's recorded thresholds illustrates the specific sounds the child can hear or the percentage of speech that is audible to the child. By counting the number of dots above the child's thresholds on the "Count-the Dot" audiogram, the audiologist will have an estimate of the child's audibility (the percentage of sounds audible).

Most school-age children are able to perform traditional pure-tone threshold auditometry reliably. Pure-tone thresholds for the octave frequencies from 250 through 8000 Hz in each ear should be established. When there is a difference of more than 20 dB HL (hearing level) in adjacent thresholds, it is also advisable to test the child's hearing at the mid-octave frequency.

Speech Thresholds

Speech thresholds are useful in providing an overall estimate of the degree of the child's hearing loss and in verifying the pure-tone threshold results. When obtaining the speech reception threshold, it is critical to use spondee words that are familiar to the child. It may, therefore, be necessary to use a modified or limited list of spondee words for younger children. Techniques for familiarization, such as word repetition or picture/written word identification, should be completed prior to formal speech threshold testing. Most often the speech threshold can be obtained using a monitored live-voice presentation. Although recorded presentations are more reliable than live-voice, the flexibility, speed, and ability to maintain rapport with the child afforded by monitored live-voice testing can be extremely beneficial when testing children. To avoid discrepancies in test results, it is important to monitor live-voice presentations carefully.

The speech reception threshold should agree with the child's three-frequency pure-tone average, unless the child has a precipitous hearing loss, in which case the speech reception threshold should approximate the two-frequency pure-tone average. If the speech reception threshold and pure-tone average do not agree, the reason for the discrepancy should be determined. Possible reasons include a lack of understanding of the directions for either the pure-tone or speech tests, not responding to either pure tones or speech at threshold levels, an unusual hearing loss configuration, a nonorganic (functional) hearing loss, or careless testing procedures.

Word Recognition Ability

Tests of word recognition ability are designed to determine the percentage of words that can be understood under ideal listening conditions. The words are usually administered at a level 30 to 40 dB above the child's speech reception threshold and may be presented using either monitored live-voice or recorded stimuli. Recorded presentations are more reliable, especially if the child will be tested by more than one audiologist. However, for younger children performance can be enhanced with a live-voice presentation, which allows more flexibility to modify the speed of presentation and the frequency of reinforcement. Scoring is most often accomplished by determining the percentage of words the child repeats or identifies correctly, but can also be done phonemically to provide more precise information for the audiologist and others working with the child.

As with the speech reception threshold assessment, it is important to use word lists that are age- and vocabulary-appropriate for the child. Table 4–2 contains a list of word recognition tests standardized for use with children, along with the minimum vocabulary age required for each test. For a child with a vocabulary age of 3 years or greater, the Northwestern University Children's Perception of Speech (NU-CHIPS) (Elliot & Katz, 1980) is appropriate. The Word Intelligibility by Picture Identification (WIPI) test (Ross & Lerman, 1970) is useful for children whose vocabulary is at a 4½-year-old level. Both of these tests use a picture-pointing response in a closed-set format. The advantage of "guessing" on closed-set tests may tend to overestimate the child's word recognition ability. Open-set lists requiring word repetition by the child include the PB-Kindergarten lists (Haskins, 1949) for ages 5 years and up, the CID W-22 lists (Hirsh, Davis et al., 1952) for ages 8 and up, and the NU-6 lists (Tillman & Carhart, 1966) for ages 12 and up. Ordering information for the NU-CHIPS and WIPI tests can be found in Appendix 16–D.

Otoscopy

Otoscopy is an important part of every audiological evaluation. The visual examination of the external ear, the ear canal, and the tympanic membrane provides observations that will often confirm the audiological findings and that may lead to a medical referral. It is critical that otoscopy be used to ensure that the ear canal is clear before beginning any procedure that requires insertion of instrumentation into the ear canal, such as immittance or otoacoustic emission testing or probe microphone measurements. For immittance testing, additional observations about the presence of ven-

Table 4–2. Word recognition tests for children.

Test	Minimum Vocabulary Age (in years)
Northwestern University Children's Perception of Speech (NU-CHIPS) (Elliot & Katz, 1980)	3
Word Intelligibility by Picture Identification (WIPI) (Ross & Lerman, 1970)	4.5
PB-Kindergarten Lists (Haskins, 1949)	5
CID W-22 Lists (Hirsh et al., 1952)	8
NU-6 Lists (Tillman & Carhart, 1966)	12

tilation tubes and the intactness of the tympanic membrane may be useful when interpreting the test results.

Immittance Testing

With the high incidence of middle ear problems in children, immittance testing becomes a particularly important component of every child's audiological evaluation. The immittance measurements are objective, require no voluntary response, and are the most sensitive audiological procedures for determining the status of the middle ear system. Complete immittance testing includes tympanometry and the measurement of static acoustic immittance, physical volume, and acoustic reflex thresholds. Although some young children, especially those who have had ear infections, may object to the probe in the ear, every effort should be made to attempt the measurement. This is especially true for young children who have abnormal hearing and for whom it may be difficult to obtain pure-tone bone-conduction results. On occasion, an extremely frightened or screaming child may remember the experience negatively, jeopardizing subsequent test sessions. However, many children are positively reinforced by watching the computer screen or by receiving a computer print-out "drawn by their ears."

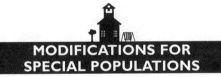

MODIFICATIONS FOR SPECIAL POPULATIONS

In an educational environment, there will be many students who will not be able to respond to standard pediatric techniques. Included in this group are infants, toddlers, preschoolers, and other children who are difficult to test because of physical, mental, or emotional disabilities. Most of these children can be successfully tested behaviorally by the educational audiologist if modified techniques are used. Children who are developmentally delayed should be tested using techniques appropriate for children at their developmental age, rather than their chronological age. An overview of the techniques that should be used with young children is provided in the ASHA *Guidelines for the Audiologic Assessment of Children From Birth Through 36 Months of Age* (1991b) (see Appendix 2–G).

Children for whom reliable or complete results cannot be obtained behaviorally should have otoacoustic emissions or other electrophysiological tests performed, either by the educational audiologist or

through an outside referral. It is important that every child suspected of having a hearing loss have an audiologic evaluation to determine the nature and degree of the hearing loss. The use of CNT (cannot test) or DNT (did not test) without additional referral should be avoided by all educational audiologists.

Pure-Tone Modifications

Behavior observation audiometry (BOA) is appropriate for infants less than approximately 6 months of age, for children whose developmental age is less than 6 months, and for those who have motoric involvement that precludes independent head control. For children whose developmental age is between 6 months and 2 years, visual reinforcement audiometry (VRA) should be attempted. This can be a highly successful technique, although children who are 2 years old may habituate to the reinforcer before a complete audiogram is obtained. Educational audiologists who use VRA should familiarize themselves with research concerning the reinforcement parameters of this technique. The design and placement of reinforcers, as well as stimulus and reinforcement schedules, significantly affect success with VRA (Diefendorf, 1988; Moore, Wilson, & Thompson, 1977; Thompson & Folsom, 1984). Conditioned play audiometry is useful for children whose developmental ages are between 2 and 5 years of age. By varying the play activity, a child's interest can typically be maintained long enough to establish complete thresholds.

Because the attention span of young and developmentally delayed children is limited, the educational audiologist should vary the order of the frequencies tested so that maximal information is obtained from the child. If only two thresholds can be obtained for the child, thresholds for a low-frequency sound (e.g., 500 Hz) and for a high-frequency sound (e.g., 4000 Hz) will provide more information about the child's hearing than if only thresholds for two mid-frequency sounds (e.g., 1000 and 2000 Hz) were obtained. It is also important to note every response made by young children because they may not continue to respond unless the stimulus is changed. Without a system for tallying these responses, such as the one found in Appendix 4–A (Arkansas Department of Health, 1978), the educational audiologist may become confused, and valuable information may be lost. Another technique for maximizing information obtained from young children is to measure thresholds in sound-field to determine the hearing in the better ear prior to attempting to measure thresholds for each ear individually. Table 4–3 contains a suggested frequency order for both sound-field and earphone/insert procedures.

Table 4–3. Suggested order for assessing young and developmentally delayed children.

Output	Frequency Order/Procedure
Sound-field:	4000 Hz; 500 Hz; 2000 Hz; 1000 Hz
Earphones/Inserts:	4000 Hz; repeat in opposite ear
	500 Hz; repeat in opposite ear
	2000 Hz; repeat in opposite ear
	1000 Hz; repeat in opposite ear
	Test other octave and mid-octave frequencies as possible, continuing to alternate ears

Although the information obtained from the child during one testing session may be limited, if audiologists select this information wisely, they can learn enough about the auditory status of the child to begin making recommendations to the parents and school personnel, especially when these results are used to complement objective findings from immittance testing. When complete thresholds cannot be measured on a child during one testing session, the child should return for additional testing on a periodic basis until complete information is obtained. Testing during subsequent sessions should focus on measuring thresholds that have not been previously obtained.

Many young and/or developmentally delayed children will not easily tolerate the use of earphones for audiometric testing. Initially, sound-field testing can be used to determine the hearing sensitivity of the better ear so that intervention can be begun. However, efforts to obtain ear-specific thresholds should be continued. Insert earphones are useful with some children, and lending parents an old set of earphones to use at home with the child may help other children overcome their fear of the earphones. Another technique that may be useful is to hold an earphone that has been detached from the headband near the ear to be tested. Although it must be recognized that thresholds cannot be measured if the earphone is not properly placed over the child's ear, the information obtained can let the audiologist know if there are any significant differences in the sensitivity of the child's two ears.

Speech Modifications

When a child cannot repeat spondee words to obtain a speech reception threshold, a task involving pointing to pictures or objects representing spondee words should be attempted. When this is not successful or possible, a speech threshold can be obtained with either visual reinforcement audiometry or conditioned play audiometry. Because the child does not have to recognize the speech

for either of these techniques, the speech threshold obtained in this manner is a speech awareness threshold or a speech detection threshold, and it will be approximately 10 dB better than the speech reception threshold. It can also be deceptively better than predicted from the pure-tone average if the child has a hearing loss with a sloping or uneven configuration.

If a child cannot repeat words intelligibly so that a word recognition score can be calculated, the point-to-the-picture tests discussed previously may be appropriate. Another, more informal way to obtain some idea of a child's ability to recognize words is to have the child point to common objects or to body parts. Some young children will wave to "bye-bye," point to "Mama," or repeat their own name. Additionally, there are several tests of auditory perception which the educational audiologist can use, depending on the child's ability. These include:

➤ Auditory Numbers Test (ANT) (Erber, 1980)
➤ Auditory Perception of Alphabet Letters (APAL) (Ross & Randolph, 1988)
➤ Children's Auditory Test (CAT) (Erber & Alencewicz, 1976)
➤ Early Speech Perception Test (ESP) (Moog & Geers, 1990)
➤ Ling Six-Sound Test (Ling & Ling, 1978)
➤ Minimal Auditory Capabilities Battery (MAC Battery) (Owens, Kessler, Raggio, & Schubert, 1985)
➤ Sound Effects Recognition Task (SERT) (Finitzo-Hieber, Matkin, Cherow-Skalka, & Gerling, 1977)

All of these tests, except the Sound Effects Recognition Task (SERT), use a limited set of words or sounds to assess the child's ability to perceive speech and its acoustic components. The SERT uses environmental sounds to assess the child's ability to discriminate among nonspeech stimuli. Most of these tests were developed for use with children with hearing impairments, but they can also be used with young or low-functioning children with normal hearing sensitivity. Table 4–4 briefly describes each of these tests, and ordering information for those commercially available can be found in Appendix 16–D.

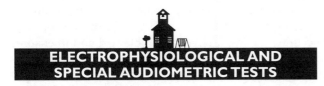

ELECTROPHYSIOLOGICAL AND SPECIAL AUDIOMETRIC TESTS

At times it is necessary to use electrophysiological and special audiometric tests to obtain audiometric information on a child. The most common reason is the inability to assess the child's hearing using behavioral techniques due to the child's developmental age or the presence of other disabilities. In addition, it may be necessary occasionally to perform site-of-lesion testing because of suspected retrocochlear involvement.

The electrophysiological tests most often used to determine the status of a child's auditory system are auditory brainstem response (ABR) and otoacoustic emissions (OAE). The advantages and limitations of these tests are discussed in more detail in Chapter 3, Identification Practices. Because both procedures require specialized equipment that may not be avail-

able in some educational settings, children are often referred to a clinical audiologist for this testing. Equipment for OAE testing is now portable and is more frequently found in educational settings, so many educational audiologists may be able to perform this testing themselves when needed. Any time a referral is made to an outside agency to determine the child's hearing status, the school has the reponsibility to pay for the assessment. It is important that educational audiologists understand the procedures that were done when an outside referral was made so that they can interpret the results to school personnel and the parents.

Tests to determine site-of-lesion may include ABR, OAE, vestibular assessment, or special behavioral audiometric tests. These tests are primarily used for medical purposes and therefore usually do not have any direct educational impact. Administration of them may therefore not be considered within the educational audiologist's scope of practice. Despite this, we must recognize that there are children within the schools who have retrocochlear hearing losses and be alert for them because of their potential life-threatening nature and the effect they can have on both the student and the family. When it is suspected that a child has a retrocochlear hearing loss, the educational audiologist must either perform the special audiometric tests or refer the child to a clinical audiologist for further assessment.

Table 4–4. Description of selected tests of auditory perception.

Test	Description of Test
Auditory Numbers Test (ANT) (Erber, 1980)	Test of ability to discriminate the numbers 1 through 5 and to identify temporal patterns for series of numbers; designed for children with hearing impairments.
Auditory Perception of Alphabet Letters (APAL) (Ross & Randolph, 1988)	Recorded test of ability to perceive the letters of the alphabet; closed-set response with 26 alternatives; score is weighted according to how acoustically close the response is to the target sound; appropriate for children with hearing impairments.
Children's Auditory Test (CAT) (Erber & Alencewicz, 1976)	Point-to-the picture test designed for students with severe or profound hearing losses; assesses ability to both identify appropriate stress patterns and recognize monosyllabic, trochaic, or spondaic words.
Early Speech Perception Test (ESP) (Moog & Geers, 1990)	Recorded test battery for young children with profound hearing losses and limited vocabulary and language skills; tests both pattern perception and simple word identification; pictures or toys used for response; standard and low-verbal versions available; appropriate for children 3 years of age and older.
Ling Six-Sound Test (Ling & Ling, 1978)	Test of ability to detect and/or recognize 6 specific speech sounds within low-, mid-, and high-frequency ranges (a, i, u, s, ʃ, m).
Minimal Auditory Capabilities Battery (MAC Battery) (Owens, Kessler, Raggio, & Schubert, 1985)	Recorded test battery with 13 subtests; two additional subtests determine benefit from visual enhancement; appropriate for students with profound, postlingual hearing impairment.
Sound Effects Recognition Task (SERT) (Finitzo-Hieber, Matkin, Cherow-Skalka, & Gerling, 1977)	Recorded test of ability to discriminate gross environmental sounds; pictured, closed-set response with 4 alternatives; appropriate for children between 3 and 6½ years.

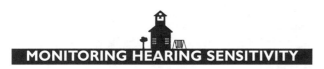

MONITORING HEARING SENSITIVITY

Once a hearing loss has been documented, it is necessary to continue to monitor the child's hearing sensitivity. The hearing of children with chronic conductive hearing losses may fluctuate frequently, and some children with sensorineural hearing losses may have a progressive or fluctuating hearing loss. Although we should be cautious to not over-amplify children with power hearing aids, additional hearing loss may sometimes occur, making it wise to monitor not only the child's hearing sensitivity, but also the amplification settings periodically.

Types of Monitoring

The monitoring of children's hearing is most often accomplished by repeating the pure-tone air-conduction thresholds at regular intervals. It is helpful to record the thresholds on a cumulative chart, such as the one shown in Appendix 4–B, so that any changes in hearing sensitivity can be easily noted. When a significant change occurs, the audiologist should work with the child's physician to determine if the change is the result of middle ear involvement, a progressive hearing loss, or the possibility of over-amplification. Additionally, the audiologist should work with school personnel to make them aware of the educational impact of the change in the child's hearing.

Immittance and OAE testing are also useful in monitoring children's auditory function, particularly for those having chronic middle ear problems or those wearing amplification. These procedures are quicker than obtaining pure-tone thresholds and are more sensitive to changes in the peripheral auditory system that may affect hearing sensitivity. When abnormal immittance or OAE results are found, pure-tone thresholds should be obtained to document any fluctuations in hearing, and the child should be referred to the physician for medical intervention, if indicated. Teachers and parents should also be notified of the changes in the child's hearing sensitivity, so that necessary educational modifications can be made until the problem (e.g., middle ear infection) is resolved.

Schedules for Monitoring

Federal law requires that all students with hearing losses have an audiologic evaluation to monitor their hearing every 3 years, unless more frequent evaluations are specified on the student's IEP. Annual audiologic evaluations are required by many states' regula-

tions for students identified as deaf or hard-of-hearing, and it may be useful for some students to have more frequent evaluations. Children with sensorineural hearing losses identified within the last 2 years should have their hearing sensitivity monitored every 4 to 6 months in order to be sure that their hearing losses remain stable. Likewise, preschool children should be evaluated every 4 to 6 months to ascertain that an accurate audiogram has been obtained and to ensure that their hearing sensitivity is stable. In addition to monitoring hearing sensitivity, these evaluations will be useful in monitoring the development of the student's auditory skills.

Children with chronic conductive hearing losses need to be monitored regularly because of the potential fluctuating nature of these conditions. Typically these children should have a hearing evaluation every 3 to 4 months with at least monthly monitoring of immittance and, if available, otoacoustic emissions to determine changes in the ear's status. Because of the transitory nature of conductive hearing losses, it may be necessary to monitor the hearing more frequently at certain times of the year (e.g., during cold and allergy seasons).

Regardless of the schedule for monitoring that we use, teachers and parents should be encouraged to stay alert for changes in the student's performance or behavior. Any time a change is noticed, the child's hearing should be checked immediately to determine if the change is related to an alteration in hearing sensitivity.

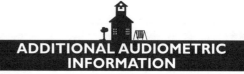

ADDITIONAL AUDIOMETRIC INFORMATION

Although the basic audiological evaluation can provide educational audiologists with a great deal of information about the nature and degree of children's hearing losses, additional testing may be useful in determining the potential educational effects of the hearing loss. Information that can easily be obtained by educational audiologists includes the determination of performance in the following areas:

➤ Speech recognition for sentences and phrases
➤ Auditory/visual speech perception
➤ Listening in noise
➤ Listening in the classroom or other environment
➤ Other auditory skills

Speech Recognition for Sentences and Phrases

The basic audiological evaluation includes measurement of children's ability to discriminate or recognize single words. Although this provides useful information, it does not represent a realistic communication situation. Children rarely listen to words in isolation; words are most often provided within the context of a phrase or sentence. Some sentence and phrase materials have been developed for children, but, as with word recognition tests, it is important to use materials that are appropriate for each child's language abilities. Most of the sentence and phrase lists that have been developed for use with children do not have normative data, but they can still provide us with information about children's use of context.

WIPI Sentences

Sentences have been written for the Word Intelligibility by Picture Identification test (WIPI Sentences) for testing young children (Weber & Reddell, 1976). The four lists of sentences, each containing 25 sentences with a key word in each sentence, are located in Appendix 15–A. These materials are useful with children 4½ years of age and older who can respond either by pointing to the appropriate picture or by repeating the entire sentence, whichever is easier for the child.

Pediatric Speech Intelligibility (PSI) Test

The Pediatric Speech Intelligibility (PSI) test (Jerger & Jerger, 1984) (see Appendix 15–B) is another sentence test that can be used with very young children. Although this test is most often used for determining the presence of central auditory processing problems, it can be used for other purposes. The test contains lists of 10 sentences which are pictured so that the child can point to the appropriate picture. The limited vocabulary and number of sentences makes the PSI appropriate for children 3 years of age and older.

Blair Sentences

Six lists of sentences appropriate for children who are in the second grade or above were developed by Blair (1976). Each list includes 25 sentences with two key words identified in each sentence. The child is required to repeat the entire sentence, and the score is based on the percentage of key words repeated correctly. The Blair Sentences are provided in Appendix 15–C.

BKB/SAE Sentences

The Standard American English version of the Bench-Koval-Bamford Sentences (BKB/SAE) are lists of syntactically and semantically equivalent sentences (Bench & Bamford, 1979; Bench, Koval, & Bamford, 1979; Kenworthy, Klee, & Tharpe, 1990). Each list contains 16 sentences (see Appendix 15–D), which were developed from language samples taken from children with hearing impairments who were between 8 and 15 years of age. They have been found to be appropriate for use with children with normal hearing as young as 5 years of age. The sentences are scored based on the percentage of the 50 key words that are repeated correctly by the child.

Speech Intelligibility in Noise (SPIN) Test

Kalikow, Stevens, and Elliott (1977) developed lists of sentences known as the Speech Intelligibility in Noise (SPIN) test (see Appendix 15–E). Although this test was designed to be administered in noise, the sentences can also be administered in quiet. The final word in each of the 50 sentences in each list is used to determine the child's score. This test is appropriate for children approximately 10 years or older and can be administered by having the child repeat the entire sentence or only the final word. An interesting feature of this test is that the key word in 25 of the sentences in each list is highly predictable from the context of the sentence, while the key word in the other 25 sentences has low predictability. Scoring of the high-predictability sentences compared to the scoring of the low-predictability sentences can give information about how children are able to use the context of the sentence to determine the key word.

Common Children's Phrases

To overcome the difficulty young children may have remembering entire sentences, Johnson and Owens (personal communication, September 22, 1996) developed the Common Children's Phrases (see Appendix 15–F). These phrases are all three or five syllables in length and are grouped into eight lists of 20 phrases each. The test is scored based on the percentage of phrases the child repeats correctly. The phrases were obtained from the language used in elementary school classrooms and are considered to be appropriate for children from 4 through 8 years of age.

Auditory/Visual Speech Perception

Most speech audiometric tests are administered using only auditory input, but it is helpful also to determine a child's ability to understand speech using a combination of auditory and visual information. This information can give the audiologist an idea of the child's use of visual speech cues and the importance of using speechreading to obtain information in the classroom. A comparison of the score the child receives using only auditory information and that from both auditory and visual information is often very helpful in convincing the teacher of the need to be sure that the child always has speechreading cues available in the classroom.

Any of the tests commonly used for speech recognition testing, including both words and sentences, can be presented using auditory and visual information. Obviously, the presenter's face needs to be seen clearly by the child when stimuli are administered via the auditory-visual mode. If there are shadows in the test booth that obscure the audiologist's face, the test score will not accurately reflect the child's ability to make use of the additional visual cues. If scores from either auditory alone or visual alone are to be compared to the combined auditory-visual score, then the auditory-visual mode should be presented last. This presentation order will avoid inflated scores for the single modes due to learning effects that could be provided if the easier (more redundant) auditory-visual mode was presented first.

Listening in Noise

It is also extremely important to measure children's ability to listen in noise. Classrooms are noisy places, and the typical word recognition scores obtained in quiet are not reflective of children's ability to understand speech in the classroom. Again, this information is useful in alerting and demonstrating to teachers the problems children may experience in the classroom, and it can also provide justification for the use of a personal or sound-field FM system for many children with auditory problems (see Chapter 6, Amplification and Classroom Hearing Technology, for additional information).

Speech recognition testing in noise can be accomplished with either words or sentences. Although it can be done under earphones, scores obtained under earphones will not be reflective of children's ability to listen in a classroom because the advantage for listening in noise provided by binaural hearing is not available. It is, therefore, best to test children's ability to listen in noise in the sound-field. The angle of presentation for the speech and noise will most likely depend on the placement of the speakers in the sound booth, but it is generally better to use separate speakers for the speech and noise signals. Rarely do the speech and competing noise come from the same source in the classroom, so separate speakers are more reflective of actual classroom listening. Additionally, the binaural advantage will not be reflected in the score unless the speech and noise come from separate speakers. Possible speaker arrangements are illustrated in Figure 4–1. Although the performance of an individual student may vary with the illustrated speaker placements, each arrangement represents situations that can occur in the classroom environment.

Various types of noise can be used for testing speech recognition in noise, but the ones most commonly used are the speech noise generated by the audiometer or a multi-talker babble. Speech noise would predict performance when there is an ongoing competing noise in the classroom, such as an air conditioner, whereas multi-talker babble is more representative of difficulties encountered when classmates and teachers talk simultaneously. The level of presentation for the speech signal is typically that of normal conversational speech, between 45 and 55 dB HL, but the level of the noise may vary depending on the audiologist's choice. Signal-to-noise ratios ranging from +10 dB to 0 dB are often used, with different levels simulating listening in a quiet or a noisy classroom. If time permits, it is helpful to obtain information from more than one level for comparison and interpretation. Because there are no normative data for sound-field listening in noise, it is important that educational audiologists use a consistent arrangement for testing in noise so that they will know the amount of decrease in the speech recognition score that is typically associated with the procedure they are using.

Listening in the Classroom or Other Environment

Recently, there has been some interest in documenting students' ability to hear in environments other than the test booth, where most audiological information is obtained. This idea has merit because the conditions in the booth are very controlled and represent an artificial listening situation, which may not adequately reflect students' ability to listen in the classroom. Johnson and Von Almen (1993, April), using a paradigm suggested by Ying (1990) and by Ross, Brackett, and Maxon (1991), developed a Functional Listening Evaluation, which can be used by audiologists to assess students' listening abilities in a variety of situations. Procedures for this evaluation are described in detail in Appendix 4–C. The Functional Listening Evaluation paradigm is designed to evaluate students in their classrooms or in rooms that are similar to their classrooms. Eight lists of sentences, phrases, or words are presented to determine the effects of noise, distance, and visual input on children's ability to understand speech. The test protocol takes approximately 30 minutes to administer if sentences are used as the speech material, and the results provide significant information about how various factors affect a particular child's performance in the classroom.

Other Auditory Skills

There are several comprehensive tests of auditory skills that may prove useful to educational audiologists.

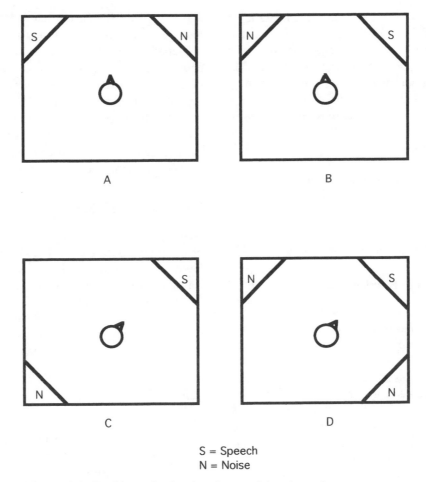

S = Speech
N = Noise

Figure 4–1. Possible speaker locations for speech-in-noise testing.

These include:

➤ Test of Auditory Comprehension (Office of Los Angeles County Superintendent of Schools, 1976)
➤ Glendonald Auditory Screening Test (Erber, 1982)
➤ Computer Assisted Speech Perception Testing and Training Program (Boothroyd, 1987)
➤ Placement Test of Developmental Approach to Successful Listening II (Stout & Winkle, 1992).

Although these tests assess children's performance on a variety of auditory tasks that differ slightly from test to test, all attempt to determine the level at which speech can be perceived auditorily (i.e., detection, discrimination, identification, or comprehension) and the linguistic level children can comprehend (i.e., isolated sounds, syllables, words, sentences, or conversation). These tests are useful in planning auditory (re)habilitation programs for children with hearing losses, but they can also be used to help teachers and parents

understand children's auditory skills. Ordering information for tests that are commercially available is provided in Appendix 16–D.

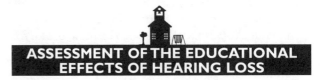

ASSESSMENT OF THE EDUCATIONAL EFFECTS OF HEARING LOSS

Perhaps one of the most distinguishing differences between clinical and educational audiologists is the educational audiologist's focus on determining the effects of children's hearing losses within a learning environment. To be effective in the schools, we must know what the ramifications of the hearing loss are expected to be in order to help parents and teachers know how to help children achieve their maximum potential. Additionally, audiologists working in the school must be aware of the educational effects of hearing loss in order to identify other conditions that may affect children's academic progress. It is not unusual for parents and school personnel, who are generally not aware of the effects of hearing losses, to assume that all of children's deficits are related to their hearing losses, when in fact there may be other conditions that need to be addressed. This section addresses the following topics:

➤ Interpretation of audiological information
➤ Need for comprehensive evaluation
➤ Use of teacher checklists

Interpretation of Audiological Information

Nature and Degree of Hearing Loss

The first step in determining the educational effects of the hearing loss is to look at the nature and degree of the child's hearing loss. Children with fluctuating conductive hearing losses, those with minimal sensorineural hearing losses, and those with unilateral hearing losses have been shown to be at risk for language and academic delays (Bess, 1985; Bess, Klee, & Culbertson, 1986; Downs, 1988; Oyler, Oyler, & Matkin, 1988). Although these delays usually are minimal, proper management is necessary for these children to achieve their potential in the classroom. As a general rule of thumb, without intervention children with bilateral sensorineural hearing losses of approximately 30 dB have a 1-year academic delay. Children with a 40 dB loss typically have a 2-year academic delay, and those with a 50 dB hearing loss may be as much as 3 years delayed (Blair, 1986). As would be expected, the primary deficit areas for children with hearing losses are in those subjects that are language-based. Anderson and Matkin (Anderson, 1991) created a chart that details the expected academic, speech-language, and psychosocial characteristics for students with various degrees of hearing losses. This chart is included in Appendix 4–D and can be quite useful for educational audiologists to share with parents, teachers, and other professionals.

Other Factors

Although the degree of hearing loss will give a general idea of children's expected performance level, we must consider additional information to determine how a specific child will function in the classroom. The age of onset of the hearing loss, the etiology, the age of amplification, prior management of the hearing loss, parental support, and the child's intelligence and personality are some of the factors that will affect the child's academic performance. Neurological functions, such as attention processing and sensory integration skills, are also important to consider. Additionally, the information obtained about the child's auditory and visual skills from any testing that was done must be included when predicting how a specific child's hearing loss will affect educational progress.

Need for Comprehensive Evaluation

It is important for educational audiologists to be aware of the total child, not just the child's auditory skills. Frequently, children with hearing losses have other conditions that may affect their academic performance. If audiologists, who are most aware of the effects that can be expected from the hearing loss, are alert to these conditions, they will be identified sooner, and appropriate, individualized intervention can begin.

PEMICS

Blair (1986) proposed the PEMICS model to ensure that children with hearing losses have a comprehensive evaluation. Using this model, educational audiologists should be sure that all children have at least a screening in each of the following areas:

➤ **P**erceptual: auditory; visual
➤ **E**motional: personality; other psychosocial factors
➤ **M**otor: gross motor; fine motor
➤ **I**ntelligence: verbal; performance (or nonverbal)
➤ **C**ommunication: receptive and expressive language; learning abilities
➤ **S**ocial maturity: adaptive skills

If the screening indicates any possible deficits, the child should then be referred for a more comprehensive evaluation of the identified areas. Blair suggested plotting the results of the PEMICS evaluation on a chart similar to the one in Figure 4–2 so that the child's strengths and limitations are highlighted for those who work with the child.

Colorado Individual Performance Profile (CIPP)

Another protocol for providing comprehensive evaluations for students with hearing losses is the Colorado Individual Performance Profile (CIPP) (Ruberry &

Diagnostic Areas	Stanine								
	1	2	3	4	5	6	7	8	9
Perceptual-Visual									
Acuity (near & far)					X				
Eye teaming					X				
Color vision					X				
Visual motor					X				
Perceptual-Auditory									
Word recognition in quiet				X					
Word recognition in noise		X							
Emotional				X					
Motor									
Gross motor					X				
Fine motor				X					
Intelligence									
Verbal		X							
Performance				X					
Communication-Lang/Speech									
Vocabulary	X								
Receptive language		X							
Expressive language		X							
Pragmatic skills					X				
Speech					X				
Communication-academic/learning									
Reading recognition					X				
Reading comprehension				X					
Math computation				X					
Math application			X						
General knowledge		X							
Memory				X					
Social Maturity				X					

Figure 4–2. PEMICS evaluation for B.B., age 10 years, 0 months.

Yoshinaga-Itano, 1993). The CIPP was designed for use with students who are 6 years or older and whose primary or secondary handicapping condition is hearing loss. Based on the results of formal and informal assessments, the student is rated on a scale of 1 to 6 for each of the following areas:

➤ Audiological acuity
➤ Communication skills
➤ English/language skills
➤ Reading comprehension
➤ Mathematics
➤ Content subject areas
➤ Social-emotional
➤ Life skills
➤ Cognitive status
➤ Special characteristics

Once a profile of the student's current functioning has been developed, the ratings can be used to assist in the identification of the appropriate intensity of services (monitoring, consultation, or direct service) for the student. A summary of the CIPP is included in Appendix 4–E.

Use of Teacher Checklists

Another useful way to determine the educational effects of students' hearing losses is to use teacher checklists. Although educational audiologists may want to develop their own checklists, there are three that are frequently used in the schools:

➤ Screening Instrument for Targeting Educational Risk (S.I.F.T.E.R.) (Anderson, 1989) and Preschool S.I.F.T.E.R. (Anderson & Matkin, 1996) (see Appendixes 3–F and 3–G)
➤ Fisher's Auditory Problems Checklist (Fisher, 1985) (see Appendix 3–D)
➤ Evaluation of Children with Suspected Listening Difficulties (Edwards, 1991) (see Appendix 4–F)

All of these checklists are brief and can be completed by the student's teacher in a relatively short period of time. They are useful when the child is first identified as having a hearing loss, as well as a tool to monitor the student's performance from year to year. Ordering information for the S.I.F.T.E.R. and the Fisher's Checklist is included in Appendix 16–D.

Screening Instrument for Targeting Educational Risk

The S.I.F.T.E.R. asks the child's teacher to rate the child in comparison to the other children in the classroom on 15 items. It is scored by taking the teacher's ratings

and plotting them on a chart which indicates pass, marginal, or fail for each of the five areas of academics, attention, communication, classroom participation, and school behavior. If children fail a specific area, they should be referred for further evaluation in that area. Children who are in the marginal category should be monitored for future difficulties. The Preschool S.I.F.T.E.R., which has been developed for use with preschool children, is similar to the S.I.F.T.E.R. and can be used with children who are not yet in school.

Fisher's Auditory Problems Checklist

The Fisher's Checklist was initially developed to screen children for central auditory processing disorders, but it can also be used for children with hearing losses. It requires the teacher to check which of 25 items are of concern for the child and is scored by determining the percentage of items not checked by the teacher. Children's scores can then be compared to the mean scores obtained by children at their grade level to determine if further testing should be recommended. It is suggested that a child scoring below 72% be referred for further evaluation.

Evaluation of Children with Suspected Listening Difficulties

This checklist provides a comprehensive description of the student's classroom listening skills and strategies. Teachers are asked to rate their overall concerns about students' listening skills, the students' current strengths and weaknesses during various listening activities, and the students' awareness of their listening problems. Additionally, teachers are asked to describe the students' listening strategies and to indicate the classroom and teaching modifications used. This checklist provides specific information that can be used to determine appropriate management techniques for students.

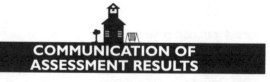

COMMUNICATION OF ASSESSMENT RESULTS

For the assessment completed by educational audiologists to be useful, the results must be communicated in a meaningful way. There are many ways that we communicate the results of our evaluations to parents, teachers, and other professionals. These include:

➤ Audiograms
➤ Written reports

➤ Teacher letters
➤ Letters to physicians or other professionals
➤ Telephone or personal conferences

These forms of communication do not stand alone. In fact, explaining test results and recommendations more than once and in more than one way is often necessary to help parents and teachers fully understand the hearing loss and its implications at home and at school.

It is important that audiologists ensure that those receiving information understand the results and are able to apply the recommendations. In a survey of teachers who had all received both a written report and a form letter about a child with a hearing loss in their classrooms, it was found that only 74% of teachers were even aware of their students' hearing losses (Blair, EuDaly, & Von Almen, 1993) . Additionally, less than half of the teachers felt that they understood all of the information contained in the report or the form letter. Ensuring that teachers and others working with the child receive and understand the results of assessments is a challenge for educational audiologists. Without this communication, the child may not be served optimally.

Audiograms

Audiologists record the results of their basic audiometric assessment on an audiogram which is frequently sent to the parents, teachers, physicians, and other professionals. Some professionals are familiar with the audiogram and will be able to use the information it provides, but audiograms are not understood by most people. To overcome this limitation, some audiologists use conventional audiograms modified to provide space for a brief interpretation of the test results and brief recommendations (see Appendix 4–G). Additionally, some of the audiograms described earlier in this chapter may provide useful information to parents and teachers. These audiograms include the "speech banana" audiogram (Watkins, 1993), the audiogram with pictures of familiar sounds (American Academy of Audiology, 1993), the audiogram containing percentages of normal conversational speech heard (Pascoe, 1980, as cited in Olsen, Hawkins, & Van Tasell, 1987), and the "Count-the-Dot" audiogram (Mueller & Killion, 1990). Regardless of the audiogram used, we should be sure that those who receive copies understand them, as well as what should be done to assist the child.

Written Reports

Written reports are one of the most common methods we use to communicate the results of our assessments. These reports are effective only if they are understood by the person who receives the report and only if the person can remember the recommendations that were made for the child. Reports to parents and teachers should typically be short, including a brief description of the hearing loss, a summary of the effects the hearing loss may have at home or in the classroom, and recommendations for management of the child. The recommendations should be specific and should be limited to no more than three or four items. Because it is often difficult to prioritize and limit the recommendations, it may be helpful to subdivide them in order to focus the teachers, parents, and other professionals on the ones they should consider first. For example, the recommendations could include the subheadings of "Audiological Recommendations," "Medical Recommendations," and "Educational Recommendations."

The reports sent to parents and teachers should also be free from professional jargon. Even terms such as "conductive hearing loss," "moderate hearing loss," and "unilateral hearing loss" may not be understood by those not familiar with audiology. If it is necessary to send information to physicians or other professionals using more technical language, it may be necessary to write a second or revised report for those persons. However, these individuals may also benefit from the interpretations and recommendations stated in less technical terms.

Teacher Letters

Form letters sent to teachers are another common way that educational audiologists communicate with educational personnel. There is a sample form letter in Appendix 4–H. Form letters typically are more useful when they are adapted to the needs of a specific child. This can be done by highlighting recommendations that are particularly important for the child or by leaving blank spaces to add handwritten notes about the child who has been evaluated. Another idea that may be more helpful to the teacher is to provide "Helpful Hearing Hints" for the child on a brightly colored 5×8 card. These hints should be limited to only three or four items which are most important for the student involved. The card can be kept by the teachers on their desks where it is a daily reminder of the things they can do to help the child in their classrooms. A sample card is provided in Figure 4–3.

As shown in Figure 4–4, a letter from the student written directly to the teacher can be an extremely powerful tool for conveying the necessary accomodations needed. This method of communication with the teacher not only demonstrates that students are responsible for identifying and managing their own accommodations, but also establishes direct communication between the students and the teachers.

HELPFUL HEARING HINTS

for _____

➤ _____ needs to be seated near the front of the classroom and away from noise sources, such as pencil sharpeners and noisy students. A seat at one side of the classroom will be helpful so he can easily turn to follow classroom discussions.

➤ Check for understanding by asking specific questions about the material (e.g., "What did I say?" or "What page will you start on?") rather than asking if _____ heard you. He may not always know if he has heard and understood correctly.

➤ The following additional suggestions will be helpful:
  —Wait until your class is quiet before speaking.
  —Maintain visual attention when speaking.
  —Write important information on the chalkboard so _____ can see it.

Figure 4–3. Helpful hearing hints.

Letters to Physicians or Other Professionals

Frequently, audiologists will need to communicate the results of the evaluation to children's physicians or other professionals. Although the audiogram and evaluation report are often appropriate for these professionals, it may at times be necessary to write a separate letter to address specific concerns and to let the professional know the educational needs of the child. These letters are often short and provide only the specific information needed by the professional involved.

Telephone or Personal Conferences

Another way to provide information to those involved with the child is through either a telephone call or personal contact. When parents are present for the child's evaluation, the audiologist explains the results to them, but conferences with teachers may occur less frequently. These conferences are time-consuming and sometimes difficult to arrange, but they are important. They allow the audiologist to review information directly with those involved with the child so that questions can be answered and recommendations can be adapted to the child's specific environment and needs. The conferences also have the advantage of providing the audiologist with information to facilitate management of the child.

When providing information to parents and teachers, we should be sure that we are understood. Techniques for enhancing understanding include the following:

➤ Asking the parents and teachers what they think about the child's hearing prior to explaining the test results. This allows the educational audiologist to use the parents' and teachers' terminology and to focus on their perceptions when explaining the audiometric results.

➤ Writing out the recommendations in simple language after the oral explanation. Parents and teachers can read over the recommendations to be sure they understand them, then sign them. Giving each participant a copy, as well as maintaining a copy in the student's file, can serve as a future reminder of recommendations made for specific concerns.

➤ Asking the parent and teacher to tell the audiologist what they plan to tell another person (i.e., spouse, relative, teacher, or principal) about the audiometric results and recommendations. Allowing them to retell the information reinforces it for them and ensures that they have understood the key points.

Although it is important that parents and teachers understand the child's hearing loss, it is also important to focus on the questions and concerns they have about the child. Providing information that is imme-

Dear _____,

    I have a hearing loss, and I want to tell you about it so you will understand the help I need in your classroom. I wear hearing aids on both ears all of the time, and I cannot hear very much without them. Although my hearing aids help me a great deal, I still have difficulty hearing and understanding when the classroom gets noisy. I read lips fairly well so it is important that I see your face when you are talking to me. Because I have had my hearing loss all of my life, my speech is not always clear.

    I want to do my best in your classroom, but will need some help from you. Things that will help me are listed below:

1. Let me sit near the front of the classroom so I can see and hear better. It will also help me to be on one side of the classroom so that I can turn to watch other students when there is a class discussion.

2. Be sure that I am watching you before you start to talk to the class.

3. Talk clearly when you speak to the class. It is not necessary to talk loudly because my hearing aids will make your speech loud enough for me. Please don't over-exaggerate your speech because that will make it hard for me to lipread you.

4. Write assignments and other important information on the chalkboard so I am sure to get it.

5. Ask me to repeat something if you do not understand me.

    I hope these suggestions will help you. If you have questions about my hearing loss, you can ask me, my parents, or my audiologist. My audiologist's name is _____; her phone number is _____. Thank you for your help.

Sincerely,

Figure 4–4. Sample student letter to teacher.

diately useful to the parents and teachers will help them be more open to other suggestions.

It is also helpful for the audiologist to meet with parents and teachers at a time that is convenient for them. Although this is often difficult for the audiologist, the parents and teachers are generally grateful for the audiologist's consideration of their time, and they are likely to be more open to the information and suggestions offered by the audiologist.

Conferences with parents and teachers should be collaborative whenever possible. To facilitate this process educational audiologists should be perceived as peers rather than as the "hearing experts." Additionally, they should be open to suggestions from others and should be willing to share in the decision-making process. When the interactions are collaborative, the parents and teachers feel that they are part of the child's program, and they will be more supportive of suggestions to enhance the management of the child.

SUMMARY

Assessment is a critical part of the educational audiologist's role. It is important not only for documenting and monitoring hearing losses, but also for determining the implications of hearing losses and the effects of various management strategies. Our assessments must never rely on electrophysiological measures to the exclusion of behavioral testing. We must go beyond traditional audiologic evaluations and seek to integrate our audiologic results with the results of other professionals to provide information that will be applicable and beneficial in the classroom. Finally, for the results of the assessment to be useful, we must be able to communicate effectively with parents, teachers, and other professionals.

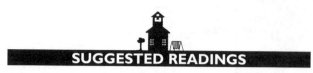

SUGGESTED READINGS

Heller, P. J. (1990). Psycho-educational assessment. In Ross, M. (Ed.), *Hearing-impaired children in the mainstream* (pp. 61–79). Parkton, MD: York Press.

Madell, J. R. (1990). Audiological evaluation of the mainstreamed hearing-impaired child. In Ross, M. (Ed.), *Hearing-impaired children in the mainstream* (pp. 27–44). Parkton, MD: York Press.

Northern, J. L., & Downs, M. P. (1991). Behavioral hearing testing of children. In *Hearing in children* (4th ed., pp. 139–187). Baltimore, MD: Williams & Wilkins.

Northern, J. L., & Downs, M. P. (1991). Physiologic hearing tests. In *Hearing in children* (4th ed., pp. 189–228). Baltimore, MD: Williams & Wilkins.

Ross, M., Brackett, D., & Maxon, A. B. (1991). Academic, psychological, social, and classroom evaluations. In *Assessment and management of mainstreamed hearing-impaired children* (pp. 141–160). Austin, TX: Pro-Ed.

Ross, M., Brackett, D., & Maxon, A. B. (1991). Audiological evaluation and amplification assessment. In *Assessment and management of mainstreamed hearing-impaired children* (pp. 85–111). Austin, TX: Pro-Ed.

Viehweg, S. (1986). Audiological considerations. In F. S. Berg, J. C. Blair, S. H. Viehweg, & A. Wilson-Vlotman, *Educational audiology for the hard of hearing child* (pp. 81–99). Orlando, FL: Grune & Stratton.

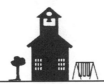

CHAPTER 5

CENTRAL AUDITORY PROCESSING DISORDERS

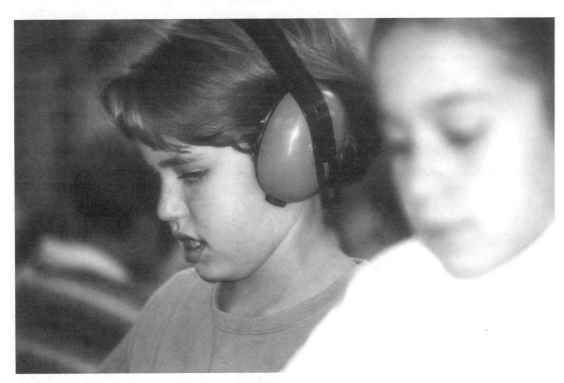

Jennifer, age 10

CONTENTS

Management of Central Auditory Processing Disorders
   Types of CAPD Management Strategies
   Selection of Most Appropriate Management Strategies
Summary
Suggested Readings

One of the most challenging areas for educational audiologists is the identification and treatment of central auditory processing disorders. Those of us who have worked with school-age children are well aware of central auditory processing problems and their educational impact, but the best way to identify and treat these problems remains controversial. This chapter discusses the following areas:

➤ Characteristics of central auditory processing disorders
➤ Screening for central auditory processing disorders
➤ Assessment of central auditory processing disorders
➤ Management of central auditory processing disorders

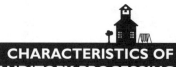

CHARACTERISTICS OF CENTRAL AUDITORY PROCESSING DISORDERS

An initial step in managing central auditory processing disorders (CAPD) is an understanding of what they are. Questions related to understanding CAPD include:

➤ What is a central auditory processing disorder?
➤ What behavioral characteristics do children with CAPD have?
➤ Are all central auditory processing disorders the same, or are there different profiles or types of disorders?

Description of Central Auditory Processing Disorders

Perhaps the uncertainty surrounding central auditory processing disorders (CAPD) is due, at least in part, to the lack of a consistent definition. Various authors have suggested that CAPD may be a language problem, a listening deficit, or a perceptual disorder. Certain children may or may not have a central auditory processing disorder, depending on the theoretical construct the educational audiologist feels underlies central auditory processing.

The definitions of central auditory processing disorders provided by the Central Auditory Processing Ad Hoc Committee of the American Speech-Language-Hearing Association (ASHA, 1990a) and the Task Force on Central Auditory Processing Consensus Development (ASHA, 1996) are provided in Appendix 5–A. These definitions are both complex and may not be easily understood by teachers and parents. A more functional definition for the educational audiologist to use may be that a central auditory processing disorder is a deficit in "what is done with what is heard."

Regardless of the definition used, there are certain characteristics and behaviors that are associated with central auditory processing disorders. Although CAPD is most often diagnosed in children with normal intelligence and normal-hearing sensitivity, it can co-exist with hearing loss or with other cognitive or neurologic impairments. Behaviors common in children with CAPD are listed in Table 5–1. Children rarely display all of these behaviors, but it is likely they will exhibit several of them.

Differences in Central Auditory Processing Disorders

Another reason for the uncertainty surrounding central auditory processing disorders is that all disorders are likely not the same and may, therefore, not benefit from similar treatment. Chermak (1992) suggested that there are three types of central auditory disorders in children, including those with a diseased central auditory nervous system (CANS), those with a maturational delay in the CANS, and those with a disorganized CANS. Currently, we are able to use various auditory site of lesion tests to identify those rare children who have a diseased CANS, but it is difficult to differentiate between those with a delayed CANS and those with a disorganized CANS. Presently, audiologists use similar recommendations and treatment strategies for all children with CAPD. The success of these management strategies is inconsistent, but in the future it may be possible to improve the success of treatment by identifying the particular type of CAPD that is present and basing remediation on what will be most effective for that type of CAPD.

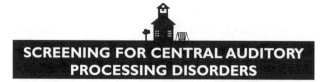

SCREENING FOR CENTRAL AUDITORY PROCESSING DISORDERS

The identification of central auditory processing disorders (CAPD) is quite complex, typically involving extensive testing prior to the final diagnosis. We feel that CAPD screening often occurs on two levels, the initial screening and a secondary screening. The ini-

Table 5–1. Characteristics of children with central auditory processing disorders.

➤ Has poor concentration/attention span
➤ Gives inconsistent responses to auditory stimuli
➤ Has difficulty following directions
➤ Gives slow or delayed responses to verbal stimuli
➤ Frequently requests repetition of what is said
➤ Often misunderstands what is said
➤ Is easily distracted by auditory and visual stimuli
➤ Has difficulty listening in presence of background noise
➤ Has memory deficits, both long-term and short-term
➤ Has language deficits
➤ Has academic difficulties, particularly with reading and spelling, despite normal intelligence
➤ Exhibits behavior problems
➤ Relies on visual cues when attempting to communicate (e.g., watches speaker's face closely)
➤ Has difficulty localizing the source of sounds
➤ Has history of chronic middle ear infections and possible fluctuating hearing loss
➤ Has lowered self-esteem

tial screening is used to identify those suspected of having CAPD, and the secondary screening determines who should be referred for an in-depth CAPD evaluation. When considering screening for central auditory processing disorders, the following questions arise:

➤ Is it efficient to provide mass screening as an initial screening for central auditory processing disorders?
➤ If not, how are children with CAPD identified?
➤ What types of instruments can be used to screen for CAPD?

Initial CAPD Screening

Mass Screening

The efficacy of screening for central auditory processing disorders has been debated a great deal. Some authors argue that mass screening is warranted because undetected central auditory processing disorders can lead to communication problems and academic failure and because there are techniques to diagnose and treat these disorders. On the other hand, others feel that mass CAPD screening should not be done because there is not a clear definition of the disorder, because there is no universally accepted way to diagnose auditory processing disorders, and because current screening tools cannot adequately separate auditory processing disorders from attention, cognition, or language deficits. Because of the concerns about CAPD screening and the time involved in providing them, mass screening for CAPD is rarely done.

CAPD Referrals

Instead of mass screening, children to be screened for central auditory processing disorders are identified most often by teacher or parent referrals. Educational audiologists can use the list of behaviors provided in Table 5–1 to educate parents and teachers about central auditory processing disorders and to encourage the referral of children with listening difficulties for a CAPD screening. Additionally, it may be advantageous to refer specific at-risk populations (e.g., children experiencing academic difficulties or children with learning disabilities) for CAPD screening.

Secondary Screening

Once a child is suspected of having a central auditory processing disorder, peripheral hearing loss must be ruled out as the reason for the concerns about the child. We believe that a more formal screening should then take place to determine if the child should be referred for an in-depth CAPD evaluation. There are basically two types of instruments used for CAPD screening: auditory processing screening tests and teacher checklists. Either or both of these instruments can be used to provide the educational audiologist with information about the child's auditory processing skills before a referral for a complete assessment is made.

Auditory Processing Screening Tests

Three of the most commonly used screening tests for central auditory processing disorders are the SCAN: A Screening Test for Auditory Processing Disorders

(Keith, 1986), the SCAN-A: A Test for Auditory Processing Disorders in Adolescents and Adults (Keith, 1993), and the Selective Auditory Attention Test (SAAT) (Cherry, 1980). Ordering information for these tests is included in Appendix 16–E. These tests are tape recorded and can be administered by audiologists, speech-language pathologists, or learning specialists. The SCAN and the SAAT are normed for administration to preschool and elementary-school children, but it should be noted that small sample sizes and the large variability in the performance of young children make these tests less valid for the preschool population. The SCAN-A is appropriate for adolescents and adults. These tests are all relatively quick to administer, with the SCAN and the SCAN-A taking about 20 minutes and the SAAT about 8 minutes.

Teacher Checklists

Another alternative for central auditory processing screening is the use of a teacher checklist, such as the Fisher's Auditory Problems Checklist (Fisher, 1985) (see Appendix 3–D) or the Children's Auditory Processing Performance Scale (CHAPPS) (Smoski, 1990) (see Appendix 5–B). Both checklists require the teacher to complete a form answering questions about the child's listening, attending, and auditory memory skills. Although the time to both complete and score these checklists must be considered, they usually take less time than the auditory processing screening tests.

ASSESSMENT OF CENTRAL AUDITORY PROCESSING DISORDERS

Once a child has failed a secondary screening for central auditory processing disorders (auditory processing test, teacher checklist, or both), the child should be referred for an in-depth assessment of his or her auditory processing skills. Questions surrounding CAPD assessment include:

➤ Are there specific questions that should be addressed during the case history interview?
➤ What specific audiometric tests can be used for central auditory assessments?
➤ Are there tests other than audiometric tests that will be useful in diagnosing central auditory processing disorders?
➤ What are some of the protocols that have been developed for use in assessing central auditory processing disorders?

➤ What are the criteria used to define the presence of a central auditory processing disorder?
➤ How are central auditory processing disorders assessed in preschoolers, in children with peripheral hearing losses, and in non-English-speaking children?

Case History

As with the assessment of any hearing loss, the assessment of central auditory processing disorders should begin with a complete case history. The history will help the educational audiologist focus on the immediate concerns of the parents and the teachers, will provide information that will supplement the more formal audiometric tests, and will prove invaluable in determining recommendations concerning the child's educational management. Although many of the questions in the history interview will be similar to those discussed in Chapter 4, Assessment Practices, the educational audiologist should also obtain information on the child's auditory behaviors, asking questions about the behaviors listed in Table 5–2. Additionally, the audiologist should focus on how the child's auditory problems are affecting his or her academic progress.

Tests Used in Central Auditory Assessments

There are many audiological tests that have been designed to test central auditory processing skills. Additionally, there are speech-language or other tests that also assess a child's auditory skills. Most often audiologists use a test battery approach to central auditory assessments to evaluate several different auditory skills of the child. This section provides a categorization of the individual tests most often used in assessing central auditory skills, including:

➤ Audiometric tests
    Monotic speech tests
    Monotic tone tests
    Dichotic speech tests
    Binaural integration/interaction tests
    Other auditory processing tests
➤ Nonaudiometric tests
    Attending
    Discrimination
    Memory
    Integration
    Language comprehension
    Other nonaudiometric tests
➤ Observation of the child

Table 5–2. Auditory behaviors to be explored in case history interview.

➤ Ability to localize sounds
➤ Ability to identify sound sources
➤ Ability to listen selectively in the presence of noise
➤ Reaction to sudden, unexpected sounds
➤ Ability to ignore environmental sounds
➤ Tolerance to loud sounds
➤ Consistency of response to sound
➤ Need to have spoken information repeated
➤ Ability to follow verbal instructions
➤ Ability to listen for appropriate length of time
➤ Ability to remember things heard
➤ Ability to pay attention to what is said
➤ Ability to comprehend words and their meaning
➤ Ability to understand multiple meanings of words
➤ Ability to understand abstract ideas
➤ Discrepancies between auditory and visual behavior

Source: Adapted from "Tests of central auditory function" by R. Keith, 1988. In R. J. Roeser & M. P. Downs (Eds.), *Auditory disorders in school children* (2nd ed., p. 88).

Ordering information for the tests listed in the following sections is included in Appendix 16–E.

In selecting specific tests to use in a central auditory processing test battery, the educational audiologist must be careful to use tests with good validity, test-retest reliability, and age-appropriate normative data. Additionally, ease of administration, administration time, availability of needed equipment, and acoustic environment must be considered when determining which tests will be used.

Audiometric Tests

MONOTIC SPEECH TESTS. Monotic speech tests include low-pass filtered speech, time-altered speech, and speech-in-noise tests. These tests are designed to determine how distortions of speech affect the child's ability to understand words or sentences with each ear separately. Tests commonly used with children include:

➤ Low-pass filtered speech
  Filtered Speech subtest of Flowers-Costello Test of Central Auditory Abilities (Flowers & Costello, 1970)
  Filtered Words subtest of SCAN (Keith, 1986) or SCAN-A (Keith, 1993)
  Low-Pass Filtered Speech subtest of the Willeford Battery (Willeford, 1977)
➤ Time-altered speech
  Compressed WIPI (Beasley, Maki, & Orchik, 1976)

Wichita Auditory Processing Test (WAPT) (McCroskey, 1984b)
➤ Speech-in-noise tests
  Clinic-made tests
  Auditory Figure Ground subtest of SCAN (Keith, 1986) or SCAN-A (Keith, 1993)
  Competing Messages subtest of Flowers-Costello Test of Central Auditory Abilities (Flowers & Costello, 1970)
  Selective Attention Test of the Goldman-Fristoe-Woodcock Auditory Skills Test Battery (Goldman, Fristoe, & Woodcock, 1974a)
  Ipsilateral Competing Message (ICM) of the Synthetic Sentence Identification (SSI) Test (Jerger & Jerger, 1974)
  Pediatric Speech Intelligibility (PSI) Test (Jerger, 1987)
  Selective Auditory Attention Test (SAAT) (Cherry, 1980)
  Speech Perception in Noise (SPIN) Test (Kalikow, Stevens, & Elliott, 1977)

MONOTIC TONE TESTS. Monotic tone tests also assess the child's ability to use each ear separately, but the stimuli for these tests are tones rather than speech. Most of these tests focus on the child's pattern perception and temporal functioning abilities. Common monotic tone tests include:

➤ Duration Pattern Test (DPT) (Baran, Musiek, & Gollegly, 1987)

➤ Pitch Pattern Sequence (PPS) Test (Pinheiro, 1978)
➤ Wichita Auditory Fusion Test (WAFT) (McCrosky, 1984a)

DICHOTIC SPEECH TESTS. Dichotic tests are tests in which a different stimulus is presented simultaneously to each ear. On these tests there is typically a right-ear advantage in younger children with the left-ear score improving as the child's auditory system matures. Tests representative of dichotic speech tests include:

➤ Competing Environmental Sounds (CES) Test (Katz, Kushner, & Pack, 1975)
➤ Competing Sentence (CS) subtest of the Willeford Battery (Willeford, 1977)
➤ Competing Sentences subtest of SCAN-A (Keith, 1993)
➤ Competing Words subtest of SCAN (Keith, 1986) or SCAN-A (Keith, 1993)
➤ Contralateral Competing Message (CCM) of the Synthetic Sentence Identification (SSI) Test (Jerger & Jerger, 1974)
➤ Dichotic C-V Test (Berlin, 1973)
➤ Dichotic Digits Test (Musiek, 1983)
➤ Dichotic Sentence Identification Test (Fifer, Jerger, Berlin, Tobey, & Campbell, 1983)
➤ Staggered Spondaic Word (SSW) Test (Katz, 1962)

BINAURAL INTEGRATION/INTERACTION TESTS. Binaural integration/interaction tests are diotic tests in that the stimuli presented to each ear is the same. These tests are effective in evaluating the integration between the two ears and include the following:

➤ Binaural Fusion (BF) subtest of the Willeford Battery (Willeford, 1977)
➤ Masking Level Difference (MLD) Test (Sweetow & Redell, 1978)
➤ Rapidly Alternating Speech Perception (RASP) subtest of the Willeford Battery (Willeford, 1977)
➤ Speech-in-Noise Tests presented binaurally through earphones or in sound-field

OTHER AUDITORY PROCESSING TESTS. Another auditory test that does not fit into the previous classification system is the Phonemic Synthesis (PS) Test (Katz, 1983). This is a test of phonemic blending skills and has been normed for children by grade level.

Additionally, both electrophysiological tests and imaging techniques have been used in the diagnosis of central auditory processing disorders. Electrophysiological tests include the brainstem, middle, late, and event-related auditory potentials and otoacoustic emissions. The auditory brainstem response (ABR) is well understood and routinely used to diagnose lesions in the brainstem. The use of the later evoked responses in diagnosing CAPD is still being investigated, but the P300 and the mismatched negativity responses seem to be particularly promising. Various imaging techniques, including magnetic resonance imaging (MRI) and positron emission tomography (PET), can also provide useful information for the diagnosis of CAPD, either alone or in combination with other techniques.

Nonaudiometric Tests

These tests are not typically administered by an audiologist, but educational audiologists may elect to administer them if they are properly trained and are allowed to do so under state laws and regulations. Alternatively, the educational audiologist may arrange for the speech-language pathologist, the psychologist, or the learning specialist to provide these tests to the child who is receiving a central auditory assessment.

Nonaudiometric tests are typically not administered in a sound booth, but should be given in a quiet, controlled environment. If the test is taped, the instructions for calibrating the tape recorder should be followed carefully.

ATTENDING. Auditory attending skills are often assessed during speech-in-noise testing. If additional testing outside the test booth is needed to provide more information, the following may be used:

➤ Observation of the child in the classroom and other situations
➤ Auditory Continuous Performance Test (Keith, 1994)
➤ Selective Attention Test of Goldman-Fristoe-Woodcock Auditory Skills Test Battery (Goldman et al., 1974a)

DISCRIMINATION. Tests of discrimination are typically administered in the audiometric test booth by the audiologist, but there are some tests that may be administered in other environments. These include:

➤ Goldman-Fristoe-Woodcock Test of Auditory Discrimination (Goldman, Fristoe, & Woodcock, 1974b)
➤ Wepman Auditory Discrimination Test (Wepman, 1973)

MEMORY. Auditory memory skills cannot be tested with traditional audiometric tests, but there are several nonaudiometric tests designed to assess both memory and sequential memory. Because this is an area in which children with central auditory processing disorders often have difficulty, it is usually advantageous to include one or more of the following tests:

➤ Auditory Sequential Memory subtest of the Illinois Test of Psycholinguistic Abilities (Kirk, McCarthy, & Kirk, 1968)
➤ Auditory Sequential Memory Test (Wepman & Morency, 1973)
➤ Memory for Sequence, Memory for Content, and Recognition Memory Tests from the Goldman-Fristoe-Woodcock Auditory Skills Test Battery (Goldman et al., 1974a)
➤ Unrelated Words, Related Words, and Sentence Repetition subtests of Detroit Tests of Learning Aptitude-2 (Hammill, 1985)
➤ Visual Aural Digit Span (VADS) (Koppitz, 1975)

INTEGRATION. Tests of auditory integration include tests that assess the child's sound blending and auditory integration skills. These skills are automatic auditory skills, and when children are deficient in these areas, they likely will have difficulty with reading and spelling. Various tests that assess auditory integration skills include:

➤ Auditory Closure and Sound Blending subtests of the Illinois Test of Psycholinguistic Abilities (Kirk et al., 1968)
➤ Lindamood Auditory Conceptualization (LAC) Test (Lindamood & Lindamood, 1975)
➤ Spelling of Symbols, Reading of Symbols, Sound Symbol, Sound Mimicry, Sound Blending, Sound Recognition, and Sound Analysis Tests from the Goldman-Fristoe-Woodcock Auditory Skills Test Battery (Goldman, et al., 1974a)

LANGUAGE COMPREHENSION. Many people would argue that tests of language comprehension should not be included in a central auditory processing assessment, noting that a language disorder may either be the result or the cause of the auditory processing problem. Although this may be true, some professionals believe that language comprehension is the highest level of auditory processing and should be evaluated. If educational audiologists choose to include tests of language comprehension in the central auditory processing test battery, they should consult with a speech-language pathologist to determine what tests would provide the necessary information. Some commonly used tests of language comprehension are:

➤ Clinical Evaluation of Language Fundamentals—Revised (Semel, Wiig, & Secord, 1987)
➤ Illinois Test of Psycholinguistic Abilities (Kirk et al., 1968)

➤ Expressive One-Word Picture Vocabulary Test—Revised (Gardner, 1990)
➤ Peabody Picture Vocabulary Test—Revised (Dunn & Dunn, 1981)
➤ Test of Auditory Comprehension of Language—Revised (Carrow-Woolfolk, 1985)
➤ Test of Language Competence—Expanded Edition (Wiig & Secord, 1989)
➤ Tests of Language Development—2 (Hammill & Newcomer, 1988)
➤ Test of Word Knowledge (Wiig & Secord, 1992)
➤ Token Test for Children (DiSimoni, 1978)

OTHER NONAUDIOMETRIC TESTS. The Test of Auditory-Perceptual Skills (Gardner, 1985) is a battery of tests that can be presented to children between the ages of 4 and 12 years of age. This test measures the auditory-perceptual skills of processing, sequential memory, interpretation of oral directions, discrimination, and word memory.

Observation of the Child

Throughout the formal assessment of the child, we believe it is important for the educational audiologist to observe the child's behaviors. Although this observation is done in a very structured situation, it may provide clues to why the child is having difficulty in the classroom and may lead to suggestions for classroom management. In addition to the observation during the assessment, the educational audiologist will find it helpful to observe the child in the classroom and other settings when this is possible. Behaviors the educational audiologist should observe include:

➤ Attention span
➤ Attention to both structured and unstructured tasks
➤ Cooperation and willingness to perform both easy and difficult tasks
➤ Response to frustration
➤ Need for praise and encouragement in order to complete a task

Protocols for Central Auditory Assessments

As mentioned earlier, educational audiologists most often use a test battery approach for assessing a child's central auditory processing skills. These test batteries are generally based on the audiologist's view of the nature of central auditory processing and are frequently modified to address concerns for an individual child. The ASHA Consensus Statement on Central Auditory Processing (ASHA, 1996) recommended that the following criteria be considered when developing a central auditory test battery:

➤ Tests should be selected based on referring complaints or other relevant information
➤ Individual tests should examine different central processes
➤ Tests selected should include both verbal and nonverbal stimuli
➤ Individual tests should be reliable, valid, and age-appropriate
➤ The duration of the test session should be appropriate for the child's attention span and motivation

Although the following list is not comprehensive, some of the authors who have suggested specific test batteries for evaluating auditory processing problems are:

➤ Bellis (1995)
➤ Chermak (1992)
➤ Colorado Department of Education (1996a)
➤ Ferre and Wilber (1986)
➤ Medwetsky (1994)
➤ Utah State University (Von Almen, Blair, & Spriet, 1990)
➤ Vanderbilt University Medical Center Audiology Clinic (Hall et al., 1993)
➤ Willeford (1977)

Bellis

Bellis (1995) has developed a central auditory assessment battery that is appropriate for children 7 years of age and older. She suggested that the battery include the following tests at a minimum:

➤ One test of temporal processing (frequency patterns; duration patterns; click fusion; two-tone ordering)
➤ Two dichotic speech tests (one linguistic; one non-linguistic) (Dichotic Digits; Dichotic C-Vs; Competing Sentences; Dichotic Rhyme; Staggered Spondaic Word; Dichotic Sentence Identification)
➤ One monaural, low-redundancy speech test (compressed speech; compressed speech and reverberation; filtered speech)
➤ One binaural interaction test (Rapidly Alternating Speech Perception; Binaural Fusion; Masking Level Differences)
➤ Electrophysiological testing, as needed

Chermak

Chermak (1992) suggested that pediatric evaluations for central auditory processing disorders include tests in the following areas:

➤ Auditory neuromaturational level
   Auditory localization
   Binaural synthesis (Masking Level Difference)
   Binaural separation (Dichotic Sentence Identification; Competing Words subtest of SCAN; Staggered Spondaic Words Test)
   Resistance to distortion (Pediatric Speech Intelligibility; Auditory Figure-Ground and Filtered Words subtests of SCAN; Synthetic Sentence Identification; Time-Compressed Speech)
➤ Tests of temporal processing (Brief Tone Audiometry; Masking Level Difference; Pitch Patterns Test)
➤ Dichotic tests (Dichotic C-V Test; Dichotic Digits; Staggered Spondaic Words Test; Competing Words subtest of SCAN; Pediatric Speech Intelligibility)
➤ Monaural low redundancy tests
   Filtered speech (Filtered Words subtest of SCAN)
   Competing messages (Pediatric Speech Intelligibility; Auditory Figure-Ground subtest of SCAN)
   Time compressed speech (Time-Compressed PBK; Time-Compressed NU-6; Time-Compressed WIPI)
   Time-compressed speech with reverberation
➤ Analysis of metalanguage (Analysis of the Language of Learning; Clinical Evaluation of Language Fundamentals—Revised; Revised Token Test; Test of Language Competence; The Language Processing Test; The Word Test; Test of Word Knowledge)
➤ Checklists of auditory performance

Chermak recommended that a central auditory processing evaluation minimally include at least one test of temporal processing, one dichotic test, and one monaural low redundancy test. If a child performs poorly in any one area, another test should be administered to evaluate that skill more completely.

Colorado Department of Education

The Colorado Department of Education (1996a) has developed a multidisciplinary approach for the assessment of central auditory processing disorders. The protocol is divided into four stages, including observation, screening and preliminary assessment, diagnostic assessment, and additional diagnostic procedures. A student may be involved in only one or two of the stages, depending on the results of intervention procedures. The complete protocol gathers input from audiology, speech-language pathology, psychology, education, and other appropriate disciplines. This is provided in Appendix 5–C. The audiological sections of the protocol recommend the use of:

➤ Observation
   Hearing sensitivity normal or cleared by an audiologist

Auditory behavior checklist (Fisher's Auditory Problems Checklist; Children's Auditory Processing Performance Scale)
Optional parent checklist or student self-checklist
➤ Screening and preliminary assessment
SCAN or SCAN-A
Test of Auditory Perceptual Skills (TAPS)
Auditory Continuous Performance Test (ACPT)
Selective Auditory Attention Test (SAAT)
Pediatric Sentence Identification Test (PSI)
➤ Diagnostic assessment—choose one from each of the following areas, unless otherwise indicated:
Dichotic (one linguistically loaded test; one non-linguistically loaded test)
—Linguistically loaded (SSW; Competing Sentences; SSI-CCM)
—Nonlinguistically loaded (Dichotic Digits; Dichotic C-Vs; Dichotic Rhyme)
Low redundancy monaural speech (Low-pass filtered speech; Time-compressed speech; Time-compressed speech with reverberation)
Temporal processing (Frequency patterns; Duration patterns)
Binaural interaction (Binaural Fusion; Masking Level Difference)
Speech-in-noise (SSI-ICM)
➤ Additional diagnostic (Electrophysiological measures when indicated)
Magnetic Resonance Imaging (MRI)
Auditory Brainstem Response (ABR) Test

Ferre and Wilber

In 1986 Ferre and Wilber proposed a test battery that was evaluated to determine the sensitivity of each test individually and of the entire battery. Their test battery included the following tests, all of which used the NU-CHIPS word list as stimuli:

➤ Low-Pass Filtered Speech
➤ Binaural Fusion
➤ Time-Compressed (60% compression ratio)
➤ Dichotic Monosyllable Test

Ferre and Wilber found that the best criteria for failure for the entire test battery was failure on three or more tests, with failure defined as one standard deviation or more below the mean.

Medwetsky

Medwetsky (1994) suggested a central auditory processing test battery for use in identifying auditory processing disorders in learning disabled students. His battery was designed to pick up weaknesses in the listening skills of students that may influence their performance in the classroom. Medwetsky suggested that the following tests be administered to all children who fail a central auditory processing screening:

➤ Visual Aural Digit Span
➤ Staggered Spondaic Word Test
➤ Lindamood Auditory Conceptualization Test
➤ Phonemic Synthesis Test
➤ Competing Sentences
➤ Pitch Pattern Sequence Test

Utah State University

Utah State University (USU) developed a central auditory assessment battery (Von Almen et al., 1990) that was based on Keith's (1988) description of central auditory processing as a composite of several auditory skills. The USU protocol uses a combination of audiometric tests, nonaudiometric tests, and observation to obtain information in each of six auditory skills areas. After an initial screening to determine whether the child may have a central auditory processing disorder, the USU protocol includes at least two tests in each of the following areas:

➤ Sound blending
➤ Discrimination/figure-ground
Words versus Sentences
Quiet versus Noise
Earphones versus Sound-field
➤ Closure
➤ Memory
Related (sentences) versus Unrelated (words)
Sequence
Length
➤ Attention: Observation
➤ Localization: Observation

The results of these tests are plotted on a chart (see Figure 5–1 and Appendix 5–D) to allow the educational audiologist to identify the child's auditory strengths and weaknesses easily. A central auditory processing disorder is present if the combined results in any one skill area are one or more standard deviations below the mean for the test.

Vanderbilt University Medical Center Audiology Clinic

The CAPD assessment battery used by the Audiology Clinic at Vanderbilt University Medical Center (Hall et al., 1993) focuses on behavioral tests with electrophysiological tests added to the test battery if request-

SUMMARY OF RESULTS OF CENTRAL AUDITORY ASSESSMENT

NAME: ___Y S___   BIRTHDATE: ___5-3-87___   CA: ___9-7___

AUDITORY SKILL	BELOW AVER						AVERAGE							ABOVE AVER				
	1	2	3	4	5	6	7	8	9	10	11	12	13	14	15	16	17	18
CAA SCREENING:																		
SCAN:																		
Filtered Words								X										
Aud Figure Ground			X															
Competing Words							X											
COMPOSITE						X												
FISHER'S						X												
TONI										X								
SOUND BLENDING:																		
LAC												X						
CAVAT #12											X							
DISCRIM/FIGURE-GROUND:																		
Right (Sent. Noise): 70%				X														
Left (Sent. Noise): 44%		X																
Both Ears:																		
Words-Quiet: 100%									X									
Words-Noise: 66%				X														
Sentences-Quiet:100%									X									
Sentences-Noise: 78%					X													
CLOSURE:																		
ITPA Auditory Closure												X						
SCAN (LP @ 1000 Hz)								X										
Willeford (LP @ 500 Hz)																		
Right Ear							X											
Left Ear				X														
MEMORY:																		
Related:																		
DTLA #2									X									
CAVAT #10										X								
Unrelated:																		
DTLA #4								X										
CAVAT #11									X									
Following Directions:																		
DTLA # 3												X						
ATTENTION:							X											
LOCALIZATION:									X									

Figure 5–1. Central auditory assessment profile.

ed or if concerns arise during the behavioral testing. The specific behavioral tests used in the Vanderbilt CAPD assessment battery are:

➤ Dichotic Digits Test
➤ Staggered Spondaic Word Test
➤ Dichotic Sentence Identification Test
➤ Competing Sentence Test (optional)
➤ Synthetic Sentence Identification—Ipsilateral Competing Message
➤ Pitch Pattern Sequence Test

Willeford

Willeford (1977) proposed a test battery that has been used by many educational audiologists. His entire test battery was tape recorded and normed for use with children between 5 and 10 years of age. The subtests of Willeford's test battery include:

➤ Competing Sentence Test
➤ Low-Pass Filtered Speech
➤ Binaural Fusion
➤ Rapidly Alternating Speech Perception

Although Willeford's test battery has received some criticism, the Competing Sentence Test and the Low-Pass Filtered Speech Test are frequently used as part of other test batteries.

Determination of Central Auditory Processing Disorders

As stated previously, we believe that it is best to use a test battery approach to diagnose central auditory processing disorders. If the determination of a central auditory processing disorder (CAPD) is based on only one test, misdiagnosis would increase dramatically because of the variable nature of CAPD and because of the large variability present with some of the auditory tests, especially in young children. Tests for CAPD batteries are chosen because they tap different auditory skills or because they provide more complete information about a skill already tested. Although the test batteries listed in the previous section provide an indication of protocols that may be used, the specific tests used by each educational audiologist will depend on the time available for evaluation, the population being tested, and the philosophy about central auditory processing disorders. In addition to the actual tests administered to the child, the educational audiologist will want to consider information obtained during the case history interview and through observation of the child.

Regardless of the test battery selected, the educational audiologist must define, in advance, what per-

formance will indicate that a central auditory processing disorder is present. The audiologist will have to consider questions such as:

➤ Must children fail a certain number of tests before they are said to have CAPD?
➤ Must children exhibit a deficiency in more than one auditory skill area to have CAPD?
➤ Is one standard deviation below the mean considered a failure? Or must the score be two standard deviations below the mean?

The exact number of tests failed and the criteria for failure may depend on whether audiologists are trying to identify *any* child who might have an auditory processing problem for preventive management or whether they want to identify only those children who *definitely* have a CAPD. Some of the protocols listed have specified criteria for failure of the test battery, but often we must rely on our own experience and intuition to diagnose central auditory processing disorders.

CAPD Assessment in Atypical Populations

Preschoolers

Some tests for assessing central auditory processing skills provide normative data for children as young as 3 years of age. Because of the extreme variability of normal auditory development in children below the age of 7 years, preschool children who have central auditory processing disorders often score within the normal range on these tests. As a result, it is difficult to diagnose central auditory processing disorders adequately in the preschool population. When asked to determine if a preschool child has an auditory processing problem, the educational audiologist can administer one or more of the tests that have age-appropriate normative data, but the possibility of a central auditory processing disorder should not be ruled out if the test results are normal. If the parents and/or teacher have strong concerns about the child's auditory skills, it is advantageous to provide management recommendations based on the behavioral characteristics of the child. The child should also have his or her auditory processing skills monitored on a regular basis to verify any long-term central auditory processing problem and to determine more specific management recommendations in the future.

Non-English-Speaking Children

There are currently no central auditory processing tests that have been standardized in languages other than English. It is therefore best to use tests with nonverbal stimuli when assessing the auditory processing skills of children who have limited proficiency in English. Tests useful with this population include:

➤ Monotic tone tests
➤ Competing Environmental Sounds Test
➤ Masking Level Difference Test
➤ Electrophysiological tests
➤ Imaging techniques

The results of these tests may not provide a complete central auditory processing assessment, but they may provide information useful in documenting and managing the child's listening difficulties.

Children with Peripheral Hearing Losses

Most of the central auditory processing tests are not normed for administration to children with peripheral hearing losses, making it difficult to assess the auditory processing skills of these children. The educational audiologist can, however, use the following tests, which are not significantly affected by peripheral hearing loss:

➤ Dichotic Digits
➤ Competing Sentences
➤ Middle Latency Response
➤ P300
➤ Otoacoustic Emissions

It is also possible for the experienced clinician to deduce information about the child's processing skills by looking at the results of monotic tone tests obtained at frequencies where the hearing sensitivity is normal or by looking for asymmetries in results of the two ears when the peripheral hearing loss is symmetrical. It must be recognized that the assessment provided for children with peripheral hearing losses will be incomplete, but the information obtained can assist in documenting auditory problems in addition to the peripheral hearing loss and can lead to improved management of the child's auditory problems.

MANAGEMENT OF CENTRAL AUDITORY PROCESSING DISORDERS

Once a central auditory processing disorder has been diagnosed, the educational audiologist must decide what can be done to manage the disorder at home and in the classroom. Questions that must be addressed include:

➤ What type of management strategies are available for children with CAPD?
➤ What classroom accommodations are most appropriate for children with CAPD?
➤ How successful is the use of amplification for children with CAPD?
➤ Is direct therapy beneficial for children with CAPD? If so, what types of remediation are most appropriate?
➤ How should the child's CAPD profile be used to determine the most appropriate management strategies?

Types of CAPD Management Strategies

Several different management strategies have been suggested for central auditory processing disorders, but unfortunately none of them will work for all children. Until techniques are available for more precise diagnosis of CAPD, the educational audiologist must work closely with the parents and classroom teachers to determine which management strategies work best for the child. Strategies that have been successful with various children are:

➤ Classroom accommodations
➤ Amplification
➤ Direct treatment
➤ Compensatory strategies

Classroom Accommodations

One of the most common management strategies used by the educational audiologist is modification of the child's learning environment. Quite often a list of suggested modifications of the classroom environment or teaching style is provided to the teacher as the only recommendation for a child with CAPD. Although the suggestions on the list are typically beneficial for the child, teachers are often overwhelmed by the number of suggestions and therefore do not consistently follow any of them. Whenever possible, the educational audiologist should limit the number of classroom modifications or prioritize them to emphasize the most critical considerations. Once the teacher has incorporated these modifications, others may be added if necessary.

Classroom suggestions often useful for children with central auditory processing disorders are provided in Table 5–3. These suggestions focus on areas such as preferential classroom seating, peer assistance, alerting, teaching techniques, and self-esteem. The educational audiologist may be able to select the most beneficial modifications based on the child's test

Table 5–3. Classroom modifications for children with CAPD.

Preferential Classroom Seating
➤ Seat student away from distracting noises
➤ Seat student near teacher's area of instruction
➤ Allow flexibility of seating if area of instruction changes
➤ Seat student so that better ear, if there is one, is favored
➤ Isolate student, using study carrels if available, for individual seatwork, tests, or tutoring
➤ Allow the student to use earmuffs or earplugs when working individually

Peer Assistance
➤ Use a "buddy system" to alert the student to attend and to be sure student has assignments and special instructions
➤ Use a notetaker to take or copy notes

Alerting: Look and Listen
➤ Gain eye contact with student before giving class instructions
➤ Touch student gently to gain attention
➤ Call student by name
➤ Use "secret sign" to remind student to listen

Teaching Techniques
➤ Speak distinctly and at a moderate rate
➤ Give clear and concise directions
➤ Use familiar vocabulary and less complex sentence structures when giving instructions
➤ Simplify information by giving it in small segments
➤ Rephrase or restate instructions in simple terms
➤ Require student to repeat instructions to ensure understanding
➤ Preview topic to be presented by introducing new vocabulary and outlining new subjects
➤ Use visual aids such as overhead projectors, illustrations, and maps
➤ Use concrete, experiential lessons when possible
➤ Write assignments on board, as well as giving them orally
➤ Be sure student writes assignments in a specific place
➤ Allow breaks between intense periods of instruction
➤ Alternate difficult instruction with simpler activities to avoid fatigue
➤ Use a consistent routine of activities to allow student to have a smoother transition from one subject to the next

Self-esteem
➤ Be positive and encouraging when working with student
➤ Provide praise for effort and successes
➤ Encourage student to pursue activities in which he or she can excel

performance, but it is often necessary to observe in the classroom to determine what should be done to improve the child's classroom environment. By giving the teacher only three or four suggestions from this list, the educational audiologist can structure the modifications to benefit the child.

Amplification

Within recent years much attention has been focused on the use of amplification for children with central auditory processing disorders. Because one of the problems often encountered by children with CAPD is difficulty attending in noisy environments, any technology that improves the signal-to-noise ratio has the possibility of benefiting the student. Both personal FM and sound-field FM systems have been used with some success to enhance students' abilities to attend in the classroom and are important strategies to consider for children who have difficulty listening in noise. We suggest that FM amplification be provided for a trial period initially so that the child, teachers, and parents can assess the benefit in the classroom before permanent use of the equipment is recommended. Additionally, if a personal FM system is recommended, the audiologist must be sure that the maximum output levels are safe for the child. The American Speech-Language-Hearing Association (1991a) addressed many of the concerns that surround the fitting of amplification on children with normal hearing sensitivity in its document *Amplification as a Remediation Technique for Children with Normal Peripheral Hearing* (see Appendix 2–H).

Direct Treatment

Most direct treatment for central auditory processing problems can be classified as one of two types:

➤ Skill-building activities
➤ Management techniques

SKILL-BUILDING ACTIVITIES. Skill-building activities seek to improve a specific auditory skill by providing repeated practice of this skill. Some skill areas that may be addressed include:

➤ Auditory memory
➤ Auditory selective attention
➤ Auditory closure
➤ Phonemic synthesis (sound blending)
➤ Auditory figure-ground (listening in noise)
➤ Auditory conceptualization
➤ Auditory discrimination
➤ Auditory temporal sequencing

Skill development may also focus on the remediation of language disorders that may be related to the central auditory processing disorder. Although these skill-building activities may prove beneficial for some children, they seem to be of little use with other children. Gillet (1993) provided a list of commercially available materials that may be useful in the treatment of these skills.

MANAGEMENT TECHNIQUES. Management techniques focus on helping students be aware of the deficits they have because of their central auditory processing disorder and teaching various compensatory strategies to manage these deficits. This treatment provides students with structured practice in the use of specific strategies, helps them identify which strategies are beneficial, and encourages the use of successful strategies in other environments.

Compensatory Strategies

Compensatory strategies are useful in helping children deal with deficits caused by central auditory processing disorders. As stated previously, they will need help in identifying successful strategies and in determining when they should be applied. Compensatory strategies that have been successful with some children who have CAPD include:

➤ Implementation of environmental modifications (e.g., preferential seating, reduction of auditory and visual distractions, etc.)

➤ Use of memory techniques (e.g., chunking, reauditorization, mnemonics, visualization, etc.)
➤ Attention to visual and nonverbal cues
➤ Use of written reminders (e.g., notebooks, calendars, etc.)
➤ Use of context and key words
➤ Use of notetakers
➤ Use of organizational techniques (diagrams, outlining, charts, etc.)

Selection of Most Appropriate Management Strategies

With the variety of strategies available for managing children with central auditory processing difficulties, it is often difficult to know which management strategy will be most successful for which child. Quite often it is a combination of management techniques that will be most beneficial. Unfortunately, the management of central auditory processing disorders is often trial-and-error because the effects of specific recommendations are not known until they have been tried. It is therefore necessary for educational audiologists to work closely with teachers and parents, as well as students themselves, to monitor the success of management and to alter or implement other management strategies when necessary.

It is obvious that not every management strategy will be effective for every child. Children with CAPD have differing patterns of auditory deficits, and it is important that CAPD management address the specific weaknesses that exist. Chermak (Chermak & Musiek, 1992) provided a chart that gives specific strategies and techniques for various deficits often experienced by children with central auditory processing disorders. This chart is reproduced in Table 5–4 and is an excellent resource for the educational audiologist who is involved in the management of these children.

SUMMARY

It is obvious that diagnosis and management of children with central auditory processing disorders is a perplexing task, but it is one that is of great concern to educational audiologists. The evaluation of central auditory processing disorders takes a great deal of time. To maximize their time, we recommend that educational audiologists use the following protocol as discussed in this chapter:

Table 5–4. Management of central auditory processing disorders.

Functional Deficit	Strategies	Techniques
Distractibility/inattention	Increase signal to noise ratio	ALD/FM system; acoustic modifications; preferential seating
Poor memory	Metalanguage	Chunking; verbal chaining; mnemonics; rehearsal; paraphrasing; summarizing
	Right hemisphere activity	Imagery; drawing
	External aids	Notebooks; calendars
Restricted vocabulary	Improve closure	Contextual derivation of word meaning
Cognitive inflex—predominantly analytic or predominantly conceptual	Diversify cognitive style	Top-down (deductive) and bottom-up (inductive) processing; inferential reasoning; questioning; critical thinking
Poor listening comprehension	Induce formal schema to aid organization, integration, and prediction	Recognize and explain connectives (additives, causal, adversative, temporal) and patterns of parallelism and correlative pairs (not only/but also, neither/nor)
Reading, spelling, and listening problems	Enhance multisensory integration	Phonemic analysis and segmentation
Maladaptive behaviors (passive, hyperactive, impulsive)	Assertiveness and cognitive behavior modification	Self-control; self-monitoring; self-evaluation; self-instruction; problem solving
Poor motivation	Attribution retraining: internal locus of control	Failure confrontation; attribution to factors under control

Source: From "Managing central auditory processing disorders in children and youth" by G. D. Chermak and F. E. Musiek, 1992, *American Journal of Audiology, 1*(3), p. 63. Reprinted by permission.

➤ Initial screening
    Teacher and parent referrals
    Screening of high-risk students
➤ Secondary screening of failures of initial screening
    Auditory processing screenings
    Teacher checklists
➤ Central auditory processing evaluation of failures of secondary screening
    Case history
    Audiometric and non-audiometric tests of central auditory functioning
    Observation of the child
➤ Management of students with CAPD
    Classroom modifications
    Amplification
    Direct treatment
    Compensatory strategies

There is a great deal of information in the literature about central auditory processing disorders, and much of it is conflicting or confusing. It may take experimentation and considerable effort, but, with persistence, we believe educational audiologists can develop a reasonable approach for identifying and managing children with central auditory processing disorders that will work in their school setting.

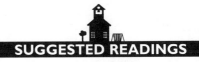

SUGGESTED READINGS

American Speech-Language-Hearing Association. (1996). Central auditory processing: Current status of research and implications for clinical practice. *American Journal of Audiology, 5*(2) 41–54.

Baran, J., & Musiek, F. (1991). Behavioral assessment of the central auditory nervous system. In W. Rintelmann (Ed.), *Hearing assessment* (pp. 549–602). Austin, TX: Pro-Ed.

Bellis, T. J. (1996). *Assessment and management of central auditory processing disorders in the educational setting.* San Diego, CA: Singular Publishing Group, Inc.

Gillet, P. (1993). *Auditory processes.* Novato, CA: Academic Therapy Publications.

Katz, J., Stecker, N., & Henderson, D. (Eds.) (1992). *Central auditory processing: A transdisciplinary view.* St. Louis, MO: Mosby-Year Book.

Keith, R. (Ed.). (1981). *Central auditory and auditory-language disorders in children.* Houston, TX: College-Hill Press.

Lasky, E. Z., & Katz, J. (Eds.). (1983). *Central auditory processing disorders—Problems in speech, language, and learning.* Baltimore, MD: University Park Press.

Levinson, P., & Sloan, C. (Eds.). (1980). *Auditory processing and language.* New York: Grune & Stratton.

Musiek, F. (Ed). (1984). Selected topics in central auditory dysfunction. *Seminars in Hearing, 5*(3), 219–352.

Pinheiro, M., & Musiek, F. (Eds.). (1985). *Assessment of central auditory dysfunction: Foundations and clinical correlates.* Baltimore, MD: Williams & Wilkins.

Sloan, C. (1991). *Treating auditory processing difficulties in children.* San Diego, CA: Singular Publishing Group, Inc.

Willeford, J. A., & Burleigh, J. M. (1985). *Handbook of central auditory processing disorders in children.* New York: Grune & Stratton.

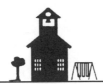

CHAPTER 6

AMPLIFICATION AND CLASSROOM HEARING TECHNOLOGY

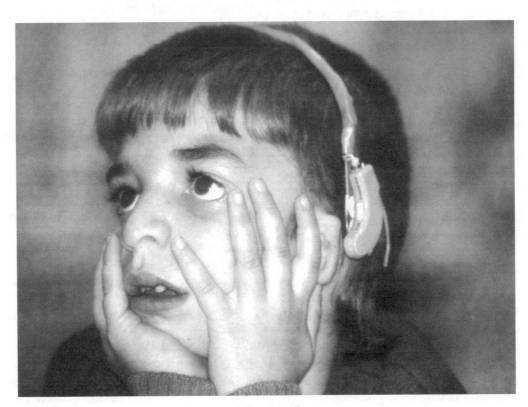

Wilson, age 7

CONTENTS

The technology explosion of the 1970s and 1980s has finally reached the amplification venue for the treatment of hearing impairment. The application of these advancements has resulted most recently from consumer demand, legislative mandates, and the increased manufacturers' awareness of the growing market of users for hearing assistance devices. Children, although they represent the smallest part of this market, are benefiting immensely from the improved technology and increased options for amplification and assistive device equipment. As a result of this improved technology, navigating the ever increasing array of choices has resulted in new challenges for audiologists. Coupled with the increase in infant hearing screening programs and the resulting earlier identification of hearing impairment, audiologists have greater potential to affect the aural development of children than ever before.

Although the benefits of amplification for children seem obvious, the complexity of the fitting process has increased significantly due to recent technological advances, as well as legal mandates. Some of the questions that now must be considered include the following:

➤ Who is a candidate for the various types of amplification and how is candidacy determined?
➤ What special considerations arise when fitting infants?
➤ Who pays for or provides devices for children in early childhood and educational programs?
➤ Are schools and other publicly funded agencies obligated to provide state of the art technology?
➤ Who dispenses, fits, maintains, and manages the devices?
➤ Can we continue to separate primary amplification, usually defined as the child's personal hearing aid or hearing instrument, from technology that provides an enhanced auditory signal, such as FM systems that are more commonly used in the schools?
➤ What role does amplification play for children who have normal hearing sensitivity but who demonstrate attention problems or central hearing deficits?
➤ What role will health care reform play in the accessibility to amplification for all children?

➤ How can we maximize the use of our audiologic services to support children and their families in both home and educational settings?

These issues are as complex as the devices themselves. This chapter considers the questions listed and provides information that is useful when making decisions regarding amplification and assistive devices for children.

RECENT TRENDS AND GOVERNMENTAL POLICIES

As most users of hearing aids and assistive listening devices will attest, the state of amplification technology has been historically dismal. Although correcting hearing function through amplification will likely remain impossible in our lifetime, significant improvement of hearing ability is attainable for most individuals. The low demand of a traditionally small market has continued to make the cost of research and resulting technological advancements in amplification systems expensive and slow to evolve. The limitations of conventional hearing aids and auditory trainers have frustrated parents and hearing professionals for years. Finally, since the late 1970s, increased consumer demand for better quality instrumentation, along with the perseverance of many physicians, electronics engineers, and audiology professionals, has resulted in a variety of devices that have begun to make a significant improvement in the hearing ability of many individuals.

Legal Mandates

The legislation that has contributed to the increased demand for amplification devices over the past two decades was discussed fully in Chapter 1, Educational Audiology: How Did We Get Here? The most notable pieces that refer specifically to assistive technology are identified below:

➤ The Individuals with Disabilities Education Act of 1990 (the Education for All Handicapped Act—PL 94-142 [1975] and the Education of the Handicapped Act Amendments—PL 99-457 [1986] combined, updated, and reauthorized).
➤ Technology Related Assistance for Individuals with Disabilities Act of 1988 (PL 100-407). This law specifically addressed the technology needs of individuals with disabilities defining "assistive technology

device" and "assistive technology service" (602(a)(25)-(26). These definitions are included verbatim in IDEA, thereby having significant implications for children in school. They deserve the attention and understanding of every educational audiologist (see handout in Appendix 1–F).

➤ The Americans with Disabilities Act of 1990 (PL 101-336). ADA extended assistive device access from children to all persons, greatly expanding the market of individuals for whom the technology could be applied. In response, the growth of companies producing and marketing assistive listening devices has mushroomed since 1990. With this growth, however, there are problems. First, because many of these devices are not classified as hearing aids, there is little regulation of their performance. Second, because of the widespread commercial availability of these instruments, audiologists may not be involved in their purchase and fitting.

The Responsibility of Education

Amplification and other classroom hearing technology are included under the assistive technology device definition of IDEA. As such, the definition is broad and the responsibility of the educational program is comprehensive. However, the use of a device and service must be determined on an individual basis as part of the development of a child's IEP and must be necessary for the child to "receive reasonable benefit" from his or her educational environment.

The Hearing Aid as Assistive Technology

In 1994, an interpretation of a hearing aid as an assistive technology device was provided by Dr. Thomas Hehir, Director of the Office of Special Education Programs, at the U.S. Department of Education. This clarification was in response to an inquiry by the Superintendent of the Illinois School for the Deaf asking if a school district was required to purchase a hearing aid, according to the requirements of IDEA, if the device was identified as a need on the student's IEP. The response of Dr. Hehir stated that a hearing aid was indeed covered under the definition of "assistive technology device" and, therefore, would be required to be provided by the district if the hearing aid was necessary for the child to receive a free and appropriate public education (FAPE) and if the child's IEP specified that the child needed the hearing aid. The implications of this interpretation are substantial because, prior to this interpretation, personal medical devices were considered exempt from educational responsibility because they were required for the child's daily living environment.

The issue of the responsibility of education to provide hearing aids has raised concern from audiologists and special education directors. For audiologists, concerns include a shortage of audiologists in the schools to meet existing needs of students, difficulty securing funds for FM and other necessary audiology-related equipment, and keeping abreast of technological advancements. Special education directors generally feel that the education system has gone too far in providing for children and have recommended, through their professional organization, the National Association of State Directors of Special Education (NASDSE), that hearing aids, eyeglasses, and wheelchairs be specifically excluded from the assistive technology device definition when IDEA is re-authorized. As of the writing of this handbook, re-authorization has been postponed and probably will not be finalized until the 1997 session of Congress.

Use of Assistive Technology Beyond the Classroom

The use of FM systems purchased by school systems outside of school is another consideration under IDEA. Again, in a Department of Education interpretation (U.S. Department of Education, September 29, 1992) reprinted in Appendix 1–B (Appendix: Analysis of Comments and Changes, Assistive Technology 300.308) the use of any assistive technology device beyond the school day is permitted provided the need is determined on an individual basis, as required by the student to receive FAPE, and is part of the student's special education services, related services, or supplementary aids and services to meet the goals of his or her IEP.

Purchasing Assistive Technology Devices

In the 1992 *Federal Register* Rules and Regulations cited above, the Secretary of Education also stated that schools "may use whatever State, local, Federal, and private sources of support that are available to provide or pay for services or devices" so long as they are "provided at no cost to the child or parent" (p. 44845). As a result, the source of funds should not prevent students from receiving assistive technology through their school systems.

Keeping up with Technological Advancements

Specificity of Equipment

Maintaining a handle on the equipment explosion has become a major challenge for audiologists in the schools. A frequently asked question concerns the school's responsibility for maintaining state-of-the-art equipment. The current legal interpretation is that the school's mandate is to provide technology or equipment that meets the child's individual needs. However, the district should not be obligated to provide specific brands of equipment, only to prove that the equipment provided works properly and meets the child's needs. Parents cannot, therefore, demand that a school purchase a certain brand of FM system for their child. This issue has become more complicated with the introduction of behind-the-ear (BTE) FM systems as cosmetic and self-esteem issues affect use of amplification in educational settings.

Common versus Experimental Equipment

With the introduction of so many different types of equipment, school audiologists must decide at what point a device is "common" or typically available in a school versus that which might be considered "experimental." It would seem that equipment available in most schools would be considered common and, therefore, be a routine recommendation for children with hearing impairments. FM systems certainly fall into this category. Although children should not be denied technology that provides reasonable access to information, schools should not be required to provide every new device that is developed. Equipment that does not carry validation data to support its effectiveness should be designated as "experimental" until proven otherwise through research and use. However, audiologists should investigate new equipment through trial placements in their schools to determine the unit's effectiveness with their students. Most manufacturers are willing to work with school-based audiologists in this manner.

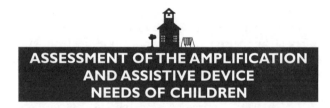

ASSESSMENT OF THE AMPLIFICATION AND ASSISTIVE DEVICE NEEDS OF CHILDREN

Although **every** child with hearing impairment, including those with mild, unilateral, and high-frequency losses, **should be considered a candidate for amplification**, the decisions regarding the type of amplification—whether hearing aids, a specialized hearing instrument, an assistive listening device, or some combination—must be based on the hearing and listening abilities and needs of the child. A thorough analysis of the child's learning and listening environments and hearing and communication patterns must be completed. Table 6–1 identifies the hear-

ing loss, physical environment, and communication environment considerations that should be included in the determination of each student's needs.

Hearing and Hearing Loss Considerations

Identification of Functional Hearing and Communication Abilities

To assess the implications of hearing loss, information must be collected that details the hearing and communication abilities of the child. Much of this information cannot be gleaned from a routine hearing evaluation. In fact, the law (IDEA, Section 300.6) states that the evaluation for assistive technology must include a functional evaluation of children in their customary environment. Therefore, a listening assessment that considers classroom listening conditions such as distant hearing ability, the effects of background noise, and the effects of visual cues (speechreading) must be performed. The Functional Listening Evaluation (Johnson & Von Almen, 1993, April) (see Appendix 4–C) utilizes a paradigm that assesses speech recognition in eight listening conditions:

➤ Auditory-quiet   ➤ Auditory-visual-quiet
➤ Auditory-noise   ➤ Auditory-visual-noise
➤ Auditory-close   ➤ Auditory-visual-close
➤ Auditory-distant   ➤ Auditory-visual-distant

Through this evaluation a comprehensive picture of a child's hearing ability emerges. Localization ability is also an important consideration due to potential difficulties with direction of sound sources that are experienced by individuals with unilateral hearing losses. Additional hearing loss from otitis media or other ear pathologies can significantly affect the hearing and listening ability of any child and may require further communication and amplification modifications.

Attention

The length of time listeners are able to focus their attention is an often overlooked, but critical, consideration. Children with hearing impairments frequently exert more effort on attending to verbally presented information than their normal-hearing peers. By late morning and mid-afternoon these children may require additional amounts or different types of hearing assistance.

Motivation

The motivation to use amplification and the individual's self-esteem are other areas that must be considered when decisions regarding the type of amplification are made. A positive attitude toward amplification is critical to the success of the fitting. Recommending an FM system for a middle school student, even though it may provide an optimal acoustic signal, will be counter-productive if the student refuses to wear it. Understanding the importance of peer acceptance and "fitting in" is a critical part of working with students to meet their hearing needs. Other compensatory alternatives may need to be explored until a student feels able to handle the extra equipment.

Multiple Disabilities

Children with multiple disabilities require extra care and sensitivity. Although hearing loss is only one aspect of their overall profile, the additional implications associated with auditory difficulties can significantly affect how these children conduct themselves in learning and social contexts. Children with cognitive impairments often have more difficulty utilizing visual and contextual cues to fill in for information that is not heard or understood. Therefore, appropriate amplification may be particularly important for some of these children. On the other hand, some developmental disabilities are so pervasive that amplification may only function as a rudimentary, but necessary, connection between these children and their environment. Validating amplification for this population often requires reliance on functional data, which should be obtained through both informal observation and formal observation with structured trial periods.

Physical Environment Considerations

Knowledge of the acoustic properties and conditions of the rooms and facilities in which children with hearing impairments live and learn is another essential component for amplification planning (see Appendix 2–K for ASHA guidelines on *Acoustics in Educational Settings* for background information). For example, if a child's home environment is relatively quiet with little TV, stereo, or other noise, and the parents use appropriate communication techniques, FM amplification may be an unnecessary addition to hearing aids. The same child, however, could spend 90 minutes each day commuting in a noisy car to daycare and greatly benefit from an FM system to capitalize on this communication opportunity with the parents. Another common situation occurs in older school buildings that often have high ceilings and concrete block walls. These rooms may be a quiet environment when empty. However, when sound is introduced, the reverberation can cause such significant distortion of speech that an FM system is required for a child to be able to participate successfully in classroom activities.

Smaldino and Crandell (1995) have developed a worksheet to use when evaluating classroom acoustic conditions as a part of determining the potential benefit of FM amplification. The worksheet is located in Appendix 6–A.

Communication Environment Considerations

The characteristics of the communication environment identified in Table 6–1 are the variables that continuously change and are, therefore, the most difficult to counteract. Without assistive listening devices, high classroom noise levels can quickly take a child with hearing impairment out of the communication loop. Factors such as distance between the student and teacher, the teacher's voice intensity and clarity, and the instructional format, are other common concerns. Picture the following typical junior high school science classroom:

> Twenty-eight students (one has a hearing loss) are seated in groups of four at lab tables; the teacher gives a brief lecture, often turning to the board to diagram chemical properties, and then gives group assignments to be completed during the remainder of the class period. The assignments generate a substantial amount of discussion among students in their groups, significantly raising the noise level of the room; the teacher continues to address the class periodically to clarify questions that are asked.

What kind of amplification, in addition to or in place of the student's hearing aids, should be recommended for this situation? How are the problems of group communication handled when the teacher is also speaking? What if the student does not want a personal FM system because of concerns about peer acceptance and being different? Sometimes the best arrangement may not be possible when the student is not willing to use it. How is a compromise reached? Often the solution may have to be the second or third option.

Considerations for Children with Normal Hearing

Assistive listening devices can improve signal-to-noise ratios, minimize distance and reverberation factors, improve attention, reduce distractibility, and improve sound awareness and discrimination skills. Many children who have normal hearing sensitivity stand to benefit from these amplification improvements. Acoustic accessibility, the access to spoken input in a manner which minimizes acoustical barriers, is an invisible and frequently overlooked variable

Table 6–1. Considerations for determining type of amplification.

Hearing Loss Variables	Physical Environment	Communication Environment
Degree of loss	Room sizes and shapes	Occupied room noise levels
Configuration of loss	Ambient noise levels	Number of occupants
Bilateral vs. unilateral	Reverberation times	Instructional format (lecture, discussion, team teaching)
High-frequency hearing ability	Outside of room noises: duration and intensity	
Fluctuating hearing levels		Distance from speaker
Distance listening abilities	Other environments (outside, home, car, daycare, work)	Speaker's voice intensity and clarity
Speech recognition skills		Use of media (audio, video, computers, movies)
Central auditory processing abilities		
Hearing and comprehension ability in noise		Lighting
Language competence		
Attention & listening fatigue		
Directionality skills		
Speechreading skills		
Motivation to use amplification		
Self-esteem of user		
Age of user		
Other disabilities		

in accessibility planning. This problem has become increasingly critical as more children with disabilities are educated in regular classrooms in their neighborhood schools. Recent investigations (Benafield, 1990; Crandell, 1991; Crandell, 1996; Flexer, Millin, & Brown, 1990) have shown that, in addition to children with hearing losses, children with central auditory processing disorders, attention deficits, language delays or disorders, phonological disorders, and English as a second language often benefit from improved ability to "hear" via assistive listening devices (ALDs). ASHA has published guidelines, *Amplification as a Remediation Technique for Children with Normal Peripheral Hearing* (1991a), in response to the growing practice of amplification with this group of children (see Appendix 2–H).

The use of amplification with normal-hearing children raises some interesting questions:

➤ How is candidacy determined?
➤ What criteria are used to determine if a child might be an amplification candidate?
➤ How is benefit defined and how is it measured?
➤ What type of ALD is most appropriate?
➤ Who pays for or provides the device?
➤ Who will manage the child and the device once provided to the child?

➤ What are possible risks to the child's hearing as a result of noise exposure from the amplification device?

Candidacy

Candidacy should require an initial screening process that identifies the hearing, listening, attention, processing, comprehension, or language concern. A commonly used screening tool is the Fisher's Auditory Problems Checklist (Fisher, 1985) (see Appendix 3–D) which considers 25 behaviors. Concerns identified through the screening process should then be evaluated by the audiologist and speech-language pathologist to determine the child's eligibility for special education services. Should the child meet eligibility requirements, a recommendation for the trial use of individual or classroom amplification would be made by the IEP (Individual Education Plan) team. **Completion of a successful trial period should always be required prior to issuing amplification to a student with normal hearing.**

Adjustment and Acceptance

Everyone who has worked with children and amplification recognizes that problems can occur getting children to wear the devices and to use them properly. Ensuring that amplification functions properly is an ongoing, aggravating, problem. Children who are active and distractible are particularly hard on equipment; at times the listening device may become a new "toy." Other children may respond initially to the novelty of the amplification and wear their devices consistently. Then, 2 or 3 weeks later, when the excitement has worn off, these children may have to be reminded to put on their equipment or may even begin to refuse it. Some children may be reluctant to use the equipment at first, fearing something new or feeling unsure of the way other children will view them with the device. Helping the student demonstrate the system to their classmates and providing time to adjust to wearing it usually helps the student adapt to the device, provided improvement in listening has been experienced. Other children may respond positively from the beginning and present no problems, but they may still want to demonstrate their amplification system to teachers and/or classmates.

Type of System

Personal walkman-style FM systems and sound-field FM systems are the most common amplification devices recommended for children with normal hearing sensitivity. Personal FM systems may provide a better signal-to-noise ratio than sound-field systems but usually require the student to wear a body-worn receiver with headsets or ear buds. Some manufacturers of behind-the-ear (BTE) FM systems now have the units available as an FM device only, providing personal FM sound transmission in a unit the size of a BTE hearing aid. However, the added expense may be difficult to justify until these units are more widely used and until research substantiates superior benefit. **Due to the wide variability in gain and output of all these systems, we recommend electroacoustic checks prior to fitting to determine appropriate volume settings, as well as frequent monitoring of the student to ensure that appropriate settings are maintained.** A major advantage of sound-field systems is that students have no equipment to wear, thereby avoiding any stigma that might be associated with using a device. Sound-field systems are also reasonably priced, available through a variety of sources, and require little maintenance. A list of sources for purchasing various types of amplification devices is located in Appendix 16–F.

Determination of Benefit

A 30- to 60-day trial period is recommended with the amplification system to demonstrate and document its effectiveness for any student who has normal hearing. Use of a pre/postlistening appraisal such as the ones developed by Anderson and Smaldino (1996) (Appendix 6–B) and VanDyke (1985)(Appendix 6–C) are very helpful for this documentation. These questionnaires are simple and quick for classroom teachers to complete, yet provide sufficient information to support or deny amplification use. The *Listening Inventory for Education: an Efficacy Tool (L.I.F.E.)* (Anderson & Smaldino, 1996) is a new instrument designed specifically for the purpose of determining amplification benefit and considers input from both the student and the teacher. The protocol also provides suggestions for intervention accommodations designed for the specific situations that are identified as problems.

Provision of Equipment

Any device necessary for children to receive reasonable benefit from their education, if written as part of the IEP, must be provided by the education agency. Therefore, following a successful trial period, the child should be provided with the system. If an educational disability resulting from the listening or language problem cannot be documented, a Section 504 meeting may be convened to consider the problem as an accessibility issue. Because Section 504 is not a special education function, the individual school becomes responsible for the equipment, if lack of access to auditory information is ruled (see Chapter 1, Educational Audiology: How Did We Get Here? for general information on Section 504 and Chapter 11, Individual Planning, for more information about IEPs and 504 Plans.)

Management of Equipment

All amplification systems utilized in schools should be managed by an audiologist, preferably one employed or contracted by the school or education agency. The type of amplification and the appropriate settings and couplings must be determined for all students who utilize amplification as part of their IEP (IDEA, Section 300.6, Assistive technology services). Additionally, fitting, maintaining, repairing, and replacing the device must be provided.

Hearing Loss Risk Considerations

Although the types of assistive listening devices recommended for children with normal hearing have output limitations minimizing the chance for hearing loss risk, a baseline audiogram should be obtained prior to use. Hearing levels should be monitored a minimum of once a year through the school's audiology or hearing screening program. Any change in hearing thresholds warrants a hearing evaluation.

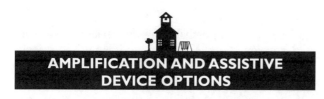

AMPLIFICATION AND ASSISTIVE DEVICE OPTIONS

The fitting and use of appropriate amplification is one of the most important initial components in the (re)habilitation process for children with hearing impairments. The array of options for amplification has increased dramatically in recent years. No longer are personal hearing aids the only amplification choice. Table 6–2 summarizes the various amplification options, including a brief description, suggested candidates, advantages, and problems associated with each type of system. Before discussing the various options, some discussion pertaining to amplification in general is necessary.

General considerations

Maintenance

Fitting amplification and assistive devices on children is only part of the audiology related service. Ensuring that the devices are functioning properly is an equally essential component of this service, clearly the responsibility of the school, and specified as such in two parts of IDEA (Assistive technology service [Sec. 300.6] and Proper function of hearing aids [Sec.300.303]). Equipment management is discussed later in this chapter.

Training in Use of Devices

Another component in the provision of assistive devices is training in the use of amplification units. The student, the classroom teacher, and other individuals who interact with the student must be knowledgeable and comfortable using the devices. Inservice training and ongoing support and technical assistance (Sec 300.6) must be included in the IEP for each child. This service should be provided as part of the audiologist's consultation time. If school -purchased amplification devices, such as an FM systems, are used at home, training for the families is also necessary. Several manufacturers include instructional booklets written for teachers and parents with their products. Although informative and helpful, they should never be substituted for face-to-face training. Chapter 7, Case Management and Aural (Re)habilitation, discusses inservice and teacher-support services related to amplification in more detail.

In addition to assistive devices, the educational audiologist may also need to provide support and training for parents of children who are first-time users of hearing aids. Home programs for hearing aid orientation and listening skill development can facilitate the adjustment to the use of hearing aids and promote proficiency with amplification. A sample Hearing Aid Adjustment Program, including basic rules for communication, can be found in Appendix 6–E.

Primary Versus Supplementary Amplification

Primary amplification is generally considered the child's personal hearing aid(s) or hearing instrument(s), whereas supplemental amplification provides the enhancement of the auditory signal, usually in connection with the primary device. Although it has been questioned whether FM as the primary device and hearing aid(s) secondary might be more appropriate (Madell, 1992; Maxon & Smaldino, 1991), the introduction of an FM circuit built into devices that are also behind-the-ear (BTE) hearing aids has resulted in the lines between the two becoming fuzzier. The issues raised by merging personal hearing aids with FM or programmable control of environmental noise include:

➤ Is the device considered a personal hearing aid?
➤ Who pays for the device when the FM component (traditionally the school's responsibility) is built into the hearing aid?
➤ Who pays for the transmitter?
➤ If the school purchases the instrument, or contributes to part of the cost, should it also be allowed for use outside of school?
➤ Who is responsible for maintenance of the device?

The options a school should consider when determining funding and responsibility for BTE-FM are discussed in the following section. The recent introduction of a snap-on FM boot for BTE hearing aids may offer schools another alternative to obtaining the cosmetic advantage without the issues introduced by the aid and FM housed in the same instrument.

SCHOOL-OWNED. The school may continue to purchase and maintain the BTE-FM as a system for school use only, just as it did for traditional FM purchases, because these systems have all the same features (FM only, FM+MIC, and MIC only). Increased cost is the most significant factor, although the advantage for older students may be justified due to the cosmetic feature of housing the FM unit behind the ear. Many of these students simply refuse to wear body-worn systems regardless of the acoustic advantages.

STUDENT-OWNED. Parents may choose to purchase the BTE-FM unit as the child's primary amplification. Certainly, the advantages of the FM capabilities are

Table 6–2. Amplification options for children

Type	Description	Candidates	Advantages	Problems
Conventional hearing aids	➤ Primary personal amplification ➤ Fit to each child's hearing impairment ➤ Usually BTE style ➤ Cros/Bicross for unilteral losses and asymmetric configurations ➤ Bone conduction style for atretic ears ➤ Fit binaural	➤ All children with permanent bilateral hearing impairment ➤ Unilateral and high-frequency hearing impairments may be considered ➤ Otitis media related hearing impairments	➤ Available in variety of sizes and colors ➤ Least obtrusive ➤ Tuned specifically to hearing loss ➤ Most common amplification device ➤ Usually compatible with assistive listening devices ➤ Directional (best for severe-profound losses) and omni (more suitable for infants) microphones available	➤ Amplifies all sound ➤ Difficulty hearing in noisy and distant listening situations ➤ Signal affected by reverberation ➤ May not provide sufficient gain, particularly in higher frequencies, to optimize residual hearing ➤ May need taupe tape, huggies, etc., to retain in place ➤ Need tamper proof battery and controls for young children ➤ Bone conduction transmission can distort acoustic signal
Programmable hearing aids	➤ Multi-channel, multi-memory or digitally adjusted hearing aids which are programmed for hearing loss specifications and different listening environments ➤ Program selection may be made by user as needed for listening environment	➤ All hearing impairments, especially unusual configurations, fluctuating hearing levels, and tolerance problems	➤ Provides more precise fitting ➤ Easier to fit unusual configurations ➤ More fitting flexibility	➤ Telecoils may be weak ➤ M-T option not always available ➤ Not always compatible with direct audio input ➤ Initial price & repair costs higher ➤ Settings usually must be changed by programmer ➤ Limited options for severe-profound hearing losses
Bone anchored hearing aid (BAHA™)	➤ Bone conduction hearing aid which couples into bone anchored abutment in skull behind the ear ➤ Vibrations are transferred from hearing aid through abutment in the bone to titanium screw in skullbone	➤ Children with atretic ear conditions ➤ Child needs to be old enough to have sufficient bone mass to accommodate implanted abutment	➤ Provides superior acoustic signal ➤ Results in near normal hearing thresholds ➤ No cumbersome headband to wear ➤ Gain requirements are minimal ➤ Relatively inexpensive procedure	➤ Hearing aid is weakest link in system & still large for young children—device will benefit from continued technological refinement
Cochlear Implants	➤ Device which includes a surgically implanted receiver and electrode array connected to an external transmitter coil, microphone, and speech processor	➤ Children with severe and profound hearing impairment who do not benefit from traditional personal hearing aids when maximum stimulation of the auditory system is desired	➤ Can provide useful stimulation for auditory speech perception when traditional hearing aids cannot ➤ Provides access to most components of the speech signal	➤ Requires family support and committment ➤ Requires intense habilitation program ➤ Costly ➤ May restrict some physical activities ➤ Requires surgery

(continued)

Table 6–2. *(continued)*

Type	Description	Candidates	Advantages	Problems
	➤ Electrode array implanted in cochlea ➤ Internal receiver and magnetic coil implanted in mastoid ➤ External headworn magnet and receiver attached by cord(s) to body-worn processor in pocket or pouch	➤ Postmeningitic children or children who lost their hearing postlingually are usually considered excellent candidates ➤ Children with additional disabilities should be considered carefully	➤ Processor can be worn under clothing and/or in a protected pouch	➤ More apparatus to wear ➤ Requires specialized knowledge and equipment to fit ➤ Difficult to interface with personal FM
Specialized personal hearing instruments (TranSonic™, EMILY™)	TranSonic™: ➤ Shifts high-frequency sounds to corresponding low-frequency sounds (real time) while retaining as much of the relative spectral information as possible (individual adjustments are made for energy above and below 2500 Hz and for additional high-frequency gain) ➤ Consists of lapel microphone, processor unit, button receiver or SLR-BTE wireless receiver ➤ Mark II model is compatible with FM systems	➤ Children with severe to profound hearing impairments, especially those whose residual hearing in the low-frequency range only ➤ Often recommended as an option prior to determining cochlear implant candidacy	➤ Provides increased access to higher frequency components of the speech signal ➤ Less costly than cochlear implant ➤ Surgery not required	➤ Significantly more expensive than conventional hearing aids ➤ More apparatus to wear ➤ Requires specialized fitting knowledge ➤ Requires habilitation program ➤ More hardware to maintain
	EMILY™ ➤ Digital signal processing detects sounds at 1000 and 2000 Hz; sounds are enhanced by adding tones that together result in more resonance and richer quality with minimized distortion ➤ Must be used in conjuction with specific Phonak hearing aids with activation from the telecoil switch	➤ Same as above and children with moderate hearing losses	➤ Same as above	➤ Same as above
Tactaid™	➤ Codes auditory information and converts it to vibro-tactile signals received on the skin	➤ Children who do not respond to auditory input	➤ Provides input of auditory signals from environment ➤ Child more responsive to speech and environmental sounds	➤ More apparatus to wear ➤ Skin has limited ability to distinguish acoustic cues ➤ Difficult to interface with personal FM system ➤ Requires intensive habilitation program

Type	Description	Candidates	Advantages	Problems
Universal Amplifiers	➤ Moderate gain, body-worn personal amplifier with head-phones or earplugs ➤ Some units have separate volume controls for each ear ➤ Considered last resort amplification for toddlers	➤ Not appropriate for infants ➤ Toddlers with temporary conductive hearing loss ➤ May be useful temporary amplifica-tion for other hearing losses depending upon degree and configuration of loss and situation of the child	➤ Inexpensive ($20–25) ➤ Readily available	➤ No tuning capabilities other than volume control ➤ Headphones large for young children ➤ Acoustic reproduction is poor ➤ Variability in gain and output
FM systems	➤ FM (frequency modulated) radio wave wireless transmitted signal ➤ FM signals can be transmitted from the remote microphones and body-worn transmitter to a variety of receiver arrangements	➤ All children with hearing impairment ➤ Selected children with other auditory learning problems and attention deficits	➤ Reduces noise, distance, and reverberation factors	➤ May eliminate input from other talkers unless environmental microphones are part of system ➤ Interference from other radio and cellular phone signals is common ➤ Additional hardware to maintain
	Personal FM: ➤ Body-worn: FM receiver is coupled to hearing aids (retaining output and frequency response characteristics of hearing aid) via tele-coil and teleloop or silhouette conductor; hearing aid and direct audio input boot, or ear microphones ➤ BTE: receiver is in BTE unit or boot which couples to BTE hearing aid; no other couplings necessary	➤ All children who wear hearing aids ➤ Direct audio input or ear microphones are preferred for infants & toddlers	➤ Maintains output and frequency response characteristics of hearing aid ➤ Useful with a variety of levels of hearing loss ➤ Very portable ➤ Several different channels available ➤ Inconspicuous (a particular benefit for older students) ➤ Fewer couplings for breakdown	➤ Cumbersome for infants and some toddlers ➤ Expensive ➤ Requires strong tele-coil to be coupled with teleloop or silhouette ➤ Malfunction common due to cords and connections ➤ Expensive
	Self-contained FM: ➤ Typically body-style auditory trainer devices which have settings for FM only, HA only, or FM/HA and operates without personal hearing aids	➤ Children with all degrees of hearing impairments	➤ Hearing aid and FM in single unit provides maximum flexibility and consistency in amplification ➤ Receiver in earmold allows for greater power due to distance from microphone	➤ Body-worn units heavy and cumbersome for small bodies—not recom-mended for infants ➤ Cord breakage and maintenance

(continued)

Table 6–2. *(continued)*

Type	Description	Candidates	Advantages	Problems
FM systems *(continued)*	➤ Separate micro-phone transmitter for FM mode ➤ Individual ear adjustments can be made for output, gain, and frequency response		➤ FM mode eliminates reception problems due to noise, distance, and reverberation factors	➤ Clothing noise ➤ Body location of microphones when used in hearing aid mode results in poor acoustic signal ➤ More expensive than hearing aids
	Walkman: ➤ All utilize a body-worn FM receiver, which may contain adjustments for output & frequency response, coupled with a headset or earbud	➤ Children with auditory processing problems, unilateral, high-frequency or intermittent (OM) hearing loss where FM signal is desirable	➤ Inexpensive ➤ Easy to operate	➤ Too cumbersome for infants & most toddlers ➤ Headsets short out easily
	Hardwire Induction Loop: ➤ Room circumference (or desired listening area) is wired for sig-nal transmission; sig-nal is received via hearing aid telecoil	➤ Children who wear hearing aids	➤ Inexpensive ➤ Easy to operate ➤ No cumbersome apparatus for small children to wear	➤ Requires strong telecoil ➤ Head position affects signal strength (hearing aid must be vertical) ➤ Limited portability
	3-D Mat: ➤ Floor of room (or desired area) is covered with an induction mat through which the signal is transmit-ted and received via hearing aid telecoil	➤ All children who wear hearing aids, especially infants and toddlers	➤ Consistent signal transmission ➤ No cumbersome apparatus to wear ➤ Durable ➤ Low maintenance	➤ Too costly for home use ➤ Not portable ➤ Requires strong tele-coil
	Soundfield: ➤ Signal is picked up by receiver/amplifier and broadcast through speakers.	➤ Children with mild, moderate, unilateral, high-frequency, or intermittent hearing losses ➤ Selected children with auditory learning problems or attention deficits.	➤ Moderate cost ➤ Easy to operate ➤ Portable ➤ No cumbersome apparatus to wear ➤ Provides signal enhancement for all students	➤ Not appropriate for severe and profound hearing losses ➤ Signal-to-noise ratio can be adversely affected by speaker placement and class-room set-up ➤ Portable speakers may be moved inadvertently

Type	Description	Candidates	Advantages	Problems
BTE Hearing aid/FM combination	➤ System contained in ear level units ➤ Available in moderate and power models ➤ Wide-band or narrow-band signal transmission	➤ Children with all degrees of hearing impairments	➤ Eliminates cords, loops, connectors, plug-in crystals, body-worn components, and receiver charging	➤ BTE/FM technology is still being refined ➤ BTE/FM combinations have large cases—may be too large for infants ➤ Wide band transmission has distance and spill-over considerations ➤ No telecoil ➤ Requires transmitter use by speaker

significant for children in many environments. With the increased accessibility available at theaters, concerts, movies, and other extracurricular events, the opportunities are much greater than in the past to benefit from the use of FM technology. In these cases, the parents would likely also purchase the transmitter so that the student could utilize the FM feature. The student would then use the unit for school just like personal hearing aids.

JOINT OWNERSHIP. Combinations and problems include:

1. The school purchasing the transmitter and the parents purchasing the receiver. In this situation each owner would likely be responsible for maintenance of the units they own. However, problems arise if the student's unit is not repaired in a timely manner or is lost. The school should have a back-up system for these situations or consider paying for repairs when parents do not or cannot afford them.
2. The cost to purchase the entire system is shared. In this case a contract or memorandum of understanding (MOU) should be drawn up to delineate each party's responsibility for purchase and maintenance of the system. Again, the school should have a back-up system to use when the unit is inoperable.

Joint ownership combinations are obviously the most complicated alternative. However, the positive aspects of a shared responsibility for meeting the amplificiation needs of the student support parent involvement and the partnership that needs to exist between school and home. Schools cannot continue to provide state-of-the-art technology by themselves; creative solutions to issues such as this one will likely become more predominant in the future.

Special Amplification Considerations for Infants

With the increase in identification of hearing loss at or shortly after birth, the fitting of hearing aids is occurring earlier. Some concerns that have arisen as a result of these fittings are discussed briefly in the following list.

➤ *Bonding.* Parents generally need time to hold, care, and talk to their infant without the intrusion of hearing aids or other devices or concern about how they are talking to their baby. If parents are so anxious that they stop holding or stop talking to their infant, normal bonding behavior could be interrupted. The time parents need with their babies could be a few weeks or several months. Most parents will guide this process, indicating when they are ready to proceed. If they do not, gentle suggestions usually work, but negligence may also eventually have to be considered.
➤ *Denial.* When hearing loss is identified near birth, many of the behaviors associated with hearing loss may not be apparent. Unless the infant has a severe or profound hearing loss, parents may still observe enough responses to sound, whether coincidental or purposeful, to question the diagnosis. Patience and understanding when working with these parents is essential to maintaining the professional relationship required to gain their respect and confidence in your diagnosis.
➤ *Multiple Disabilities.* Extra sensitivity should be given to parents of infants with multiple disabilities. Acute medical problems may override the auditory and amplification needs for a time. Issues of quality of life, comfort, and developmental potential, as well as scheduling and coordinating the various therapists and professionals, can overwhelm parents, leaving little time for themselves and their other children. For some of these families, amplification decisions may need to be deferred until a later time or not at all.

➤ *FM Systems.* The advantage of FM amplification is clear. Yet for infants, who are usually in close proximity to their caregivers, the benefits of the addition of an FM system may be minimal. An analysis of the child's listening and communication environment should occur frequently and be used to help determine when FM is appropriate and beneficial. The ASHA document *The Use of FM Amplification Instruments for Infants and Preschool Children with Hearing Impairment* (1991c) in Appendix 2–J provides some additional information in this area.

Hearing Aids

Although hearing aids are generally considered a child's primary amplification system, they may not be the preferred choice for very mild, unilateral, high-frequency, or profound hearing losses. Hearing aids, though improving technologically, still cannot offset the effects of background noise, high reverberation, and distance listening. Features such as multi-channel and multi-memory capacities and digital processing offer significant advantages for children, but are still not routinely utilized due to cost and management issues. Certainly for infants, hearing aids are the first amplification used, primarily due to their small size and fitting flexibility. Additionally, most interactions with infants are at close range and in the home where distance listening, noise, and reverberation can be minimized.

Although BTE hearing aids are most common, several other styles may be utilized with children. With improving technology, the use of in-the-ear (ITE) and completely-in-the-canal (CIC) fittings are increasing popular, particularly for older students. Considerations for determining the appropriateness of fitting of these styles include FM capability (size and strength of telecoil), the child's ability to manipulate the controls, and the possibility that the hearing aid may be lost due to the smaller size.

Bone conduction hearing aids are also common with many children who have microtic or atretic malformations which prohibit BTE fittings. It is most practical to fit bone conduction units with headbands or, for young children, with exercise headbands. A bone anchored hearing aid (BAHA™) has recently been approved by the FDA for use in the United States and offers a significant new option for individuals requiring bone conducted amplification (Nobelpharma, 1993). These instruments provide significant improvement in hearing over traditional bone conduction hearing aids and the surgical procedure is simple and problem free (N. Pashley, September 29, 1996, personal communication). The bone anchored ear prosthesis also warrants attention and should

prove to be a viable alternative to the extensive surgeries of ear construction, and other less-appealing prosthetic ears.

Although some children are still being fit with body style hearing aids, there seems little reason for their continued used unless all other alternatives have been exhausted. Although body style aids may provide a broader frequency response, with reduced feedback, the actual functional benefit of the added frequencies may be questionable. Use of body style hearing aids with Y-cords should not be considered an appropriate binaural fitting for any child.

Certain hearing aid manufacturers have begun programs to specifically market their hearing aids to children. Part of their goal is to improve the image of hearing aids for children. The use of various colors for the cases have given children an important option in the selection of their aid(s). Whether parents agree or not, children should be allowed to select their own colors and be reinforced for developing pride in their hearing aid(s). As children mature, they may decide to switch to more neutral tones, but again in a way that allows them to determine their own cosmetic needs.

Cochlear Implants

Recommendations for cochlear implant use in children have become increasingly more common since the Nucleus 22, manufactured by Cochlear Corporation, was approved in 1990 by the FDA for children who have profound hearing loss and who do not benefit from more traditional types of amplification. A second device, the CLARION, manufactured by Advanced Bionics Corporation, was approved for investigational status in children by the FDA in 1995, but clinical trials with this device are still incomplete. Both the Nucleus 22 and the CLARION devices consist of internal and external parts, which are summarized in Figure 6–1. Each device changes acoustical energy into electrical signals through a computerized strategy programmed within the speech processor. These signals are then sent through a transcutaneous magnet system to an electrode array surgically implanted within the cochlea. Each electrode is also programmed (mapped) to receive a portion of the signal and provide direct stimulation to the auditory nerve.

Results of early and ongoing research clearly show that appropriately selected candidates derive significant benefit in the areas of speech perception and speech production from the use of cochlear implants, and that the importance of emphasizing auditory skill development within the child's (re)habilitation and/or educational program is becoming increasingly apparent (NIH, 1995). Although significant performance changes have been documented for children

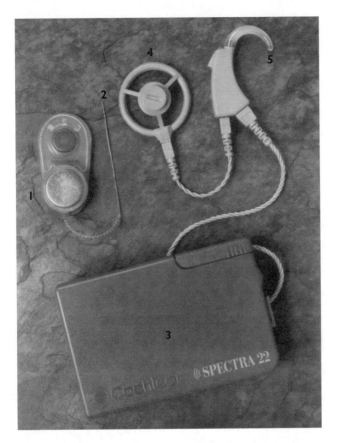

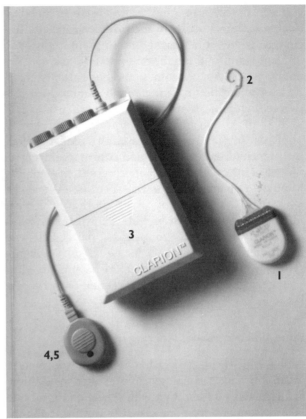

A   **B**

Figure 6–1. Component parts of (A), the Nucleus 22 Channel Cochlear Implant System and (B), the CLARION™ Multi-Strategy Cochlear Implant. **Key:** 1 = Receiver/Stimulator, 2 = Electrode Array, 3 = Speech Processor, 4 = Transmitter Coil, 5 = Microphone. (From Cochlear Corporation, 61 Inverness Drive East, Denver, CO 80112; Advance Bionics Corporation, 12740 San Fernando Rd., Sylmar, CA 91342. Reprinted by permission.)

enrolled in programs using an auditory-oral approach (Geers & Moog, 1994), children who use total communication have also been shown to demonstrate improved speech recognition and intelligibility over time (Tye-Murray & Woodworth, 1995). Postlingually deafened children demonstrate the most rapid benefit, but improved performance for children with congenital and acquired prelingual deafness after 5 years of implant use has also been reported (Gantz, Tyler, Woodworth, Tye-Murray, Fryauf-Bertschy, 1994). Children implanted at an earlier age also tend to show more rapid improvement in speech perception and production than those implanted at a later age (Waltzman et al., 1994). Recent data (Robbins, Svirsky, & Kirk, 1996) has also shown that language development in implanted children improves significantly regardless of communication methodolgy.

Controversy continues to exist over the use of cochlear implants in children, especially focused on clarifying eligibility, expectations, and the need for intensive aural (re)habilitation within the child's edu-

cational program. Children under 2 years of age are not currently eligible for cochlear implants, and clearly the process of identifying those very young children who cannot benefit from traditional amplification is not an easy process. Initial implant eligibility requires a period of at least 6 months' full-time use of appropriate hearing aids while receiving intensive auditory training, and this should be stressed when providing information to parents and educators about implant candidacy. Although data concerning language development of children using a variety of communication methodologies is not clear-cut, the educational environment of children has been reported to affect the use of cochlear implants, especially for adolescents. Rose (1994) cited survey results of implanted children living in residential schools as indicating that 73% of those implanted children no longer use their implants. Clearly, there are some children who do reject use of cochlear implants, but reasons for this disuse have not been carefully documented. The Deaf community, as well, continues to decry the implant as an effort to "fix" those who are deaf.

Cost, surgery risks, and the intensive (re)habilitation program are usually the primary concerns discussed when considering an implant. However, implant teams and families need to understand thoroughly all aspects of deafness and have clear expectations of what the implant can and cannot do before proceeding. Educational audiologists can help to provide accurate and unbiased information concerning implants, implant use, and auditory skill development in children to families and educators during all phases of the cochlear implant process-from eligibility through (re)habilitation. A fact sheet (see Appendix 6–F) was developed by the Colorado Cochlear Implant Consortium to provide information regarding cochlear implants to parents, physicians, and other interested individuals. As the research evidence grows, we can expect children to be implanted at younger ages and with greater flexibility in hearing loss criteria.

Specialized Personal Hearing Instruments

Along with cochlear implants, recent advancements in amplification technology have resulted in additional alternatives for children with severe and profound hearing impairments. These are the TranSonic and the EMILY, which are described in the following section along with the TACTAID.

TranSonic

The TranSonic, developed by AVR Communications LTD in Israel, has refined frequency-transposition technology in a product that alters high-frequency sounds by compressing them into the lower frequency range of usable hearing that is characteristic of severe-to-profound impairments. Unique to this device is the "perceptual real time" speed of this transmission—only a 9 to 13 msec delay, depending upon the transposition coefficient settings. These two coefficient settings control acoustic energy above 2500 Hz (ZC—unvoiced phonemes) and below 2500 Hz (ZV—voiced phonemes), allowing the response to be customized to each child's hearing loss. The instrument can be used with body-worn or ear-level receivers in conjunction with the lapel microphone and body-worn transposer. The transposed sound varies from "Darth Vaderish" to fairly traditional, though high-pitched, amplified sound depending on the degree of transposition.

The reported improvement in sound and speech reception with the TranSonic has been remarkable (Johnson & Rees, 1995). However, as with any amplification device, improvement in auditory and communication skills is only achieved through an intensive treatment program. Determining the degree of transposition and learning to code the sounds that are now within the hearing range of these children are the first habilitation steps with this instrument. The TranSonic does not appear to provide sufficient auditory input for most individuals who use sign language as their primary communication mode to participate in complex and lengthy oral conversations. For children who communicate primarily through audition, however, the TranSonic has provided a significant enhancement of the auditory signal. The cost of this instrument is high depending on options, over twice the usual price of two conventional hearing aids, but comparable to many of the hearing aids incorporating programmable and digital technologies. The TranSonic has been used as an alternative to a cochlear implant device for some children.

EMILY

A lesser known device, the EMILY, was developed in France and named for the child for whom it was designed. Recently approved by the FDA, the EMILY utilizes digital signal processing to enhance the frequencies of 1000 and 2000 Hz to produce amplifiation with greater resonance and less distortion. The instrument was designed to be booted with Phonak Super-Front hearing aids and is activated by the telecoil switch. At present, there have been little reported data on the EMILY's benefits, but now that a more powerful model is being distributed in the United States, its use is increasing. Both the EMILY and the TranSonic are devices which may be used "on loan" during the period of time when a cochlear implant is being considered.

TACTAID

Vibro-tactile devices have been used as an alternative to auditory stimulation for some time. These devices receive acoustical energy and convert it to vibro-tactile signals in a body-worn processor, which then sends the information through a cord to a stimulator array worn on the skin, typically the chest or the wrist. The TACTAID is the most common vibro-tactile device and is available in both two-channel (TACTAID II+) and seven-channel (TACTAID 7) models, the latter designed to provide a more complex reproduction of the auditory signal. Complete descriptions of the TACTAID models can be obtained from the manufacturer, Audiological Engineering Corporation (see Appendix 16–G for address). Again, training is required to learn to utilize the device for meaningful discrimination and comprehension of the vibrations or tactile patterns (see Appendix 16–J for relevant curricula). The TACTAID has been useful with some children who have multiple disabilities including hearing loss, or who are deaf-blind, connecting them to their surroundings. Other children are distracted by the addition of tactile input. The TACTAID may also be valuable as a therapy tool for speech development, providing tactile representation of segmental and suprasegmental features as a supplement to auditory input.

Universal Amplifiers

These devices provide generic, moderate-gain, broadband amplification. Although there may be some ability to adjust the loudness to each ear in the stereo versions, and some simple Hi-Lo tone settings, they are not known for their sound reproductive quality. Mostly available through Radio Shack and mail-order catalogues, these units are usually body-worn with walkman-style headphones or earbuds. Most recently, a behind-the-ear version has been advertised in magazines. These units may be useful as a last resort, temporary amplification for children with mild or moderate hearing losses such as those associated with otitis media. The fact that they are so inexpensive ($20 to $30) and that they are readily available should not justify their use for any individual's permanent, primary amplification. **Universal amplifiers have been shown to have extreme variability in gain and output and should only be used after electroacoustic analysis demonstrates that the amplification is appropriate for the individual using it.**

FM Systems

FM (frequency-modulated) signal transmission continues to represent the most successful and the largest market of assistive listening devices for children. The FM advantage of an improved signal-to-noise ratio (15–20 dB according to Hawkins, 1984) has a domino effect on other behaviors. The benefits, as discussed earlier for children with normal hearing, include improved attention, reduced distractibility, and improved sound awareness and recognition skills. Compared to other wireless systems, such as infrared, FM transmission offers the best sound quality and greatest resistance to interference (Boothroyd, 1992). There are currently 40 narrow-band channels allocated by the Federal Communication Commission (FCC) for educational use. Figure 6–2 identifies these frequencies by narrow-band, wide-band, and color codes as used by various manufacturers. For narrow-band transmission, each channel is .05 MHz wide while wide-band channels are .20 MHz wide. Although the wider channel allows for improved quality of the signal, it also reduces the number of channels available to 10. Wider channels also increase signal spillover problems and reduce the distance the signal can be transmitted. General problems with FM signal transmission are primarily due to signal interference and set-up difficulties when two or more concurrent transmissions are desired (common with team-teaching situations).

FM systems provide a direct, wireless signal from the teacher, or individual wearing the transmitter, to the child wearing the receiver. The transmitter, coupling, and output options provide considerable flexibility for a variety of situations and individual children's needs. The cost of the systems vary significantly for the different FM arrangements which are described in the following sections. The FM microphone/transmitter options are identified in Figure 6–3 and the FM coupling options for self-contained and personal FM systems in Figure 6–4.

Personal FM

The personal FM system coupled with hearing aids is probably the most frequently used of all FM transmission arrangements. The receiver may be used with a teleloop or silhouette unit that is activated with the hearing aid telecoil or directly connected to the hearing aid(s) with an audio input cord and boot. The FM signal should maintain the same acoustical characteristics as the hearing aid(s). Before the teleloop/T-coil option is chosen, the telecoil strength must be checked.

The receiver of the personal FM can also be used with walkman-style headsets for children who do not wear hearing aids. This arrangement works well for children with central auditory processing problems, very mild, unilateral, or high-frequency hearing losses, and intermittent hearing problems (e.g., otitis media) and is also fairly reasonable. Another derivation of the personal FM system is the use of the transmitter in a "conference style" arrangement. In this situation an omnidirectional microphone is placed in the center of a space or table so that it can pick up the voices of the individuals near the microphone, such as a group of students sitting around a table during a discussion.

Self-contained Receiver FM

Another widely used FM application is the self-contained receiver. These FM units are coupled with BTE ("ear mics") or button receiver transducers and contain internal controls for output and frequency setting adjustments functioning both as a hearing aid and FM. This option is necessary for children who do not have appropriate personal hearing aids or whose reliability for bringing their aids to school are poor.

Sound-field FM

Another arrangement, which continues to gain popularity, is the sound-field system. Using the same

FREQ MHz	COLOR CODE	FREQUENCY CODE NUMBER
72.025	Red/Gray	1
72.075	Brown/Gray	2
72.125	Red/Brown	3
72.175	Brown/Red	4
72.225	Orange/Gray	5
72.275	Brown/Orange	6
72.325	Orange/Brown	7
72.375	Brown/Yellow	8
72.425	Yellow/Gray	9
72.475	Brown/Green	10
72.525	Yellow/Pink	11
72.575	Brown/Blue	12
72.625	Yellow/White	13
72.675	Brown/Pink	14
72.725	Green/Gray	15
72.775	Brown/White	16
72.825	Green/Brown	17
72.875	Black/Gray	18
72.925	Green/Red	19
72.975	Black/Brown	20
75.425	Black/Orange	21
75.475	Green/Yellow	22
75.525	Black/Yellow	23
75.575	Green/Blue	24
75.625	Black/Green	25
75.675	Green/Pink	26
75.725	Black/Blue	27
75.775	Green/Black	28
75.825	Black/Pink	29
75.875	Pink/Gray	30
75.925	Black/White	31
75.975	Pink/Yellow	32
74.625	White/Brown	33
74.675	White/Red	34
74.725	White/Orange	35
74.775	White/Yellow	36
75.225	White/Green	37
75.275	White/Blue	38
75.325	White/Pink	39
75.375	White/Black	40

10 WIDE BAND CHANNELS

FREQ MHz	COLOR CODE	FREQUENCY CODE LETTER
72.100	RED	A
72.300	BROWN	B
72.500	WHITE	C
72.700	ORANGE	D
72.900	YELLOW	E
75.500	GREEN	F
75.700	BLACK	G
75.900	BLUE	H
74.700	GRAY	I
75.300	PINK	J

Figure 6–2. Narrow-band and wide-band FM frequency comparisons. (From Phonic Ear Inc. [1993]. *Phonic Ear Frequency Reference Chart.* Phonic Ear Inc., 3880 Cypress Drive, Petaluma, CA 94954-7600. Reprinted by permission.) *Note:* The FCC recently approved the spectrum between 216–217 MHz for auditory assistance devices and other low power users. This will create more interference-free channels for FM use.

transmitter, the signal is sent to speakers strategically placed in the classroom via an amplifier. Because there are so many benefits from this type of arrangement, it is surprising that sound-field systems are not more widely

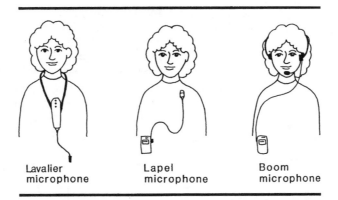

Figure 6–3. FM microphone/transmitter options. (From "Assistive Devices for Classroom Listening" by D. Lewis, 1994, *American Journal of Audiology*, 3[1], p. 62. Copyright 1994, by Asha. Reprinted by permission.)

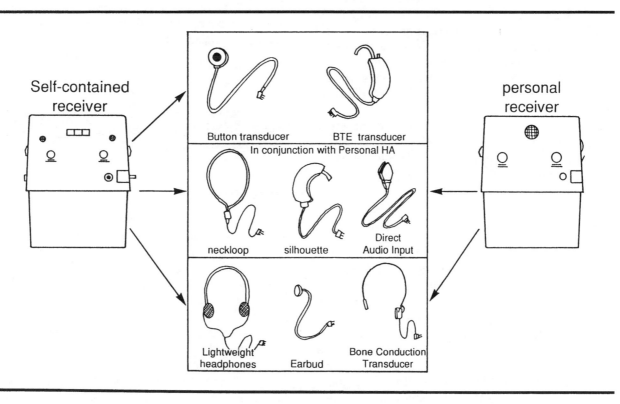

Figure 6–4. Coupling options for self-contained and personal FM systems. (From "Assistive Devices for Classroom Listening" by D. Lewis, 1994, *American Journal of Audiology*, 3[1], p. 62. Copyright 1994, by Asha. Reprinted by permission.)

used. Perhaps the greatest advantage to this arrangement is that there is no equipment for the student to wear. As a result, students are not seen as being different from their peers, and there are fewer maintenance problems.

There is clear evidence (Rosenberg & Blake-Rahter, 1995) that a variety of problems common among children can be improved through the use of these sound-field listening systems. Even children with more significant hearing impairments who refuse to wear hearing aids or other types of amplification will derive some benefit from this arrangement. Candidates, in addition to those mentioned previously under Personal FM, include children with normal hearing and those who use cochlear implants (Hanin & Adams, 1996).

Care as to the speaker positioning and arrangement must be given in the installation of the systems. The room acoustics and composition and the teacher's structure of the class and teaching style are considerations when installing the system. Systems are currently available with one or more portable speakers, as well as systems which incorporate multiple speakers into a single ceiling-mounted unit. This type of system is the least "technological" of the FM group and often the least expensive. As more units become available, price, ease of installation, and durability may become the factors which determine choice of model. Purchase of sound-field FM systems is a good project for school parent organizations or service clubs, because so many students have the potential to benefit from them.

Hardwire Induction Loop

This FM set-up operates with an induction loop that encircles an area or room like an over-sized neckloop. The signal is transmitted to an amplifier and then, via the induction loop, to the student through the T-coil of the hearing aid. To be effective, this system requires a good T-coil on the student's hearing aid(s). The induction loop system is relatively portable, fairly inexpensive, and can have some interesting applications, such as looping the inside of a car. The best feature, again, is that students do not wear any device except their own hearing aid(s). The biggest problem is set-up time if the system needs to be portable.

3-D Mat

Another application of FM signal transmission is through a special floor mat that is installed beneath carpeting or a rug. The signal is picked up through the hearing aid telecoil. This system is advantageous for all students but particularly for preschool children. Since there is no apparatus to wear other than their hearing aids, there are no FM systems on little bodies, no receivers to keep working, and no cords that can be chewed or tripped over. The telecoil position on the child's hearing aid can be in any direction without interruption of the signal, hence the name 3-D. As with the other set-ups not "worn" by the student, there are far fewer maintenance problems with the 3-D mat. The powerful signal capability of this system makes it particularly beneficial for children who have more severe and profound hearing impairments, and most hearing aids have more than sufficient telecoil strength to function well in this capacity. Due to cost, this system is most often recommended for resource rooms or classrooms where there are at least eight students.

Hearing Aid/FM Combinations

The goal for every individual with hearing impairment should be total access to all information within their environment. A major step was taken toward this goal with the introduction of the FM system built into the BTE hearing aid. Our dream is that individuals with hearing impairment in the future will be able to attend any function, turn their hearing aid switches to the appropriate setting (FM), and be "on-line."

The hearing aid/FM systems combine the benefits of hearing aid and FM technology in one unit at the ear. In the past, these features were available in what have traditionally been called "auditory trainers" or "self-contained systems." At this time, manufacturers of these devices produce moderate gain and power models which together are suitable for most hearing losses. When these devices are also used as the student's primary amplification, that is, for home as well as school, the responsibility for purchase and maintenance can be complicated and, therefore, must be worked out ahead of time.

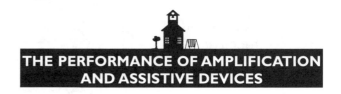

THE PERFORMANCE OF AMPLIFICATION AND ASSISTIVE DEVICES

Fitting Issues

The fitting of appropriate amplification for children may be the most critical step in the (re)habilitation process. The Pediatric Working Group, an outgrowth of the October 1994 conference co-sponsored by the Vanderbilt University Bill Wilkerson Center and the Academy of Dispensing Audiologists on amplification for children with auditory deficits, has recently published a Position Statement on amplification for infants and children with hearing loss (1996). This statement contains excellent guidelines for assessment and fitting pediatric amplification and is included as Appendix 2–N. The discussion following is a cursory overview of fitting considerations.

The Use of Probe Microphone Measurements

Fitting procedures for hearing aids, FM, and other amplification systems should include real-ear measurements. Whether conducted by the dispensing audiologist, the school-based audiologist, or both as a team, the information obtained from probe microphone measurements is essential. This procedure allows the matching of the outputs (real-ear gain/frequency response and maximum output) of hearing aids and FM systems so that together they function as a more effective unit for the child. Portable equipment makes this job even easier. Standard real-ear measurements may include insertion gain, in situ gain, in situ frequency response, output limiting characteristics, input/output functions, and harmonic distortion.

With young children, the fitting of hearing aids or other assistive devices is often subjective. Probe microphone measurements, when obtainable, can help to validate fittings based on estimated thresholds from ABR, OAE, and behavioral assessments. Use of a prescriptive fitting procedure designed for children, such as the Desired Sensation Level (DSL) (Seewald, Ramji, Sinclair, Moodoe, & Jamieson, 1993), the comparison of unaided and aided sound awareness thresholds for speech and nonspeech stimuli, as well as behavioral observations of the child at the test facility, in preschool, and in the home, can provide adequate, and often quite accurate, information for the amplification selection and fitting process.

Electroacoustic Measures

Electroacoustic measures are a necessary part of any hearing aid and assistive device fitting and management program. These measures assess the device to determine that it is functioning according to the manufacturer's specifications. A hearing aid analyzer that meets ANSI S3.22-1987 specifications is necessary to perform the measures which include gain, SSPL, frequency response, harmonic distortion, internal noise level, and telecoil function. While it is assumed that new instruments, as well as those returning from repair, are working properly, it is crucial to check their functioning prior to fitting them.

Behavioral and Functional Measures

For all children, behavioral measures must remain part of every amplification fitting procedure. Although a trend to include less behavioral assessment seems to be apparent, the information obtained from behavioral audiological assessment, observation of the child, anecdotal reports, auditory development checklists, amplification performance rating scales or questionnaires, and functional assessments is critical to validate the amplification fitting (see Chapter 4, Assessment Practices, for more information about behavioral measures). In addition, these strategies provide ongoing evaluation and monitoring of the equipment as well as information documenting the child's auditory performance. In fact, the assistive technology legislation requires "a functional evaluation of the child in the child's customary environment" (Sec.300.6) for determination of appropriate equipment. Amplification rating scales and fitting protocols, such as those in Appendixes 6–B, 6–C, and 6–D are particularly useful as part of a trial period in helping to determine whether a child benefits from amplification or which type or combination of amplification is most effective. The *Guidelines for Fitting and Monitoring FM Systems* (ASHA, 1994b), reprinted in Appendix 2–I, is an excellent policy and procedural source for the use of real-ear measurements for fitting and adjusting FM systems, for electroacoustic measures of FM systems, and for speech recognition measures.

Earmold Considerations

Earmolds play a significant role in how hearing aids and certain assistive device couplings function. Modifications in canal length, bore size, tubing diameter and length, vents, and damping materials can make important modifications in the output characteristics of the instrument. The major implications of these variables are summarized in Table 6–3. Other earmold considerations include:

➤ **Earmold materials:** Most children should use a soft material mold that provides pliability and comfort for play and other physical activities as well as a better seal; lucite, while durable, is not appropriate for young children. Some children will need nonallergenic materials due to allergic reactions. Current earmold impression materials are primarily silicone-based but vary individually to provide faster curing, greater detail, or other specific functions. Silicone-based materials also hold their shape better than other types of materials.
➤ **Earmold styles:** Most children use a shell or shell variation-style mold. Many children with hearing losses in the mild to moderate range may be able to use a silhouette or skeleton-style mold. The addition of a helix lock may offer better ear retention but can also cause problems with maintaining a tight seal for young children whose external ears are still growing.
➤ **Earmold color:** Colors have finally become a routine option in earmold selection for children. Allowing the child (or parent, if an infant) to choose the earmold color gives the child pride in the ownership of their hearing aid(s).

THE SCHOOL'S ROLE REGARDING EARMOLDS. The audiologist's role with earmolds will vary depending on the individual school's involvement with hearing aids and other amplification devices. School districts are responsible for providing earmolds necessary for FM or other school-owned devices. Some school-based audiologists also provide a service to parents by mak-

Table 6–3. Effects of earmold/tubing modifications.

Modification	Effect
Canal depth	➤ Lengthen the canal (or tubing), to achieve greater mid-frequency emphasis ➤ Shorten canal for greater high-frequency emphasis
Bore size	➤ Increase bore diameter for more high-frequency emphasis including above 3000 Hz ➤ Decrease bore diameter for more low-frequency emphasis down to 750 Hz ➤ Increase bore length for more low frequency emphasis down to 750 Hz ➤ Decrease bore length for more high-frequency emphasis up to 3000 Hz
Tubing diameter	➤ Larger internal diameter increases high-frequency emphasis up to 3000 Hz ➤ Smaller internal diameter increases low-frequency emphasis down to 1000 Hz
Tubing length	➤ Increase length for greater low-frequency emphasis including below 750 Hz ➤ Decrease length for greater high-frequency emphasis including above 3000 Hz
Venting	➤ Increase vent size to decrease low frequencies between 20–1000 Hz without reducing high frequencies
Damping	➤ Filters in earhooks smooth out entire frequency response ➤ Can also reduce output ➤ Mainly affects 1000–3000 Hz
Horns	➤ High-frequency emphasis ➤ Smooths response between 3000–5000 Hz

ing earmolds for personal devices worn for school. Parents, or third party payors, may be billed for these molds depending on the schools' policies. There are several benefits to providing this earmold service including the following:

➤ Increased efficiency as a result of eliminating the time involved scheduling children with their private audiologist to take impressions and returning to pick up the mold(s)
➤ Decreased absenteeism because of these appointments
➤ Diminished fear regarding the impression process because earmolds can be made for several children within their preschool room
➤ Lower cost to parents

Re-evaluation

For most children an evaluation of amplification performance is recommended annually, at the same time as the child's routine hearing evaluation. As with fitting amplification initially, the annual assessment needs to consider children's amplification devices as a unit and re-evaluate their relevance to each child's learning environment and communication needs. Although the need for annual evaluations is often questioned by nonaudiologists, particularly when the child's hearing is stable, it must be understood that auditory skills and listening needs change, even when hearing thresholds remain stable. There is always the potential for hearing sensitivity levels to decrease or

fluctuate, a situation that requires immediate medical attention, as well as concern regarding the possibility of over-amplification and the subsequent potential for further hearing loss. The following components should be considered for the initial and annual evaluations of amplification:

Behavioral audiologic assessment
➤ Speech audiometry (quiet and noise, auditory and auditory-visual)
➤ Functional gain measurement (frequency-specific)
➤ Listening check and Ling 6-sound test

Nonbehavioral assessment
➤ Electroacoustic measurements
➤ Real-ear probe-microphone measurements

Functional assessment (non-sound-booth)
➤ Auditory skill development measures
➤ Classroom amplification appraisals
➤ Listening evaluation

Monitoring and Equipment Management

Equipment monitoring and management can be one of our greatest challenges as educational audiologists. As the numbers of pieces of equipment and their variety increases, the time required to monitor, troubleshoot, repair, test-check, clean, and catalogue also increases. The assistance of a technician or aide can be invaluable in the management of equipment.

Monitoring

The monitoring of hearing aids and amplification is not an option. Verification procedures to determine that proper fittings have been made are essential for all amplification devices worn by children. While the law (IDEA, 34 CFR 300.303) requires schools to "ensure that the hearing aids worn by children with hearing impairments . . . are functioning properly," it does not state the frequency with which monitoring should occur. Reports continue to show that hearing aid and FM system malfunctions are frequent, which certainly points to the need for daily amplification checks. In addition, more comprehensive monitoring may be warranted for certain students who are younger or who are prone to more problems. Monitoring carries long-term consequences, because the process demonstrates to the student the value of working amplification and the importance of the daily listening checks. In the interest of promoting individual independence and responsibility, all children with personally worn amplification having an IEP, regardless of age, should have a goal regarding the use of their equipment. Table 6–4 illustrates an example of appropriate goals and objectives.

DAILY MONITORING. Until students reach a level of independence with their amplification instruments that meets their long-term amplification goal, a plan will be necessary for some level of regular monitoring. The monitoring frequency may be determined by the performance of the child's equipment and the ability of the child to identify problems. For most children this monitoring will need to occur daily, at least through preschool and the early elementary school years. The audiologist should not have the direct responsibility of daily amplification monitoring, but rather should assume responsibility for providing instruction and support to a designated staff member who is in the building on a daily basis (e.g., the special education teacher, the regular classroom teacher, an aide, a school nurse, or a speech-language pathologist). A hearing aid/amplification test kit (see sample Hearing Aid Check in Appendix 6–G) should be available for the student which includes:

➤ Battery tester
➤ Listening stethoscope
➤ Extra batteries
➤ Cleaning brush
➤ Wax loop
➤ Directions for conducting a physical and listening check
➤ Who to call when a problem is identified

Younger students tend to enjoy using a charting system with a reward plan when they conduct their checks (see Appendix 6–H for a sample amplification monitoring chart).

The daily check should include the following components (see Appendix 6–G for instructions for hearing aid checks):

Table 6–4. Sample IEP long-term goal and short-term objectives for amplification.

Long-term Goal:
(Name of student) will be to be able manage his/her own (hearing aids and/or FM system).

Short-term Objectives (use one or more of the following as appropriate):

Objective 1. *To identify when hearing aids and FM system are nonfunctioning by having student conduct a self-check and record results on a chart with 75% accuracy.*
  ➤ identify when hearing aids are not producing sound
  ➤ identify when FM system is transmitting teacher's voice

Objective 2. *To conduct simple troubleshooting to determine cause of problem by having student conduct a self-check and record results on a chart with 75% accuracy .*
  ➤ check earmold to see if it is plugged with wax
  ➤ check hearing aid battery to see if it is dead
  ➤ check FM receiver light to see if FM battery is dead

Objective 3. *To correct simple problems with hearing aid and FM by having student conduct activities to correct problem with 75% accuracy.*
  ➤ clean earmold
  ➤ replace hearing aid battery
  ➤ charge FM receiver

Objective 4. *To contact the audiologist when additional assistance and support is required with 75% acuracy as determined by contacts made and spot checks of amplification devices.*
  ➤ use telephone or TDD to call audiologist to report problem and explain the troubleshooting and correction steps that have been tried

➤ Visual Check
  ✔ Are aid(s)/FM worn?
  ✔ Are aid(s)/FM turned on and set appropriately?
  ✔ Are there defects or problems with the earmold, tubing, or case?
➤ Listening Check
  ✔ Is there amplification of sound?
  ✔ Is volume set correctly?
  ✔ Is the FM signal present?
  ✔ Conduct Ling 6-sound test while listening for the following:
       satisfactory sound quality
       intermittent sound
       interference from another source (FM only)

Comments and actions taken should be recorded on the monitoring form. Parents need to be notified when problems exist that require repairs by the dispensing audiologist (see Appendix 6–I for a sample form).

COMPREHENSIVE MONITORING. More comprehensive monitoring may be necessary when there is a need to analyze the type of equipment problems, or to collect data. This level of monitoring usually requires a greater degree of sophistication and knowledge of the equipment and may be reserved for the audiologist, teacher of the hearing impaired, or a specially trained aide or technician. This level of monitoring may be done less frequently than the daily monitoring and may include probe-microphone and electroacoustic measurements done on-site to identify specific amplification problems and to verify amplification settings. A sample comprehensive monitoring form is in located in Appendix 6–J.

Equipment Management

In addition to monitoring equipment, there must be a method for cataloging the equipment to track all pieces by serial number, date of purchase, funding source, service contract data, repair history, and current location. The procedure can be done simply with an index card file system or in a more sophisticated, computer data base. As a school district audiology program acquires more equipment, it is increasingly more important that a good system be developed. Loss from theft or damage, inventory for insurance purposes, tracking repair histories, and separating equipment purchased by regular education versus special education, are common issues that can benefit from data contained in such a management system. Information concerning date of purchase, amount of purchase, and repair history is invaluable for budget proposals that specify additional or replacement equipment and that address the need for repair contracts through extended warranties.

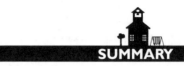

SUMMARY

This chapter has provided the essential information necessary to set up amplification procedures and practices in a school setting. The decisions that must be made for children regarding amplification provide some of the most compelling justification for the necessity of school-based audiology services.

Technology growth will continue to result in more options for children. But, without appropriate audiological services and technological supports, these children will not have the opportunity to access information and participate in learning as they deserve. As school-based audiologists, we must do our part by actively advocating for the amplification needs of these children.

SUGGESTED READINGS

Berg, F. (1993). *Acoustics and sound systems in schools.* San Diego: Singular Publishing Group, Inc.

Crandell, C., Smaldino, J., & Flexer, C. (1995). *Sound-field FM amplification: Theory and practical applications.* San Diego: Singular Publishing Group, Inc.

Flexer, C. (1994). *Facilitating hearing and listening in young children.* San Diego: Singular Publishing Group, Inc.

Lewis, D. (1995). Assistive devices for classroom listening: FM systems. *American Journal of Audiology.*

Nevins, M., & Chute, P. (1995). *Children with cochlear implants in educational settings.* San Diego: Singular Publishing Group, Inc.

Ross, M. (Ed.). (1992). *FM auditory training systems: Characteristics, selection, and use.* Timonium, MD: York Press.

Seewald, R., Ramji, K., Sinclair, S., Moodie, K., & Jamieson, D. (1993). *Computer-assisted implementation of the desired sensation level method for electroacoustic selection and fitting in children: User's manual.* London, Ontario: University of Western Ontario.

Staller, S. (Ed.). (1991). Multi-channel cochlear implants in children. *Ear & Hearing,* Supple. 12.

Tye-Murray, N. (1992). *Cochlear implants and children: A handbook for parents, teachers, and speech and hearing professionals.* Washington, DC: Alexander Graham Bell Association for the Deaf.

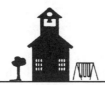

CHAPTER 7

CASE MANAGEMENT AND AURAL (RE)HABILITATION

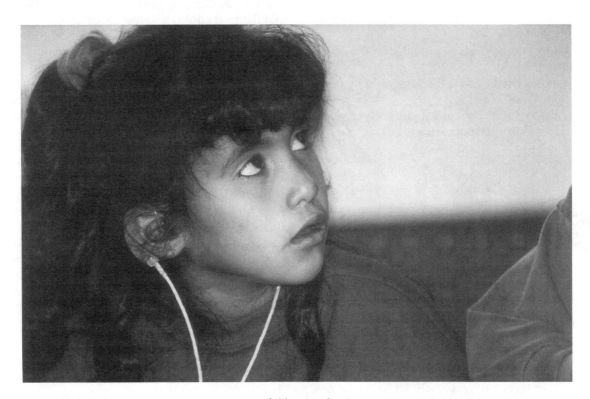

Ashley, age 6

CONTENTS

The educational audiologist's role in case management and service delivery will be affected by a number of factors and may not be the same for each student who is deaf or hard-of-hearing. The availability and qualifications of additional service providers, characteristics and needs of individual students, school schedules, and locations to be served all impact on the determination of the most cost-effective plan for case management and service delivery. In addition, all of these factors change over time and can cause modification of the educational audiologist's role as new resources become available, as student needs are met, and as different needs arise. Flexibility is the key if the educational audiologist is to be most effective in the areas of case management and service delivery for students with hearing impairments.

This chapter addresses the following questions:

➤ What strategies can be used to facilitate case management?
➤ What direct services can be provided by the educational audiologist?
➤ What indirect services are the responsibility of the educational audiologist?
➤ What is the educational audiologist's responsibility in services for special populations, infants, and toddlers?

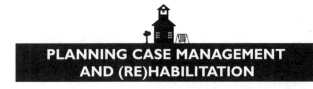

PLANNING CASE MANAGEMENT AND (RE)HABILITATION

The Importance of Service Coordination

The educational audiologist is in a unique position to act as the service coordinator for students with hearing impairments. Case management by definition implies communication and coordination with more than one service or service provider, which is often the case with students who are hearing impaired. We, as educational audiologists, have knowledge and training that covers the medical, audiological, educational, communication, social-emotional, and vocational impact of hearing loss. This knowledge and experience can help facilitate communication between service providers, as well as with family members and the students themselves. Communication breakdown often occurs between medical professionals and educators when family members are used to transmit information from one to the other. Similar to the old "telephone game," information gets lost and/or modified

each time an additional person attempts to receive, remember, then transmit the information. Individuals tend to focus on information they understand, and this is the content that is remembered and transmitted most accurately. The educational audiologist can facilitate communication by clarifying medical terminology for educators and family members, as well as by providing the educational context for medical or clinical personnel to incorporate in their evaluations and recommendations.

The educational audiologist can also facilitate decision making by anticipating future difficulties and helping to prevent their occurrence. For example, providing information concerning technological advances to parents and students could change the direction of an anticipated vocational choice and allow scheduling of more relevant or necessary coursework. Educational audiologists who build flexibility into their schedules also have greater opportunity to facilitate communication between service providers. For example, we may be able to accompany families to medical appointments and help explain educational needs or schedule meetings with teachers to help interpret medical reports when they are received. The educational audiologist often has better access to a telephone than other educational service providers, as well as office time for contacts with service providers who are not school-based. Knowledge of school schedules can often lead to more efficient scheduling of medical/clinical appointments for students. Parents should be encouraged to ask for appointments after school, on a teacher work-day, or during a vacation break, so no school time needs to be missed. In addition, many physician offices and clinics are happy to see siblings on the same day. If the school is providing transportation, a single appointment date for siblings is more cost-effective. These logistical issues make the educational audiologist the logical contact person between the educational and medical personnel who are involved with students who have hearing impairments.

Facilitating Effective Case Management

Strategies recommended for initiating and implementing case management include the following activities:

➤ Clarification of the needs and services for the student who is hearing impaired
➤ Identification of currently available school personnel
➤ Arrangements for effective collaboration between service providers
➤ Development and implementation of a written communication system

Clarification of Needs and Services

Begin by identifying the student's needs and the individuals currently addressing these needs. Areas to include are listed in Table 7–1. Although this information typically is included on the school district's individual education plan (IEP), it can be useful to design a form specifically for needs of students with hearing impairments (see Appendix 7–A). It is also helpful to have this information available in an organized format for each IEP meeting to facilitate the discussion of options to address each area of potential need.

Identification of Personnel

Although educational audiologists are trained and certified to provide direct habilitative services, other demands often preclude their availability to provide these services on more than a consult basis. At best, most school-based audiology schedules do not permit direct student service more frequently than once a week or bi-weekly. If other service providers (e.g., certified teachers of the hearing impaired, speech-language pathologists, counselors, interpreters, tutors) could address some of the direct service needs of the student who is hearing impaired on a daily or collaborative basis, the case manager can coordinate student needs with service provider expertise and availability. Viewing a list of all potential direct and support personnel and their schedules can sensitize service providers and administrators to the need for service coordination. Maintaining such a list also can help to facilitate case management decisions. The development of positive attitudes toward collaborative planning and service delivery should lead to more flexibility on the part of individual service providers when unplanned change is needed.

Arrangements for Effective Collaboration

Team coordination should be completed during the pre-planning process. However, schedules often change as new students enroll, resulting in an ongoing need for service coordination. The educational audiologist, as case manager, should help service providers determine how they can work most efficiently as a team throughout the school year. Each team member should be asked for input, and an attempt should be made to incorporate any input received. Service time and schedules are tight, thus alternate ways to provide input should be made available for those who cannot attend meetings. Effective team collaboration requires that the service coordinator clarify and disseminate in writing how and when team members will communicate.

Efficient Written Communication

One of the most critical responsibilities for a service coordinator is to facilitate the development of a workable system for *simple* written communication among team members. When forms are devised, draft copies must be given to team members for input. Credit those who provide input by including their names on any form utilized. This practice helps to formalize their commitment to using this written communication system. Make time at team meetings for modification of either the oral or written communication system, especially if the process does not appear to be facilitating effective interchanges among staff and support personnel. Be flexible when attempting to meet the needs of service providers, as well as students. *Clear, concise communication is critical for effective coordination of multiple service providers* (see Appendix 7–B for a sample communication form between school and nonschool providers).

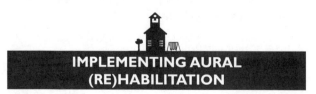

IMPLEMENTING AURAL (RE)HABILITATION

The educational audiologist's primary purpose for being involved in the habilitation of students with hearing impairment is to facilitate the maximum use of auditory input during the learning process. (Re)habilitation includes involvement with equipment, involvement with teaching and learning strategies, and knowledge of environmental acoustics (both classroom and nonclassroom) in any situation where learning takes place. Although other educational service

Table 7–1. Areas of potential need for students who are hearing impaired.

➤ Medical
➤ Audiological
➤ Educational
➤ Communication
➤ Amplification
➤ Visual Technology
➤ Special Transportation
➤ Interpreting
➤ Notetaking
➤ Tutoring
➤ Counseling
➤ Vocational

providers may address auditory input, only educational audiologists have audition as their primary focus. The educational audiologist may assume this role in the form of direct service, indirect service, or in some combination of these two.

Direct Services

When the educational audiologist provides direct services to students who are deaf or hard-of-hearing, these usually are delivered on a regularly scheduled basis. However, the length of time for these services may vary, depending on the content to be covered, long- and short-term objectives, and the availability of other personnel to assist with some or all of these services. The following areas encompass the most typical direct services provided by a school-based audiologist:

➤ Management of amplification
➤ Development of listening/auditory skills
➤ Speechreading
➤ Communication repair training
➤ Development of skills to overcome environmental barriers
➤ Informational counseling
➤ Psychosocial development

Management of Amplification

Most curricula now include a section on developing students' independence in managing their own amplification devices. The educational audiologist may want to utilize or modify one of these published programs or develop and implement a more individualized program of hearing aid maintenance, such as the one described in Lipscomb, Von Almen, and Blair (1992). Either approach should include the following objectives for each student, depending on his or her needs and developmental ability:

➤ insertion of earmold(s)
➤ basic power and volume control operation
➤ battery care
➤ identification of when unit is or is not providing amplification
➤ trouble-shooting techniques and solutions as appropriate for age-level

For younger students, appropriate trouble-shooting activities might include checking and changing batteries, earmold cleaning and maintenance, and acting out situations where a responsible adult is advised of a possible problem. The educational audiologist may want to arrange for older students to contact their hearing aid dispenser by phone (voice or TDD) from school to describe the problem and to determine possible solutions. The more independent a student can become with his or her own amplification (including FMs or other assistive devices), the more likely this equipment will be monitored and, as a result, be working on a regular basis. (See Chapter 6, Amplification and Classroom Hearing Technology, for a more detailed discussion of daily monitoring of amplification.)

Taking earmold impressions, electroacoustic and/or real ear measurement of hearing aid(s) or other assistive devices at the student's school facility, and on-site adjustment of amplification parameters can also be considered direct service by the educational audiologist, even though they may be provided on a less frequent basis.

Development of Listening/Auditory Skills

For students who are deaf or hard-of-hearing to develop functional and automatic use of their auditory potential, attention must be focussed on auditory development throughout each day, and audition must be integrated into the child's communication environment by all participants. In addition, direct skill training must be provided on a regular basis if significant progress in auditory development is to occur. Whether provided by the educational audiologist, speech-language pathologist, or teacher of the hearing impaired, auditory training should be included in any specific oral language and speech (re)habilitation. The school-based audiologist may work in collaboration with other designated personnel to enhance the auditory focus, when time for direct instruction is limited. An example might be for the educational audiologist to team teach a lesson with the teacher of the hearing impaired and/or the speech-language pathologist to model the emphasis on auditory skill development within the classroom or therapy room environment. The direct service role of the educational audiologist should be to focus on the following areas:

➤ development of objectives
➤ introduction of training activities for specific skills (e.g., awareness of environmental sounds, following two-step directions from auditory cues alone)
➤ monitoring and measurement of the use of specific skills in unstructured and structured settings
➤ development of techniques and strategies that would address these objectives on a daily basis

There are a number of good auditory curricula available that list auditory skills in developmental sequence, along with suggested activities for each skill level. A listing of currently available curriculum guides and ordering information is included in Appendix 16–G. Although the educational audiologist may initiate use of one or more of these curricula, additional copies should be made available to all other personnel working with the student, as well as family members when requested (see section on Indirect Services). Appropriate goals should also be included on the IEP. Examples of audiology goals and objectives for IEPs are included in Appendix 11–B. A Listening Development Profile, a checklist that includes student outcomes and performance indicators of progress in functional listening, is included as Appendix 7–C.

Speechreading

Although there is no question of the importance of visual cues to supplement audition for students with hearing impairment, agreement is not unanimous concerning the acquisition of visual skills in individuals who are deaf and hard-of-hearing. The emphasis placed on the use of visual training in oral and auditory-verbal programs varies according to their program philosophy. In some programs the curricula includes speechreading activities, while in others it is assumed that the skill will be acquired naturally. The most common practice is to integrate speechreading activities with language or combined auditory/visual activities, rather than to work on speechreading in isolation. Three situations where speechreading instruction might enhance learning are described below:

1. If the student is involved in a phonically based reading program, the educational audiologist may want to encourage an emphasis on the visual aspects of specific speech sounds as an aid to decoding written material.
2. If a student does not make good eye contact during one-to-one conversation, work on visual attention could be beneficial.
3. If a student is not aware of ways to enhance visual cues during communication, instruction for these skills could enhance communication understanding.

Some of the objectives for these situations might fall under the area of communication repair training or environmental management strategies (see next two sections for a discussion of these areas). In addition, it is critical that specific skill training be reinforced in all other communication settings and activities. A coordinated effort of all team members, including parents, is necessary to determine appropriate daily opportunities for learning. A sample letter to parents describing speechreading is included as Appendix 7–D. Published speechreading materials for children are listed in Appendix 16–H.

Communication Repair Training

Frequently, students who are deaf or hard-of-hearing are not aware of communication breakdowns that occur during the school day, and they are uncomfortable with or unaware of a variety of repair strategies. Stone (1988), Elfenbein (1992), and Tye-Murray (1994) have addressed this area in recent publications, and each publication gives specific suggestions for strategies to teach children. Elfenbein (1993) also has developed a program for use with students in a school environment that includes the following five steps:

1. Understanding basic communication processes
2. Understanding communication breakdowns
3. Message formulation
4. Introduction of communication repair strategies
5. Practice using communication repair strategies

This program helps students to acknowledge that communication breakdowns occur and assists them in developing appropriate ways to cope independently with these breakdowns.

Development of Skills to Overcome Environmental Barriers

The educational audiologist has specific expertise for teaching students about communication barriers that arise in a variety of environments. Information concerning the effects of noise, distance, reverberation, and poor lighting should be provided to students with hearing impairments, as well as to teachers. The sections covering teacher consultation in this chapter and in Chapter 12, Inservice, provide more detailed information regarding suggestions for environmental modifications. Students and teachers should be made aware of the significant effect of fatigue that results from straining to listen in noise and/or attend visually to speakers or interpreters for extended periods of time. Suggested student activities for these areas include the following ideas:

➤ Students can be helped to identify noise sources through drawing diagrams of their classrooms and measuring noise using a sound-level meter for specific classroom areas during different classroom activities.
➤ Students can identify surface materials found in their classrooms and determine which surfaces help to decrease unwanted noise.
➤ Older students can actually calculate reverberation time for their individual classrooms (English, 1995, pp. 154–155).
➤ A schedule of noisy times/activities can be made, followed by the development of strategies for the

student to use when noisy or poor visual conditions occur

➤ Students can participate in discussions about which classes require more energy for attending to instruction (both visual and auditory) and make recommendations about class schedules.

Another approach described by Morlock (1995) is the development of a self-advocacy checklist for use by students who are deaf or hard-of-hearing. Sample letters are included in Appendix 7–E, and in Table 4–5 in Chapter 4, Assessment Practices. Again, the overriding goal for providing direct service in this area is to empower the student by increasing his or her independence in communication during the school day.

Informational Counseling

Marttila and Mills (1993) and Greenblatt and Daar (1994) have developed programs to provide students with information concerning their own hearing losses and ways to manage environmental barriers. This information fosters independence and promotes self-esteem and should be provided as an ongoing component of direct services to students who are deaf and hard-of-hearing at all educational levels. Students feel empowered by having information related to their own hearing status and by making the decision about how much to share and what strategies to use when sharing this information with others. This process can begin early by simply showing one's hearing aid or assistive device during a preschool or kindergarten "Show and Tell" activity and progress to written and oral reports, science projects, student interviews, and so on. The curricula that are available make good material for a teaching module on "Understanding Your Hearing," which, when developmentally appropriate, helps students acquire knowledge related to the following topics:

➤ Etiology of the student's own hearing loss
➤ Personalized hearing test results
➤ Equipment utilized for assessment
➤ Different types of amplification for different individuals and varying environments
➤ Current and future technology other than amplification

Topics may be taught in groups, if enough students of similar ages are in the same facility. If done individually, often necessary when there is only one student with hearing impairment in a school, allowing the student to bring a friend to the sessions facilitates a peer support system and helps the student feel less isolated. Whatever the approach, this knowledge not only employers

the students but allows them to make more informed decisions about amplification use, both within and outside of the educational environment.

Psychosocial Development

Often addressed as counseling related to the impact of hearing loss, the educational audiologist's role in this area of counseling is more often one of a resource, rather than a direct service provider. Counseling is a much more complex process that requires knowledge and training outside the preparation for educational audiology. However, there are some informational supports that we, as school-based audiologists, can use to assist students with hearing loss. These include the following:

➤ Bringing in adults who are deaf or hard-of-hearing for "rap sessions"
➤ Providing written materials, such as *Hip Magazine* (ordering information in Appendix 16–I), and facilitating group discussions about social situations and barriers resulting from hearing loss
➤ Maintaining and making available to students a file of news articles or stories concerning children and adults who are hearing impaired
➤ Encouraging and helping to arrange participation in the PC Pals Deaf Teen Chat (Appendix 16–I) or other appropriate computer networks or chat rooms

Additional suggestions for activities to facilitate social growth can be found in Schum and Gfeller (1994). Provision of information concerning legal rights and future vocational options may also be considered under the umbrella of couseling students with hearing impairments (Marttila, 1994). The educational audiologist may be the team member who identifies a need for more in-depth counseling for some students, and, therefore, may serve as the referral source for these individuals. Knowledge of counselors with hearing impairments and those with particular expertise in working with individuals who are deaf and hard-of-hearing should be acquired by each educational audiologist for his or her particular geographic area.

Indirect Services

Indirect services, usually identified as consultation, may be regularly scheduled by the educational audiologist, delivered on an as-needed basis, or provided as a combination of the two. The latter option is usually preferred, because regularly scheduled visits may not address problems as they develop, and consultation on an as-needed basis frequently is perceived as "not being there very often or at all."

Administrators may question the amount of time allocated for indirect services by the educational audiologist, especially when funding is tied to reimbursement for direct services to identified students who are deaf or hard of hearing. Figure 7–1 describes factors that should be considered when building consultation time into the educational audiology program.

The following six primary areas of consultation and collaboration are those in which the educational audiologist has specific expertise:

➤ Classroom amplification and other assistive devices
➤ Teacher collaboration regarding strategies for the classroom
➤ Selection of classrooms and teachers
➤ Selection of auditory curricula and materials
➤ Facilitation of auditory skill development with sign language use
➤ Information concerning student hearing loss and auditory function

Classroom Amplification and Other Assistive Devices

The educational audiologist is the staff member in the educational environment who has the expertise to recommend the purchase and facilitate the use of current technology available for students with hearing impairments in the educational setting. Although clinical audiologists may have knowledge of the technology available, they cannot "match" the device(s) to specific classroom environments without being on-site. This selection should be based not only on physical characteristics of the classroom (see Chapter 6, Amplification and Hearing Technology), but also on personal characteristics of the student(s) and teacher(s) involved.

The educational audiologist should have knowledge of the budget and time-lines for equipment requisition. Frequently, manufacturers will provide short-term loan of equipment if payment must be delayed for budgetary reasons, and lease-purchase agreements are another option available to school systems who prefer to space out payments over an extended period of time. A good relationship between the educational audiologist and the manufacturers' representatives can lead to trials of new equipment and devices before release to the general public.

When classroom amplification is introduced for the first time, the educational audiologist needs to be available more often to facilitate its use. Frequently, the initial orientation is not sufficient, because daily use can lead to problems that were not anticipated. For example, one of our first experiences with rechargeable batteries in FM systems led to learning that the maintenance personnel had been instructed to turn off all appliances when they left the building overnight, resulting in uncharged units the next morning. Although an orientation should be provided at the beginning of each school year, once a classroom amplification system has been used successfully, the teachers may feel more comfortable helping one another with problems that occur. One of Murphy's laws for audiology is that equipment that is used *will* break down; thus, the educational audiologist serves as an invaluable link between the classroom teacher and the manufacturer of any classroom equipment used in support of students who are hearing impaired. Regular monitoring and maintenance of classroom equipment, together with the development and modification of quick and simple ways to verify that this is done, is discussed in Chapter 6, Amplification and Classroom Hearing Technology.

Technology and assistive devices that can enhance the visual environment for students who are hearing impaired are listed in Table 7–2. Although the educational audiologists may not be the designated managers for visual assistive devices, they can often provide valuable input concerning sources for funding and purchase.

Teacher Collaboration Regarding Strategies for the Classroom

Although strategies such as "preferential seating" appear routinely in audiological reports, there is no substitute for classroom observation to pinpoint suggestions appropriate for each teacher, classroom, and student. Questions to ask include the following:

➤ Where is the best location for the student's desk?
➤ Is this seating the best location for all types of teaching activities?
➤ When there is lighting glare from one direction and competing noise from another, how do you reconcile the two for the best advantage of the student?
➤ How well is the student following not only teacher instruction but also classroom discussion?
➤ Does the teacher alert the student with hearing impairment to changes in topic and supplement group instruction with individual checks to assess the student's comprehension of assignments and material covered?
➤ Would a student "buddy" be helpful?
➤ Would an oral or sign interpreter be helpful, and for which classes?
➤ If an interpreter is used, is the student totally dependent on him or her for one-to-one instruction, or does the student make an attempt to follow what is happening in the classroom? (Educational inter-

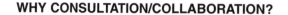

WHY CONSULTATION/COLLABORATION?

- Emphasis on regular classroom programming continues to increase
- Services go directly to the child rather than child having to go to the program
- Expanded at-risk preschool placements within community daycare and preschools create more need for on-site supports
- More children with mild/moderate hearing losses and otitis media require services
- The number of children with neurological or developmental disorders of which hearing impairment is only one component has increased

SKILLS NECESSARY TO PROVIDE CONSULTATION SERVICES

- Effective interpersonal communication skills
- Accurate, current knowledge of all areas of hearing and hearing impairments, including implications of hearing loss
- Ability to troubleshoot amplification equipment
- Possess an understanding of the classroom teacher's teaching perspective
- Ability to accept different cultural backgrounds
- Ability to relate with a variety of ages and situations
- Ability to understand the student's perspective
- Permission to say "I don't know. Let's find out"
- Ability to work with administrators for support and program development
- Ability to share certain tasks that may have only been done by the audiologist in the past

ROLE OF EDUCATIONAL AUDIOLOGIST AS A CONSULTANT

1. Advocacy for hearing for all students and particularly for those with hearing impairments.
2. Direct efforts to those responsible for educating child rather than to the child
3. Provide support (information, planning, training,) to staff, students, and parents in collaborative manner, including:
   - hearing processes
   - auditory learning development
   - development of speech-language
   - cognition
   - social-emotional issues
   - hearing aids
   - assistive listening & other technologies
   - classroom acoustics
   - environmental adaptations
   - instructional modifications
   - motivational strategies
   - organizational strategies
   - delivery modifications
   - curricular modifications
4. Facilitate continued placement in most appropriate setting
   - teacher collaboration
   - classroom and teacher selection

OUTCOMES OF EDUCATIONAL AUDIOLOGY CONSULTING SERVICES

- Responsibility for meeting students' needs is shared with teachers and other school support staff
- Supports for students in classroom settings increase
- Opportunities to have an impact on more students increase

Figure 7–1. Factors to consider in the delivery of educational audiology consultation.

Table 7–2. Visual technology to enhance the visual classroom environment.

➤ Signaling and alerting devices
➤ Telecommunication Devices for the Deaf (TDDs)
➤ Captioned television monitors
➤ Captioned films and videos
➤ LCD information displays which inform students of daily schedule of events
➤ Real-time captioning
➤ Electronic mail and bulletin boards
➤ Computers with software appropriate for students with hearing loss

preters vary in their skill levels, and their physical location relative to the teacher and/or student may benefit from modification.)

➤ Would a notetaker be helpful? If so, the educational audiologist may be able to help in the selection and instruction of an appropriate student. Written materials covering the use of notetakers can be obtained from Alexander Graham Bell Association and Clarke School for the Deaf (see Appendix 16–I).

Teachers and program philosophies vary in their approach to support services in the mainstream. The current trend for full inclusion has been perceived by many to imply that students should adjust to the classroom without special supports or instruction (see section on Inclusion in this chapter). In reality, however, there may be many times when the content is totally missed or misunderstood by the student who is deaf or hard-of-hearing because visual supports, such as interpreters or notetakers, were not requested or made available.

If a student with hearing impairment is included in the mainstream without assistance, observation by the educational audiologist can lead to valuable input that could help alleviate academic problems before failure occurs. In these cases, observations should be scheduled throughout the day to assess performance in a variety of instructional settings. Classroom observations will be required more frequently during the beginning of a school year, but should be scheduled no less than once a month throughout the year. A classroom observation checklist (see Appendix 7–F) can make these observations more efficient by pinpointing areas of difficulty, documenting progress, and clarifying the need for additional classroom modifications. It can also be useful for teachers to complete the same checklist and compare observations with those of the educational audiologist.

Selection of Classrooms and Teachers

There is no substitute for on-site observation to match teachers and classroom environments with the needs of each student who is hearing impaired. Questions to be answered during the observation include the following:

➤ What type of informal sound treatment is present? Are there multiple uncovered windows, or will reverberation be lessened because of walls covered with bulletin boards?
➤ How many students are there in each classroom, and are there any others who may require instructional modifications?
➤ Is there a class available where the teacher might be able to give more one-to-one instruction and/or one that is farther from the cafeteria or band room?
➤ What is the teacher's traditional teaching style? Does the teacher stand in the front and lecture most of the day, or does he or she move around a great deal? A moving instructor may be more difficult for the student with a hearing impairment to follow, but on the other hand, this type of teaching style may lead to more individual instruction.
➤ Does the teacher routinely use supplementary visual aids, such as pictures, instructions on the board, written outlines, and assignments? Is he or she flexible enough to use equipment that will probably break at the most inopportune time, and does he or she have a sense of humor?
➤ Does the teacher express herself or himself with whole-body cues, and does he or she frequently give "mixed messages" by these cues?
➤ Is the teacher willing to take a risk, and does he or she reinforce and help students who take the initiative?
➤ Did these teachers volunteer to have students with special needs in their classrooms?

There are no absolute rules to follow in teacher selection for students with hearing impairments, but a teacher who has natural instincts to simplify material that is not easily understood and who routinely uses a lot of visual aids in teaching will usually be more effective in communicating with these students. A classroom observation form that addresses these areas is included in Appendix 7–F, and a sample checklist for parents is located in Appendix 10–C. Teachers who have a sensitivity and focus on developing self-esteem in all of their students will also make students who are deaf or hard-of-hearing feel more comfortable in acknowledging when they have missed or misunderstood communication in the classroom.

Facilitating Selection and Use of Auditory Curricula and Materials

The advent of cochlear implant use in children has led to the development of several good auditory curricula, which are listed in Appendix 16–G. This list should be updated annually, as costs change and new materials are published. Individual and classroom activities are incorporated with each curriculum guide, and most are available on 30-day trial prior to purchase. If school personnel have access to a regional resource library, requests can be made to order specific curricula for review prior to individual school or district purchase.

Educational audiologists can make suggestions for specific curriculum guides based on their experience with auditory goals and objectives. Whenever possible, we should also suggest how these objectives can phase into the regular or special education curricula in use for specific students. Examples include use of vocabulary lists for listening exercises, taping sounds around the school facility for recognition of environmental sounds, and use of classroom directions for auditory comprehension activities. Additional suggestions for incorporating auditory goals into academic lessons are described in Firszt and Reeder (1996).

Implementation of Auditory Skill Development Together with Sign Language Use

Auditory skill development can be fostered within programs that use a total communication approach, that is, an approach that encourages use of whatever sensory input is necessary for the specific activity at hand. If American Sign Language (ASL) is used, rather than a Manually Coded English system, there is an inherent conflict during simultaneous communication using sign and speech. Therefore, students in most ASL programs may not make use of auditory input during the majority of communication situations throughout the school day. Under these conditions, auditory skill development may be very slow and laborious and should be discussed thoroughly by parents, teachers, and the students to see if auditory learning is a desired goal. Appendix 7–G includes an overview of communication options most commonly used to communicate with and educate children who are deaf and hard-of-hearing, and the

emphasis on audition is addressed within this overview for each option. If the decision is made to continue with the development of auditory skills, a discussion should follow with clear recommendations for ways that use of audition can be integrated into the student's communication system, both within and outside the formal classroom environment. In addition to the traditional IEP forms, a written statement of commitment to an auditory learning program may help to clarify each participant's desire to be involved in this program. A sample statement of commitment is included as Appendix 7–H.

If a program uses a total communication approach, auditory input without supplementary visual cues (speechreading or sign language) should be incorporated into informal communication, as well as instruction, throughout the school day if maximum progress is to be expected. The educational audiologist can assist with facilitating this approach by sitting in on an activity suggested by the classroom teacher and demonstrating how to incorporate each student's auditory goals (see suggested readings by Cole & Gregory, 1986; Erber, 1982; Tye-Murray, 1992). The educational audiologist should be sensitive to potential goals for visual language input for other children in the class and collaborate with the classroom teacher in devising creative strategies for facilitating the use of audition for each student. Without multiple opportunities for meaningful practice, use of the auditory channel for learning will be secondary for most students with significant hearing impairments.

Information Concerning Student Hearing Loss and Auditory Function

A final area where the educational audiologist has a primary role is in the provision of information concerning the specifics of the hearing loss for each student with hearing impairment and how it impacts on his or her ability to communicate within the classroom setting. This information should be communicated to all educational personnel who come in contact with the student during the school day and should be made relevant to each person's role with the student involved. For example, a school-wide inservice might be held prior to the enrollment of a student who is deaf or hard-of-hearing to outline basic information on hearing loss, personal amplification, classroom amplification systems, and relevant communication performance in academic and social situations. Questions addressed during this inservice might include the following:

➤ Will the students be able to order for themselves in the cafeteria, or will they have a full-time sign language interpreter?

➤ Will the student be using specialized equipment on the playground that will require explanations for other students in the school?

➤ Should the student be wearing amplification on the bus, and, if so, who will be responsible for its management?

Chapter 12, Inservice, provides additional discussion of this topic.

When providing information concerning specific students, it is important to discuss the information with both the student and his or her parents before the presentation. This, again, empowers students by allowing them to have the opportunity to select the type of information they want to have provided to others. Parents may have specific ideas concerning areas they would like to have covered and may also want to attend and/or participate in discussions concerning the specifics of their child's hearing loss. The educational audiologist is responsible for providing this information in the IEP meeting, but specific communication situations within the classroom and/or school environment may require additional collaboration between teacher and audiologist. For example, the child with a mild hearing loss may demonstrate no difficulty communicating with peers on the playground but could have major problems hearing and following teacher instruction in a noisy computer lab. Materials from the Clarke Mainstream Center (see Appendix 16–I) can be easily adapted for individual student/teacher collaboration, as well as for a general inservice. A brightly colored 5″ × 8″ index card for placement on the teacher's desk (see Figure 4–3 in Chapter 4, Assessment Practices, for a sample card), can be a helpful reminder of the primary recommendations for a student who is hearing impaired. Include the educational audiologist's name, address, and phone number on the back of this card for easy reference, and ask the student involved to sign the card to indicate awareness of suggestions that have been given to the teacher. As stated in Chapter 4, this card should include only the three or four most important considerations for classroom communication.

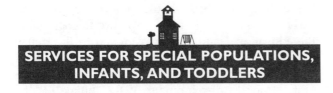

SERVICES FOR SPECIAL POPULATIONS, INFANTS, AND TODDLERS

(Re)habilitation of Special Populations

The educational audiologist usually serves as an indirect service provider or consultant for students not placed in a program for students who are deaf or hard-of-hearing or those whose hearing disability is not considered to be their primary learning difficulty. This population might include students with unilateral hearing losses, those with minimal or high-frequency losses, students with fluctuating hearing problems, those with central auditory processing difficulties, and students who have multiple disabilities. The educational audiologist's role with special populations may include any or all of the indirect services listed previously, but will usually focus on the following four primary areas:

➤ Equipment recommendations
➤ Strategies for classroom management and auditory development
➤ Development of auditory goals and objectives
➤ Monitoring student progress in auditory function

Equipment Recommendations

Students with unilateral hearing losses, central auditory processing disorders, minimal or high-frequency losses, and fluctuating losses due to otitis media may benefit from classroom amplification, especially for large group instruction. If these students are not classified as hearing impaired, equipment may need to be funded from an alternate source (see Chapter 6, Amplification and Classroom Hearing Technology, and Chapter 9, Community Collaboration, for nontraditional funding sources). The educational audiologist can often be a resource for funding options and should be involved in the selection and operation of classroom amplification systems.

Noise can be particularly detrimental to auditory learning for these students and can make the regular classroom inaccessible to them on a daily basis. For students who have multiple disabilities, it is especially critical for the educational audiologist to be involved in the selection and evaluation of personal or group amplification, because these children frequently do not give their best responses during a single clinical assessment.

Strategies for Classroom Management and Auditory Development

Strategies to reduce noise levels in the classroom should be a primary focus of the educational audiologist for children with unilateral, mild, or fluctuating hearing losses. Classroom modifications for all children with listening difficulties regardless of the etiology are listed in Table 5–4, Chapter 5, Central Auditory Processing Disorders, and these modifications are summarized again in Table 7–3. As

Table 7–3. Classroom modifications for children with listening difficulties.

➤ Environmental modifications
➤ Seating arrangements
➤ Peer assistance
➤ Alerting techniques
➤ Teaching strategies

---

mentioned previously, use of a classroom observation checklist, such as the one included as Appendix 7–F, is helpful in determining which modifications are currently in use and which ones may need to be recommended.

Frequently, information on normal auditory development is helpful to teachers of children with multiple disabilities, along with suggestions for activities in this area. Appendix 7–I is a sample handout for teachers covering developmental auditory skills with classroom strategies for each developmental stage.

Development of Goals and Objectives

The educational audiologist can assist in the development of the IEP for children who have multiple disabilities by helping to clarify goals and objectives for these students. Questions that will help to structure development of appropriate goals and objectives include the following:

➤ If a student who has limited cognitive ability also has a hearing loss, what should his or her teacher expect in the area of auditory performance?
➤ If a student has major motor involvement, is it realistic to expect that student to insert his or her own earmold, or is there another strategy that will help to achieve independence in hearing aid use?
➤ If the child with multiple disabilities has a severe-to-profound hearing loss, should an alternate or augmentative communication device be utilized instead of speech or sign language?
➤ Can this student respond appropriately to an emergency situation (e.g., a tornado drill) if a visual alerting signal is incorporated into the classroom?
➤ What technology is available that might assist in developing independent living skills for this student?

The development of appropriate goals and objectives for these students must take into account overall developmental level in nonauditory areas, as well as hearing levels and auditory performance. If a student has an identified etiology that includes the possibility of a progressive or fluctuating hearing loss, these fac-

tors should also be considered when developing auditory goals and objectives.

Monitoring Auditory Function

Monitoring auditory performance is a critical role for the educational audiologist with students who have multiple disabilities. Frequently these students' progress cannot be monitored through traditional clinical assessment techniques. Therefore, the monitoring of auditory goals, as well as response to and management of amplification, becomes an important factor in decisions regarding communication mode, placement options, and future development of realistic, yet challenging, educational goals and objectives. These students should receive monthly consultation from the educational audiologist, with careful written records maintained concerning their performance. A simple daily checklist should be devised in collaboration with the classroom teacher to monitor auditory responses and to ensure that amplification is working if it is utilized. Performance indicators, especially those included in the beginning and intermediate states of the Listening Development Profile (Appendix 7–C), can be used as a method of comparing student behavior with and without amplification. Auditory responses such as those typically noted in behavioral observation audiometry can be incorporated into a chart to assist in monitoring students with severe disabilities, both with and without amplification (see Appendix 7–J).

(Re)habilitation of Infants and Toddlers

The educational audiologist's role with this population will vary with each state's rules and regulations. (See Chapter 1, Educational Audiology: How Did We Get Here?, for more specific information on legislation covering infants and toddlers.) If the responsible agency for birth to 3 years of age is not the Department of Education, the educational audiologist can still be the individual who initiates and facilitates communication for a smooth transition to a school-based program. There should be a contact with the early intervention service coordinator to ensure that the educational audiologist is invited to the transition meeting required to be held at least 90 days prior to placement within the educational agency program. Prior to development of the initial IEP, the educational audiologist should collect and evaluate assessment information on functional listening skills, and obtain and review available assessment information necessary for considering placement options. If possible, the educational audiologist should arrange to attend and/or assist with audiological assessments completed during the 90-day transition period. This will help facilitate communication between service providers, even before the child is enrolled in a school setting.

ASHA and the Council on Education of the Deaf have published a technical report, *Service Provision to Children Who Are Deaf and Hard of Hearing, Birth to 36 Months* (see Appendix 2–L). This report details knowledge and skills needed by those individuals who are involved in the assessment and management of the auditory potential of this population, as well as the provision and management of sensory devices. Although the educational audiologist may not be the primary service provider in all of these areas, we can disseminate these best practice guidelines to all relevant individuals. This will help ensure that these guidelines are followed for infants and toddlers with hearing impairment.

If the infant or toddler is placed in a daycare or other nonpublic preschool setting, the educational audiologist should, at a minimum, observe the child's functioning for relevant acoustical information and functional listening skills (see previous section on classroom management strategies). If the child's placement is to fill a federally funded slot for students with disabilities or a state funded at-risk program placement in a regular daycare or preschool setting, the educational program is required to provide the necessary support services. The educational audiologist can serve as a resource for preschool programs for amplification equipment (both personal and classroom), appropriate curricula and materials for maximizing auditory learning, and other habilitation needs (see prior section on Indirect Service).

INCLUSION

We cannot conclude this chapter without a brief discussion of the inclusion philosophy as it applies to students who are deaf and hard-of-hearing. The term was *mainstreaming* in the 1970s and *integration* in the 1980s when discussing academic placements for children with disabilities. The importance of including all children in academic and social activities cannot be overlooked, but the effect of communication on true participation also needs to be recognized. Not every person perceives inclusion of students who are deaf and hard-of-hearing in the same way (Johnson & Cohen, 1994), and a thorough discussion of this topic is beyond the scope of this handbook (see Chapter 1, Educational Audiology, How Did We Get Here?

and Chapter 11, Individual Planning, for discussion of the legal history of inclusion and the least restrictive environment). Regardless of our personal philosophies, it is important to assist students who are placed in a mainstream environment to function as effectively and independently as possible within that setting.

Earlier in this chapter some strategies for student empowerment were discussed in the sections Development of Skills to Overcome Environmental Barriers, Informational Counseling, and Psychosocial Development. Knowledge about school and classroom rules can also help students assume responsibility for their own behavior and avoid unnecessary conflicts with teachers or peers. Often these classroom requirements are communicated incidentally, and the student who is hearing impaired misses this information. Answers to the following questions can assist the student in acting appropriately without calling attention to himself or herself, a prerequisite for inclusion:

➤ What are the most important rules in your classroom(s)?
➤ What are the rules for the cafeteria?
➤ What are the playground or school campus rules?
➤ What is the first thing you should do when you get to school?
➤ What is the last thing you should do before you go home at the end of the day?
➤ How do you know when your teacher wants you to be quiet?
➤ How do you know when your teacher is annoyed?
➤ How do you know your homework assignment?
➤ How do you know when you are allowed to talk in class?

Inclusion is important for all children, and the educational audiologist can be an important resource for facilitating the inclusion of students who are deaf or hard-of-hearing.

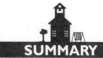

SUMMARY

In summary, the educational audiologist's focus in case management and aural (re)habilitation, whether service is direct or indirect, is on facilitating maximum use of auditory input during the learning process. This involves knowledge and dissemination of information regarding current technology, school operations, learning environments, teaching strategies, and content to be learned, as well as knowledge of individual students who are hearing impaired within this school system.

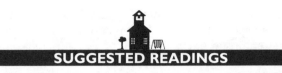

SUGGESTED READINGS

Berg, F. (1987). *Facilitating classroom listening: A handbook for teachers of normal and hard-of-hearing students.* Boston, MA: College-Hill Press.

Cole, E., & Gregory, H. (1986). *Auditory learning.* Washington, DC: AG Bell Association.

Davis, D. (1989). Otitis media: *Coping with the effects in the classroom.* Stanhope, NJ: Hear You Are, Inc.

Erber, N. (1982). *Auditory training.* Washington, DC: AG Bell Association.

Flexer, C. (1994). *Facilitating hearing and listening in young children.* San Diego, CA: Singular Publishing Group.

Luetke-Stahlman, B., & Luckner, J. (1991). *Effectively educating students with hearing impairment.* New York: Longman Publishing Company.

Maxon, A., & Brackett, D. (1992). *The hearing-impaired child: Infancy through high-school years.* Washington, DC: AG Bell Association.

National Association of State Directors of Special Education, Inc. (1994). *Deaf and hard of hearing students: Educational service guidelines.* Alexandria, VA: Author.

Ross, M. (1990). *Hearing impaired children in the mainstream.* Parkton, MD: York Press.

Tye-Murray, N. (Ed.) (1992). *Cochlear implants and children: A handbook for parents teachers and speech and hearing professionals.* Washington, DC: AG Bell Association.

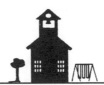

CHAPTER 8

HEARING CONSERVATION

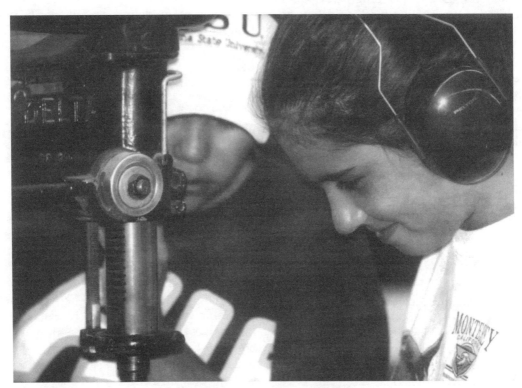

Lindsey and Jacob—Shop Class

CONTENTS

Many educational audiology job descriptions and standards documents include the area of hearing loss prevention and/or hearing conservation, but, in reality, this topic is often the one given lowest priority in the busy day-to-day schedule of the school-based audiologist. Although "prevention" comes before problem identification and remediation in the natural scheme of things, many factors contribute to the low position of prevention activities on the totem-pole of educational audiology duties and competencies.

First and foremost is the budget or funding of educational audiology personnel and materials. Most, if not all, school-based audiology positions stem from public laws that mandate services to students with *identified* disabilities, usually including participation in the identification process as a funded related service area (see Chapter 1, Educational Audiology: How Did We Get Here?). This practice leaves little or no time for attending to the prevention of these disabilities (i.e., hearing conservation programs).

In addition, school-based audiologists always seem to be in short supply, and personnel to design and deliver programs appropriate for preschool, elementary, and secondary school students may not be available. Creative materials and approaches may have been developed for specific projects, such as for a class or thesis, but the sharing of these materials is often not completed, due to both time and financial constraints.

On the positive side, the recent emphasis on *recreational audiology* has resulted in workshops and the development and dissemination of materials not previously available. One enterprising audiologist has implemented a program incorporating the use of customized hearing protection devices for professional football players (Gitlin, 1995), and individuals in the music industry are increasingly involved in programs designed to prevent hearing loss (Hall & Santucci, 1995). Many professional musicians have "gone public" with their own hearing difficulties, thus providing role models for many teens to acknowledge the potential for permanent damage from loud music.

Finally, the debate for health care reform has increased public awareness of the need for wellness programs that emphasize prevention of disease and disabilities. It is well known that exposure to high-intensity levels of sound may result in permanent hearing impairment, and, therefore, early education to prevent hearing loss from noise exposure is becoming more of a priority. As a result, the time is ripe for school-based audiologists to take advantage of new funding sources and commercially developed materials in the areas of hearing conservation, as well as to pursue the development and use of strate-

gies and materials that might be unique to individual school environments.

This chapter begins with general guidelines for developing a hearing conservation program for student populations of any age. Questions addressed in the first section include the following:

➤ What should be considered to plan an effective hearing conservation program?
➤ How can I make the most efficient use of materials and information?
➤ How can this program be funded?
➤ How should I provide for the inclusion of students with hearing impairments?

The general guidelines are followed by outlines for hearing conservation curricula that target four educational levels—preschool, elementary, middle, and high school.

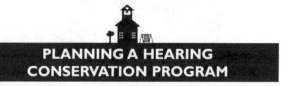

PLANNING A HEARING CONSERVATION PROGRAM

Ongoing Programming

Although many commercial materials lend themselves to one-shot opportunities (lectures, special productions, or videos), the emphasis in planning for a school-based audiologist should be follow-up to these introductions, if prevention is truly to occur. Designing activities that can be done later by the classroom teacher, paraprofessionals, or by students themselves—as independent study activities or homework—may be time-consuming initially, but will lead to the educational audiologist becoming an integral part of the curricular planning process, as opposed to a one-time "invited guest." For example, developing a handout to stimulate science fair projects takes time to complete but can lead to the school-based audiologist becoming routinely consulted for any project involving sound or acoustics in the future. Designing a curricular sequence from preschool through high school also increases the probability of retention of knowledge and skills for target student populations.

Curricular Interface

Suggestions specific to each educational level are given in the suggested hearing conservation curricula included later in this chapter, but, as a general rule, school-based audiologists need to become familiar with their individual schools' curricula and objectives and to learn the time-lines for interfacing recommended activities into these curricula. Serving on a school's curriculum committee is one approach to consider, but this can be a time-consuming strategy. Reading the curricula on one's own time, learning when the committee meets, and requesting time at a specific meeting to present suggestions orally and in writing can be less time-consuming and achieve the same results. Schedule a day or two prior to a curricular meeting to prepare materials to present to the committee; be prepared to state how much class time the program would require, but be ready to modify this time, if necessary. In situations where hearing conservation has not been included previously in the curriculum, even a minimal amount of time is a beginning. If there is documentation showing that such a program has been successful, there is a higher probability that additional time will be allocated in the future.

Teacher Involvement

It is important that all materials developed by the educational audiologist be reviewed by teachers at targeted grade levels prior to use. This practice ensures the developmental appropriateness of the materials, as well as increasing teacher support. Teachers' names should be included on handouts they have reviewed; they are more likely to feel compelled to use these handouts if they have some publicly acknowledged ownership. Feedback should be requested when handouts are distributed initially, but a follow-up request can be helpful before using a handout a second time.

Targeting the School Environment

Attention should be drawn to noise produced within the school environment at each educational level. One immediately thinks of industrial arts, band, and music classes as sources of excessive noise, but gymnasiums, cafeterias, and heating and cooling equipment produce noise levels that are also a major concern in the schools. Noise levels in classes can range from 85 dB to 115 dB (Lankford & West, 1993), and one of the current authors (JS) has measured intensity as high as 128 dB in a woodworking class. State industrial arts curricula should be reviewed for information concerning hearing loss. Most, if not all, include the use of safety glasses but rarely mention hearing protection devices. Student organizations can be alerted to the existence of potentially dangerous noise sources and encouraged to sponsor and promote projects such as limiting music levels at school functions. Additional ideas for activities are included in the suggested hearing conservation curricula sections later in this chapter.

Additional Architectural Information

The school-based audiologist should collect and disseminate information concerning architectural modifications that can reduce noise levels in school buildings. Sound reverberation is a major concern for students who have hearing impairments, as well as for those who have additional auditory learning problems (See Chapter 5, Central Auditory Processing Disorders, and Chapter 7, Case Management and Aural (Re)habilitation for additional information). When new buildings are being proposed and designed for school districts, information should be considered prior to construction concerning the potential adverse effects of various ceiling, floor, and wall materials, as well as the overall room design.

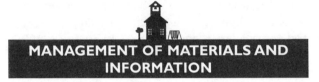

MANAGEMENT OF MATERIALS AND INFORMATION

Information Dissemination

Frequently, the educational audiologist will be asked to participate in inservice programs dealing with disabilities, specifically to provide information concerning referrals, assessment, hearing impairment, and assistive devices. Although the specified topic may not be hearing conservation, an attempt should be made to incorporate information on materials and activities that are related to the prevention of hearing loss. This information should be personalized with the educational audiologist's name and phone number for additional information, and a tear-off request form to be returned as individuals leave the inservice can lead to immediate opportunities for follow-up contacts.

Resource Material Availability

It is important for the educational audiologist to identify all commercial materials with the date they were received. In reviewing files and boxes that belong to the authors and their school-based audiology colleagues, many materials and programs were identified as no longer available. If there is no major demand for a program or product, it may be sold to another producer or donated to another source after a specified time period. By the time this book is in print, some of the resources available today undoubtedly will no longer be accessible, or will be available from a different source. Sources for materials or programs more than 3 years old should be contacted prior to recommending their order or use.

Copyright Laws

It is important to observe copyright laws for videos and written materials. This practice certainly applies to any material disseminated by the educational audiologist, but the temptation to copy published material in the area of hearing conservation can be great, especially when certain materials are not easily available.

Sharing with Peers

Several states have groups of educational audiologists who meet regularly for support, inservice, and sharing. If you can form or access such a peer group, this is an excellent way to exchange creative ideas and costly materials in the area of hearing conservation. Schedule a session at your state audiology or speech and hearing association meeting to share programs and materials that have been developed and/or used (successfully or unsuccessfully) in the schools.

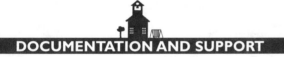

DOCUMENTATION AND SUPPORT

Recordkeeping

Following the completion of any activities that address hearing conservation, the educational audiologist should document what was done in order to enlist support for program continuation and expansion. A brief summary of goals, activities, time, and cost will help to inform the necessary school administrators. Specify all curricular objectives that were addressed, especially if these objectives are mandated by local or state curricula. Short letters of support from teachers and students will add to a positive view of the hearing conservation program, but letters of support from students' parents may have the most impact at budget-setting time. This material can be included in the educational audiologist's marketing information for use with administrators, teachers, parents, and the public (see Chapter 13, Marketing).

Funding

As mentioned in the introductory section to this chapter, traditional financial support for educational audiology programs rarely provides money for pre-

vention activities. As a result, school-based audiologists often need to access nontraditional funding sources for commercial materials and programs. Although some programs, such as the "Good Vibes" project by the Sertoma Foundation (see Elementary Hearing Conservation Program section for information), require involvement of a service club, other local service clubs may be willing to purchase materials, programs, and equipment for hearing conservation (especially if a program can be provided for one of their club meetings; see Chapter 9, Community Collaboration). In Colorado, hearing conservation efforts are supported through the Colorado Hearing Coalition, a consortium including the Colorado Speech-Language-Hearing Association, Colorado Academy of Audiology, Center for Hearing, Speech and Language, Colorado Hearing Foundation, Denver Ear Institute, the Listen Foundation, and Hear Now. Professional organizations and nonprofit agencies can be a resource to individual educational audiologists if there are not enough peers to develop a hearing consortium in your area. University programs and regional special education resource libraries are additional sources for current materials that can be loaned out to public schools.

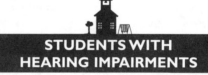

STUDENTS WITH HEARING IMPAIRMENTS

One final caution is for educational audiologists to be aware of the potential impact of a hearing conservation program on students who are deaf or hard-of-hearing. Hearing conservation programs place a positive value on hearing and a negative value on not hearing. If one or more students who are deaf or hard-of-hearing are included in the classes, activities may need to be modified to reflect sensitivity regarding students' self-esteem, diversity, and/or Deaf culture issues (see Chapter 7, Case Management and Aural (Re)habilitation). Although the goal of a hearing conservation program is to provide education regarding preventable hearing loss, care should be taken not to imply that individuals with hearing impairments are in any way inferior because of their hearing disability or that they are to blame in some way for having a hearing loss. Comments such as, "If you don't take care of your ears, you may have to wear a hearing aid," increase negative perceptions of amplification and may have the opposite effect of that intended for those students who do need auditory assistance in school. Involvement of these students in planning classroom presentations and activities can have a positive outcome, as students with hearing impairments can increase their awareness of potential damage from noise that could result in increased hearing loss for them as well.

All of the suggestions in the initial section may apply to areas covered in other chapters in this handbook, but they appear particularly appropriate for the area of hearing conservation, as educational audiologists increasingly promote hearing conservation within the school setting.

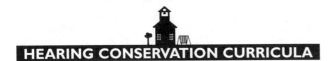

HEARING CONSERVATION CURRICULA

The following section provides outlines for hearing conservation programs that target four educational levels (preschool, elementary, middle, and high school). Outlines for each academic level address the following questions:

➤ What objectives should be covered?
➤ What content should be included?
➤ What individual and classroom activities are appropriate for the objectives?
➤ What commercial materials are currently available to supplement this program?

Specific ordering information for commercial materials is included in Appendix 16–J.

Preschool Hearing Conservation Program

Objective

Initial exposure to concepts about hearing and noise.

1. We hear with our ears.
2. We need to take care of our ears in order to hear.
3. Loud sounds can hurt our ears.

Content

1. Location and number of ears.
2. Sources of sound; loud versus soft.
3. Causes of damaging noise most common in this age group (fireworks, toys, race cars, tractors, motorcycles, snowmobiles).
4. Ways to avoid noise damage for preschoolers (stay away from use; move if sound hurts your ears).

Sample Activities

1. Find your ears; draw a person with ears; find/match pictures of ears; hold your ears while listening to music; cover your ears and listen again.
2. Draw/find/cut out/paste pictures of things that make loud sounds; same with soft sounds. Make a poster of each.
3. Group sound making toys in the class by loud versus soft.
4. Have group name things you like to hear; choose what you would miss hearing most if you could not hear.
5. Place poster of loud sounds and/or loud sound-making toys out of reach; soft sound close or within easy reach.
6. Distribute letters to parents suggesting activities to do at home (see Appendix 8–A).

Commercial Materials (See Appendix 16–J for ordering information)

1. Cartoon Poster on Healthy Hearing—features cartoon lion and elephant teaching lessons about hearing. Includes one 17″ × 22″ full color poster, 25 black and white posters for coloring, and classroom guide.

Elementary Hearing Conservation Program

Objective

Expand knowledge of concepts introduced in preschool.

1. Interface with school's curricular objectives on hearing (one of five senses, parts of the ear, how sound is transmitted, etc.). Grade level will determine specific objectives.
2. Loud noises can damage hearing.
3. We can help protect our ears from loud noises.

Content

1. How the ear transmits sound—specific content will be determined by curricula/grade level.
2. Damage to the ear from noise cannot be seen but can be temporary or permanent.

3. Causes of damaging noise (toys, fireworks, transportation, recreation activities, personal stereo headphones)—modify by grade level and personal observations.
4. Some rooms and locations are noisier than others.
5. Ways to avoid noise damage—see preschool program, and introduce earplugs; differentiate noise plugs versus swim plugs versus use of cotton.

Sample Activities

1. Poster contest (possible topics—what I like to hear; sounds that hurt your ears; ways to protect your ears)—top three winners win a set of earplugs.
2. Screen hearing (especially valuable if this is a grade not normally screened).
3. Show and Tell—bring something from home that makes noise.
4. Hide sound making object—locate and/or identify by sound only.
5. Walk on grass to demonstrate temporary versus permanent damage.
6. Identify noisy rooms and activities in school environment.
7. Discuss/draw how noisy rooms and quiet rooms make you feel.
8. Make a chart illustrating relative loudness of everyday sounds.
9. Distribute letter/handouts to parents (see Appendix 8–A).

Commercial Materials (See Appendix 16–J for ordering information)

1. Quiet Pleases III, "Listen Up for the Sounds of Your Life." Teaching module includes 28-minute video, brochures, poster, and five lesson plans for Grades 4–6.
2. "Operation SHHH." A program centered around an automatic sound-operated traffic light to be mounted in the school where the program is presented. Basic classroom package includes the light, 8 color posters, and 15 teacher kits (Teacher's Guide, 2 information booklets, 2 student activity charts, student workbook).
3. "Good Vibes." Newspaper tabloid on hearing that includes articles on hearing loss and noise appropriate for upper elementary. Materials are produced by Sertoma, who will furnish generic copies or masters that can be adapted for local use.

4. "I Love What I Hear!" Program includes eight-minute video and teachers guide for grades three through six. Produced by the National Institute on Deafness and Other Communication Disorders.
5. "Have you ever wondered about . . . The Ear and Hearing?" Informational pamphlet on the ear, hearing loss and steps to hearing health.
6. "Know Noise." Program includes 13-minute video, 2 audiotapes including the Unfair Hearing Test, 140-page instructor's manual including 26 lesson plans, supporting learning activities and transparencies. Targets students in grades 3–6.

Middle School Hearing Conservation Program

Objective

Understanding implications of damaging noise exposure and active use of ear protection when needed.

1. The inner ear is susceptible to permanent damage from noise.
2. Specific strategies can prevent this noise damage from occurring or from increasing.

Content

1. How the ear works and what part is damaged by noise exposure.
2. Noise damage can be permanent but can be prevented; can also prevent increased loss if problem already there.
3. Sources of damaging noise exposure (emphasize music and recreational sources).
4. Symptoms of excessive noise levels.
5. Ways to prevent damage from noise (avoidance, moving away from speakers, using ear plugs, temporary breaks).
6. Different surfaces reflect or absorb sound waves, affecting the intensity of noise.

Sample Activities

1. Screen hearing.
2. Facilitate interactive lectures, supplemented by videos.
3. Demonstrate/distribute earplugs for use.
4. Distribute articles by rock stars, sports figures regarding noise-induced loss; have class review

teen magazines for references to hearing loss caused by noise; suggest that individuals or entire class write to rock stars/sports figures/other idols who have hearing loss and ask how it has affected them.
6. Talk with science teacher regarding possible science fair projects, if school is involved.
7. Measure noise levels in various locations in school environment. Discuss reasons for excessive noise (e.g., structural considerations) and ways to modify.
8. Write article for school publication regarding noise sources in school environment.
9. Provide handout for students (see Appendix 8–B).

Commercial Materials (See Appendix 16–J for ordering information)

1. "Hip Talk." Program includes 34-minute video, curriculum guide, ear plugs, and HIP buttons.
2. "Say What . . .?" Program includes 12-minute audio cassette discussing hearing and hearing loss (demonstrates simulated high-frequency loss) and two noise-related posters.
3. "Stop That Noise." Program in 12-minute video, plus a curriculum targeting students in grades 4–7.

High School Hearing Conservation Program

Objective:

Knowledge necessary for prevention of hearing loss caused by occupational and/or recreational noise.

1. Damaging noise levels can occur in the workplace.
2. There are laws that require employers to protect employees from noise-induced hearing loss.
3. Individuals can and should take their own measures to prevent noise-induced hearing loss from recreational sources.

Content (interface with vocational and health curricula)

1. Expand information regarding anatomy of the ear with specific attention to cochlea and cochlear damage.
2. Audiogram and configuration associated with noise-induced loss.

3. Sources/levels for damage from noise exposure (occupational; recreational).
4. Temporary threshold shift (TTS) vs. permanent threshold shift (PTS).
5. Symptoms of noise damage.
6. Strategies for prevention; concepts of duration of exposure and distance from source—how they interact with potential for damage.
7. Expand concept of reverberation introduced in middle school.
8. Occupational Safety and Health Administration regulations in the workplace (OSHA, 1983).

Sample Activities

1. Videos.
2. Fit students with earplugs; review use and maintenance.
3. Measure vocational environments (e.g., transportation, woodworking) with sound-level meter; figure length of time allowed at sound levels recorded.
4. Measure concert/dance music and develop sample regulations for school activities.
5. Measure sound levels from car speaker with windows up vs. down.
6. Provide information to science coordinator for science fair projects.
7. Invite health/safety officer from local manufacturing plant to discuss their procedures for hearing protection.
8. Provide handout for students (see Appendix 8–B).
9. Write research paper and/or give oral presentation on noise exposure concerns (see Appendix 8–C for periodical reference list).

Commercial Materials (see Appendix 16–J for ordering information)

1. "HIP Talk." See Middle School Materials for description.
2. "People vs. Noise." Fifteen-minute video featuring famous Americans testifying in a simulated court situation about their own hearing losses caused by noise.
3. "Can't Hear You Knocking." Program includes 17-minute video featuring well-known musicians telling how their hearing has been damaged through loud music. Also includes brochures, earplugs, and lesson plans.
4. Additional H.E.A.R. materials (Hearing Education and Awareness for Rockers). Information packet

consisting of two sample brochures, "What Do These Musicians Know?" and "Noise, Ears, and Hearing Protection" (prepared by the American Academy of Otolaryngology); information on musicians' earplugs; copies of articles from periodicals such as *Rolling Stone, Modern Drummer, Rider,* and *Guitar Player.* T-Shirts, posters, postcards, and earplugs also available.

5. "An Earful of Sound Advice About Hearing Protection." Twelve-page illustrated pamphlet describing hearing conservation and various ear protection devices.

6. National Hearing Conservation Association educational materials. A set of four photos of the inner ear featured in three slides (cross sections of healthy and damaged cochleas, and side by side magnified images of healthy and damaged hair cells); "Noise Destroys" poster depicting a healthy inner ear and an inner ear damaged from repeated noise exposure.

SUGGESTED READINGS

Allonen-Allie, N., & Florentine, M. (1990). Hearing conservation programs in Massachusetts' vocational/technical schools. *Ear and Hearing, 11,* 237–239.

Anderson, K. (1991). Hearing conservation in the public schools revisited. *Seminars in Hearing, 12,* 340–364.

Chermak, G., Curtis, L., & Seikel, J. (1996). The effectiveness of an interactive hearing conservation program for elementary school children. *Language, Speech and Hearing Services in Schools, 27,* 29–39.

Chermak, G., & Peters-McCarthy, E. (1991). The effectiveness of an educational hearing conservation program for elementary school children. *Language, Speech and Hearing Services in Schools, 22,* 308–312.

Clark, W. (1991). Noise exposure from leisure activities: A review. *Journal of Acoustical Society of America, 90,* 175–181.

Danenber, M., Loos-Cosgrowe, M., & LoVerde, M. (1987). Temporary hearing loss and rock music. *Language, Speech and Hearing Services in Schools, 18,* 267–274.

Florentine, M. (1990). Education as a tool to prevent noise induced hearing loss. *Hearing Instruments, 41,* 33–34.

Frager, A., & Kahn, A. (1988). How useful are elementary school health text books for teaching about hearing health and protection? *Language, Speech and Hearing Services in Schools, 19,* 175–181.

Hardegree, D. (1992). *The necessity and effectiveness of a hearing conservation program for third grade students.* Unpublished Ed.S. Thesis, Utah State University, Logan, UT.

Lass, N., Woodford, C., Lundeen, D., & Everly-Myers, S. (1986). The prevention of noise-induced hearing loss in the school-aged population: A school educational hearing conservation program. *Journal of Auditory Research, 26,* 247–254.

Lass, N., Woodford, C., Lundeen, C., Lundeen, D., Everly-Myers, S., McGuire, K., Mason, D., Patnik, L., & Phillips, R. (1987). A hearing conservation program for a junior high school. *The Hearing Journal, 40,* 32–40.

Lewis, D. (1989). A hearing conservation program for high-school-level students. *The Hearing Journal, 42,* 19–24.

Pelson, R., & Trestik, J. (1987). Public school hearing conservation in Oregon. *Language, Speech, and Hearing Services in Schools, 18,* 241–249.

Peppard, A., & Peppard, S. (1992). Noise-induced hearing loss: A study of children at risk. *The Hearing Journal, 45,* 33–35.

Plakke, B. (1991). Hearing conservation training of industrial technology teachers. *Language, Speech and Hearing Services in Schools, 22,* 134–138.

Roeser, R. (1980). Industrial hearing conservation programs in the high schools. *Ear and Hearing, 1,* 119–120.

COLLABORATION AND PLANNING

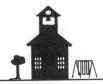

CHAPTER 9

COMMUNITY COLLABORATION

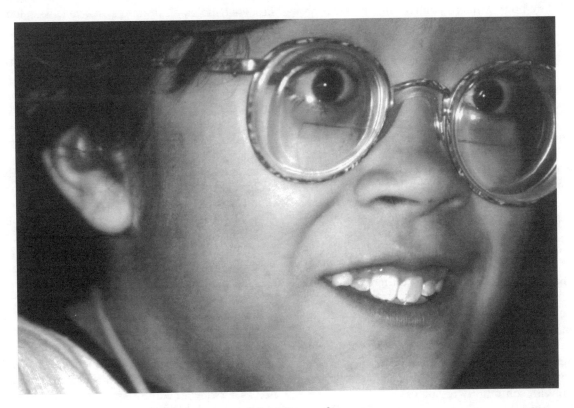

Samantha, age 8

CONTENTS

Providing community leadership through collaboration can help to ensure that all infants, toddlers, and youth with impaired hearing are promptly identified, evaluated, and provided with appropriate intervention services. Reasons for developing and maintaining community collaboration are listed below:

➤ Establishing good community relationships leads to more efficient service-delivery for the consumers who are students, families, and the local school system.
➤ Knowledge of what is available in the community can prevent duplication of services and lead to more cost-effective delivery of services.
➤ Collaboration with community members results in a better exchange of information, thus easing the referral process for medical, audiological, and educational follow-up for students with hearing problems.
➤ Families have improved access to identification information, support, and appropriate services for their children through a collaborative system.
➤ Community collaboration can result in support from community leaders, parents, and other service providers when funding crises occur (see Table 9–1).

Community members can also assist in establishing priorities when services must be cut or altered. Knowledge of what community resources currently exist and how to access them and obtain their support in the design and delivery of school-based audiology service is invaluable to the educational audiologist. Questions to be asked during this process include the following:

➤ What audiology services are currently available within this community?
➤ Are there gaps in the audiology services that currently exist?
➤ Could the school-based audiology program fill gaps that have been identified?
➤ What strategies can be used to facilitate collaboration with community resources?
➤ How can community and school-based audiology programs support and enhance each other?

Table 9–1. Target areas for community support during funding crises.

➤ Advocacy
➤ Lobbying
➤ Financial contributions
➤ Assistance with fund-raising activities
➤ Ideas for alternate funding sources

This chapter will attempt to answer these questions by suggesting strategies to identify and interface with existing community resources. In addition, techniques will be described to assist the educational audiologist in the development of relationships with community resources that can foster ongoing collaboration.

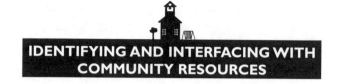

IDENTIFYING AND INTERFACING WITH COMMUNITY RESOURCES

Community Needs Assessment Overview

Completion of an initial needs assessment that identifies what audiologic resources are available in the community at present and the population(s) for whom these services are available is a critical first step in developing a network for community collaboration. (More detail concerning the content and design of this needs assessment is provided in the following section.) As this needs assessment is completed, gaps in services should be identified, and gaps that the educational audiology program can address should be highlighted. Whenever possible, these activities should be completed prior to initiating any school-based audiology service, because it is much more difficult to modify or drop a service (even one that is a duplication) once it has been delivered. For example, if a hearing aid bank already exists in the community and can be made accessible to students who need loaner hearing aids, it may require less time and/or expense to phase into this existing bank than it would to establish a duplicate bank within the school facility. If no hearing aid bank exists, this is a gap in services that the school-based audiologist may wish to make a top priority.

If the educational audiology program already exists and a community needs assessment has never been completed, the time spent on this activity can be justified as a review of current services to see if costly and unnecessary duplication exists. Once the information is documented, it becomes obvious when services, such as measuring functional listening skills or classroom observation/collaboration, are not available. This documentation can help when promoting the development of a school-based audiology program that does include these services.

Designing the Initial Community Needs Assessment

A community needs assessment should list all of the programs and agencies who deliver audiology services in the community, as well as potential resources for financial and volunteer support for a school-based audiology program. Questions that should be answered through a needs assessment format include the following:

➤ What specific individuals and agencies deliver audiology services?
➤ What services are currently offered by each individual and agency?
➤ What do these services cost?
➤ When and where are these services available?
➤ Who offers related medical services? Where, and at what cost?
➤ How does one make referrals to these individuals and agencies?
➤ How is information obtained from these individuals and agencies?
➤ What agencies or organizations might provide support for additional audiology services?

At a minimum, the needs assessment should include the previous information for the areas and community resources listed in Table 9–2. A more detailed description of each target area follows, and a sample format for compiling the needs assessment information is included as Appendix 9–A.

Newborn Screening Programs

Newborn screening programs have increased in both number and scope as technology has improved and become more readily accessible in local communities. It is critical for educational audiologists to be aware of screening programs that identify children within the local school districts and to obtain current information on these programs. Suggested strategies and questions for the educational audiologist include the following:

Table 9–2. Target areas for educational audiology community needs assessment.

➤ Newborn screening programs
➤ Child find programs
➤ Hospital services
➤ Physicians
➤ Community-based audiologists
➤ Public health clinics
➤ University training programs
➤ Service clubs
➤ Parent support groups
➤ Advocacy organizations
➤ Child care agencies
➤ Recreation services
➤ Other funding sources

➤ List and describe each program and identify the test method or high risk registry approach that is utilized.
➤ Identify the funding source and current fees that are charged, noting that rates are subject to change and should be verified.
➤ Identify the contact person who is in charge of the screening and follow-up portions of the program.
➤ Identify what information is given to parents at the time of the initial screening and in what form this information is given.

How can the school-based audiologist and/or parent obtain results (either pass or fail), and what method should be used by the school system to access this program for referrals? Most neonatal screening programs report difficulty with family compliance for follow-up (re-screening or diagnostic testing), and this may be a gap that the school-based audiologist can help to fill. The educational audiologist also can assist in providing additional information concerning educational risks resulting from hearing loss, as well as other information designed for parents about hearing and hearing loss. (See Chapter 10, Relationships with Families, for suggested content for a resource booklet for parents.)

Other Child Find Programs

If additional programs within the community include the identification of hearing loss in children, the educational audiologist's community needs assessment should provide for the following:

➤ List and identify any program, such as Headstart, that is not included in any other category but which screens children for hearing in the community.
➤ Identify the name, address, and phone number of the contact person.
➤ List screening method and personnel utilized.
➤ Identify what happens to children who fail community or agency screenings.

For example, the local mall may sponsor an annual health screening day that includes pure-tone hearing screening administered by local Kiwanis Club members. Is information kept in a master file, given to parents, or available for service providers? Are parents given a list of referral sources in the community, as well as notified that free screenings and audiologic assessments can be obtained through their child's school? Is this a program that has one or more gaps that the school-based audiologist could fill (e.g., assistance in training and supervision of those who screen hearing, provision of written information about hearing loss and school audiology program, referral forms, etc.)? Best practice calls for the school-based audiologist to be involved in the design and/or implementation of any community screening project that includes children.

Hospital Services

Most community hospitals provide services related to hearing in the pediatric population. Relevant information for the educational audiologist can be obtained through the following activities:

➤ List and describe each program provided through the local hospital(s) on an outpatient basis.
➤ Cross-reference any newborn screening program provided by the hospital, if it has already been described.
➤ Identify the contact person for program services.
➤ Identify the individual to contact for reimbursement questions.
➤ Clarify the schedule and any restrictions for services.
➤ Identify the most efficient way for the school system to access written reports and recommendations.
➤ Identify the individual in charge of receiving and disseminating information from the educational setting.

Services for children may include (but are not limited to) those identified in Table 9–3.

Are there specific days of the weeks that certain services are not available? Are there any services that are available only for certain age groups? How does medical treatment interface with community physician or clinic treatment?

Table 9–3. Potential pediatric hearing services available from hospital programs.

➤ Hearing screening
➤ Behavioral auditory assessment
➤ Electrophysiologic auditory assessment
➤ Assessment of vestibular function
➤ Otologic assessment
➤ Otologic treatment
➤ Personal amplification
  Evaluation
  Fitting
  Dispensing
➤ Assistive devices
  Evaluation
  Fitting
  Dispensing
➤ Aural (re)habilitation

Answers to these questions are critical to the educational audiologist, who may be involved in communicating this information to parents and school personnel.

Physicians

Physicians are a key resource for both referral and treatment of pediatric hearing loss. Activities that target these professionals include the following:

➤ Develop a current list of otologists (identifying those who specialize in pediatric or neuro-otology), pediatricians, general practitioners, and any other physicians who assess and/or treat hearing problems in children that are within a reasonable geographic distance for families.
➤ List each physician's primary office, address and phone number, as well as any satellite offices and the days available.
➤ List audiologist(s), if employed in physician office, but specify audiology services under private practice audiologist category.
➤ If third party payments (such as Medicaid) are not universally accepted in the community, this information should be noted for each physician.

Community Audiologists

Information about services provided by local audiologists is vital to include in a community needs assessment completed by the educational audiologist. The following strategies can be helpful in obtaining accurate information:

➤ List each audiologist's name, address(es), phone number(s) and schedule, if not full time in one office.
➤ Identify physician by name only, with day(s) available at this site.
➤ Describe audiology services and any specialized equipment/facilities for children (e.g., VRA, otoacoustic emissions, sedated ABR).
➤ Identify options for reimbursement and fees for services, if available.
➤ Include audiologists in private practice, as well as those in private or nonprofit clinics in this section.

Public Health Clinic Options

It is critical to know if public health is designated by state law as the responsible agency for hearing screening in children (see Chapter 3, Identification Practices). In some states there is a legal mandate for state-managed health department involvement, but in other cases their responsibility has been taken on "by default." Questions to be answered include the following:

➤ Are there now duplicate mandates for school-age children resulting in program duplication?
➤ Are all residents eligible, with some differentiation between those who can pay and those who cannot?
➤ What are the hours, and do they schedule appointments?
➤ Is there a fee schedule and is every service available during all hours of operation?
➤ What is the method used for screening hearing, who are the personnel involved, and at what ages are screenings completed? (See Chapter 3, Identification Practices, for more information on screening methods and follow-up.)
➤ Do health clinic personnel come to the schools to do health screenings?

For each community there is a need to identify the pediatric population eligible for assessment/treatment through the local public health clinic. Clarify what information is provided to parents of children who fail the hearing screening and what recommendations are made. Finally, list a primary contact person for child health within each community clinic serving children from the local school system.

University Training Programs

Post-secondary training programs in speech-language pathology and audiology often provide hearing services for the community at large. The school-based audiologist should obtain and summarize information about any college or university program within the local community by completing the following tasks:

➤ List audiology services provided for children and cost, if available.
➤ Identify advantages versus restrictions related to obtaining services through a training program. (For example, do they have access to the latest equipment and technology? Do assessments take longer, but cost less? Do they require fees in a lump sum, or can payment schedules be arranged? Can they provide services off-campus and what is their availability during university vacation schedules?).
➤ List a contact person with phone number, and identify if this is the same contact person for the general public. If not, list the public access phone number as well.

Service Clubs

Service Clubs can provide significant support to school-based audiology programs. Listed below are suggestions for collecting relevant information for this community resource:

➤ List all service clubs with chapters in the local community that have hearing or hearing loss as an official club focus. A list of national organizations that currently emphasize hearing is included in Appendix 16–K.
➤ Identify the contact person and phone number for information about current projects and potential funds for school-based audiology and students with hearing impairments.
➤ Note the fiscal year for each club, and the procedure for making financial requests
➤ Identify the program chair, club meeting day and time, and dates for program planning for the year.

Other Community Resources

Any other categories of community resources available to the educational audiology program should be included, with information concerning the type of support, personnel involved, and ways to contact for collaboration. These might include, but are not limited to parent support groups, parent or professional advocacy groups, hearing aid funding sources, sign language classes, child care, churches, and recreation services designed to include students with hearing disabilities.

Updating the Community Needs Assessment

The community needs assessment requires annual updating, because community services and personnel change frequently. Once a functional format has been devised, updating previously listed resources should take a brief telephone call, with more time required only for new resources. Updating can be completed by mail, but return rates will vary when this method is used. If no response is received, a follow-up telephone call will be necessary; therefore, updating initially by telephone may turn out to be a more efficient use of time and money. If pertinent questions are listed beforehand, updating a list of community resources is an activity that can be handled by a volunteer or paraprofessional, unless direct contact with the school-based audiologist will promote the relationship with resource personnel. Annual needs assessment information should be summarized in a format that lends itself to presentations. Useful presentation formats include transparancies and/or slides, but whenever possible the layout and content should be computerized, so that modifications can be made quickly. Information on audiologic services available in the community can be included in presentations to parent groups, community service clubs, or government groups, and is most useful in presentations to school administrators who are responsible for funding school services. A visual graphic that clearly demonstrates that school-based audiology services do not duplicate other services in the community promotes good will among professionals and helps in lobbying for financial support for the educational audiology program.

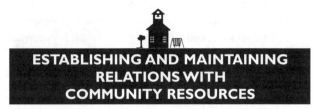

ESTABLISHING AND MAINTAINING RELATIONS WITH COMMUNITY RESOURCES

Providing Community Education

Whether the school-based audiology program has been in place or just begun services, it is critical to educate the community resources about the program. Members of the community frequently are not aware that audiology services are mandated and available free of charge to children through the school system. As a result they often do not know how to access or support these services.

Community collaboration requires communication. When a new program or service is available within a community, information should be disseminated, both in writing and in person, at every opportunity. Updates should be made available when program changes occur and/or on an annual basis. Use of a consumer survey for program effectiveness can assist in increasing awareness of educational audiology services by those who receive this inquiry (see Appendix 13–E for a sample consumer survey). High visibility leads to increased utilization of services and promotes better understanding when attempting to expand or change services. Some specific strategies that can be used to increase community awareness about the school-based audiology program and services are identified in Table 9–4 and described in more detail in Chapter 13, Marketing. Although many of the suggestions listed in Table 9–4 appear simple or self-evident and require minimal time to implement, they can pay off in increased opportunities for collaboration with a variety of community resources.

Table 9–4. Strategies to increase community awareness of educational audiology.

> ➤ Writing letters
> ➤ Developing and disseminating brochures
> ➤ Giving presentations
> ➤ Writing articles
> ➤ Giving radio/TV interviews
> ➤ Providing public acknowledgments
> ➤ Using business cards and stationery

Letters

Take time to write a letter to all potential referral sources briefly describing the educational audiology program and how to access services. A written update that identifies new personnel and any modification of prior services should be sent at the beginning of each school year to all potential referral sources. This update should also repeat specific referral information (e.g., who is eligible, services provided, contact person, address, and phone number). Include referral forms if they are required. (See Appendix 9–B for sample letter.)

Brochures

Development of a brochure for the educational audiology program is an efficient way to disseminate information. Now that desktop publishing is readily available, brochures are much less costly to produce. If funds are not available through the school, brochures can be funded by specific grants from parent groups, community organizations, or professional organizations. If the community includes a college or technical school, talk with the instructors of journalism or business education classes to see if a brochure could be a class project. Some larger high schools may also have the computer capability to design and/or print brochures, and they will learn about the educational audiology program if it is included in class assignments. Brochures should be as timeless as possible. List job titles, rather than individual names, and describe services in terms that will not be dated by changes in funding or legislation. Photographs can be eye-catching, but graphic illustrations tend to be less dated. The educational audiologist should carry a few brochures with him or her at all times and distribute them at any presentation. In addition, a brochure should be included in the annual update sent to community professionals and agencies who are potential referral sources.

Presentations

Presentations to parent, professional, and other community groups are very useful for educating residents of the community. Many service clubs have hearing as their primary or secondary focus (see Appendix 16–K), and these clubs are always looking for interesting programs. As recommended in the section that described the design of a needs assessment, find out who is in charge of the service club schedule at the beginning of the year and offer to speak at one of their meetings. Local physician, nursing, speech and hearing, early intervention, and other professional groups may also meet on a regular basis with scheduled programs or presentations.

Keep visual aids, such as slides, videos, and transparencies, on hand in order to respond to "unscheduled" requests for programs for community groups. Topics of interest to community service clubs and the public are listed in Appendix 9–C, and resources for topic information are identified in Appendix 16–L. In an ever-changing field such as audiology, it is important to maintain current topic information. A quick call or form letter to a national resource can be completed by a volunteer during pre-planning, to insure that resource material is still available. Always supplement any general information with local information, brochures, slides, or videos. Joint presentations with another professional or a family who has received services frequently draw and maintain high interest.

Articles

Submit an article for the local newspaper or a letter to the editor concerning pediatric hearing loss. Offer to be interviewed by a local journalist. Children always make good subjects for pictures, and hearing loss has broad appeal as a topic. Professional organizations, such as ASHA, disseminate news bulletins over the national wire when newsworthy items concerning communication disorders occur. These bulletins can be leads for stories about local programs. Include a name and phone number for additional information somewhere in the article or letter. Cultivate a local contact for the paper who will be receptive to information about the educational audiology program and the students and families served.

Radio or TV Interviews

If there is a local radio or television talk show, pick a topic with which you feel comfortable and offer to participate in a broadcast. Most local stations are looking for new topics to present, and when provided with interesting written information, they may be willing to present or moderate a program for the public. If a collaborative program already exists, arrange for a person representing the community agency or service club to participate in the interview. Offer to be a resource on hearing and hearing loss for any local radio or TV station. Be sure to have any radio or television interview taped for future use—these can be great supplements to formal presentations.

Public Acknowledgments

Public acknowledgment of support from community organizations or agencies serves not only to promote goodwill with members of these organizations, but it can also serve as another way to raise community awareness of the school-based audiology program. Local publications frequently print pictures of community leaders receiving awards. Letters to the editor of the local newspaper can also acknowledge support, and a story about a specific project or piece of equipment funded by a community organization might be printed. If such stories are not easily outdated, the publication may use it on a day when the news is slow. Copies of any such publicity should be collected and maintained in a format (such as a scrapbook) that can be displayed during any meeting or presentation.

Business Cards and Professional Stationery

For any of the previously mentioned written correspondence, use stationery and a signature that identifies your educational audiology program by name. Always carry business cards that identify you as an educational audiologist and that give your business address and phone number. Sign your letters to the editor with your title and program name, or include this in the body of the letter so that they will be published.

Facilitating Professional Collaboration

School-based audiology can be perceived as a duplication of and, therefore, in competition with other services provided in the community. Portraying the roles and responsibilities of the school program and their relationship to community resources will clarify how the programs support one another and preserve their uniqueness. Each professional contacted should be asked for his or her input concerning gaps in audiological services within the community and for ways the educational audiologist can support their program so that all services can best complement each other. By seeking input directly from the other audiologists in the community, the fear that school-based audiologic services are meant to replace private services can be alleviated. If a concern is expressed (e.g., no one follows up on neonatal screening failures), it should be addressed as quickly as possible—especially if the program is just beginning. The incorporation of a service not currently available or referal to an existing source that has been identified are both ways of addressing concerns. Send a note to the professional who expressed the concern describing how it was addressed. As mentioned in the previous section, joint professional presentations can help to clarify audiology options within the community for the presenters, as well as the audience.

Take every opportunity to emphasize that a priority of the school-based audiology program is to avoid duplication of services. This point can lead to an expanded client base, because the educational audiologist can and should serve as a "bridge" between clinical audiology and educational services, rather than replacing or duplicating clinical assessment and follow-up. Even when the educational audiology program includes opportunities for similar or identical assessments, parents often choose to utilize both resources, and thus continued collaboration will be required.

It is important that all parties—students, parents, clinical audiologists, and other professionals—understand the responsibility of the school to focus on the educational part of audiology, that is the impact of hearing and auditory function on learning and communication within the educational environment. For students with hearing disabilities, this includes determining the additional impact of noise, distance, auditory-visual factors, type and use of hearing aids and other assistive devices, appropriate classroom accommodations and modifications, as well as direct instructional services. For services to be most appropriate for students assessed by nonschool-based audiologists, ongoing communication regarding individual students is essential (Seaton, 1991).

When schools contract for services from community audiologists, services should be delineated in the contract and duplication avoided (ASHA, 1993). If community audiologists are not under contract, the school-based audiologist can help to clarify the responsibilities each professional can take. For example, on-site amplification management is necessary for optimum use of residual hearing in the classroom. When this is a designated responsibility of the educational audiologist, monitoring and maintenance are implemented more often, repairs can often be completed without the student missing school, replacement parts can be obtained more quickly, and appropriate loaner aids can be provided when necessary (Bollella-Sample, 1994). In this way the amplification follow-up program becomes more efficient and cost-effective for everyone involved.

Fostering Creative Collaborative Efforts

There are as many ways to collaborate creatively as there are individuals attempting to do so. Suggestions listed in Table 9–5 and discussed in the following sections represent a few ideas that might work for some communities. This list is not exhaustive and should be expanded and updated for each school population.

Otology Clinics

Arrange for monthly otologic clinics to be held at public health facilities or another central location. As

Table 9–5. Areas for creative community collaboration.

> Otology clinics
> Leasing facilities and equipment
> Student practicum
> Research
> Special projects
> Vocational opportunities
> Newborn screening
> Unique community needs
> Contractual services
> Producing public or parent information
> Monthly interagency staffings

health care delivery systems change in the future (see Chapter 15, Contemporary Issues: Where are We Going?), this may be a cost-effective way to obtain medical examinations for children who do not have access through other means.

Leasing Facilities and Equipment

The school system may want to consider renting audiologic facilities from a university program or an audiology private practice for assessment of students closer to their school or for access to equipment not available within the school program. University training programs, in particular, may offer state-of-the-art technology that a local school district cannot afford to purchase, and many training programs are required to document community service to earn a portion of their funding. Cost savings can occur by avoiding large expenditures for audiologic equipment, but input may or may not be requested from the educational audiologist when additional equipment is being purchased. Also, when arranging such agreements, school systems need to be made aware of the expense of maintaining audiologic equipment, because additional use by the educational audiologist could result in increased repair cost.

Student Practicum Sites

Another option for collaboration with university training programs is to establish on-campus or off-campus opportunities for students to obtain practicum hours under the supervision of the school-based audiologist. Training programs often need both patients with hearing impairments and additional supervisory personnel. All professional organizations, including the Educational Audiology Association, support increased practicum experiences for students in actual work environments. This option is not viable, however, unless the educational audiologist has the current credential required for audiology supervision. Practicum may include screening, assessment, management of hearing aids and assistive devices, as well as all phases of classroom management. Chapter 2, Roles and Responsibilities of the Educational Audiologist, provides a more detailed discussion of areas that could be included in such a practicum experience.

Assistance with Research

Development of grant proposals is a third way to collaborate with audiology training programs that can benefit both the school-based audiology program and the higher education setting. Assisting with research subjects can result in access to additional personnel and equipment that school districts are unable to fund.

Joint Projects with Service Clubs

Collaboration with local service clubs can result in the development and maintenance of a loaner hearing aid bank for student use. Where possible, this bank should involve community audiologists and be accessible to consumers of all ages who need hearing aids but cannot afford their purchase. Group amplification systems (e.g., sound-field FM), packaged hearing conservation programs, program brochures, and videos can also result from collaboration with community resources. These clubs are not only a source of funding, but also many club members have connections for publishing at a discount fee, resources for photography and illustrations, and additional ideas and options for inexpensive dissemination of materials.

Vocational Opportunities

Collaboration with local service club members can also result in invaluable vocational connections for secondary students looking for job information or job placements. Often community members are willing and eager to be available for presentations to classes or be interviewed by students. Vocational placements can be facilitated and result in an opportunity for the educational audiologist to increase awareness of methods for achieving accessibility in work sites.

Newborn Hearing Screening

Collaboration of community resources can lead to the creation and implementation of a newborn screening program and follow-up process, if not already in place within the community. Participation in this activity promotes increased awareness of the need for earlier identification of hearing loss and resulting intervention services, facilitates continuity between community-based and school-based programming, and can lower the age of identification within a targeted community.

Solutions for Unique Community Needs

Community resources can be brought together to brainstorm and propose solutions to specific problems, such as special transportation needs, interpreter requests, and the provision of mental health and other services delivered outside the school setting. The sharing of community resources usually results in the most efficient and cost-effective solutions so that all citizens benefit.

Contractual Services

Another avenue for community collaboration, contracting with community-based audiologists for school services, has been discussed in Chapter 2, Roles and Responsibilities of the Educational Audiologist. As stated in the *ASHA Guidelines for Audiology Services in the Schools* (see Appendix 2–B), contracts should include staff development activities that pertain to associated educational issues. Participation in these activities will result in increased awareness of educational policies and procedures, as well as the design and scope of the school-based audiology program.

Producing Public or Parent Information

Chapter 10, Relationships with Families, describes the development of a parent resource packet that resulted from a collaborative effort in Colorado. Community audiologists worked together to develop the contents, initial production and mailing costs were underwritten by the Colorado Department of Education, and duplication costs were absorbed by individual audiologists who disseminated information to their clients. This is an excellent example of a product that can be the result of effective community collaboration.

Monthly Interagency Staffings

In New York City, Albert Einstein Hospital now collaborates with the local school for the deaf through monthly interagency staffings (J.Gravel, April 19, 1996, personal communication). Although these meetings were initiated to discuss specific students shared by the two facilities, collaboration now occurs for many of the current and proposed educational audiology services for all students enrolled in this educational program.

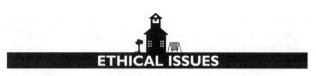

ETHICAL ISSUES

It is important to recognize potential conflict of interest issues if community resources are utilized for services and/or equipment as a part of the school-based audiology program. All appropriate community resources must be given the opportunity to participate in programs, such as otologic clinics and community hearing aid banks, to avoid the perception of referral bias. On the other hand, school responsibility versus private responsibility for audiology services must be spelled out in the contract to avoid conflict-of-interest situations that arise when the same audiologist fulfills the school contract as well as the private audiology services in a community (ASHA, 1993). In any situation where educational audiology services are provided through a collaborative agreement with resources from the community, familiarity with current profes-

sional guidelines regarding ethical standards and conflicts of interest is of utmost importance.

SUMMARY

In summary, community collaboration is an essential component of any comprehensive educational audiology program. Programs can be enhanced by increased awareness of services, leading to a greater variety of available resources. From decreasing the age of identification to increasing the number and extent of opportunities for secondary students with hearing impairments, results from community involvement in the school-based audiology program are only as limited as one's willingness and ability to collaborate with school, parents, teachers, special support personnel, relevant community agencies, organizations, and other professionals.

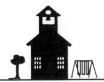

CHAPTER 10

RELATIONSHIPS WITH FAMILIES

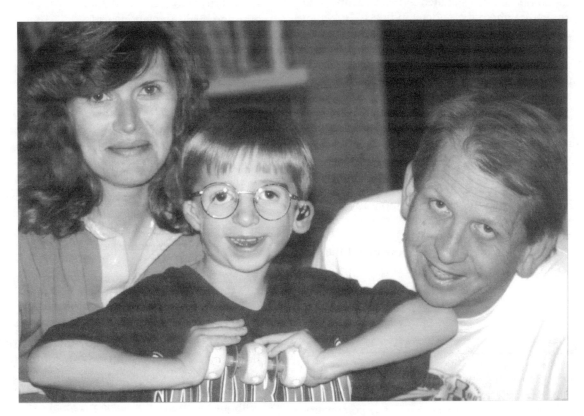

MaryAnn, Erich, and Kyle

CONTENTS

Balancing the desires of parents and the opinions of professionals may be one of the most difficult challenges facing those of us in education. As parents have acquired greater knowledge and interest in their children's educations, they have demanded more accountability and pushed "individualization" to obtain services that more specifically address their desires. PL 99-457 (now Part H of IDEA), more than any other single cause, has heightened our awareness of the needs and roles of families. The shift from being *the* specialist to becoming *multi-* and *inter*disciplinary has not always been easy for audiologists or other professionals. Yet the power and impact of collaboration by a team of specialists which includes parents as equal partners cannot be overestimated. A relationship based on partnership where the understanding is "together we can" goes a lot further in supporting a successful educational process than a "we-they" one.

This chapter addresses the following questions to emphasize conditions crucial to establishing and maintaining positive relationships with parents:

➤ How can positive attitudes be developed and maintained with families?
➤ How can effective communication be established with families?
➤ How should information be provided to families?
➤ What can parents do to become more involved in school activities and support the specific needs of deaf and hard-of-hearing children?
➤ When difficult situations arise, how might they be handled?

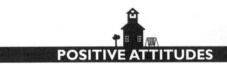

POSITIVE ATTITUDES

Effective relationships with parents begin with healthy attitudes. The attitudes that people develop are, for the most part, shaped by experience and personality. Some people have more pessimistic viewpoints, tending to expect the worst from a situation, while others have outlooks that are more hopeful. As audiologists, we must work with a variety of people. In public education, where there is no option of choosing whether to provide services for children and their families, the attitudes of some parents can be very counterproductive. Establishing effective relationships with parents requires a reciprocal understanding where both parties share respect and trust to sustain their partnership. Rapport, respect, and trust are considered in the following sections as important steps when building effective relationships with families. The use of these strategies should have a positive influence on the attitudes of the individuals involved.

Rapport

Establishing rapport with a family is the first step toward building a healthy relationship.

1. We should attempt to understand how the family functions, their resources, and interaction style. Using this understanding can help us adopt an interaction style which is compatible with the family's style and respond to them accordingly. Although a professional atmosphere must always be maintained, it is possible to be relaxed with some families, formal with others, frank with some, and gentle with others. Attitudes of intimidation or superiority have no constructive purpose when building healthy relationships.

2. One effective approach for developing rapport is called "joining the family" (Haley, 1976). Haley suggested that interventionists become part of the family system as a way to be a more integral part of the support structure and, in the end, achieve more effective services for young children. Although home programming is not a routine activity for many audiologists, there are several advantages to "house calls." A visit to the home to meet the family members can not only help to establish the relationship, but also will provide the audiologist with valuable insights and information that facilitate intervention efforts during the diagnostic, (re)habilitative, and educational process. The visit provides an opportunity to assess the home environment informally, resulting in information regarding such factors as house and room size, communication styles between family members, structure of communication, functional use of hearing, discipline, daily routines, and available toys and materials.

3. Empathy is another important component to building a relationship. Despite what some individuals believe, audiologists can be empathetic without having had similar personal experiences. The development of good reflective listening skills is the most important characteristic of being empathetic. The audiologist should also learn what questions to ask, when to ask them, and how to interact in a nondomineering and nonjudgmental manner. This demonstration of genuine care and commitment to assisting the family is essential. The ability to put oneself in the family's situation and to look outward from their perspective often provides a more realistic understanding of the family's concerns and needs and results in a stronger partnership with the family. The letter *Welcome to Holland* (see Appendix 10–A), has often been used as an example of how parents feel on learning of their child's disability. In addition to being a beneficial

resource to share with parents, it should be read by all professionals who work with children.

Respect

To continue to develop a strong relationship, all parties should respect one another. Respect does not mean agreement. Rather, it describes how people are treated and the honor they hold for one another's beliefs.

1. Recognition of the importance of the parents and family in the diagnostic and (re)habilitative phases of hearing impairment is essential. Audiologists, regardless of their own personal biases, must maintain an open attitude and acceptance of the options a family may choose. Respect for the family's time, their need to understand all information clearly, including the audiology services and intervention program, and their need to make decisions for their child's current and future needs reinforces their role as the primary caregiver and case manager in the long-term process. Likewise, the parents and family should also be respectful of the audiologist's time, efforts, and support to them.
2. A sensitivity for socio-economic, family constellation, and cultural differences and acceptance of the unique characteristics that may be associated with them is also a component of respect. Services need to be responsive to family values and beliefs. If audiologists are uncomfortable with certain cultural issues or working with disadvantaged economic conditions, they should remove themselves from the case.
3. Maintain confidentiality at all times; the world of hearing impairment is surprisingly small.

Trust

Once rapport and respect have been established, trust should be inherent. The passage of time continues to strengthen good relationships.

1. Credibility is a critical feature of the trust component. Professional competence must be demonstrated before trust with the audiologist can be established. The audiologist's expertise should be exhibited in the technical aspects of diagnostics and (re)habilitation, communication skills, networks with other agencies, and follow-through. Audiologists should be careful to make only commitments that they can fulfill.
2. Recognize when referrals to other individuals should be made for services that are either outside the purview of audiology or beyond the audiologist's level of expertise (just as educational audiol-

ogists specialize in pediatric habilitation, other audiologists may provide more expertise when fitting certain types of hearing aids).
3. Trust in a relationship evolves and, therefore, is strengthened over time as the interactions between the parties continue to reinforce the initial foundation on which it was begun.

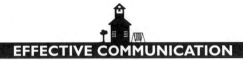

EFFECTIVE COMMUNICATION

Parents deserve open, honest communication. This means that professionals must take time to listen, and must set aside prejudices and biases to work as a member of a team for the best interests of the child and the family. In the age of multidisciplinary assessment and collaborative planning, communication is even more critical because of the increase in numbers of people and services involved.

Effective communication with families is not always easy. Many parents have little motivation or understanding of the real consequences of hearing impairment, regardless of our efforts. For others, language and cultural barriers distance families from participating in the school environment. In addition, the transition from family-focused early intervention to school-based education can also be a difficult adjustment for parents. The extra time and effort we invest, however, should result in more productive and stronger partnerships over time. Some strategies for communicating with families include:

1. Listen first; begin by asking the parents about their concerns and their observations of their child. Completing a history form with the parents is a good opportunity to obtain this information.
2. Include parents in the assessment of the child and describe each step of the evaluation. Their participation will help them understand the results more easily. Do not let parents leave until they have at least a basic understanding of the outcome of the evaluation.
3. Acknowledge when information or answers to questions are not known or when additional information would be helpful. Let parents know when they can expect the information being sought.
4. Provide parents with written information to review and share with other family members, as well as other professionals. Provide parents a report (use accurate but simple language) including a description of the implications of the hearing loss and recommendations. Obtain parent permission to share information and to copy the report to

appropriate school, private practice, medical, and other professionals.

5. Conduct follow-up phone calls to inquire how the child is doing. These calls are indicative of the audiologist's care and concern; the unsolicited contact goes a long way to building and sustaining an effective relationship.

6. Remember to use these strategies for developing rapport, respect, and trust in all communications.

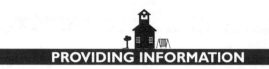

PROVIDING INFORMATION

We practice audiology in the schools to provide a service to children. With children who are deaf or hard-of-hearing, our primary role is to identify and advocate for their needs. However, consistent, strong parent support often affects the way a student performs more than the work of the audiologist and school team. As we continue to emphasize, even better results can be achieved when the parents and the school are working together. A major step in developing effective relationships is to provide families with information. Information is powerful; it can enable and empower parents to make choices for their child and family. Unfortunately, information can also be used incorrectly, often leading the parent down a path of stress and problems.

To be effective, information must be presented in a manner that parents and family members can easily understand, and must be individualized for each family, child, and situation. Many parents need multiple opportunities to hear and discuss information, especially when it addresses a topic that is new for them. In addition, *there must be ample discussion time with the audiologist to provide clarification of the information, to respond to questions, and to provide objective guidance.*

Quantity of Information

It is often difficult to decide how much information parents should be given and under what time frame. Each parent has a different capacity to absorb various quantities of materials. The degree of information necessary is usually a function of where a family is in the diagnostic or treatment phases of intervention. Obviously, the parent of a newly diagnosed infant or child will require a great deal more general information than the family of a child diagnosed 5 years previously.

In the early stages after identification, we believe it is best to give parents enough information to provide an introduction to the basic areas they will need to be aware of. Some audiologists may feel this amount of information is too much for parents to process, but this strategy allows the family to decide how much they want to read, review, or access and on what timetable. It also gives parents adequate information in the event they move or are not seen again by an audiologist for some time. Additional information can also be given at each appointment, provided that there are sufficient opportunities for discussion with the audiologist.

When providing large packets of information to parents, always identify the materials that require their immediate review. Further reading can be suggested for follow-up visits. Some parents respond to these "assignments" in a formal way; for others, a suggestion to read an article may be more appropriate.

Generally, let parents determine when they are ready for more detailed information. Their questions should be indicators of when they are ready for more information and the type of information they want.

Types of Information

There are many types of information and formats that are effective with families. Information is most commonly provided in written and verbal formats, but, as computers and technology are increasingly used in homes, computer programs, the Internet and Web sites, and CD-ROMs will become more popular. Additionally, the increased variety of informational videotapes, sign language instructional videotapes, and videtape stories provides improved access to parents. Appendix 16–A contains a list of materials, books, and videotapes available for parents, as well as information about national resources and programs. The types of information provided to families will differ depending on whether the child has a recently identified hearing loss or if the family has already been involved with an intervention program.

Information for Families: Phase I—Newly Identified or Recently Identified Hearing Impairment

The most immediate and critical information to be provided to parents at this stage targets understanding of the hearing loss, the possible cause, the implications, connections to intervention programs, and the necessity of amplification. Whatever time is necessary must be taken to complete this phase of the process. Depending on the diagnostic situation, this responsibility could belong to the educational audiologist, to the dispensing audiologist, or, even better, to both working together to support the family in both home and school environments. We have found this collaboration to benefit all parties because it uses each audiologist's time more efficiently, shares the responsibility, and demonstrates to parents that the audiologists work together for their child. As part of the information conveyed, parents need to learn about amplification options and gain a realistic expectation of what each provides. Once the fitting process begins, a written home hearing aid program can be particularly helpful in supporting parents during the hearing aid adjustment period. This program should include charts for recording wearing time and activities to do when the child is wearing the hearing aid(s). An example of a program for parents is contained in Appendix 6–E.

Information for families of children new and recently diagnosed is usually more general but still should provide the breadth necessary to touch on most of the critical topics parents immediately face. One of the most helpful activities the audiologist can do is to compile a resource booklet to provide for parents when hearing loss is diagnosed. Our experience with this type of information has been extremely positive. Audiologists (educational and private) within a community should meet to devise such a booklet and to develop a list of local resources. Production and duplication costs can be shared between the school district (often production) and the private providers (duplication of copies for their clients). By involving all area audiologists, an ownership in the product is attained, and audiologists are given the opportunity to improve communication between themselves as they share in the development of the booklet. The following topics are suggested for the content of a booklet:

➤ An introductory page: a description of the contents, the purpose, and how to use the manual
➤ Communication Choices: a definition and description of each communication method in an straightforward, nonbiased manner
➤ The Effects of Hearing Loss: a description of the implications of the varying degrees of hearing loss, including a picture of an audiogram
➤ Glossary: a complete listing of terminology and definitions common to audiology and deaf education
➤ Reading and Resource List: a compilation of books, videotapes, national organizations and resources, and state organizations, resources and providers
➤ Local Resources: a listing of city or county resources, including:
  ✓ General information regarding community services for children (Part H agency should be included here)
  ✓ Financial resources (SST, Medicaid, state disability services for children, etc.)
  ✓ Hearing and speech services (audiology and hearing aids, hearing therapy, speech therapy, hearing aid bank program if available, etc.)
  ✓ Health-medical resources (county health department, health and medical clinics that serve chil-

dren, Early Periodic Screening, Diagnosis, and Treatment [EPSDT], Women, Infants & Children [WIC], ear, nose and throat physicians, etc.)
  ✓ Public schools: Child Find and specialized programs for deaf and hard-of-hearing, Head Start, etc.
  ✓ Parent/family supports (parent groups for disabilities and deaf/hard-of-hearing, preschool support groups)
  ✓ Child care and respite services
  ✓ Transportation
  ✓ Housing (transition, homeless, abuse protection)
  ✓ Counseling
  ✓ Emergency (poison control, suicide hotline, fire-police-ambulance)

In Colorado, a group of professionals (audiologists, deaf educators, habilitation specialists, Deaf adults, and State Departments of Health and Education representatives) and parents developed a booklet entitled, *RESOURCES for Families of Children with Hearing Loss in Colorado* (Colorado Department of Education, 1995). After a year of meetings to develop the booklet, the Colorado Department of Education funded production and mailing to every audiologist in the state with a cover letter regarding its use. Within each community, audiologists were instructed to develop a list of "local resources" that would be added to the main booklet, to distribute and reproduce copies for each audiologist, and then to provide them to parents whenever hearing loss was diagnosed. This process attempts to ensure that all parents are provided the same basic information and options throughout the state.

Parents also need information that addresses the specific type and degree of hearing impairment of their child. The audiologist (or groups of audiologists) may wish to develop packets of information that are specific to certain types of hearing loss populations such as hard-of-hearing, deaf, otitis media, unilateral, noise-related, or central auditory processing. Information specific to genetic types of hearing loss is also important (National Institute on Deafness and other Communication Disorders and the Hereditary Hearing Impaired Resource Registry is an excellent resource for parents, address is in Appendix 16–A). Additional resources parents can order through the mail include videotapes, books for parents on hearing loss, and intervention programs (see Appendix 16–A). A Family Needs Survey, such as the one adapted from Bailey and Simeonsson (1988) located in Appendix 10–B, can also be given to families periodically to determine areas in which the family may need more information or support.

Another need for parents is information about their rights and the IFSP or IEP process. This information should be provided in writing as well as explained. Most parents are now involved with the IFSP process first. Because there is so much flexibility in how IFSPs are conducted and written, and because the parent is more "in charge," the IFSP is much less intimidating that the IEP (see Chapter 11, Individual Planning, for more information on development of the IFSP and IEP and transition between them).

Information for Families: Phase II— Living with the Diagnosis

Once a family has spent several months adjusting to the diagnosis of their child's hearing impairment, they should be ready for more detailed information about education, options, and the future for their child. The first phase of adjustment is often more internal, that is, understanding and meeting the immediate needs of the child and family. The following years include many external activities, such as parent groups, workshops, and deaf adult or Deaf culture activities. The benefit of early childhood home intervention programs is that the parent education process is ongoing and can proceed at the parents' pace as they are ready to explore new areas. For preschool and school-age children, home programming is not as readily available usually because of time and travel limitations of public school program staff. As a result, special efforts must be made to keep parents informed.

Information about workshops, parent groups, and signing classes are all important to families. If an otology consultation was not scheduled to evaluate the etiology of the hearing loss, this exam should be recommended.

This phase is also a good time to meet deaf or hard-of-hearing adults. Their insight and experience can be helpful to parents and provide a perspective that we, as normal-hearing individuals, cannot convey. There are several books written by parents for parents and by adults who are deaf or hard-of-hearing that are included in Appendix 16–A. Often a book or a videotape can serve as a starting point for ongoing discussions to help parents adjust to changing family dynamics which often follow diagnosis of hearing loss.

The grief process for parents does not end once the diagnosis has been made and intervention begun. Rather, the feelings of loss resurface each time certain milestones are reached that cause the impact of the hearing impairment to be particularly apparent. The most difficult times are often entry into kindergarten, puberty, high school graduation, and independent living. As audiologists, we must be understanding of these circumstances and be prepared to offer parents supports through counseling, meetings with other parents who have been through these difficult times, and parent support groups.

A Word about Counseling

This discussion is primarily about the audiologist's role in accepting parents, providing them with information, helping them make decisions, and offering support. Although these activities may be considered part of the counseling process, we should be careful how counseling activities are defined. Providing information and support to parents as they make decisions about methodology and programs is more of a guidance than counseling function. Specific counseling services are usually directed to helping parents deal with the grieving process or to help their children with personal problems associated with their hearing impairment or deafness. Whether preventative or prescriptive, counseling should be left to individuals who are appropriately trained and who have specific training or experience working with deaf and hard-of-hearing individuals. When situations arise that require counseling, and they often do, refer the child and family to the appropriate school counselor or psychologist. If an appropriately trained counselor or psychologist is not available, work with the school to identify and contract with one. The value of understanding hearing loss and deafness, and direct communication with the student cannot be minimized.

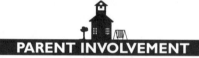

PARENT INVOLVEMENT

Parents generally want to work with their children's teachers and other professionals. However, in some situations and particularly once their child enters formal schooling, they may feel they have less control and that they are not kept informed or given enough time to discuss their child's progress. The parent questions in Table 10–1 may be helpful for parents when trying to determine what they need and want from their relationships with professionals.

Committee/Task Force Work

All parents should be welcome participants in school programs. Whether it is planning workshops, curriculum development, parent programs, or hiring a new teacher or staff member, parents should be involved in the process. Not only is it often a challenge to include parents, but it is also difficult to find different parents who are willing to give of their time to participate actively on a committee or task force. When parent participation does occur, however, the outcome is stronger and has greater credibility. Furthermore, in the process, parents learn about school issues and

Table 10–1. Parent checklist of questions to ask when working with professionals.

➤ Do I believe I am an equal partner with professionals, and accept my share of the responsibility for solving problems and making plans on behalf of my child?

➤ Do I clearly express my own needs and the needs of my family to professionals in an assertive manner?

➤ Do I treat each professional as an individual and avoid letting past negative experiences or negative attitudes get in the way of establishing a good working relationship?

➤ Do I communicate quickly with professionals serving my child when significant changes or notable events occur?

➤ When I make a commitment to a professional for a plan of action, do I follow through and complete that commitment?

➤ Do I maintain realistic expectations of professionals, myself, and my child?

Source: From *Focal Point,* 2(2), 1988. Research and Training Center, Regional Research Institute for Human Services, Portland State University, Portland, OR 97207-0751; (503) 725-4040. Reprinted by permission.

increase their understanding of the problems teachers and staff face.

Some parents participate because they have an agenda of their own that needs attention. Although they are not necessarily disruptive to the process, their focus is set narrowly on their own issues, rather than on what is best for the group. To avoid, or at least minimize these actions, screening of parents who have volunteered or selection of an alternative representative may be necessary. In addition, a set of operating rules for the participants of the group is essential. The goal or purpose of the group needs to be stated clearly, with timelines and outcomes set. All members should be respected for the perspective they bring to the task, but refocused when they stray too far from the objective.

Classroom Support

It is helpful to involve parents in day-to-day classroom activities. Parents can often be much more instrumental in accomplishing certain tasks than teachers. When accompanied by knowledge and direct experience, their input is more credible. When parents have options regarding classroom placements, one area in which they may choose to advocate for their child is in selecting the best classroom environment, including teacher style and provision for appropriate accommodations. Appendix 10–C contains a classroom observation checklist that parents can use when considering options for classrooms, teaching styles, and facilities for their child.

Parent Activities

One of our biggest challenges with families is keeping them active in parent groups. It often seems that it is the same parents who participate and that parents of younger children participate more frequently than parents of older ones. Some strategies to increase parent involvement include the following:

➤ Try to have as many parents as possible involved in the planning of parent activities. The intent should be to have the activities developed and run by parents for parents. Keep the role of teachers or staff as support.

➤ Have operating rules for parent planning meetings as well. Care needs to be practiced so that all participants are heard and their opinions respected.

➤ Stay on task at the meeting; parents' time is valuable and they need to feel personal accomplishment to continue to participate.

➤ Offer child care whenever possible; many parents do not participate due to the cost of baby-sitting.

➤ Develop a carpool for parents who do not have transportation.

➤ Provide refreshments when appropriate (not essential); if possible, either have a fund to purchase snacks or ask participants to rotate bringing them. Some parents may prefer potluck dinners—let them choose.

➤ Provide interpreters for non-English-speaking parents or for Deaf participants. This should be paid for by the school because it is an accessibility issue (504, ADA).

➤ Solicit input from all parents when developing programs, workshops, or events. Try a calling tree to keep all parents informed of activities.

➤ Rotate the meeting times and days. Different meeting times may permit more parent involvement in the long run, even if their attendance cannot be consistent.

➤ Establish a parent welcome group that calls on families who are new to the school or who have a newly identified child. A parent-to-parent chat can often mean as much, or more, to the parent than a professional's support. Be cautious that parents who make these visits and calls are good representatives of the program and have a thorough understanding of the school and services. They also must have good communication skills. Avoid using parents who are dissatisfied with the school's services or experiencing other significant problems.

HANDLING DIFFICULT SITUATIONS

Not all families are easy to work with. Unfortunately we have to deal with these difficult families and situations more often than we want. There are no specific solutions to these problems because each family and the dynamics of the situation are different. We will share some of the common problems we have encountered with some suggestions for handling them.

Generally, disputes should be dealt with carefully, maintaining sensitivity and respect for all participants involved. Sometimes they cannot be resolved, and mediation or due process proceedings are necessary. Although schools are often inclined to give in to parents to avoid lengthy and costly due process hearings, they may find mediation, which has been used successfully in the last few years to resolve differences, as a viable alternative. However, even these meetings can take many hours, and when the financial impact of the time of the parties involved is calculated, the cost is still quite high. Ultimately, if differences remain unresolved, due process may be the only alternative.

Parent/School Disagreement Over IEP Services

A common problem that occurs is when the parents and school are in disagreement over services. A frequent scenario is parents who want more speech therapy than the school is able to provide. The issue of the educational relevance of speech production is a little confusing for all of us, particularly because the problem occurs most frequently with students who are deaf or who have very severe hearing losses. Often these children also use sign language so that they do have a system of communication established. Although our desire is for children to have the best speech possible, we must ask the question how does speech production rank as an educational priority?

One tactic is to acknowledge the importance of speech therapy by providing a reasonable amount of small group or individual time with the speech-language pathologist and to look at how activities that promote speech production can be implemented throughout the school day and at home. If parents still desire additional services, they should be encouraged to look at options outside of the school setting. Parents often have the perception that more speech therapy is always better. One question to be asked concerns the potential benefit of shorter sessions provided more often versus longer sessions less often. Also, the integration of the skill development activities into the

child's school and home environment must be emphasized. One early mistake that special education made was to try to assume the total responsibility for education and related services for children with disabilities. Now as we backstep, we have learned to be more realistic about the services that special education is able to reasonably provide.

Request for a Specific Brand of Amplification

As the variety of amplification devices increases, there are more options for the type and style used. Parents occasionally request a certain brand of FM or, more recently, a BTE-style FM for their child. Although school audiologists make every effort to accommodate parents, the schools are under no obligation to provide a specific brand or style, provided that the equipment used by the school performs the necessary functions and is appropriate for the student's needs as designated in the IEP. One argument that parents have used successfully to justify the BTE FM has been their child's willingness to wear the BTE-style when they would not wear the body-style FM.

Influence of Private Provider on School Services

Private providers often make recommendations for services with which the school does not agree. This problem occurs in a variety of situations, including specific services and types of (re)habilitation, the recommendation of specific amplification devices, and different interpretations of a diagnosis.

When a private provider recommends a specific type of therapy approach (such as an Auditory-Verbal method for children with cochlear implants), schools should make every effort to provide appropriate, individualized services. This effort might include the implant center providing the therapist with extra training in the specialized treatment techniques. It does not mean, however, that the school has to provide a specially certified Auditory-Verbal therapist as the only qualified individual to conduct the therapies. Services are directed by the IEP and must describe the needs of the student, the annual goals, and the short-term objectives, including the individual(s) responsible for providing the services and evaluating progress.

Another area of conflict that often arises between schools and private providers is the diagnosis of central auditory processing disorders (CAPD) and the resulting recommendation for amplification. Most schools conduct assessments in a multidisciplinary manner. When CAPD is diagnosed by a private provider, academic, health, psychological, and speech-language assessment information may be missing. Without regard for information which might reflect the impact of the CAPD in these other areas, it is difficult to ascertain the significance of the disorder. Many audiologists who conduct CAPD assessments privately, utilize extensive test batteries that may ultimately detect an abnormal finding. However, difficulty on only one subtest of a larger battery may not have enough significance to warrant special education intervention or amplification. Furthermore, the recommendation for a service, such as the use of amplification within the school environment, is the IEP team's decision determined during the IEP or Section 504 process. Furthermore, best practices recommend that amplification for a child with CAPD should first be preceded by a successful trial period to determine the actual benefits of the system.

Many of the problems that occur between the private provider/parent and the school could be remedied if all individuals worked together to develop IEP services. As has been emphasized, relationships are much more effective when all parties work together and have ongoing communication already established. It is also critical that the audiologist or individual coordinating these meetings have accurate information on school legal obligations and current case law.

Uninvolved Families

Families who either do not provide supports for their children in the home or who do not follow through on recommendations made by the school are challenging for all of us. Whether the families are noncompliant, willing but unable, or dysfunctional, their children are often left to the schools for education and support.

Completing audiological assessments, obtaining medical treatment, getting hearing aids fit, and completing financial aid applications are all necessary but difficult steps when families are unable or unmotivated to follow through on needed services. It is for these children that we must rally and work together so that they are able to receive the services to which they are entitled. Audiologists need to be connected to their community interagency network for assistance in arranging transportation to appointments or obtaining home visitors who can help parents with appointments and completing financial assistance paperwork. Often these are the children who truly benefit from the school's ability to provide comprehensive audiology services.

An additional concern is poor hearing aid use outside of the school. These are usually children whose families either do not encourage hearing aid use at home or are afraid that the hearing aid will be broken or lost if used during out of school activities. Our efforts to maintain the hearing aids at school and to demonstrate the advantages of amplification in all aspects of the child's life are important in instilling future self-responsibility for hearing aid use on the part of the student.

Differing Methodology Opinions

Methodology remains a controversial topic in deaf education. With controversy comes a variety of opinions. Although this is not the place for a discussion of methodology issues, the impact on deaf education programs continue. In addition to the continuing oral-manual debate, we now have heated discussions over types of sign systems, with the bilingual/bicultural (ASL) and English-based signs most prevalent.

Another interesting situation often occurs with families who start their young children with a total communication philosophy. As parents struggle with the often slow progress of speech production, they may reconsider their choice of communication methods and decide to discontinue sign language due to the opinion that it detracts from oral skill development. These decisions are very difficult for education staff because of the potential harmful emotional effects that could occur by removing the child's primary language mode. Again, any decisions made regarding methodology should be made only when based on sound evaluation data.

The educational audiologist is a critical team member who can help in the discussion by providing objective data on the status and progress of auditory development and the need for additional visual input. Additionally, we should always support the necessity of objective evaluation data to monitor language and other development when guiding methodology decisions. Generally, the more delayed the child's language is, the greater the consideration for providing additional inputs, accommodations, or curricular modifications. Regardless of communication methods selected by families, we need to continue to emphasize that their children's successes with the choosen method is affected by the intensity with which the family embraces and integrates the communication system into their every day routines.

SUMMARY

This chapter has discussed the multiple facets involved when building relationships with families. Because each family is different and each situation unique, audiologists should rely on their own professional judgment along with other members of the professional team when working with families. Suggestions on how to develop and maintain partnerships, how to talk with families, and what to talk with them about have been discussed. Matkin (1994) suggested eight essential characteristics that should be practiced when working with families who have children who are deaf or hard-of-hearing. These are presented in Table 10–2 and summarize this chapter well. In the end, however, there is one primary rule to remember: treat families as you would want yours to be treated.

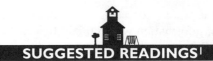

SUGGESTED READINGS[1]

Clark, J.G., & Martin, F. (1994). *Effective counseling in audiology.* Englewood Cliffs, NJ: Prentice Hall, Inc.

Luterman, D. (1979). *Counseling parents of hearing-impaired children.* Boston: Little, Brown & Co.

Moses, K. (1985). Infant deafness and parent grief: Psychosocial early intervention. In F. Powell, T. Finitzo-Hieber, S. Friel-Patti, & D. Henderson (Eds.), *Education of the hearing impaired child* (pp. 86–102). San Diego: College-Hill Press.

Ogden, P. (1996). *The silent garden: Raising your deaf child.* Washington D.C: Gallaudet University Press.

Rousch, J., & Matkin, N. (1994). *Infants and toddlers with hearing loss.* Baltimore: York Press.

Table 10–2. Eight essential characteristics for individuals working with parents of children with hearing impairments.

1. Possess a basic conviction that, given an appropriate support system, people can grow and change if they so desire.
2. Possess a nonjudgmental attitude regarding cultural and life style differences.
3. Possess an empathetic—not sympathetic—attitude (feel "with" vs. feel "for").
4. Be a perceptive listener regarding nonverbal as well as verbal messages.
5. Possess the basic conviction that parents can and do directly influence the outcomes of intervention; time and effort now will pay off later.
6. Be able to accept parental expression of a variety of emotions without personalizing and becoming defensive.
7. Be able to develop a warm, caring relationship, while retaining a professional role.
8. Respect privacy of parents.

Source: From "Key considerations in the provision of family centered services" by Noel D. Matkin, 1994. Paper presented at the Colorado State Symposium on Deafness, Colorado Springs, CO. Reprinted by permission.

---

[1]See Appendix 16–A, Part II, Articles, Books, and Videotapes for additional reading sources.

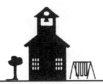

CHAPTER 11

INDIVIDUAL PLANNING

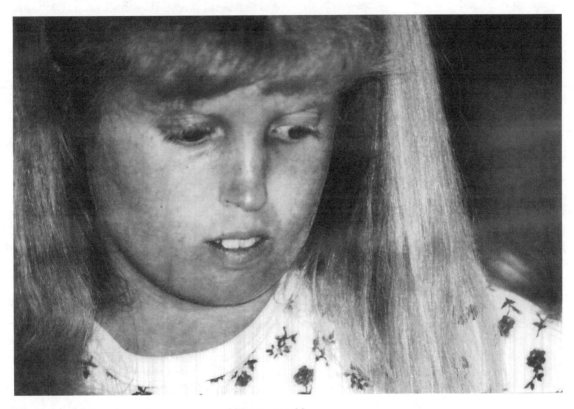

Maggie, age 11

CONTENTS

The role of the audiologist in the development of Individual Education Programs (IEPs), Individual Family Service Plans (IFSPs), 504 Plans, and Transition Plans has not been well defined and is often misunderstood or overlooked. Because audiology is classified as a related service in the federal law, this demarcation tends to blur audiologists' perceptions of their role in planning meetings and in the provision of services to children with auditory disorders. Teachers are typically looked on as the primary service providers for children with disabilities. In reality, many children with auditory disorders have the combined services of a teacher, a speech-language pathologist, and an audiologist. However, there are also many children who only require specialized support services such as audiology, speech-language therapy, or counseling to meet their needs. Although each type of planning meeting (IEP, IFSP, Transition, and 504) has a slightly different purpose, each includes an important role for the audiologist.

Training programs have also contributed to the lack of clarity surrounding the role of audiologists in the educational planning process. The (re)habilitative aspects of audiology training programs tend to put more emphasis on amplification than on any other type of intervention. Because the parameters of long-term treatment are much more individualized, more complicated, and less well defined, this part of (re)habilitation is more difficult to teach, as well as learn. Furthermore, therapy does not provide much immediate gratification because of the long-term persistence required by the audiologist, the individual who is treated, and the individual's family members to achieve meaningful results. Audiologists, because of the independent nature of much of our work, are often not trained in collaborative strategies and the nuances of working as part of a team to provide services. Bridging treatment between the family's supports and the child's education program and collaborating with other agencies, service providers, and community resources are elements of the intervention process that are usually more time-intensive than the therapy itself. Yet, the absence of these elements can impede an optimal treatment program.

Management of hearing impairment and central auditory processing disorders (CAPD) extends well beyond the auditory disorder itself. For planning and services to be effective, audiologists must have knowledge of the issues surrounding the hearing impairment and of the resources available for support and intervention and, most important, must exhibit a sensitivity for dealing with them. The focus of this chapter is to provide an understanding of individual planning and the audiologist's specific role within each of the following areas:

➤ The placement process
➤ The Individual Education Program
➤ The Individual Transition Plan
➤ The Individual Family Service Plan
➤ The 504 plan

A review of legal definitions and terminology for IDEA and 504 (see Chapter 1, Educational Audiology: How Did We Get Here?) may be helpful prior to reading this section.

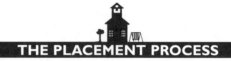

THE PLACEMENT PROCESS

Prior to the development of individual service programs, appropriate assessment for determination of disability and eligibility must occur. The assessment and placement component is represented in Figure 11–1. This section will refer primarily to the special education process for 3- to 21-year-olds (IDEA, Part B and 504).

Step 1: Concern About the Child

The process begins with a concern about the child, which may be identified by the parent, the teacher, school nurse, physician, or other individual or agency. With hearing impairment, concern typically is followed by a screening or audiological assessment to confirm or rule out hearing as the problem. Depending on the individual school district, agency, and state policy, the concern may or may not require a formal special education referral prior to audiologic assessment. However, due to the high incidence of otitis media as a cause of many parent and teacher concerns regarding hearing, most programs screen or conduct an initial evaluation to determine the nature of the impairment and the appropriateness of a special education referral.

The audiologist may also identify a concern based on findings from hearing screening and/or subsequent assessment. Children with previously undiagnosed hearing losses continue to be identified by school hearing screening programs. Community-based early childhood screening programs, which screen children in all areas of development to identify those who may have disabilities or who are at risk for learning problems, are very common at present. These screening programs are usually provided under federal and state Part H and Child Find programs and involve school district early childhood personnel. School-based audiologists often participate, either by training and supervising nurses, speech-language pathologists,

PLACEMENT PROCESS

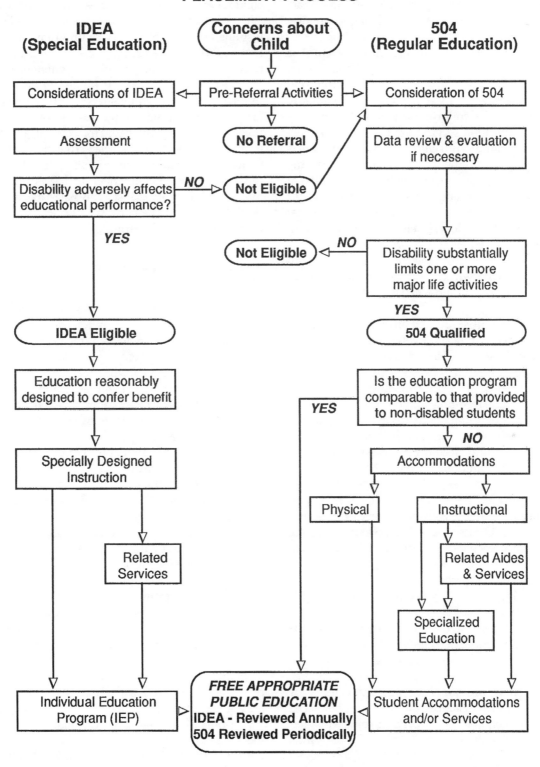

Figure 11–1. The IDEA and 504 placement process. (From *Planning and Preparing Quality Individualized Education Programs* (Section 1, p. 6), 1996b, Colorado Department of Education, Denver.

or technicians or by screening children whose age and developmental abilities prevent the use of traditional screening methods (see Chapter 3, Identification Practices, for specific information on screening techniques and programs).

For the IEP process, a pre-referral conference[1] is usually held with the teacher and other school special education providers prior to making the formal special education referral. Exceptions to this conference may be justified for children for whom it is obvious that special education services are necessary (usually children with significant sensory disabilities). Generally, the purpose of the meeting is to discuss the child's disorder, resulting problems, and needs in order to determine strategies and supports that could be implemented to assist the child prior to a referral and multidisciplinary assessment. If the team recommends a special education referral, the conference may also be used to determine what assessments will be conducted, who will conduct them, who will obtain parent permission, and when the IEP meeting will be held.

For a child with hearing impairment, the audiologist should have significant involvement in this meeting. Because the group of individuals who work with the child are present, it is a good opportunity to explain the audiological test results and their implications and to make recommendations for accommodations that will help compensate for the hearing loss.

The process may be slightly different for children suspected of central auditory processing disorders (CAPDs). Because audiologists are not usually routine members of the pre-referral conference committee, audiologic referrals are usually recommended as part of the multidisciplinary assessment for special education when CAPD is suspected. However, there are more and more teachers who recognize the symptoms of CAPD and include the audiologist in the early stages of the referral process.

If the hearing impairment is not considered significant (e.g., very mild, unilateral, or high-frequency hearing loss) and if there are no concerns expressed by the teacher or other school personnel regarding academic, speech/language, or social/behavioral status, the accommodations recommended by the educational audiologist may provide adequate intervention by themselves. In such instances, the child may be placed on a monitor status to be checked at some predetermined interval, without any direct special education involvement. The responsibility of the monitor roster may lie with the audiologist, speech-language pathologist, itinerant teacher of the deaf/hard-of-hearing, or

some other special service provider, depending on how responsibility is delineated for these individuals. These children may also be candidates for a 504 referral.

Other children will require the accommodations as just one aspect of their service program and will still require the special education referral for multidisciplinary assessment. The pre-referral conference committee must decide on the basis of the significance of the problem and interventions recommended whether to (a) reconvene to discuss the success of the interventions and subsequent need for referral, (b) proceed immediately with the special education referral, or (c) make a referral for consideration of 504. Decisions regarding children with hearing losses may not be made without a specialist who has expertise in this disability present (usually the audiologist or teacher of the deaf/hard-of-hearing).

Step 2: Referral to Special Education and Assessment

A referral is made for a multidisciplinary assessment on recommendation of the prereferral conference participants. The assessment requires parent permission and notification of parent rights. Referral paperwork should indicate the specific areas of assessment, the assessments that will be completed, and the individuals who will conduct them. Rarely, parents refuse permission to have their child assessed. If this occurs, the local educational team must decide if the concerns that exist are significant enough to pursue the referral through legal channels.

The purpose of the assessment is to obtain information regarding how the child is functioning in order to determine eligibility for special education. Information gathered may be through formal and informal measures in areas which include health, communication, academics, cognition, and social/emotional functioning. Specific disability areas require formal tests in certain areas: for example, to be identified with a hearing disability, a formal hearing evaluation must be completed, and to be labeled with a cognitive disability, a formal intelligence test must be administered. Each state education agency will have its own assessment criteria. The IEP team interprets the assessment results and implications to determine if the child is eligible to receive special education and related services.

A group of Colorado professionals, supported by the Colorado Department of Education, developed the Colorado Individual Performance Profile (CIPP) (Ruberry & Yoshinaga-Itano, 1993) for use with students who are deaf and hard-of-hearing. This instru-

[1]Different terms are used in each state to describe these meetings; examples include pre-assessment, student support team meeting, and child study meetings.

ment is used statewide to address the areas of assessment, student needs, and appropriate service and placement options systematically. Portions of this instrument are excerpted in Appendix 4–E. This instrument has been invaluable when making placement recommendations and justifying services for students.

The Educational Audiology Assessment

Appropriate assessment must always be the foundation of disability and eligibility determination. Measures must include standardized diagnostic audiologic procedures as well as functional measures of auditory performance. Assessment procedures and options that should be included in the educational audiology evaluation of children are discussed fully in Chapter 4, Assessment Practices. A well written, concise report that includes background information, test results, implications of hearing loss within the educational environment, and recommendations should accompany all initial evaluations. Care should be taken so that the information is understandable to those for whom it is written, including parents, teachers, and other educational personnel.

Hearing Loss and Eligibility

Criteria for an educationally significant hearing loss vary from state to state. Within the continuum of hearing loss levels, mild losses in the high-frequency range, mild unilateral losses, or bilateral ones with a pure tone average (PTA) in the 20 to 25 dB range may have questionable impact on hearing for learning. Therefore, these losses might not be considered educationally significant, that is, known to interfere with the child's potential ability to obtain reasonable benefit from regular education alone. For eligibility under IDEA, the hearing loss must adversely affect educational performance. Examples of adverse effects include poor auditory discrimination, language delay, articulation, voice or fluency problems, reading comprehension delay, poor academic achievement, or social-emotional problems. At least one of these effects of hearing loss must be documented.

Although the federal definition of hearing loss is not specific to any decibel criteria, the number of states that have established specific decibel levels is growing. A survey in 1990 (Johnson, 1991) found seven states with bilateral hearing loss criteria, two states with unilateral criteria, and two with high-frequency hearing loss criteria. Anderson and Whalen (1996) conducted a survey in 1995 and found 20 states with bilateral criteria, six with unilateral, and seven with high-frequency. In states without criteria, referrals are generally based on local interpretation and include

any child with a hearing loss that appears to have caused adverse educational effects.

Step 3: Determination of Disability and Eligibility

Disability and eligibility are somewhat confusing terms. The presence of a *disability* is determined from the assessments that are completed and the resulting needs of the child. Once a disability is diagnosed, *eligibility* for special education and related services is considered by ascertaining if the *disability* adversely affects educational performance (i.e., the child's ability to obtain reasonable benefit from regular education alone). For children with hearing impairments, the question of how much loss constitutes a *disability* cannot be determined by audiometrics alone. Many factors affect the relationship of hearing impairment and the ability to compensate for it. Age of onset, age of intervention, intellectual capacity, neurological function, central auditory processing ability, environment, other health factors, and the effects of otitis media are all variables which impact the disabling effects of hearing impairment. For some children, a minimal loss can have significant implications, whereas for others, the same impairment may present no consequences.

Cause and Effect with Other Disabilities

The relationship between hearing impairment, especially when it is mild, and speech/language delays, learning disabilities, emotional or behavioral problems, and a limited capacity to learn is difficult, and often impossible, to delineate. Each factor affects the other so that determination of the *primary* disability, or cause of the child's problems, may not be clear. However, if the child has enough difficulties to result in a disability under any one area, and the combined effects meet eligibility requirements for special education, then the focus should be on designing a program to meet his or her needs, rather than on the particular label that was used to qualify the student. In other words, a label of hearing impairment, while used to meet disability and eligibility requirements, does not mean the student necessarily has to be served by a provider who is a specialist in hearing disorders. For example, if the student's primary manifestations are behavior and social problems, a behavior specialist might be the most appropriate and effective service provider.

Definition of Hearing Loss

It is our opinion that for a child to be considered as disabled due to hearing loss, one of the following audiometric criteria should be met:

➤ A bilateral hearing loss of at least 20 dB PTA in the better ear

➤ A unilateral hearing loss of at least 35 dB PTA in the affected ear

➤ A bilateral high-frequency hearing loss averaging at least 35 dB at any two frequencies for 2000Hz, 4000Hz, or 6000Hz

➤ A fluctuating conductive hearing loss that meets one of the above criteria for at least 3 months (cumulative) during the school year or 4 months annually

Children (ages 3 to 21 years) who have minimal hearing losses not covered by these criteria generally should not be considered for special education based solely on their hearing ability. If they exhibit learning problems, other disability areas should be explored to determine the cause of the problem. Likewise, these children should also not be considered for 504 services on the basis of their hearing losses alone.

Central Auditory Processing Disorders

Children with CAPD may be eligible for special education or 504 services depending on the severity and implications of the problem. Disability and eligibility requirements vary from state to state, but usually students with significant CAPD qualify for eligibility consideration with either a hearing, speech-language, or learning disability.

Special Education or 504?

To determine the category of services for which a child may be eligible, (i.e., special education or 504), the IEP team or eligibility committee[2] must review all of the assessment results, determine the child's strengths and needs, and then ask the following questions:

1. *Have sufficient assessments been completed, documented, and considered to determine the student's current level of functioning, achievement, and performance and to determine the student's educational needs?*

If "NO," the meeting must be rescheduled so that all necessary assessments are completed.

2. *Can the student receive reasonable educational benefit from regular education alone?*

If "YES," the child does not meet special education criteria and the meeting is terminated; the child may then be referred for 504 consideration, if appropriate.

If "NO," ask . . .

3. *Does the child have a disability which adversely affects educational performance (as defined by state Rules to Administer the Individuals with Disabilities Education Act)?*

If "NO," the special education meeting is terminated; the child may then may be referred for 504 consideration.

If "YES," proceed with development of goals and objectives for the IEP.

Eligibility for 504, (i.e., determining if *the disability substantially limits one or more major life activities*) is a function of regular education. The eligibility team may include an administrator from the school, the child's teacher(s), the parents, and a specialist who understands the impact of the disability. If the student meets the disability criteria, then 504 needs are identified and a plan developed (see 504 plan section of this chapter). If there are no limitations determined, then the child is not eligible for any services. It is also possible that children could receive services under both IDEA and 504 if they are eligible as disabled under IDEA. The relationship between regular education, 504, and special education is illustrated in Figure 11–2.

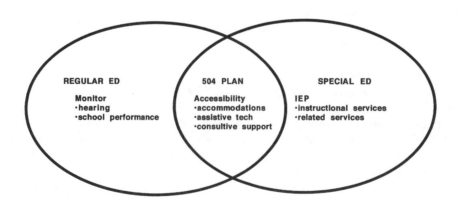

Figure 11–2. The Regular Education—504 Plan—Special Education relationship

[2]States and local education agencies have the option of holding the eligibility meeting separate from the meeting to develop the IEP; placement decisions are made at the IEP meeting, although placement options could be discussed at the eligibility meeting.[IDEA Regulations, Appendix C to Part 300—Notice of Interpretation]

Adaptations, Accommodations, and Modifications

Although theses terms are often used interchangeably, it is important to understand their distinctive meanings because they are used so frequently with reference to deaf and hard-of-hearing students as well as all students in special education. Adaptations are changes made to the environment, curriculum, instruction, and/or assessment practices in order for a student to be a successful learner. Adaptations include accommodations and modifications defined below:

Accommodations are provisions in how a student accesses information and demonstrates learning and do not substantially change the instructional level, content, and/or performance criteria. The changes are made in order to provide a student equal access to learning and equal opportunity to demonstrate what is known. Accommodations include changes in and/or provision of the following:

➤ Presentation and/or response format and procedures
➤ Instructional strategies
➤ Time and scheduling
➤ Attitudes
➤ Architectural features
➤ Environmental features
➤ Equipment

Modifications are substantial changes in what a student is expected to learn and demonstrate. These changes are made to provide a student the opportunity to participate meaningfully and productively in learning experiences and environments. Modifications include changes in the following:

➤ Instructional level
➤ Content
➤ Performance criteria

Adaptations are increasingly important as more schools and states adopt academic standards which students must meet in order to pass to the next level or graduate. In some states, students must have IEPs to qualify for modifications to established standards. A checklist for identifying necessary accommodations and modifications is located in Appendix 11–A.

Step 4: Development of the Individual Plan

Individual plans or programs are written documents which define the content and parameters of appropriate educational services for each student. These plans, which include certain legal rights and due process, are actually contracts between the school and/or other agencies and the child's parents. Fulfillment rights of the plan or program pertain to parameters of the document such as how often, by whom, or the amount of time services are scheduled rather than the amount of progress made by the child. School or agency personnel are not held accountable when students do not achieve the growth projected in the annual goals stated in their individual plans when all other aspects of the plans are met (IDEA Regulations Section 300.350 Individual Education Program—Accountability).

Individual plans were first implemented with the Individual Education Program (IEP) defined in PL 94-142 for school-age children. The provisions of the IEP have since been extended to eligible 3- and 4-year-olds. They also serve as the basis for the Individual Family Service Plan (IFSP), the corollary document serving infants and toddlers defined under Part H of IDEA. A more recent addition to the IEP has been the Individual Transition Plan (ITP) designed to prepare students 16 years and older for life after high school. Transition planning is also Used to bridge early childhood/Part H services with special education/Part B services (see Chapter 1, Educational Audiology: How Did We Get Here, for a more thorough discussion of past and current regulations).

The 504 Plan, as discussed previously, is actually a component of regular education programming. It defines what a school must provide to the student who has been identified with a disability to ensure equal access to educational services and the opportunity to benefit from those services.

The Audiologist's Role in the Placement and Planning Process

The following list describes activities which the audiologist should complete as part of the placement and planning process for children with auditory disorders:

1. Refer for consideration of special education and related services any child with hearing loss or CAPD that is potentially educationally significant (i.e., the hearing loss or CAPD could interfere with the child's ability to obtain reasonable benefit from regular education)
2. Participate in the pre-referral conference in order to conduct the following activities:

➤ Explain the parameters of the auditory disorder, including whether the hearing impairment meets established criteria to qualify as a hearing disability

➤ Explain the implications of the auditory disorder for communication and learning
➤ Provide recommendations for educational management and amplification
➤ Provide recommendations for medical intervention if appropriate
➤ Provide additional follow-up needs, when indicated
➤ Collaborate with the team to determine:

Adaptations, management strategies, and supports to assist the child

Follow-up steps to monitor the child (if no other concerns are present and the child is performing well in academic, behavior, and social areas)

If a referral to special education for multidisciplinary assessment is appropriate

If a referral to 504 is appropriate (if the student's auditory disorder constitutes a disability, but it is clear that the child would not be eligible for special education and related services)

3. Conduct additional audiological assessments, if not completed as part of the initial assessment, to:

➤ Provide information regarding the child's auditory skill development and functional abilities (e.g., recognition and comprehension of speech in noise, at a distance, with auditory only, and with auditory/visual input),
➤ Evaluate candidacy for amplification
➤ Determine the most appropriate type of amplification for the educational setting

4. Prepare a written report which details background information, audiologic findings, implications of hearing impairment or CAPD, needs, recommendations for audiologic follow-up, and classroom management (see Chapter 4, Assessment Practices) for information on specific components of the written report); provide copies to parents, teachers, nurse, special education personnel, the child's physician, dispensing or private audiologist, and others as appropriate

5. Participate in the meeting to discuss the team's assessment results, integrating audiologic findings and recommendations into the discussion of the child's needs, determination of disability, and eligibility options (special education, 504)

6. Participate in the planning meeting to develop the child's individual plan, advocating for appropriate services including necessary adaptations, accommodations, and modifications

These activities are summarized in Table 11–1.

Table 11–1. The audiologist's role in the placement and planning process.

---

1. Refer child for consideration of special education and related services
2. Participate in pre-referral conference
3. Conduct appropriate educational audiology assessments
4. Prepare a written report
5. Participate in meeting to determine disability and discuss eligibility options
6. Participate in development of individual plan

THE INDIVIDUAL EDUCATION PROGRAM

There are two parts of the Individual Education Program (IEP): the IEP meeting and the IEP document. The IEP meeting is where the parents and school personnel make decisions about the education program, and the IEP document is the contract or written record of the decisions made. Important clarifications of the purpose of the IEP are indicated below (U.S. Department of Education, September 29, 1992, 34 CFR 300; Appendix C to Part 300—Notice of Interpretation, p. 44833).

➤ The *IEP meeting* serves as a *communication* vehicle between parents and school personnel, and enables them, as equal participants, to decide jointly what the child's needs are, what services will be provided to meet those needs, and what the anticipated outcomes may be.
➤ The *IEP process* provides an *opportunity for resolving any differences* between the parents and the agency concerning the special education needs of a child with a disability; first, through the IEP meeting, and second, if necessary, through the procedural protections that are available to the parents.
➤ The *IEP document* sets forth in writing a *commitment of resources* necessary to enable a child with a disability to receive needed special education and related services.
➤ The *IEP* is a *management tool* that is used to ensure that each child with a disability is provided special education and related services appropriate to the child's special learning needs.
➤ The *IEP* is a *compliance/monitoring document* that may be used by authorized monitoring personnel from each governmental level to determine whether a child with a disability is actually receiving the FAPE (free and appropriate public education) agreed to by the parents and the school.

➤ The *IEP* serves as an *evaluation device* for use in determining the extent of the child's progress toward meeting the projected outcomes.

To complete the IEP certain decisions must be made and included as statements in the document. The audiologist has a direct role in some of these discussions and decisions and a more peripheral role in others. Care must be taken to present information in a sensitive way that invites or includes parent input, as well as input from the teachers and other professionals who work with the child. It should always be remembered that *IEP development is a team process*. Information required for the IEP [34CFR300.345(a)] and the audiologist's role in providing that information are presented in Table 11–2.

Goals on the IEP that promote auditory development, independence with amplification, and self-advocacy for hearing needs should always be included. Depending on the specialists in hearing and their individual roles, these goals might be the responsibility of the speech-language specialist, the audiologist, or the teacher of the deaf/hard-of-hearing or a combi-

nation of these. Sample goals and objectives for these audiology related needs are located in Appendix 11–B.

Planning the Eligibility And IEP Meeting

Eligibility for special education services must be determined within 45 days of the signing of the referral for assessment; the IEP must be developed within 30 days of the determination that the student qualifies for special education and related services. The IEP process usually involves a number of school specialists, teachers, administrators, representatives of other agencies, and the parents. In addition, a trained facilitator can help the discussion in order for the meeting to proceed smoothly. The meeting outline in Table 11–3 is a sample of how such a meeting can be structured. This particular example includes eligibility determination and the IEP as one meeting.

Least Restrictive Environment Considerations

Least restrictive environment (LRE) issues have been controversial when applied to the education of chil-

Table 11–2. Required information for the IEP and the audiologist's role in contributing to that information.

Required Information	*Audiologist's Role*
Statements which describe the child's present levels of functioning.	Present functional information regarding the impact of the hearing impairment or CAPD on communication, learning, and social/emotional development.
Statements of annual goals and short-term objectives.	Present annual goals for the development of auditory skills, use and independence with amplification, determination of appropriate compensatory strategies, or other areas as appropriate for the child's age and hearing or processing needs.
Statement of the specific special education and related services to be provided to the child and the extent to which the child will participate in regular education.	Present recommendations for necessary audiology services, which may include an annual hearing evaluation, use of an FM system, monitoring the functioning of the hearing aids and FM system, specific auditory training or skill development, training on assistive devices, and appropriate environmental and instructional accommodations.
Projected dates for initiation and anticipated duration of services.	Present recommendations based on services needed.
Appropriate objective criteria for evaluation procedures and schedules for determining, on at least an annual basis whether the short-term instructional objectives are being achieved.	Present criteria for auditory-related goals.
For children who are 16 or older, a statement of the needed transition services.	Present relevant information regarding community linkages necessary to continue hearing or processing-related services once the child graduates. These may include establishing a relationship with a community audiologist for hearing and hearing aid services, working with vocational rehabilitation for support services, and connecting with the Center on Deafness or other community programs for individuals who are deaf/hard-of-hearing or who have learning disabilities.

Table 11–3. Outline for eligibility/IEP meeting.

I.	Introductions:	*Facilitator introduces the individuals present.*
II.	Purpose of meeting:	*The purpose of the meeting is stated (i.e,. "We are meeting today to discuss the findings of the assessments, discuss strengths, and identify problems which may require special help. We will together determine if (child's name) has a disability and if the disability causes a significant problem which makes him/her eligible to receive special education and related services"). In addition to the purpose, all participants should be told that each person is an important member of the IEP team and that all discussion, comments, and questions are welcome.*
III.	Process for the meeting:	*Explain the process for discussion, reaching consensus, and for closure on issues.*
IV.	Begin the formal part of the meeting:	A. Present Levels of Functioning *Identify the student's strengths and needs in each functioning area on the basis of the assessments.* B. Statement of Educational Needs *Identify and prioritize the areas of need on which the IEP will focus.* C. Determination of eligibility *Determine if the student can receive reasonable benefit from general education alone, without special education services. If not, determine if the student has a disability.* D. Goals and Objectives *Identify annual goals, short-term instructional objectives and objective criteria, evaluation procedures, and schedules for determining whether each short-term objective has been accomplished.* E. Special Education and Related Services *Identify the specific special education and related services that will be provided and the extent to which the student will participate in regular education programs; identify the projected starting date and length of service; determine whether the student is eligible for services beyond the school year; and determine if modifications are necessary for the student to participate in regular education programs.* F. Recommended Placement in the Least Restrictive Environment *Determine the settings in which special education and services will be provided.*
V.	Signatures	*Obtain signatures of participants indicating their involvement in the development of the IEP; if it is the initial meeting to determine eligibility, obtain the signature(s) of the parent(s) for placement of their child in special education.*

Source: From Planning and Preparing Quality Individualized Education Programs (Section 1, pp. 9–10), 1996b, Colorado Department of Education, Denver.

dren with hearing losses. Although historically these children were most often educated in separate classrooms and facilities, the trend for mainstreaming in the 1970s resulted in more frequent participation of these students in regular education. The inclusion movement in the 1980s, however, advocated full participation, challenging our philosophical biases regarding the extent to which participation in regular education could really provide an appropriate education for children who were deaf or hard-of-hearing. Although the inclusion proponents were primarily parents and professionals of children with severe disabilities, the movement has affected all special education populations. For deaf students, where inclusion often meant regular classrooms, noncenter-based programs, fewer supports, and virtual isolation from peers with hearing impairment, this practice may have resulted in more harm than benefit. The role of state residential schools for the Deaf was, and still is, questioned in several states. Skepticism on the part of deaf educators slowed the practice of total inclusion for students with hearing impairments in many parts of

the country. The 1988 Report of the Commission on Education of the Deaf raised multiple concerns, and a special Policy Guidance was issued by the U.S. Department of Education in October, 1992 to clarify LRE issues related to the education of students who are deaf or hard-of-hearing (see Appendix 1–G).

The extent to which a student who is deaf or hard-of-hearing can reasonably benefit from regular education classes can be determined more objectively by addressing the following:

1. Determination of the subjects and activities in regular education in which the student can participate:

   ➤ with no modifications or adaptations,
   ➤ with specific accommodations or modifications, or
   ➤ with alternative curriculum, instruction, or assistive technology.

2. Determination of the alternative curriculum, instruction, or assistive technology when needed.

3. Determination of type and amount of supportive training needed in deficit areas.
4. Determination of strategies needed to be carried out consistently by all service providers and parents.

For children who are deaf and hard-of-hearing, the primary issue in the LRE discussion continues to be the role that Deaf culture and deaf or hard-of-hearing peer-group experiences play in their education. We know that the socialization aspects of education have significant consequences for academic as well as non-academic development. Each child should have access to a continuum of placement options from home school, regular education to center-based programs to regional and state schools for the Deaf. With a growing movement back to center-based and multi-district shared programs, the pendulum seems to be balancing as parents and professionals have realized that *inclusion for students who are deaf or hard-of-hearing equates to an environment that understands, accepts, challenges, and supports each student while ensuring that all communication is accessible.* Most important, the realization that every disability group has different characteristics and needs, and that within each group each child has unique characteristics and needs as well, is finally occurring. The operational tenant must continue to be "individualized" education.

Due Process and Lack of Consensus

When parents are not in agreement with services as part of IEP planning, an interim course of action should be taken (see Appendixes 1–B and 1–C for IDEA regulations). When an agreement cannot be reached, the child's last IEP remains in effect in the areas in which the disagreement occurred. Differences can also be resolved through due process procedures as described under IDEA, Part B, or through mediation or some other informal procedure for resolving the differences without going to a due process hearing.

Annual Review and Triennial Evaluations

Current IDEA regulations require that the goals and short-term instructional objectives be reviewed and evaluated annually. Parents and regular and special education personnel directly involved with the student should attend the IEP review meeting which includes:

1. Review of previously identified needs with revisions made as necessary
2. Review of performance on the previous year's goals and objectives
3. Development of new annual goals and objectives including evaluation criteria

4. Identification of the special education and related services to be provided and the extent to which the student will participate in regular education programs, including starting date and duration, and eligibility for services beyond the regular school year
5. Determination of modifications necessary to participate in the regular education programs
6. Identification of settings where special education and related services will be provided
7. Signatures of those in attendance indicating involvement in the development of the IEP

Triennial evaluations (every 3 years) are required to fully re-evaluate students in all areas of functioning. The evaluation and IEP meeting process is the same as for initial placement with the exception of signatures. If the disability and eligibility requirements do not change, then parent permission is not necessary to continue services. However, if the child's disability status changes, parent permission is required to change categories or remove the child from special education.

The audiologist's role in annual review meetings is to provide any new or additional information obtained from the student's annual hearing evaluation. Often audiologists' caseloads are high and prohibit attendance at every annual review. If there are no changes in the status or needs of the student, attendance is usually not necessary. However, if the audiologist provides direct (re)habilitation services, attendance is required as a service provider. Generally, audiologists should use their professional judgment of the situation when deciding the need to attend the annual review. If unable to attend, a current written report or "update" should be provided.

Triennial evaluations do require full assessment of the student, as well as attendance at the IEP meeting. Functional, as well as standard audiologic assessments, should be completed, including a written "update" report for the student's file. Information should also contain a summary of the child's performance in the classroom relative to hearing. The IEP/triennial meeting functions in the same way as the initial placement meeting except that parent permission to continue services is not required.

THE INDIVIDUAL TRANSITION PLAN

Transition services were added to the federal legislation as part of the 1990 and 1991 Amendments to IDEA (PL 101-476, PL 102-119). The law specifies that the addition of transition services to IEPs for all students in special education must occur no later than age 16. This part of the IEP is often set up separately and called an Individual Transition Plan (ITP). As stated in 34 CFR Section 300.18:

(a) Transition services means a coordinated set of activities for a student, designed within an outcome-oriented process, that promotes movement from school to post-school activities, including postsecondary education, vocational training, integrated employment (including supported employment), continuing and adult education, adult services, independent living, or community participation.

(b) The coordinated set of activities described in paragraph (a) must [1] be based on the individual student's needs, taking into account the student's preferences and interests; and [2] include needed activities in the areas of (i) instruction; (ii) community experiences; (iii) the development of employment and other post-school adult living objectives; and (iv) if appropriate, acquisition of daily living and functional vocational evaluation.

Additional requirements for the content of the IEP or ITP are the inclusion of a statement of each public agency's and each participating agency's responsibilities before the student leaves the school setting. Schools are encouraged to begin transition planning at age 14, or even younger if necessary, due to the high number of drop-outs by the age of 16. The transition planning meeting must be attended by the student involved.

General areas which should be addressed in transition planning for deaf and hard-of-hearing students include:

➤ Postsecondary educational options
➤ Vocational training options
➤ Living arrangements
➤ Personal management
➤ Job training
➤ Financial management and planning
➤ Transportation
➤ Medical services and resources
➤ Legal services and advocacy resources
➤ Recreation and leisure activities
➤ Cultural awareness

The audiologist's specific role in transition planning was described in Table 11–2.

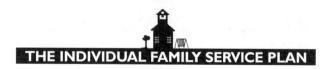

THE INDIVIDUAL FAMILY SERVICE PLAN

The IFSP defines services for infants and toddlers (birth through age 2). Services to this age group are specified under Part H of IDEA (34CFR Part 303, 1993). The most significant difference between IEPs and IFSPs is that the IEP is more child-centered and school-directed, while the IFSP is family-focused and parent-driven. The family-centered philosophy was promoted in response to recognition of the importance of the family's role in (a) supporting the development of their child, (b) determining the services needed by their child and their family, and (c) determining how their child's needs might best be met relative to their specific family context. The designation of the family as the central agent for the development and coordination of services has resulted in the need for audiologists and other professionals to rethink their role with families. Rather than a directive approach of telling parents what to do, the challenge is to provide families with information and options that enable them to make their own decisions for their child. In theory, this concept is laudable; in reality, the coordination of services when multiple agencies are involved requires a significant amount of time and effort. Despite these efforts to empower parents, many families still require a great deal of professional support to coordinate services for their child.

The components that must be included in each state's system for early intervention services include (34 CFR Part 303.300–512):

➤ State eligibility criteria and procedures
➤ A central directory of services
➤ A public awareness program
➤ A comprehensive child find system, including designation of a lead agency
➤ An evaluation and assessment component which incorporates nondiscriminatory procedures, is timely, is comprehensive and multidisciplinary, is conducted by a qualified provider, and includes assessment activities related to the child and the child's family
➤ Case management
➤ An Individual Family Service Plan, including procedural safeguards

Eligibility Criteria

Infants and toddlers from birth through age 2 are eligible for early intervention services because they [34CFR300.16(a-b)]:

(1) Are experiencing developmental delays, as measured by appropriate diagnostic instruments and procedures, in one or more of the following areas:

(i) Cognitive development
(ii) Physical development, including vision and hearing
(iii) Communication development
(iv) Social or emotional development
(v) Adaptive development; or

(2) Have a diagnosed physical or mental condition that has a high probability of resulting in developmental delay.

States may also choose to include infants and toddlers who are at risk of having substantial developmental delays if early intervention services are not provided. Infants and toddlers who are deaf or hard-of-hearing qualify under either part (1) or (2) of the definition. Unlike Part B of IDEA (ages 3 to 21), infants and toddlers may qualify for services solely based on the presence of a hearing impairment.

Audiologists are often the professionals who begin the IFSP referral process. With the increase in newborn hearing screening programs, audiologists are identifying more hearing impairments shortly after birth, before parents have suspicions about hearing development. As a result, audiologists who work with pediatric populations have a responsibility to know and be connected with early childhood Part H services in their communities (see Chapter 9, Community Collaboration, for more information).

Purpose of the IFSP

The IFSP should be a working, fluid document that identifies and organizes the formal and informal community resources that are available to help families achieve the goals they have established for their child and themselves. The IFSP process should:

➤ Be flexible, family-focused, and nonintrusive for families
➤ Reflect a variety of services and supports that provide options for the delivery of services for families
➤ Support, enable, and empower families to coordinate and utilize local community resources

IFSP Requirements

The IFSP must be developed within 45 days of receiving the referral, be reviewed at least every 6 months with an annual meeting to evaluate progress, be accessible and convenient for families, and include parental consent for services. The specific content requirements of the IFSP [34CFR303.344(a–h)] and the audiologist's role in providing that content are described in Table 11–4. Transition plans should be developed about 6 months prior to the third birthday for children moving from services on IFSPs to preschool special education services and IEPs. The plan should state the activities to be completed and the individual responsible during the transition period. Examples of activities include meeting school special education personnel and visiting potential preschool or other service programs.

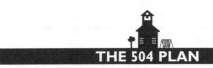

THE 504 PLAN

Under Section 504, schools must make adequate provisions so that students with disabilities are not "excluded from participation in, denied the benefits of, or otherwise subjected to discrimination under any program or activity because facilities are inaccessible or unusable" (29 U.S.C. Sec 794, 1977). It is further the responsibility of the school and staff to develop and implement the delivery of all needed services. The determination of necessary services and accommodations must be made by a group of persons knowledgeable about the student, with the parents included in the process whenever possible. This group must review the nature of the disability and how it affects the student's accessibility to education. The decisions about Section 504 eligibility and services should be documented in the student's file and reviewed periodically. A formal 504 Plan is often used to document this information. A sample form is located in Appendix 11–C.

Most children with hearing impairments (at least those who meet the recommended audiometric criteria discussed earlier) should meet 504 disability requirements; that is, they have a physiological impairment, hearing, which impacts education by "substantially limiting major life functioning in the areas of hearing, speaking, and learning." Although 504 is a regular education program, the audiologist is the individual most likely to present the evidence and make the 504 recommendation. The blurring of roles between special education and regular education are evident in this process. Although 504 eligibility determination occurs independently of special education, 504 consideration may occur at the IEP meeting if enough regular education personnel are present. The parent, the teacher, and an administrative representative such as the principal are typical members of the team that makes the eligibility determination and develops the 504 plan.

Athough 504 is civil rights legislation that governs all education programs, the audiologist is usually the consulting specialist when hearing impairment is involved. As a result, the audiologist is typically the primary support to the student with a hearing disability when hearing impairment is the concern. The audiologist's role in 504 includes the following:

1. Provide evidence to support disability and eligibility for 504
2. Recommend necessary accommodations and services based on the hearing loss and its implications. These may include:

Table 11–4. Required information for the IFSP and the audiologist's role in contributing to that information.

Required Information	Audiologist's Role
A statement of present levels of development in the areas of physical(including vision, hearing and health), cognitive, language and speech, social-emotional, self-help.	Present results of audiological assessments, including information regarding the child's auditory development and functional use of hearing; describe the impact of the hearing impairment on communication, language, learning, and social/emotional development.
A statement of the family's resources, priorities, and concerns related to enhancing the development of the child.	Provide additional information or clarification when appropriate to support the parents and supplement the group discussion.
A statement of the major outcomes expected to be achieved for the child and the family, and the criteria, procedures, and timelines used to determine the degree to which progress toward achieving the outcomes is being made, and whether or not revisions of the outcomes or services are necessary.	Assist the family in the development of the outcomes and evaluation components, especially those relevant to the child's hearing
A statement of specific early intervention services necessary to meet the unique needs of the child and the family. This statement should reflect that there was a discussion about the options and array of community services available for the child and family.	Provide specific recommendations for intervention and treatment of the child related to the hearing impairment and the supports needed and desired by the family. Include all service and program options discussed with the family.
The projected dates for initiation of the services and the anticipated duration of the services.	Assist the family in determining these dates.
The name of the person responsible for implementing the service plan and coordinating the process among other agencies and/or persons.	Assist the family in determining who this individual will be.
The steps to be taken to support the child's transition to preschool services, if appropriate.	Help bridge the family between clinical and school-based audiology services; schedule a meeting with both audiologists and parents present to determine roles and responsibilities related to the child's audiology services needs.

➤ Amplification
➤ A notetaker or interpreter
➤ Classroom and environmental accommodations
➤ Instructional modifications
➤ Assistive technology (captioner, TDD)

3. Conduct annual hearing evaluations and update hearing needs when appropriate
4. Monitor amplification and provide inservice to teachers on correct usage of equipment
5. Monitor academic performance

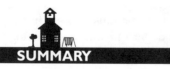

SUMMARY

Individual planning serves a variety of purposes for children with disabilities. For the past two decades federal legislation has served these children well, providing them access to the quality education, services,

and supports that is deserved by each one. Audiologists have a critical role in planning for these services because it is the individual plan, whether the IFSP, the IEP, or the ITP, that is the defining legal document which determines the services and supports for these children. Audiologists must use this avenue to advocate for the needs and services that children with hearing impairments are entitled.

SUGGESTED READINGS

Luetke-Stahlman, B., & Luckner, J. (1991). *Effectively educating students with hearing impairments.* New York: Longman.

National Association of State Directors of Special Education, Inc. (1993). *Deaf and hard of hearing students educational service guidelines.* Alexandria, VA: Author.

Roush, J., & Matkin, N. (1994). *Infants and toddlers with hearing loss,* Baltimore: York Press.

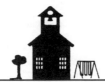

CHAPTER 12

INSERVICE

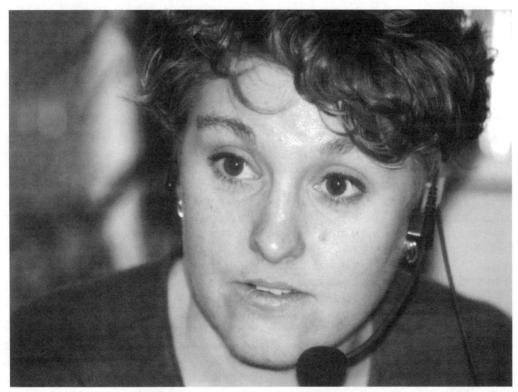

Ann, teacher, deaf and hard of hearing students

CONTENTS

The word *inservice* typically is used within the field of American education to refer to training or education provided to school personnel after they have accepted or are already working in a specific job. Inservice usually targets job-specific information or skills related to needs in the present job situation which were not adequately addressed in the employee's preservice education, that is, that which took place before the individual was hired. Although inservice was initially used as an adjective in conjunction with the word *training,* common usage has been shortened to the single word, inservice, which will be used throughout this handbook.

Inservice should be provided for all educational staff working with one or more students who are deaf or hard-of-hearing. In addition, all school personnel can benefit from inservice to increase their awareness of pediatric hearing loss, prevention strategies, and referral procedures. The importance of auditory function in traditional learning environments and children's social development is often overlooked, and inservice can be a relevant reminder of these factors, even if there are no identified students with hearing impairment within a specific school building or district.

Frequent conferences and numerous publications are available to assist individuals in developing and improving the skills needed to present information in workshop or inservice formats. This chapter gives suggestions specifically for educational audiologists whose role includes the provision of inservice. Three major phases that should be considered critical to the development and delivery of inservice for school personnel include preparation, presentation, and follow-up. Questions to be addressed in each phase include the following:

➤ Preparation—What activities should be completed when planning an inservice?
➤ Presentation—What techniques make inservice presentations interesting and effective?
➤ Follow-up—What strategies are helpful in maximizing carryover of information and strategies that have been presented?

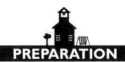

PREPARATION

Most educational audiologists have a wealth of information to share with their colleagues. Preparation of materials is often not as important as deciding what, when, and how much information to share within a given inservice session. These decisions should be based on knowledge of inservice schedules, target audiences, and current student needs. Once this knowledge is obtained, the organization of materials and equipment, and preparation of the facility can help to make more efficient use of inservice time. Some specific strategies to facilitate planning for the educational audiologist are described in the following sections.

Scheduling

The educational audiologist should find out if the school building or district has a formal inservice schedule. If so, identify the person who is in charge of this schedule, and ask him or her what procedure needs to be followed for educational audiology to be included on the schedule. Preplanning days are often used for inservice, but teachers may not have much available time or interest in formal presentations during this period. Individual or small group inservice may be more effective, if this time slot is all that is available.

If the educational audiology topic cannot be scheduled for the entire time allotted to a scheduled teacher inservice (often 1–2 hours, half a day, or a full day), determine if 15 minutes could be allocated with the entire school faculty. If so, a brief description of educational audiology services, student characteristics that suggest a need for referral, and current referral procedures might be more useful than an overview of specific effects of varying degrees of hearing loss or information on hearing conservation.

Targeting the Audience

Know the audience beforehand, if possible. What are their reasons for attending the inservice? Learning depends on motivation, and if the audience consists of teachers who are required to be there, the educational audiologist will need to plan a technique to involve them or pique their interest in the topic prior to presenting key information.

Has this group of teachers or administrators listened to information on hearing loss previously and have most of them been involved with students who are deaf or hard-of-hearing? If so, the information provided would be much different than that given to an audience who was receiving material for the first time. If the educational audiologist is new to the school system, or if there has been a significant change in school personnel, a brief needs assessment of the target audience can help to describe prior knowledge of and experience with the topic(s) being considered before preparing for an upcoming inservice.

How many people will be in the audience? A group of 12–15 people is excellent for audience participation, and smaller groups can have relevant discussions and problem-solve while completing hands-on activities (e.g., setting up an audiometer). Larger groups can cause presenters to lose focus with personal questions and comments, and it is much more difficult to make each audience member feel closely involved in the topic. Problem solving in a large group requires a method of quickly recording proposed solutions (e.g., chalkboard, chart paper) and a recorder with legible writing who can synthesize information on the spot.

Selecting Content

Knowledge of the target audience, together with current student needs, can help in selecting content to be covered during an inservice presentation. Information given during an inservice should be practical and personalized as much as possible. If limited time is available, the educational audiologist must prioritize the information and determine what is critical to present to the group orally and what information could be given in writing for later review and follow-up. For example, if an FM system will be used for the first time immediately following the inservice, it would be critical that all school staff see and listen to this system in order to recognize it and to understand its purpose. Only those teachers directly involved in using the system might need to have information on operation and maintenance, if time precludes presenting this information to the entire group. Appendix 12–A includes a list of suggested inservice topics for educational audiologists.

Organizing the Presentation

Develop an Outline

Once the topic has been selected, the audience is known, and the time has been defined, the educational audiologist should write down the objectives and develop an outline for the presentation. The time alloted for each subtopic or activity should be determined; this is especially crucial if time is of the essence, as it always seems to be in a school system. The longer the inservice, the more need for a variety of presentation methods. A general rule of thumb to consider when planning is that there should be interaction and activity every 15 to 30 minutes for maximum involvement in adult learning. Because many participants in inservice sessions like to have an outline of the presentation with space to take notes, consider this as a possible handout. Additional information on techniques and strategies to maximize adult learning can be found in Brundage, Keane, and Macknesen (1993) and Moore (1988). Sample outlines for inservice for teachers, administrators, and paraprofessionals can be found in Appendix 12–B.

Select Materials

Collect more materials than you plan to use, then divide them into materials that are critical to show or disseminate and those that can be put aside to refer to if there is extra time. Materials, equipment, and supplementary videos can also be shown or made available for individual perusal during a break. In our experience extra materials are rarely looked through after the inservice session has concluded.

Review any videos in advance, and have them set to begin exactly where needed to illustrate a point. Keep video segments brief, and provide the audience with oral or written instructions concerning what they should be looking for during each segment.

Overheads should be easy to read and have minimal information contained on each one. If the information on an overhead is crucial, consider providing it in a handout as well.

A listing of currently available commercial materials that are useful for inservice presentations is included in Appendix 16–M. However, it should be emphasized again that inservice for school personnel should be personalized as much as possible to the current educational environment, as illustrated by the students presently enrolled and the equipment in use or proposed for use within the participating school system(s). Commercial materials should only be used to introduce topics or illustrate specific points.

Preparing Equipment and Facilities

Equipment

Immediately preceding the inservice session, make sure any audio-visual equipment is working and positioned for easy use. A variety of media can help maintain attention during an inservice, but multiple pieces of equipment can lead to awkward body positions and occasional trips over extension cords. If amplification or assistive devices are to be demonstrated, they should be checked just prior to the session, and plans for troubleshooting should also be available just in case. Equipment malfunction can be a great reinforcement for teachers whose FM equipment always seems to break down just before the educational audiologist is scheduled to arrive, but spare devices should be available for an inservice if audience members have not experienced their use before.

The Room

Structure the room so that participants can both see and hear. Poor seating arrangements can dramatically illustrate difficulties faced by students who are hearing impaired, but time should be available for participants to change their seating arrangement(s), if that is the point being emphasized. Any time the audience is required to move around, a period of 10 to 15 minutes is required before they can come back together as a group.

Teachers always appreciate a table for taking notes and spreading out, especially after a full day in the classroom. If there are extra materials to peruse, arrange them on a separate table for easy access. Check the temperature and the lighting, and know where the controls are so that each can be modified, if necessary, during the inservice session.

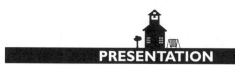

PRESENTATION

Audience Effects

Personalize Information

Reinforce the participants' current knowledge, and make information presented as specific to their situation as possible. During an hour presentation, leave the audience with no more than two or three key points to remember and, whenever possible, use within the next 24 hours. The prevalence of hearing loss is such that almost all participants will know someone (child or adult) who has a hearing problem. If it is possible to trigger thoughts of that person, any information provided immediately becomes more personalized and more likely to be remembered.

If the audience is small (less than 15 individuals) and their background is unfamiliar to the educational audiologist, have each participant give one or two pieces of information about an individual with hearing impairment they have known or worked with in the past. Record this information on chart paper to incorporate in later discussion. For example, gender, age, and amount of hearing loss could be incorporated into a presentation on incidence of hearing loss (does this audience's experience match local, state, or national demographic information?). This technique can be especially useful when participants do not know each other well, because they can immediately identify those with whom they share a common background.

Another familiarizing technique is to have participants take the first 2 or 3 minutes to write one question they have about hearing or hearing loss on index cards that are provided when they arrive. These cards can be collected and reviewed by the presenter during the first break to see if the information being presented is on target for this audience. Another use for these

question cards would be to have participants answer relevant questions as a group during the wrap-up of the session, especially for key points that have been addressed. Always have extra cards available for questions that may arise during the inservice session.

Be Flexible

Allow time for questions throughout the presentation. Questions are invaluable for identifying issues of concern and the focus of audience members. Questions can let the presenter know if the information presented has been understood and when the information has already been personalized to individual participants' teaching situations. If the answer is not known (or inaccessible during the stress of a formal presentation), arrange to follow up with the participant at school. This, again, not only personalizes the information, but is a good marketing tool for the educational audiology program.

Postpone questions if they will be more relevant during a later portion of the presentation, but remember to answer them and identify the person who asked, whenever possible. One technique that can be helpful for remembering questions is use of a chart or section of blackboard for recording or "parking" deferred questions in full view of both presenter and audience. This technique can be especially helpful in preventing a discussion from going off on a tangent, while still reinforcing questioners who asked something that was important to them.

Be Alert to Physical and Mental Limits

Respect the participants' time and energy. No one likes to sit and listen for lengthy periods of time after a full school day. Let audience members specify or choose time for break(s)—that empowers them to allocate their attention in the way they feel is most productive. Encourage participants to move for better viewing or listening, or just to change position when needed. Again, this can be a relevant demonstration of the recommendation for flexible seating often given for students with hearing impairment.

Consider placing bowls of candy or other food energizers on each table. Sugar and chocolate can increase attention after a long day. Sensory toys, such as soft squishy balls, can also help the urge to fidget while listening.

Use Ice Breakers and Humor

If the inservice session is scheduled for a half or full day, consider taking time for a warm-up activity. Break up into pairs or small groups and have each person introduce another participant, giving name plus one piece of personal information—hobby, children's ages, pets, or travel fantasy. Small groups can also be used to generate specific questions or concerns about hearing loss brought to the session. As stated previously, familiarity among participants usually increases the comfort level of the audience, and knowledge of audience interests and motivations can be invaluable for the presenter.

Humor has many benefits during inservice, as well as life. Humor can reduce stress, facilitate learning, enhance creativity, diffuse anger and feelings of frustration, and improve communication. Strategic use of cartoons on slides or overheads can illustrate key points, as well as serve as a break from processing auditory and/or written information. Daily comic strips often deal with pertinent points (competing noise, multiple word meanings, idioms), and these can be laminated and passed around during a presentation. Another display strategy is to tape various cartoons around the room to be viewed during break time. Cartoons and jokes should be used judiciously, however, as they can become a distraction when too many or irrelevant ones are included.

Equipment Demonstration

If equipment is demonstrated, make sure all participants have hands-on experience before they leave the inservice. For example, the easiest way to demonstrate a classroom amplification system is to use it during a presentation. This technique is especially effective at the end of a school day, when everyone appreciates improved signal-to-noise conditions. Passing around a personal hearing aid and an FM receiver on separate stethoscopes can be a dramatic demonstration of the difference in the auditory signal available to the student. Use captioned videos whenever possible. If not specifically included in the formal presentation time, have a captioned video available for viewing during a break. Participants are also usually eager to have their own hearing screened and/or experience tympanometry, if they have not done so previously, and these are easily done during break times. If a telecommunications device for the deaf (TDD) is being shown, arrange for a call to another site where an actual conversation can be experienced. Again, as with lecture information, incorporate practical applications into equipment demonstrations.

Use of Handouts

Handouts can be used as outlines to follow during a presentation and/or as follow-up information. Either use requires at least a mention and some direction

during an inservice presentation—for example, under what circumstances the handout might be useful, or highlights for specific information on a reference list. Handouts should be easy to read and use (double or triple-spaced, bulleted, highlighted by different fonts, etc.). If the inservice covers several different areas (e.g., equipment use and maintenance, teaching strategies, referral procedures), consider color-coding them for easy future reference for participants.

Always provide a handout restating the critical points to be taken away from the inservice, and include name, office address, phone number, and hours the educational audiologist can be reached. If office hours are not an option, make sure there is a way messages can be accessed at the phone number provided. As stated earlier, information on overhead transparancies should be considered as handouts.

Permission should be obtained for copyrighted material prior to dissemination as a handout. Sources should always be credited on each page of a handout.

Commercial brochures and other written materials may contain useful information, but they are frequently not personalized and too general for immediate use. Although they usually look good, they are more likely to be placed on a shelf or in a file without being read.

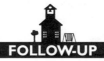

FOLLOW-UP

Follow-up activities are a critical part of any inservice program designed and delivered by the educational audiologist. Evaluation of materials and formal presentations help to ensure that future inservice programs are informative and relevant. Follow-up with individual participants helps to ensure that information is retained and implemented for the benefit of the students being served. Different follow-up activities can help achieve each of these objectives.

Evaluation

Participants should have the opportunity to evaluate an inservice presentation at its conclusion. Most individuals do not return a form later if they take it with them intending to do so. If a form is not already required for use in the school district, the educational audiologist should design one which will elicit the maximum information in a format which is quickly completed. A sample inservice evaluation form is included in Appendix 12–C. If the educational audiology presentation was a part of a larger course or inservice program, request a copy of the portion of the course evaluation that applies to audiology.

Review the outline and objectives developed during the preparation phase. Were the objectives appropriate to this audience? Were the anticipated times realistic? Which activities were successful, and which ones did not go well? Why? What should be changed for future presentations?

Re-evaluate all handouts before disseminating again. Were they read? Were they used? This re-evaluation can take the form of a brief follow-up questionnaire for inservice participants or can be as informal as a glance around the teachers' rooms the next day to see what happened to the materials that were distributed.

If handouts contain necessary information but were not read or used, try to rephrase and/or illustrate the point in a more meaningful fashion for the next inservice.

Continuing Contact with Participants

Large-group inservice sessions can serve several useful purposes, such as dissemination of general information, increasing awareness concerning the scope of school-based audiology services, and provision of specific information regarding educational audiology procedures or individual student needs. It is critical to provide follow-up information on specific students with small group or individual conferences to insure that relevant information has been understood. Techniques that can facilitate individual follow-up include scheduling small group sessions, classroom observations, individual consultations, and specific activities related to hearing and hearing loss.

Small Group Sessions

Use of a small group session as a follow-up to an educational audiology inservice is an efficient way to help school personnel implement information on troubleshooting of personal hearing aids and classroom amplification. Individuals attending might include the regular classroom teachers, teacher assistants, tutor, interpreter, speech-language pathologist, building administrators, and any other adults involved in extracurricular activities. When appropriate, students could also be involved, although they would be considered as an assistant to the educational audiologist rather than an inservice participant during this activity. Staff and student responsibilities could be assigned during this session, and a workable form for daily recording for equipment function could be developed or modified at this time.

Classroom Observations

Teachers might request classroom observations as a follow-up to an inservice when they think they may have a student appropriate for referral. If time is available, this request should be quickly followed up, because individual interactions with referring teachers can facilitate more appropriate future referrals without classroom observation. When a teacher is given a referral form and advised to refer the student without observation, the benefits of face-to-face interaction between the educational audiologist and classroom teacher are lost. Suggestions for classroom modifications and interim teaching strategies can also be reinforced when appropriate.

Individual Consultation

Chapter 2, Roles and Responsibilities of the Educational Audiologist, and Chapter 7, Case Management and Aural (Re)habilitation, of this handbook cover the role of the educational audiologist in case management and consultation and serve to illustrate the importance of proficiency and flexibility when delivering information which will provide for the maximum benefit of each individual student who is hearing impaired. It is imperative that teacher requests for consultation for students with hearing loss be addressed by the educational audiologist as quickly as possible, even if the information requested has been given previously in writing or during a prior face-to-face contact.

Special Activities on Request

Other requests that may result from an initial inservice presentation by the educational audiologist include measurement of classroom noise levels, lecture/classroom teaching on anatomy of the ear or the hearing process, screening of children of inservice participants, information for spouse or other relatives concerning hearing assessment and amplification, and classroom lessons on ear protection. Although some of these activities may not be listed as a priority in the educational audiologist's job description, each affords an opportunity to build credibility and improve communication with individual school staff members. For this reason, whenever a request follows an inservice, it should be addressed by the educational audiologist as quickly as possible.

One way to elicit and remember specific staff requests is to provide a sign-up list for participants during the initial inservice presentation. Sending a follow-up letter through school mail identifying activities that can be requested is another way to elicit opportunities to interact individually with inservice participants after a formal presentation. Attach a request form and referral sheet to this letter. In addition to observing which handouts seem to be used by inservice participants, the educational audiologist should request selected teacher critique of handouts before using these again. If equipment such as TDDs, tele-captioners, or classroom amplification systems are available for loan, provide a sign-up sheet for such equipment or other materials identified during the inservice presentation. Even if directions for installation and use are not required, another opportunity for face-to-face interaction can occur if the educational audiologist can deliver the requested equipment or material in person.

successful techniques used in meetings previously attended and adapt these whenever possible for use in a school-based inservice. Information on successful techniques and relevant materials should be shared during peer group meetings, as well as through professional newsletters and conferences. Thoughtful planning and rapid follow-up can help to improve skills and expand opportunities for inservice by the school-based audiologist.

SUMMARY

Inservice needs to be an integral and ongoing part of an educational audiology program. Too often, students with hearing impairment remain unidentified or underserved because school staff are not given information in an interesting and usable format. The educational audiologist should develop an ongoing list of

SUGGESTED READINGS

Kemp, J.E.,& Smellie, D.C. (1994). *Planning, producing, and using instructional media* (7th ed.). New York: Harper & Row.

Rosenberg, G., & Blake-Rahter, P. (1995). Inservice training for the classroom teacher. In C. Crandell, J. Smaldino, & C. Flexer. *Sound-field FM amplification: Theory and practical applications*. San Diego: Singular Publishing Group, Inc.

PROGRAM EFFECTIVENESS

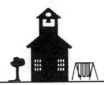

CHAPTER 13

MARKETING

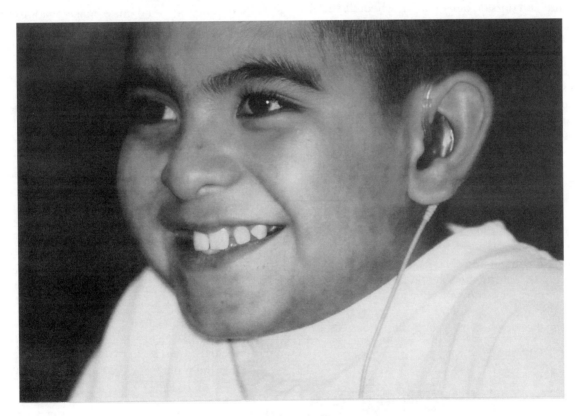

Luke, age 9

CONTENTS

Historically, marketing has been perceived as selling, and most of us did not select the profession of educational audiology because of a desire to sell either ourselves or a product. More recently, we have begun to understand that the provision of information concerning our programs and services is considered a form of marketing, and this information dissemination is vital if educational audiology programs are to continue. In today's climate of reduced governmental budgets and health care cost containment, it is critical that educational audiologists be clear about who we are, what we do, and the value of these services within the educational setting. In addition, for school-based audiology to remain a vital part of education, educational audiologists must continually market their programs both within and outside of individual school districts.

All communication by educational audiologists serves the two purposes of marketing identified by English (1995)—increasing the visibility of educational audiology services and educating specific target audiences concerning the implementation as well as importance of those services. This chapter elaborates on the concept of marketing through communication to target both internal and external audiences, and, further, details ways to enhance communication with other school-based personnel, parents, and the community at large. Specific questions addressed in this chapter include the following:

➤ What are the goals for marketing educational audiology?
➤ Who are the target audiences?
➤ What type of information should be disseminated?
➤ What strategies are most effective for disseminating information?
➤ How can the success of marketing efforts be assessed?

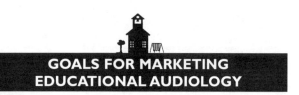

GOALS FOR MARKETING EDUCATIONAL AUDIOLOGY

Marketing goals for educational audiologists can be summarized under three broad areas of increased name recognition, increased visibility of services, and increased knowledge of program outcomes (see Table 13–1).

Increased Name Recognition

In traditional marketing, name recognition gives the perception that a product is better because more peo-

Table 13–1. Primary marketing goals for educational audiology.

➤ Increased name recognition
➤ Increased visibility of services
➤ Increased knowledge of program outcomes

ple are familiar with its name. If buyers do not know a product's name, how will they know to buy it or even take a look at it? Similarly, if school administrators are not familiar with the term educational audiology, they will have difficulty assessing the program's value to their school system. If teachers do not know what services are available through the educational audiology program, they may make inappropriate referrals or not utilize the program at all. If community resources have not heard or seen the title "Educational Audiologist," service coordination can be more time consuming. Clearly, a top goal for marketing educational audiology is increasing name recognition both within and outside of the educational community.

Increased Visibility of Services

A second goal that is an integral part of increasing name recognition is increased visibility of services. What services fall under the scope of educational audiology, and what services are provided in the current program? Although we may focus initially on making our present services more visible, it is important to educate school personnel and the community at large about additional services that should be included in a comprehensive educational audiology program. If a comprehensive school-based audiology program is in place, the educational audiologist's marketing goal would be to maintain visibility of services so that the program will continue.

Increased Knowledge of Program Outcomes

A third goal for an educational audiology marketing program is increased awareness and understanding of the results and outcomes for educational audiology services. It often seems that our programs are justified by the number of students tested, the number of assessments completed, and/or the number of hearing aids analyzed. There is an ongoing need for disseminating information that clarifies the benefits that students and school systems receive from a comprehensive educational audiology program.

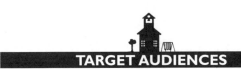

TARGET AUDIENCES

Internal Marketing

Although Hampton (1992) restricts his description of an internal marketing population to a practice's own clients (e.g., individuals with identified hearing losses), internal marketing efforts for an educational audiology practice should target all individuals who are employed by or operate within the school system. These individuals include teachers, support personnel, building administrators, central office personnel, School Board members, and other district employees, as well as students and parent volunteers. Each audience will dictate the content and strategies used, depending on audience members' specific job responsibilities. For example, the educational audiologist might include more fiscal data when giving a presentation to administrators responsible for budget approval, while listing referral information in a handout prepared for classroom teachers.

Internal marketing by the educational audiologist frequently takes place through the provision of inservices to school employees and during teacher conferences on specific students. Strategies to use during these activities are discussed in Chapter 7, Case Management and Aural (Re)Habilitation, and Chapter 12, Inservice. One target audience frequently overlooked consists of the students themselves. Although students who are hard-of-hearing would be considered our consumers, do they know us as educational audiologists? Are their parents aware that an educational audiologist is located within the school to assist with the assessment and management of the classroom environment?

There are differences in school employee responsibilities, but each of these individuals could serve as a potential referral and advocacy resource. For this reason, each of the three goals listed in Table 13–1 should be addressed during all internal marketing efforts by the educational audiologist.

External Marketing

External marketing targets audiences made up of those individuals in the community who are not employees of the school system. These may include community service clubs, parent support groups, professional organizations, private or public agencies, other educational institutions, and the news media.

External audience members may serve as referral sources, political advocates, and financial supporters, as well as assist with public relations and collaborative service provision. Reasons for targeting these external audiences are discussed in more detail in Chapter 9, Community Collaboration.

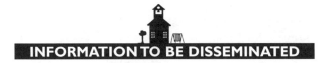

INFORMATION TO BE DISSEMINATED

Although the detail and the format of the educational audiologist's message will vary with the particular audience targeted, there are a few essential pieces of information that should be disseminated at every opportunity:

➤ The words educational audiology and educational audiologist
➤ A listing of services currently available from the educational audiologist
➤ A contact name, address, and phone number for further information

Additional topics of interest to community groups are listed in Appendix 9–C, and inservice topic suggestions are included in Appendix 12–A. Program demographic data, as well as fiscal and budget information, are critical in planning marketing efforts targeted at program administrators. Specific information on this topic is discussed in Chapter 14, Program Development, Evaluation, and Management.

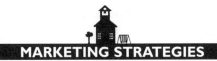

MARKETING STRATEGIES

Develop a Plan

Most marketing authorities recommend developing a marketing plan prior to launching a marketing campaign, and English (1995) described an approach for educational audiologists to use in developing this plan. She suggested developing goals or objectives from questions that reflect information the educational audiologist wishes to disseminate. Once these questions have been developed, the educational audiologist can determine if specific target audiences have the information reflected in the question. Using a chart, such as the one displayed in Figure 13–1, the educational audiologist can quickly

Questions To Be Answered	Teachers	Administrators	PTA	Students
Does audience know educational audiologist serving XYZ district?				
Does audience know services available in XYZ district?				
Does audience know referral procedures for educational audiology services in XYZ district?				
Does audience know effects of hearing loss on learning?				
Does audience know projected incidence of hearing loss in XYZ district?				
Is audience familiar with amplification equipment used by students with hearing impairment?				
Does audience know strategies to prevent hearing loss?				
Has audience had experience with hearing loss?				

Figure 13–1. Use of questions to develop objectives for target audiences. (From *Educational audiology across the lifespan*, by K.M. English, 1995, p. 54. Baltimore: Paul H. Brookes Publishing Company. Adapted by permission.)

determine objectives for each target audience. The plan is then completed by identifying strategies to get the necessary information to the target audience.

Marketing Prior to Completion of a Formal Plan

Although planning is essential to an ongoing marketing effort, many of us have had unexpected opportunities for marketing presented to us. If the educational audiologist is already doing some or all of the activities listed below, a formal marketing plan can be completed quickly and then updated as needed.

1. Begin a collection of slides, transparencies, and other visual aids that would augment a presentation when the opportunity arises. Obtain permission from parents to use photographs of students whenever these pictures are taken. Slides, videos, and photographs personalize your message, which helps it to be remembered.

2. Develop a one-page handout or brochure identifying the services provided and a contact name, address, and phone number. This activity should be a priority for every educational audiology program. Additional suggestions for developing a brochure can be found in Chapter 9, Community Collaboration.

3. Maintain a listing of current research that supports educational audiology programs and the services you now provide or would like to include in the future. This information can then be readily accessed for a handout to program administrators such as that described by English (1995, p. 56).

4. Use the handout, "18 Reasons Why Your School Needs An Educational Audiologist," developed by the Educational Audiology Association, that is included as Appendix 13–A. Keep a few copies with you at all times; it can be used in response to questions during many types of meetings.

5. Incorporate the words *educational audiology* or *educational audiologist* into each presentation you give. Our experience suggests that sooner or later an audience member will ask, "What's an educational audiologist?" Responding to this question will give you a golden opportunity to market the profession informally on the spot.

6. Use stationery and a signature that identifies your educational audiology program by name for all written correspondence, including reports on student assessment.

7. Purchase business cards as an inexpensive marketing tool—they are easily carried and disseminated, and they should identify you as an educational audiologist for increased name/title recognition.

Written Marketing Materials

Written Techniques

It may be obvious by now that any written material disseminated by the educational audiologist can and should serve the purpose of marketing. A list of written communication techniques is included in Table 13–2, but it is by no means exhaustive.

Brochures and business cards have been discussed previously, as well as letterhead and professional signatures for reports. A sample letter to parents and teachers is included in Appendix 13–B, and a sample student letter is included in Appendix 13–C. Laminated index cards with information on program services and demographics (see Appendix 13–D) are useful for dissemination both within and outside of the school system. A written consumer survey, such as the one included in Appendix 13–E, can also serve to market an educational audiology program by bringing attention to those services that may be available, but have not been utilized.

Letters to the editor of local newspapers are an excellent cost-free method of written marketing (see Chapter 9, Community Collaboration), and if there is a newsletter or other ongoing written communication within the local Deaf community, consider submitting a brief column for each issue. If there are several students served through a local or regional hearing-impaired program, consider developing a monthly or quarterly newsletter for both students and parents including "Tips From Your Educational Audiologist." Teachers of students who are deaf or hard-of-hearing may want to participate in this project as a way to address written language development. In today's era of computers and desktop publishing, newsletters are much easier to produce than in the past.

Many manufacturers and professional organizations now provide marketing information that can be adapted for use by educational audiologists. A partial listing of these resources is included in Appendix 16–L, but it will be important for the reader to update this listing, because it may change frequently.

Table 13–2. Written marketing techniques.

➤ Brochures
➤ Business cards
➤ Professional stationery
➤ Information letters to parents, teachers, students
➤ Laminated index cards
➤ Consumer surveys
➤ Letters to the Editor
➤ Newsletter columns and articles

Style and Content

It is important to remember that written materials designed for marketing should be brief, eye-catching, and highlight the primary information to be conveyed. Decide on no more than three bits of information to be remembered; then print the most important information in larger, bolder, or a different color or style of writing. Another way to approach the development of any written marketing information is to target one bottom-line message and a small number of points to support it. As stated in Chapter 9, Community Collaboration, photographs are eye-catching but they can date your written material. If this is something you might find useful for more than 1 year, critically evaluate any current data and illustrations with the future in mind.

Before mass-producing and disseminating any written material, show it to one or two individuals who could be members of your target audience and ask them to tell you what they remember about what they just read. As professionals, we bring a different level of expectancy-reading to materials we produce, and an unfamiliar eye can be very helpful.

Tips for Presentations

The suggestions given for developing and giving inservice presentations that are described in Chapter 12, Inservice, can be applied to any formal talk given by the educational audiologist. Consider the following when organizing your presentation:

1. Depending on the length of time alloted for presenting, determine the primary message and no more than two additional pieces of information for your audience to remember by the end of the session.
2. It is critical to know the background and motivation of the audience and to tailor your intended message to their interest level as much as possible. If you do not know much about your audience, ask one or two questions in the beginning that will help to shape your presentation. Sample questions are listed below, but it is important to remember to target your questions to the information you want to provide:

   ➤ How many of you have children (or grandchildren) in XYZ school district?
   ➤ How many of you have heard the title "Educational Audiologist?"
   ➤ How many of you know someone who uses hearing aids?
   ➤ How many of you have a child with a hearing problem?
   ➤ How many of you have ever seen captioned TV?

3. Involve your audience in your presentations by personalizing the information you want to provide. If the audience is a service club whose members have participated in community projects in the past, thank them for these efforts before mentioning how they might provide support for the educational audiology program you represent. If spontaneous audience questions tend to distract you from your intended message, define a time and strategy for the listeners to ask questions. For example, tell the audience you will allot the last 5 minutes to questions, and provide index cards for them to jot down these questions as they occur.
4. Supplement oral presentations with visual materials, for example, videotapes or slides, whenever possible. A picture of a baby turning to look at a sound will be remembered far better than a description of testing techniques used by the educational audiologist. One name recognition technique would be to begin your presentation by showing a videotaped segment of a student who is deaf or hard-of-hearing saying, "This is Ms. X, my educational audiologist." The same activity could be done without videotape, by showing a slide of the student while playing the same tape-recorded message.
5. Send a notice of any community presentation to the local news media, and invite them to attend. Include your business card, program brochure, and offer to write a brief article on the topic you plan to cover.
6. Always repeat your primary message at the end of your presentation, and provide written material (described previously) that reiterates target information for the audience to take with them.

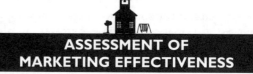

ASSESSMENT OF MARKETING EFFECTIVENESS

Assessment of marketing effectiveness is a critical component of any marketing plan. Did you achieve your goals? Which techniques were most successful and which were not productive?

Including a question on the consumer survey asking how the community respondent learned of the educational audiology program is one evaluation technique that is easy to incorporate into this strategy. Remember to include a statement offering to provide more business cards or brochures; if they take you up on it, they are assisting in your marketing efforts. Asking new referral sources how they heard of the program or service can also be a way to assess response to a marketing effort.

Pre- and post-tests can be used to document an increase in knowledge, but these are often difficult to incorporate into a marketing campaign. Following a targeted mailing or a presentation, a log of your telephone and written inquiries and referrals for a period of 2 weeks my be more useful in assessing the effectiveness of these efforts. Appendix 13–F includes a sample format of such a follow-up log.

Documenting the time spent on developing written marketing material or putting together a presentation can also help the educational audiologist decide if this particular activity was worth the effort. Financial support is easy to document, but at times other benefits can be less tangible. Did the news media print an announcement of your presentation, and did they cover it in person? An ongoing file of any media coverage provides resource material for future marketing efforts.

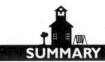

SUMMARY

There is no better person to educate about a service than the person providing that service. Creative marketing is only limited by our perception of how we can and do disseminate information. English (1996) described marketing as just another word for sharing excitement about an important and meaningful profession. If educational audiology is to survive, we, as educational audiologists, should take advantage of every opportunity offered to let others know who we are, what we do, and why we need to continue doing it.

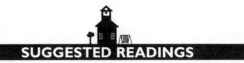

SUGGESTED READINGS

Bloom, S. (1996). High-power marketing ideas for a low-voltage budget. *The Hearing Journal, 49*, 23–28.

Levinson, J. (1994). *Guerrilla marketing.* Boston: Houghton Mifflin.

Matthew, C. (1993). *Marketing speech-language pathology and audiology services: A how-to guide.* San Diego: Singular Publishing Group, Inc.

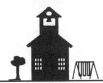

CHAPTER 14

PROGRAM DEVELOPMENT, EVALUATION, AND MANAGEMENT

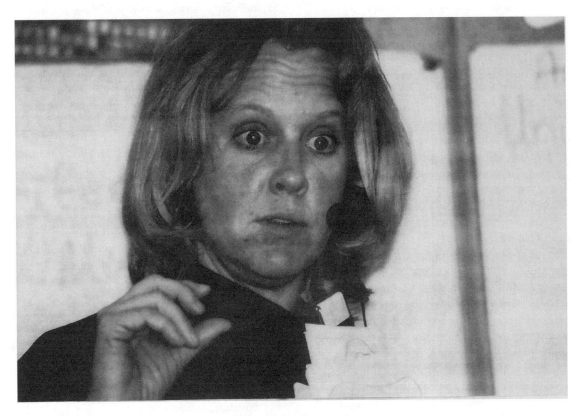

Sheila, classroom teacher

CONTENTS

183

Educational audiologists have been employed in school systems for over 20 years, yet there are still many areas in which educational audiology services are minimal or nonexistent. Few states have developed specific guidelines that ensure there is at least one educational audiologist for every 12,000 students in a school system, as recommended by ASHA's *Guidelines for Audiology Services in the Schools* (1993).

When developing new educational audiology services or expanding existing ones, the educational audiologist must have a clear idea of what needs to be changed and how these changes can be accomplished. Therefore, one of the most important aspects of the practice of audiology, or for that matter, any business, is the evaluation of the effectiveness of the services that are provided and the planning process to determine modifications or additions to the program. Likewise, the day-to-day program management is also critical to the efficiency of services. Unfortunately, due to time limitations, most of us typically make decisions based on immediate needs without thoughtful regard for their impact on our total service package. The formal evaluation and planning process can be thought of much like an Individual Education Program (IEP). The resulting long-range plan (usually a 3–5 year plan) can provide a systematic method for developing and improving services and be extremely helpful when working with school administrators to request equipment or personnel or to enhance services.

This chapter is divided into three components: program development, program evaluation, and program management. While management is on–going (i.e., day-to-day program operations), the sequence of development and evaluation may vary depending on the current status of the audiology program. For example, if the audiologist is just setting up a program, it would be appropriate to start with program development activities. On the other hand, if there is an existing program, an evaluation process should occur first to shape the development phase.

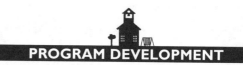

PROGRAM DEVELOPMENT

Program development begins with building a support base and conducting a needs assessment. Once the results of the needs assessment are summarized, a plan for services can be developed.

Laying the Foundation

Building the foundation for program development should include collecting evidence that supports the need for services, developing effective leadership skills, and garnering support for services.

Gathering Supporting Documentation

Guidelines of existing professional standards related to audiology services in the schools should be gathered as the first step in program development. These may include the *Guidelines for Audiology Services in the Schools* (ASHA, 1993) (see Appendix 2–B), other professional guidelines in specific areas such as screening and amplification (see Appendix Section 2—Guidelines), as well as any guidelines developed by local state departments of education. These documents are the evidence for standards of care that each local school district audiology program should follow.

Leadership Skills

Effective leadership skills are an important feature in the development and implementation of any program. A good leader should have the ability to motivate, stimulate, facilitate, and influence. The following characteristics are found in effective leaders:

➤ Good communication skills—written, oral, and listening
➤ Knowledge of administrative issues, including budget
➤ An understanding of the bigger pictures of special education and regular education, including current trends and issues
➤ Knowledge of audiology, health, and deaf education issues
➤ An ability to project future program directions (visioning)
➤ Knowledge of the community
➤ An ability to run effective meetings, synthesize information, and build consensus
➤ Flexibility

➤ Good organization
➤ Sense of humor
➤ Trusted reputation and credibility within the educational and medical communities
➤ Ability to learn quickly

Although there may only be one audiologist in a school district, his or her role must fit into the larger plan for services which involve screening programs for identification of potential disabilities (Child Find) and direct services to children with disabilities (deaf/hard-of-hearing programs). For either screening or direct services, the larger team may include nurses, teachers, early childhood specialists, speech language specialists, and other support service staff such as psychologists, counselors, and social workers. Within these teams, the audiologist must be able to garner support for the importance of comprehensive audiology services so that the support of the entire team can be used to advocate for audiology. Although educational audiologists may be independent and autonomous for decisions about specific audiology components, they must be able to work effectively as team members while providing leadership for audiology.

Support from Key Decision Makers

WITHIN THE SCHOOL DISTRICT. Perhaps the most critical element when establishing or expanding the educational audiology program is gaining support from the key decision makers, particularly the school's administration. During the steps of program development, planning, and evaluation, it is important that local administrators be aware of the activities. As a result, they will feel involved in the process and will more likely support the recommendations. Any activities the audiologist can do to make the local administrators aware of needed services or changes will be beneficial. Every opportunity to capitalize on specific situations that arise should be used as examples for reinforcing or modifying the program. Examples of activities to promote awareness of the educational audiology program include:

➤ Providing formal presentations
➤ Having informal discussions over a period of time
➤ Providing information on the mandates of the federal and state laws
➤ Sharing articles and other printed information
➤ Arranging for visits to neighboring districts
➤ Inviting principals, supervisors, school board members, or others to accompany the audiologist during all or part of the school day, including the provision of a courtesy hearing evaluation

➤ Encouraging parents to express their support, both orally and in writing

It is important that the administrators endorse the specific plans made by the educational audiologist for changes to occur. Administrators should feel that the recommended changes are possible and that they can help facilitate them. They need data concerning cost-effectiveness and information documenting that the changes will improve services to the students in their district.

STATE DEPARTMENT OF EDUCATION. In addition to support within the district, it is helpful to contact state department of education representatives who have responsibility for audiology as a related service within special education. If no one has specific audiology responsibility, the educational audiologist should identify a consistent contact person at the state department to discuss questions, concerns, and needs. If significant numbers of inquiries occur over a period of time, state department officials may begin to recognize the need for a specific person with audiology expertise to be part of the staff. Once an educational audiologist joins the state special education department team, the leadership of that individual should result in significant improvements statewide through policy development and monitoring activities.

STATE PROFESSIONAL ORGANIZATIONS AND UNIVERSITY TRAINING PROGRAMS. Support must also come from state professional organizations and from university training programs. State speech-language-hearing associations, Academy of Audiology state affiliates, and state educational audiology organizations can work together to create a professional task force on audiology services in the schools. University training program faculty should also be involved in developing and supporting school-based audiology services. Faculty member's expertise and their role in training future educational audiologists for the state should more than justify their participation in the task force. Recommendations that are presented from a body of professionals representing these various areas should provide substantial support toward the development of audiology services in the schools.

Needs Assessment

A needs assessment has a variety of functions, which are delineated below. The educational audiology needs assessment is conducted to:

➤ Determine current status of audiology program components
➤ Determine existing resources (equipment, staff, budget) necessary for audiology services
➤ Determine perceived strengths and problems of the existing services by school-based and community-based consumers and parents
➤ Help educate school, community, and parents on issues related to audiology services
➤ Obtain input on strategies to deal with the issues
➤ Stimulate discussion, consensus, and actions to address the identified program needs

A needs assessment should include:

➤ Data on national and local demographics, including incidence of hearing loss and a description of the hearing characteristics of the existing population
➤ Performance data on existing components of audiology services
➤ Opinion surveys for school-based consumers (nurses, teachers, regular education, and special education administrators—usually principals and special education coordinators), community-based consumers (agencies, physicians, and audiology and speech-language clinics), and parents
➤ Evaluation of community resources for needs related to hearing loss

The type of needs assessment conducted should be determined by the type of information required and how it will be used. There may also be different formats for the various groups that are queried. For example, a parent needs assessment may be a survey and contain less specific information than one completed by school staff. For audiology services, both specific program components and the service-delivery system should be assessed. The systems-related areas include:

➤ Comprehensiveness of services
➤ Accessibility of services
➤ Coordination of services
➤ Continuity of services
➤ Accountability for services
➤ Efficiency of services
➤ Collaboration with school and community

The protocol, Self Assessment: Effectiveness Indicators for Audiology Services in the Schools (see Appendix 14–A) can be used for both needs assessment and program evaluation. This tool is based on specific program components and service-delivery systems for educational audiology, identified as effectiveness indicators, in a self-assessment format. The rating status

for each component can be identified as "accomplished," "emerging," "a goal," or "not applicable at this time." There is also space on the form for comments and action plan activities. Another tool, Consumer Survey of Audiology Services (see Appendix 13–E), can be used to survey other groups from whom less specific information is required.

Once completed, the needs assessment should be compiled and shared with appropriate groups. These should include members of teams with whom the audiologist works most closely (e.g., nurses, teachers of the deaf/hard-of-hearing, and speech language-pathologists) as well as immediate supervisors. The results should then be used to guide the planning phase.

Planning

The planning process is a time to dream about what should be, that is, to think about optimal services and situations. Planning should begin with a vision, specifically, what a reasonable program of audiology services should be like, based on legal mandates and local needs. The vision may include several components which more specifically describe the program. An example of a vision for educational audiology services might be:

All children in ("your town" School District) will have access to comprehensive audiology services that promote early identification of hearing loss, maximal use of residual hearing, and appropriate accommodations for adapting the communication and learning environment. Specifically, children will receive audiology services that will reflect:

➤ *Sufficient resources (staff, equipment, materials, budget, and space) to provide consistent services and meet equipment needs of students*
➤ *A partnership between parents and school to maximize benefits of audiology services*
➤ *Collaborative efforts with community agencies, clinics, and services that support children with hearing impairments*
➤ *Current audiologic assessment and intervention practices*
➤ *Access to appropriate equipment*

Along with the vision, a goal is needed to provide direction for the plan. An example of a goal might be:

Implementation of a comprehensive audiology program for all children birth through 21 years old, within 2 years.

The plan for audiology services is like the short-term objectives of an IEP. We find that plans are best laid out for 3 to 5 years with specific yearly activities. As part of the development of the plan, any parameters that might affect or limit the ability to conduct certain activities should be identified. Insufficient financial resources is a common limitation to program development. Inclusion of an administrator during the planning not only facilitates the process, but may also help engender support for the activities. The plan should also include an introduction summarizing demographic and needs assessment data, as well as a brief historical overview of past and current audiology services, staff, and resources if the program currently exists.

Activities should be prioritized to determine which ones can be achieved immediately, or within a reasonable period of time (1st-year goals), and which fit into the longer term plan (2nd, 3rd, 4th, and 5th years). A sample worksheet for prioritizing goals based on a rating system is presented in Figure 14–1 (see Appendix 14–B for a blank worksheet). Activities should be determined for each component of the audiology services program. Figure 14–2 contains a sample format for a 3- to 5-year plan (only 2 years are shown in this sample) including potential audiology components (see Appendix 14–C for a blank worksheet).

Long-range plans must be reviewed at least annually to evaluate progress and determine the appropriateness of the activities as they were laid out. Revisions should occur as part of the evaluation activity. Like IEPs and IFSPs, the plans should always be considered working documents.

To summarize, the program development activities should:

1. Lay the foundation by providing standards and guidelines for audiology services in the schools and developing a support base of key individuals and groups.
2. Include data from a needs assessment including surveys of various potential consumers of the school's audiology services.
3. Develop a program vision and goal(s) based on needs assessment results.
4. Develop a long-range plan that identifies specific activities in each of the program component areas.
5. Determine budget implications and any other limiting parameters to the activities planned.
6. Prioritize activities for determination of placement within the plan (1st year vs. 2nd, etc.)
7. Provide for annual evaluation with implementation of necessary adjustments.

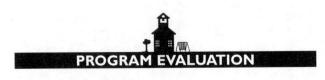

PROGRAM EVALUATION

Periodic evaluation of existing audiology services is a necessary process for all audiology programs. A comprehensive evaluation should occur at least every 3 years with annual reviews conducted at the end of each school year. Evaluation promotes change in a systematic fashion where areas of concern are identified and appropriate planning occurs to facilitate the change. The program evaluation process overlaps with program development in many areas as described in Figure 14–3.

Assessment of Existing Audiology Services

The first step in an evaluation is to consider all components of the existing program to determine potential gaps or weak areas. The self-assessment should include all necessary services for children within the school system, whether currently part of the program or as suggested in national or state guidelines. Current resources and systems information (accessibility, coordination, continuity, accountability, and efficiency of services; collaboration between the school and community) should be included. The self-assessment tool contained in Appendix 14–A can be used for this purpose as well as the survey in Appendix 13–E. Data should be collected as follows:

Self-assessment:

➤ School audiologist(s)

Consumer Survey of Audiological Services:

➤ Teachers(regular and special education)
➤ Other special education providers, (e.g., nurses, speech-language pathologists, psychologists)
➤ Administrators (principals and special education coordinators or supervisors)
➤ Community agencies
➤ Community audiology and communication disorders clinics
➤ Physicians
➤ Parents

Once all data are collected, they should be summarized in a report that includes a brief synopsis of the program, resources, demographic data, and any other appropriate supporting information. The results should be shared with the audiologist's immediate supervisor and any other appropriate individuals.

Planning for Improvement

As with program development, improvement planning should begin with a vision of what the audiologist believes services should be like, followed by a goal or goals, activities to meet the goals, and a timeline for accomplishing them. As with the program develop-

In the boxes across the top, write the goals or objectives that are under consideration. Rate them using the listed criteria. The higher the total score, the more likely that the objective is appropriate.

Goals/Objectives 1　2　3　4　5 Little　　Great	Increase communication with other audiologists in community.	Increase PE teachers' awareness to potential fistula problems associated with weight lifting	Improve identification of otitis media in preschoolers.	Increase knowledge of use of OAEs in school setting.	Increase use of sound-field amplification systems.
Importance What is the urgency or impact?	5	3	4	3	4
Control To what extent do you have control?	4	3	4	4	3
Difficulty What is the relative dificulty of achieving it?	2	3	4	3	3
Time Required How much time is required to achieve it?	3	3	4	3	2
Return on Investment What is the expected pay-off?	4	4	4	3	5
Resource Requirement What skills, space, etc. are needed?	3	3	4	5	4
Total Points	21	19	24	18	21

Figure 14–1. Sample Goal Prioritization worksheet. (From Academy for Team Leadership. A project of the University of Colorado, Denver. Adapted by permission.)

PROGRAM COMPONENT	GOALS	1ST YEAR		2ND YEAR	
		ACTIVITIES	BUDGET/RESOURCES	ACTIVITIES	BUDGET/RESOURCES
Community/Family Collaboration	Increase communication with other audiologists in the community.	1. Facilitate 2–3 lunch meetings with audiologists to discuss school and private service relationships.	1 1/2 hrs/lunch	1. Continue periodic lunches. 2. Invite private audiologists to visit school clinic facility.	1. 1 1/2 hr/lunch 2. 1 hr/audiology visit
Prevention	Increase PE teachers' awareness to potential fistula risks associated with weight lifting.	1. Conduct inservice for high school PE teachers.	2 hrs (1 hr prep & 1 hr inservice)	1. Conduct inservice for junior high PE teachers.	2 hrs
Identification	Improve identification of otitis media in preschoolers.	1. Identify screening sites 2. Purchase tympanometer. 3. Train nurse(s) to do tympanometry screening. 4. Implement tympanometry screening & referral criteria.	1. $1800 for tympanometer 2. 2 hrs training 3. Time for screening.	1. Expand tympanometry screening to all preschool sites.	1. Increased time for screening
Assessment	Implement OAE screening in school settings.	1. Attend one OAE workshop.	1. 8 hrs to attend workshop. 2. $200 workshop registration fee	1. Purchase OAE screening equipment. 2. Implement screening program for difficult to assess students.	$5000.00
Amplification	Increase use of sound-field amplification systems.	1. Target 2 classrooms, purchase 2 systems, & set up. 2. Conduct pre- & postlistening evaluations on targeted students in classrooms.	$1200.00	1. Target 2 additional classrooms, purchase systems, and conduct pre- & postlistening evaluations.	$1200.00
Management and (Re)habilitation	Increase accountability for development of auditory skills in HI students.	1. Develop auditory development profile.	20 hrs	1. Implement use of auditory development profile for 10 HI students.	20 hrs (2 hrs/student)
Program Development & Management	Use time to provide most critical audiology services.	1. Review & prioritize audiology services. 2. Provide essential services according to priority list.	8 hrs	1. Review priority list of services; make necessary adjustments.	4 hrs

Figure 14–2. Sample long-range planning format.

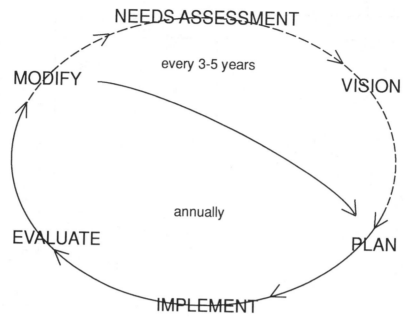

Figure 14–3. The program development, planning, and evaluation cycle.

ment, the plan should contain both long-and short-term activities that can be contained in a three to five year plan (see Table 14–2 for a sample long-range planning format). Development of the components and activities for the plan should be based on the needs that were identified in the assessment and the comparison of existing services to those required or desired. Particular attention should be paid to including a plan for purchase of new equipment and replacement of old items. The high costs of equipment often require at least 1 to 2 years of advance budget planning. When developing and prioritizing goals (see Table 14–1 for a sample prioritizing worksheet) and activities, the following questions should be considered:

➤ How will the goal/activity be accomplished?
➤ Who will be responsible for implementing the goal/activity?
➤ What current resources can be used to accomplish the goal/activity?
➤ What additional resources, especially financial, will be needed?
➤ How will the goal/activity be implemented?
➤ When will the goal/activity be completed, or will it be on-going?
➤ How will achievement of the goal/activity be measured?

Implementation of New Services

Once the administrators have approved the plans for improving the educational audiology services in

their district, the audiologist can begin to implement the changes in the program. It is important to remember that these changes will be effective only if they are supported by other members of the educational staff. The audiologist must be careful to educate all personnel and parents about the services and why they are important for the students. Changes in the educational audiology program should be implemented in a systematic manner as determined in the 3- to 5-year plan to ensure adequate resources and necessary support to promote the program's success. Administrators should always be kept informed of program developments and the effects of the changes. Their support will be continued only if they feel informed and can see the benefits in services for children. This requires ongoing attention to marketing on the part of each educational audiologist, which should be included in the long-range plan (see Chapter 13, Marketing, for more specific information on marketing educational audiology programs).

Measuring Effectiveness

Effectiveness and outcome measures tell us whether program goals have been accomplished. The major questions to ask when determining effectiveness are (1) "Does the program make a difference?" and (2) "What would have happened in the absence of the program?" To determine effectiveness accurately, the relationship between cause and effect should be as close as possible. As program efficacy becomes more of an issue in the justification of services, we will need

Table 14–1. Outcomes for Educational Audiology Services

1. Audiology services are coordinated with community-based services.

2. Audiology services support community resources in the development of a high-risk registry, newborn screening, and follow-up services to identify and manage infants and toddlers with hearing loss.

3. Audiology services, using audiometric technicians or other trained personnel, provide hearing screening programs that identify preschool and school-aged students with hearing loss.

4. Audiology services use both traditional and functional measures to provide comprehensive, developmentally appropriate, hearing evaluations that are educationally relevant.

5. Audiology services provide identification and assessment of students with central auditory processing disorders.

6. Audiology services provide medical, educational, and community referrals for students with hearing loss.

7. Audiology services report and interpret assessment results for parents, school personnel, and others involved with the student.

8. Audiology services are coordinated with other educational services and make specific recommendations for auditory and communication needs to assist with the determination of program placement.

9. Audiology services provide inservice training to students, parents, and school personnel concerning hearing, hearing impairment, and the implications of hearing impairment.

10. Audiology services educate students and school personnel about noise exposure and hearing loss prevention.

11. Audiology services provide recommendations for the use of hearing aids, cochlear implants, group and classroom amplification, and assistive listening devices.

12. Audiology services evaluate and monitor the proper fit, functioning, and use of hearing aids and other auditory devices.

13. Audiology services analyze classroom acoustics and make recommendations for improving listening environments.

14. Audiology services manage the calibration and use of audiometric equipment.

15. Audiology services are coordinated with services provided by school, parents, teachers, special support personnel, and relevant community professionals.

16. Audiology services provide the necessary assistive devices for students with hearing loss.

17. Audiology services provide direct services to students with hearing impairments, including speechreading, listening, communication strategies, use and care of amplification, including cochlear implants, and self-management of hearing needs.

to monitor effectiveness more closely. Outcome measures are one way to determine program effectiveness. Some outcomes for educational audiology services are listed in Table 14–1. These outcomes are included as part of a program effectiveness evaluation which is described in Figure 14–4. This process considers evaluation in two phases: (1) process or formative measures (monitoring of daily tasks and assessment of program activities) and (2) outcome or summative measures (identifying outcomes, measuring their effectiveness, and assessing the impact of the audiology services program).

In summary, the program evaluation process includes the following steps:

1. Look at school/community needs for audiology services.
2. Evaluate the various models that might be used to provide the services (see Chapter 2, Roles and Responsibilities of the Educational Audiologist, for information on service delivery models).
3. Determine the services that presently exist.
4. Determine the services that are needed.
5. Determine how to get the services that are needed.

6. Evaluate the services and their effectiveness based on prevailing standards and best practices.

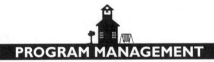

PROGRAM MANAGEMENT

The day-to-day operation of school audiology programs requires good organization and management. This section addresses many of the operational aspects of the program, including scheduling, office support, data management, and budgeting.

Annual/Monthly Schedule

It is helpful to lay out an annual schedule of monthly activities so that necessary advance preparation and scheduling can occur. This schedule should include the months of the year that certain activities should be completed. Table 14–2 shows a sample monthly schedule of activities. This schedule should be provided to the audiologist's immediate supervisor so that the supervisor is aware of what will be accomplished at certain points during the year.

Process/Formative Evaluations	Outcome/Summative Evaluation
I. *Monitoring Daily Tasks* • Are audiology service obligations being met? • Are audiology services taking place how and when they should? • Are audiologists and support personnel working when they should? • Is the audiology program administered soundly? • Are daily audiology activities carried out efficiently? • Are audiologists and support personnel adequately trained for their duties? II. *Assessing Audiology Program Activities* • What is done to whom? What audiology activities are occurring? • Who is the target of each activity: numbers and types of individuals (students/staff/parents etc.)? • How well is the audiology activity implemented? • How could the activity be done more efficiently? • Were students, teachers, parents, physicians, and other consumers satisfied with the audiology services? • Does the audiology program have a favorable image?	III. *Enumerating Audiology Program Outcomes* • What are the results of the audiology activities described in II? • Should different audiology activities be substituted? • Have audiology program goals and objectives been achieved? • What happened to students with auditory disorders? How do students function differently from before? • Have unanticipated outcomes also occurred and are they desirable? • What audiology activities might be continued to insure their future occurrence? IV. *Measuring Effectiveness of Audiology Services* • What would have happened to students/staff/parents in the absence of the audiology service? • What are all the factors that may have contributed to the changes documented in II? • How cost effective is the audiology program? V. *Assessing Impact of Services on the Prevention, Identification, and Management of Children with Auditory Disorders* • What changes are evident as a result of the audiology services? • Have the students' ability to function improved as a result of the program? • What new knowledge has been generated for the field of audiology or deaf education as a result of these services?

Figure 14–4. Evaluation of audiology program effectiveness: the sequence of program implementation and evaluation activities.

Table 14–2. Sample monthly schedule of activities.

Month	Activity
July	1. Calibrate all audiometers, tympanometers, and conduct other equipment maintenance
August	1. Review events calendar and make additions and changes for year. 2. Prepare FM and assistive equipment for distribution. 3. Schedule classroom inservices for students with equipment. 4. Prepare classroom accommodation cards for teachers. 5. Distribute equipment to students and classrooms. 6. Set evaluation schedule for year. 7. Set meeting schedule for year (triennials, annual evals, staff meetings). 8. Coordinate and set schedule for monthly preschool and community screenings.
September	1. Continue to conduct inservices for teachers. 2. Hearing screenings begin. 3. Attend state audiology conference.
October	1. Send out S.I.F.T.E.R.s to monitor elementary HI students. 2. Begin 4–6 week follow-up screenings.
November	1. Conduct first monitor of secondary HI students.
December	RELAX AND ENJOY HOLIDAYS
January	1. Review program vision, goals, and activities; make necessary modifications; meet with supervisor or administrator to discuss changes, need for increased resources, budget issues, etc. 2. Conduct second monitor of secondary HI students (at end of 1st semester).
February	1. Send out S.I.F.T.E.R.s to monitor elementary HI students. 2. Complete school hearing screenings.
March	1. Submit preliminary budget needs (equipment and staff) for following school year.
April	1. Review student records for assessments and classroom observations needed before end of current year. 2. Update PR materials and make contacts for *May is Better Speech & Hearing Month* activities.
May	1. Determine final FM and assistive device needs for coming year and submit request. 2. Submit final equipment and staff needs for coming year.
June	1. Check in, clean, and test check all FM systems, loaner hearing aids, and other assistive equipment. 2. Send in equipment for annual service. 3. Prepare FM and assistive equipment for summer school programs. 4. Order new FM and assistive equipment for coming school year. 5. Prepare school hearing screening schedule for coming year.

Day-to-Day Scheduling

A monthly calendar should be completed for daily events. Many educational audiologists schedule certain days of the week for "in-house" operations (e.g., hearing evaluations, central auditory processing evaluations, hearing aid evaluations, and report writing) and "on-site" activities (e.g., follow-up hearing screenings and monitoring of otitis media children). Because other activities, (e.g., equipment set-ups, initial IEP meetings, classroom observations, functional assessments, and teacher consultations) occur on an as-needed basis, it is recommended that at least one-half day per week be set aside for these "unscheduled" activities.

Another scheduling component concerns flexible work schedules. Many school-based audiologists have implemented work schedules that must accommodate parent's work schedules, extended school year schedules, as well as their own personal needs. Setting up appointments that include evening or Saturday hours may result in days in which work hours are between 12:00 and 8:00 PM, or trading a weekday for work on a Saturday. Other options may include summer work days that are paid either through additional contract time or by trading days during the regular school year for work days during the summer (known as "comp" time). The latter option provides summer coverage without increasing work days and, therefore, has no budget implications for the school district.

Office Support

Secretarial support and other assistants can make the day-to-day and overall operations of the program run efficiently. Activities that consume a great deal of time and that can easily be handled by a secretary include:

➤ Scheduling appointments
➤ Data entry and management
➤ Computer assistance
➤ Sending out reports and letters
➤ Filing
➤ Fielding requests for information

Without this support, the audiologist's time to conduct "audiology business" may be limited and does not demonstrate wise budgeting and delegation of program resources.

Data Management

Another area demonstrating increasing value is the use of computers for data management. Data are important to the evaluation of our services and may be cumbersome to track without computer assistance. Data management systems can be used effectively for the following activities:

➤ Managing school hearing screening results
➤ Tracking students with hearing problems
➤ Maintaining reports
➤ Collecting data on numbers of students screened, types of hearing losses, other demographics, and follow-up recommendations
➤ Scheduling timely re-evaluations

Forms

Forms help the management process by keeping track of data and other information in a consistent manner. Most audiologists now use forms that are in the computer so that information can simply be entered and then printed. Forms for various aspects of an educational audiology program can be found in the Appendixes.

Budget and Finances

Once a budget is established for the program operation and equipment outlay (due to its high cost, a specific plan for equipment acquisition and replacement should be developed), a mechanism needs to be set up to track expenditures. Purchases of equipment, repairs and maintenance, as well as incidentals and consumables (e.g., batteries, toys for the sound booth and conditioning activities, cleaning materials, earmold materials, probe tips, and paper for real ear and immittance measures) should all be tracked. Separate budget codes usually are maintained for major equipment purchases, equipment repairs and maintenance, equipment supplies, office supplies, copying and postage, and other operational expenses. The audiologist needs to work with local school finance personnel and special education administration to determine his or her responsibility as well as the method for tracking these expenses.

Facilitating Meetings

The audiologist will often need to facilitate meetings with teachers and other support personnel to provide information regarding a student's hearing needs. Additional meetings might be necessary to set up or review hearing screening programs or to develop program guidelines. Because time is valued by most school personnel, the audiologist should be mindful of all the participants' time. The following suggestions for facilitating effective meetings are important:

➤ Provide ample notification of the meeting and be mindful of participants' specific schedule limitations
➤ Clearly identify the meeting's purpose
➤ Have a function for each participant
➤ Maintain a definite pace
➤ Specify the task(s) to be completed
➤ Summarize the results of the meeting orally and in writing (if appropriate) so that all participants are clear in their understanding of the outcomes and their responsibilities for follow-up if tasks are assigned

Challenges

Regardless of our efforts to include and inform administrators of our purpose and rationale in program development, attitudes, philosophies, and budget constraints or cuts often impede our ability to provide or improve services. If the barriers can be anticipated, the problems may be easier to handle. Consensus building and conflict resolution are two strategies currently used for problem solving. Other strategies for reducing conflict include:

➤ Establishing a relationship with the individual(s) presenting the conflict
➤ Stating your concern
➤ Requesting permission to explore options for solving the problem
➤ Receiving permission to explore those options

When sharing the concern, it is helpful to be specific, brief, and to listen carefully to the individual's responses.

Information that clarifies the implications of decisions for all participants is also helpful. The Outcome Evaluation chart in Table 14–1 may provide a useful format for presenting various components of the program and how they might be affected by reducing or eliminating certain services.

Unfortunately, it is not possible to control all factors that affect the delivery of services in schools. Social value changes, alterations in public policies, and fluctuations in economic conditions are often out of our control. The challenges will continue.

SUMMARY

Developing and improving program services is essential. Although this aspect of school audiology programs often receives little attention due to our time limitations, the effort spent can be productive. Furthermore, as resources dwindle, we are experiencing increased scrutiny regarding every aspect of the services we provide. The information gathered and used for measuring program effectiveness can help provide the necessary justification for continuation of audiology services in the schools.

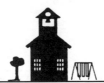

CHAPTER 15

CONTEMPORARY ISSUES

Where Are We Going?

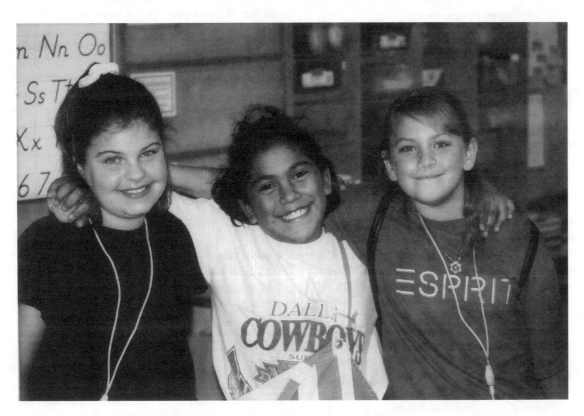

Sarah, Sadie, and Courtney . . . Friends

CONTENTS

Although none of us is a futurist, active planning for the future is critical for educational audiology. We have tried to include state-of-the-art information in this handbook, but we know that change is inevitable. Our challenge as educational audiologists is to maintain flexibility as change occurs without sacrificing our professional standards of care. The questions that follow identify issues of primary concern to educational audiologists as we look to the future:

➤ What legislation will govern our services?
➤ How will our services be delivered and paid for?
➤ What technological advances will impact our services in the schools?
➤ Who will we serve, and where will services be delivered?
➤ What training will be required for professionals to provide educational audiology services?

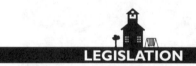

LEGISLATION

Although the current trend is toward a return to local control and away from federal regulation, it is a fact that educational audiology and educational audiologists will continue to be impacted by legislation on some level—local, state, federal, or a combination of these. Chapter 1, Educational Audiology: How Did We Get Here?, provides a thorough discussion of our legislative history and reviews current regulations that impact audiology services in the schools. A review of this information reinforces the need for educational audiologists to increase their involvement in the political process by committing to being heard on issues that affect educational audiology and students who are deaf and hard-of-hearing. We hope that the legislative changes looming in the near future retain the spirit of the current law and do not weaken the accomplishments that have been achieved for children and their families. To make this happen, however, we as educational audiologists must continually market our services through the education of legislators, as well as school personnel and other members of our communities, about who we are and what we do.

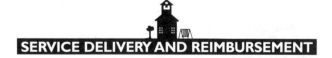

SERVICE DELIVERY AND REIMBURSEMENT

Managed Care

Just as school systems are beginning to access Medicaid and other third-party payors for educational audi-

ology services, *managed care* comes to the forefront. Publications refer to managed care as the current concept for medical cost containment, as a nationwide initiative, and as the primary focus of health care reform. As state Medicaid programs are merging with state managed health care systems, more Medicaid clients, including children enrolled in special education, are receiving services through managed health care. A whole new vocabulary, including terms such as preferred provider, fee for service, prior approval, over- and under-utilization, is seen and heard more and more often. Although the managed care emphasis on prevention is attractive and could allow funding for additional audiology services not presently covered under special education formulas, the impact of a shift to a state-operated managed care approach for all related services (including educational audiology) is not currently known and will likely not be the same for every state.

What we do know is that cost-containment is a goal in the educational arena, as well as in the arena of health care, and that whatever plans are adopted will impact what we do and how we do it. Educational audiologists must stay informed about the state and national trends in health care and work closely with the school administration to ensure that educational audiology services are included in future program plans.

Public/Private Coalitions

Collaboration with parents and the community have been discussed at length in this handbook, but the importance of working together now and in the future cannot be over-emphasized. Public/private coalitions may become more necessary for the delivery of comprehensive educational audiology services in the future, and we should begin now to plan for the intermeshing of values and philosophies that successful collaboration requires. Effective collaboration results from shared power, shared decision making, shared resources, and shared responsibility. Educational audiologists must help to build partnerships and coalitions that will ensure appropriate and seamless services for children with hearing impairments. Increasingly, the involvement of families as equal partners in coalitions that target the needs of children who are deaf and hard-of-hearing should continue to be promoted and supported by educational audiologists.

Cost-Effectiveness and Outcome Measures

Educational audiologists have become accustomed to accountability through the special education process of initiating, developing, and evaluating appropriate individual educational programs. As trends toward group managed health care plans emerge, we need to develop and use outcome measures to support the utilization and cost-effectiveness of our services. Documenting positive outcomes from the additional time required to complete a functional listening assessment or consultation with a teacher is not an easy task, but a necessary one if these services are to continue.

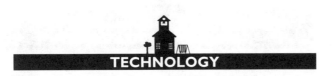

TECHNOLOGY

It almost goes without saying that keeping up with the technology explosion in audiology is an enormous challenge for all of us. There are three primary areas related to technology that educational audiologists should target now and in the future:

➤ Practice management
➤ Assessment and Amplification
➤ Educational technology

Practice Management

Computers are indispensable in the management of records required for educational audiology, as well as for other school services. This handbook contains a disk with sample forms that can be adapted for individual school systems and printed on school district letterhead. Why reinvent the wheel, if a form someone else has designed can work for you? We hope this method of sharing information will become even more common in the future.

Tracking goals, objectives, and outcome measures is much less time-consuming once the appropriate information is incorporated into a computerized student file. Data concerning students screened, assessed, results, and follow-up can be quickly obtained for administrators who always seem to need this information yesterday. Newborn hearing screening programs offer an opportunity for us to track progressive hearing losses more accurately, and computerized records will allow us to complete this task more efficiently.

The Internet includes listservs and web sites that offer a wonderful way to network with colleagues across the country about individual student needs, as well as professional issues. Recently, referral information was requested and provided through the Educational Audiology Association listserv network for a newly identified student who is hard-of-hearing whose family was moving to another state. This student did not fall through the cracks during a change of school districts because timely and accurate information concerning services, as well as the name of a per-

sonal contact, was provided to the family before their move. Educational audiologists in remote areas can access the latest information related to diagnosis and (re)habilitation for students who are deaf and hard-of-hearing through a variety of Internet web sites. Computer programs to assist in screening, diagnosis, and (re)habilitation are now on the market, and their availability will increase in the future. Tsantis and Keefe (1996) reported that 14 million workers will have access to the Internet at work by the year 2000. It is no longer debatable that computer literacy is a requirement for professional survival in the 21st century.

Assessment and Amplification

The technology available for assessment of hearing loss has expanded our options for identification of hearing loss in the school population. Increased use of otoacoustic emissions for screening cochlear function, new computer systems that operate our traditional audiometers, and automated visual reinforcement audiometry for screening younger and more involved students are just a few of the ways technology currently is affecting our role in the identification and assessment of hearing loss. Assessment technology will continue to grow and expand in the next century, and we, as educational audiologists, need to access accurate and timely information to achieve effective integration of new technology into our practices in the schools.

Amplification has changed dramatically since most of us entered the field of educational audiology, and it is difficult to envision what will be available in the near future. Educational audiologists must strive to have a working knowledge of all personal amplification that is available for pediatric fittings, even if the expertise or equipment to fit and program some of the more complex devices is not available in every educational program. True digital hearing aids are on the horizon, and this will have a vast impact on personal amplification recommended for and used by children (imagine manageable feedback!).

Personal and group FM systems have been around for a long time, but their application has increased enormously, as knowledge about the detrimental effects of noise and reverberation on auditory learning has increased. It is expected that these devices will continue to become smaller, more flexible, and routinely incorporated into personal hearing aids. Educational amplification is the educational audiologist's area of expertise, and we must continue to work closely with the manufacturers of FM and other wide-area systems to bring about solutions to problems that occur as new devices are used in a greater variety of educational settings.

Educational Technology

The expansion and increased variety of technology being utilized in learning environments for all children will impact the practice of educational audiology in the future. As computers become available for every student and teacher, and as satellite transmissions alter traditional instructional styles, educational audiologists need to be alert to changes that might affect the accessibility of classrooms and equipment for students who are deaf or hard-of-hearing. With a greater number and variety of signals being transmitted within school facilities, interference could be an even more significant problem in the future. Successful use of visual enhancement technology, such as real-time captioning and voice-activated computers, will undoubtedly result in requests to incorporate this technology into the schools of the future.

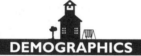

DEMOGRAPHICS

We can only speculate about school populations in the 21st century, but our past and present experiences give us some clues that can help us to anticipate future students and their accompanying needs. Increasing numbers of children from other cultures are entering the public schools, and the Goals 2000: Educate America Act (U.S. Department of Education, 1994a) refers to the need for school personnel to acquire the knowledge and skills necessary to teach an increasingly diverse student population. We have already seen changes that widened the age range of students requiring our services to include preschoolers and individuals up to 21 years of age. Again, Goals 2000 targets adult literacy and lifelong learning, so the inclusion of adult learners as consumers of educational audiology services is not beyond the realm of possibility.

And what about our primary target population—students with hearing impairment? The major known cause of childhood hearing loss when many of us entered this field was rubella, a disease that can now be prevented. Genetic research continues to identify a greater number and variety of etiologies, and vaccines in various stages of development will, we hope, eradicate some of the diseases with accompanying hearing loss in the next century.

Many students with hearing impairments attended residential schools without the services of an educational audiologist prior to the passage of PL 94-142. Now adults who are deaf or hard-of-hearing are bringing an awareness of Deaf culture to all educa-tional settings, and the resulting social and methodology issues continue to remain controversial. Never has the need for individualizing programs for students who are hearing impaired *using objective data* been greater.

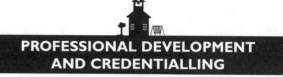

PROFESSIONAL DEVELOPMENT AND CREDENTIALLING

Finally, who will control our professional development and determine the competencies needed to practice educational audiology? We must be proactive in our approach to the issues of professional development and credentialling. The competency list compiled by the Educational Audiology Association (see Appendix 2–M) is a beginning, but these competencies need to be built into curricula used by the colleges and universities who are teaching future educational audiologists. We can break the cycle of inadequate training in many areas if we are more assertive in informing our colleagues about our practice settings, our expertise, and our training needs.

Use of support personnel within all audiology settings is a hot topic as we write this handbook. Educational audiologists must be involved in discussions on this issue because effective use of support personnel within school practices may be critical to our professional survival. Who should decide the qualifications, competencies, and scope of practice for educational audiology support personnel? If there is a national credential for audiology support personnel, how can we ensure that school systems will not hire these individuals without appropriate supervision by educational audiologists? How would the availability of support personnel impact our current services? As we review the roles and responsibilities of educational audiologists (discussed in Chapter 2, Roles and Responsibilities of the Educational Audiologist), we should strive for agreement concerning which tasks might be effectively completed by support personnel and determine which responsibilities will continue to require our direct professional expertise.

The credential on audiology's horizon is the Au.D. Although we cannot be sure of the impact of a professional doctorate on the practice of educational audiology, we do know that the development of new and expanded programs will give us the opportunity to include educational audiology as a specialized practice arena—something that is not available in many training programs at present. As a result, all audiologists should have more knowledge of the skills and competencies required to address the special hearing needs of children in schools.

The push for a new advanced-level credential has led to the development of a greater number and variety of distance learning opportunities. Continuing education has always been necessary to maintain our professional competence as educational audiologists. Expanding information and the technology explosion make ongoing professional learning even more critical, and the future will offer us more diverse ways to achieve new knowledge than ever before.

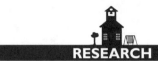

RESEARCH

One final area we must briefly address is that of research. We all know there is much to be done in the schools, but research that impacts what we do and how we do it often is not completed within the actual school environment. Research projects can offer educational audiologists another way to access new technology. For example, several school districts in Ohio and Florida received sound-field FM units from equipment manufacturers to collect data on student performance with and without these systems. Once school districts have evidence that their own students benefit from such equipment, they are more likely to provide for purchase and maintenance in future budgets.

Currently, information on transient-evoked and distortion product otoacoustic emissions as screening tools for the school-age population is limited. Who could better provide this information than educational audiologists who are incorporating TEOAEs or DPOAEs into their present screening protocols? Do we have sufficient data to justify which grade levels should be included and which should be eliminated for a cost-effective mass screening program? Private foundations and service clubs are also potential resources for funding research projects, and educational audiologists need to tap these resources and participate in the research that will affect our future and the future of our students.

SUMMARY

Although change is inevitable, there are some things that do not change over time. As educational audiologists look to the future, we should remember our roots. Most of us entered this profession because of a

commitment to children who experienced difficulty learning because of hearing impairments. Our commitment can best be illustrated by a bill of rights for children who are deaf and hard-of-hearing, developed by the Council of Organizational Representatives (COR,1992), and outlined below. These rights can and should continue to serve as our central focus as we look to the challenges and opportunities that will be presented to future educational audiologists.

COR BILL OF RIGHTS FOR CHILDREN WHO ARE DEAF AND HARD-OF-HEARING

➤ Children who are deaf or hard-of-hearing are entitled to appropriate screening and assessment of hearing and vision capabilities and communication and language needs at the earliest possible age and to the continuation of screening services throughout the educational experience.

➤ Children who are deaf or hard-of-hearing are entitled to early intervention to provide for acquisition of solid language base(s) developed at the earliest possible age.

➤ Children who are deaf or hard-of-hearing are entitled to their parents'/guardians' full informed participation in their educational planning.

➤ Children who are deaf or hard-of-hearing are entitled to adult role models who are deaf or hard-of-hearing.

➤ Children who are deaf or hard-of-hearing are entitled to meet and associate with their peers.

➤ Children who are deaf or hard-of-hearing are entitled to qualified teachers, interpreters, and resource personnel who communicate effectively with the child in the child's mode of communication.

➤ Children who are deaf or hard-of-hearing are entitled to placement best suited to their individual needs including, but not limited to, social, emotional, and cultural needs; age; hearing loss; academic level; mode(s) of communication; styles of learning; motivational level; and family support.

➤ Children who are deaf or hard-of-hearing are entitled to individual considerations for free, appropriate education across a full spectrum of education programs.

➤ Children who are deaf or hard-of-hearing are entitled to full support services provided by qualified professionals in their educational settings.

➤ Children who are deaf or hard-of-hearing are entitled to full access to all programs in their educational setting.

➤ Children who are deaf or hard-of-hearing are entitled to have the public fully informed concerning medical, cultural, and linguistic issues of deafness and hearing loss.

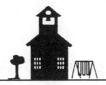

SECTION I

APPENDIXES

Federal Documents and Legal Information

CONTENTS

*Appendixes marked with an asterisk are available on a companion computer disk, which allows users to customize these forms.

Appendix I–A

FEDERAL REGULATIONS FOR SECTION 504: SUBPART D— PRESCHOOL, ELEMENTARY, AND SECONDARY EDUCATION

Subpart D applies to preschool, elementary, secondary, and adult education programs and activities that receive or benefit from federal financial assistance and to recipients that operate, or that receive or benefit from federal financial assistance for the operation of such programs or activities.

Section 104.3(j) Handicapped person.

The Section 504 regulation defines a "handicapped person" as follows:

(1) "Handicapped persons" means any person who (i) has a physical or mental impairment which substantially limits one or more major life activities; (ii) has a record of such an impairment, or (iii) is regarded as having such an impairment . . .

(2)(ii) "Major life activities" means functions such as caring for one's self, performing manual tasks, walking, seeing, hearing, speaking, breathing, learning, and working.

Section 104.32 Location and notification.

A recipient that operates a public elementary or secondary education program shall annually:

(a) undertake to identify and locate every qualified handicapped person residing in the recipient's jurisdiction who is not receiving a public education; and

(b) take appropriate steps to notify handicapped persons and their parents or guardians of the recipient's duty under this subpart.

Section 104.33 Free appropriate public education.

(a) **General**. A recipient that operates a public elementary or secondary education program shall provide a free appropriate public education to each qualified handicapped person who is in the recipient's jurisdiction, regardless of the nature or severity of the person's handicap.

(b) **Appropriate education**. (1) For the purpose of this subpart, the provision of an appropriate education is the provision of regular or special education and related aids and services that: (i) are designed to meet individual educational needs of handicapped persons as adequately as the needs of nonhandicapped persons are met and (ii) are based upon adherence to procedures that satisfy the requirements of Sections 104.34, 104.35, and 104.36.

(2) Implementation of an individualized education program developed in accordance with the Education of the Handicapped Act is one means of meeting the standard established in paragraph (b)(1)(i) of this section.

(3) A recipient may place a handicapped person in or refer such person to a program other than the one that it operates as its means of carrying out the requirements of this subpart. If so, the recipient remains responsible for ensuring that the requirements of this subpart are met with respect to any handicapped person so placed or referred.

(c) **Free education**. (1) General. For the purpose of this section, the provision of a free education is the provision of educational and related services without cost to the handicapped person or to his or her parents or guardian, except for those fees that are imposed on nonhandicapped persons or their parents or guardian. It may consist either of the provision of free services or, if a recipient places a handicapped person in or refers such person to a program not operated by the recipient as its means of carrying out the requirements of this subpart, of payment for the costs of the program. Funds available from any public or private agency may be used to meet the requirements of this subpart. Nothing in this section shall be construed to relieve an insurer or similar third party from an otherwise valid obligation to provide or pay for services provided to a handicapped person.

(2) **Transportation.** If a recipient places a handicapped person in or refers such person to a program not operated by the recipient as its means of carrying out the requirements of this subpart, the recipient shall ensure that adequate transportation to and from the program is provided at no greater cost than would be incurred by the person or his or her parents (a guardian if the person were placed in the program operated by the recipient).

(3) **Residential placement**. If placement in a public or private residential program is necessary to provide a free appropriate public education to a handicapped person because of his or her handicap, the program, including nonmedical care and room and board, shall be provided at no cost to the person or his or her parents or guardian.

(4) **Placement of handicapped person by parents**. If a recipient has made available, in conformance with the requirements of this section and Section 104.34, a free appropriate public education to a handicapped person and the person's parents or guardian choose to place the person in a private school, the recipient is not required to pay for the person's education in the private school. Disagreements between a parent or guardian and a recipient regarding whether the recipient has made such a program available or otherwise regarding the question of financial responsibility are subject to due process procedures of Section 104.36.

(d) **Compliance**. A recipient may not exclude any qualified handicapped person from a public elementary or secondary education after the effective date of this part. A recipient that is not, on the effective date of this regulation, in full compliance with the other requirements of the preceding paragraphs of this section shall meet such requirements at the earliest practicable time and in event later than September 1, 1978.

Section 104.34 Educational setting.

(a) **Academic setting**. A recipient to which this subpart applies shall educate, or shall provide for the education of, each qualified handicapped person in its jurisdiction with persons who are not handicapped to the maximum extent appropriate to the needs of the handicapped person. A recipient shall place a handicapped person in the regular educational environment operated by the recipient unless it is demonstrated by the recipient that the education of the person in the regular environment with the use of supplementary aids and services cannot be achieved satisfactorily. Whenever a recipient places a person in a setting other than the regular educational environment pursuant to this paragraph, it shall take into account the proximity of the alternate setting to the person's home.

(b) **Nonacademic settings**. In providing or arranging for the provision of nonacademic and extracurricular services and activities, including meals, recess periods, and the services and activities set forth in Section 104.37(a)(2), a recipient shall ensure that handicapped persons participate with nonhandicapped persons in such activities and services to the maximum extent appropriate to the needs of the handicapped person in question.

(c) **Comparable facilities**. If a recipient, in compliance with paragraph (a) of this section, operates a facility that is identifiable as being for handicapped persons, the recipient shall ensure that the facility and the services and activities provided therein are comparable to other facilities, services, and activities of the recipient.

Section 104.35 Evaluation and placement.

(a) **Preplacement evaluation**. A recipient that operates a public elementary or secondary education program shall conduct an evaluation in accordance with the requirements of paragraph (b) of this section of any person who, because of handicap, needs or is believed to need special education or related services before taking any action with respect to the initial placement of the person in a regular or special education program and any subsequent significant change in placement.

(b) **Evaluation procedures**. A recipient to which this subpart applies shall establish standards and procedures for the evaluation and placement of person who, because of handicap, need or are believed to need special education or related services which ensure that:

(1) Test and other evaluation materials have been validated for the specific purpose for which they are used and are administered by trained personnel in conformance with the instructions provided by their producer;

(2) Tests and other evaluation materials include those tailored to assess specific areas of educational need and not merely those which are designed to provide a single general intelligence quotient; and

(3) Tests are selected and administered so as best to ensure that, when a test is administered to a student with impaired sensory, manual, or speaking skills, the test results accurately reflect the student's aptitude or achievement level or whatever other factor the test purports to measure, rather than reflecting the student's impaired sensory, manual, or speaking skills (except where those skills are the factors that the test purports to measure).

(c) **Placement procedures**. In interpreting evaluation data and in making placement decisions, a recipient shall (1) draw upon information from a variety of sources, including aptitude and achievement tests, teacher recommendations, physical condition, social or cultural background, and adaptive behavior, (2) establish procedures to ensure that information obtained from all such sources is documented and carefully considered, (3) ensure that the placement decision is made by a group of persons, including persons knowledgeable about the child, the meaning of the evaluation data, and the placement options, and (4) ensure that the placement decision is made in conformity with Section 104.34.

(d) **Reevaluation**. A recipient to which this section applies shall establish paragraph (b) of this section, for periodic reevaluation of students who have been provided special education and related services. A reevaluation procedure consistent with the Education for the Handicapped Act is one means of meeting this requirement.

Section 104.36 Procedural safeguards.

A recipient that operates a public elementary or secondary education program shall establish and implement, with to actions regarding the identification, evaluation, or educational placement of persons who, because of handicap, need or are believed to need special instruction or related services, a system of procedural safeguards that includes notice, an opportunity for the parents or guardian of the person to examine relevant records, an impartial hearing with opportunity for participation by the person's parents or guardian and representation by counsel, and a review procedure. Compliance with the procedural safeguards of section 615 of the Education of the Handicapped Act is one means of meeting this requirement.

Section 104.37 Nonacademic services.

(a) **General.** (1) A recipient to which this subpart applies shall provide nonacademic and extracurricular services and activities in such a manner as is necessary to afford handicapped students an equal opportunity for participation in such services and activities.

(2) Nonacademic and extracurricular services and activities may include counseling services, physical recreational athletics, transportation, health services, recreational activities, special interest groups or clubs sponsored by the recipients, referrals to agencies which provide assistance to handicapped persons, and employment of students, including both employment by the recipient and assistance in making available outside employment.

(b) **Counseling services.** A recipient to which this subpart applies that provides personal, academic, or vocational counseling, guidance, or placement services to its students shall provide these services without discrimination on the basis of handicap. The recipient shall ensure that qualified handicapped students are not counseled toward more restrictive career objectives that are nonhandicapped students with similar interests and abilities.

(c) **Physical education and athletics.** (1) In providing physical education courses and athletics and similar programs and activities to any of its students, a recipient to which this subpart applies may not discriminate on the basis of handicap. A recipient that offers physical education courses or that operates or supports interscholastic, club, or intramural athletics shall provide to qualified handicapped students an equal opportunity for participation in these activities.

(2) A recipient may offer to handicapped students physical education and athletic activities that are separate or different from those offered to nonhandicapped students only if separation or differentiation is consistent with the requirements of Section 104.34 and only if no qualified handicapped student is denied the opportunity to compete for teams or to participate in courses that are not separate or different.

Section 104.38 Preschool and adult education programs.

A recipient to which this subpart applies that operates a preschool education or day care program or activity or an adult education program or activity may not, on the basis of handicap, exclude qualified handicapped persons from the program or activity and shall take into account the needs of such persons in determining the aid, benefits, or services to be provided under the program or activity.

Section 104.39 Private education programs.

(a) A recipient that operates a private elementary or secondary education program may not, on the basis of handicap, exclude a qualified handicapped person from such program if the person can, with minor adjustments, be provided an appropriate education, as defined in Section 104.33(b)(1), with the recipient's program.

(b) A recipient to which this section applies may not charge more for the provision of an appropriate education to handicapped persons than to nonhandicapped persons except to the extent that any additional charge is justified by a substantial increase in cost to the recipient.

(c) A recipient to which this section applies that operates special education programs shall operate such programs in accordance with the provisions of Sections 104.35 and 104.36. Each recipient to which this section applies is subject to the provisions of Sections 104.34, 104.37, and 104.38.

Source: From Code of Federal Regulations (CFR), Title 34; Education; Parts 1–299, July 1988.

Appendix I–B

PERTINENT EXCERPTS FROM THE INDIVIDUALS WITH DISABILITIES EDUCATION ACT: ASSISTANCE TO STATES FOR THE EDUCATION OF CHILDREN WITH DISABILITIES PROGRAM AND PRESCHOOL GRANTS FOR CHILDREN WITH DISABILITIES, FINAL RULE

Section 300.4 Act.

As used in this part, "Act" means the Individuals with Disabilities Education Act, formerly the Education of the Handicapped Act.

(Authority: 30 U.S.C 1400)

Section 300.5 Assistive technology device.

As used in this part, "assistive technology device" means any item, piece of equipment, or product system, whether acquired commercially off the shelf, modified, or customized, that is used to increase, maintain, or improve the functional capabilities of children with disabilities.

[Authority: 20 U.S.C. 1401(a)(25)]

Section 300.6. Assistive technology service.

As used in this part, "assistive technology service" means any service that directly assists a child with a disability in the selection, acquisition, or use of an assistive technology device. The term includes—

(a) The evaluation of the needs of a child with a disability, including a functional evaluation of the child in the child's customary environment;

(b) Purchasing, leasing, or otherwise providing for the acquisition of assistive technology devices by children with disabilities;

(c) Selecting, designing, fitting, customizing, adapting, applying, retaining, repairing, or replacing assistive technology devices;

(d) Coordinating and using other therapies, interventions, or services with assistive technology, such as those associated with existing education and rehabilitation plans and programs;

(e) Training or technical assistance for a child with a disability or, if appropriate, that child's family; and

(f) Training or technical assistance for professionals (including individuals providing education or rehabilitation services), employers, or other individuals who provide services to, employ, or are otherwise substantially involved in the major life functions of children with disabilities.

[Authority: 20 U.S.C. 1401(a)(26)]

Section 300.7 Children with disabilities.

(2) "Deaf-blindness" means concomitant hearing and visual impairments, the combination of which causes such severe communication and other developmental and educational problems that they cannot be accommodated in special education programs solely for children with deafness or children with blindness.

(3) "Deafness" means a hearing impairment that is so severe that the child is impaired in processing linguistic information through hearing, with or without amplification, that adversely affects a child's educational performance.

(4) "Hearing impairment" means an impairment in hearing, whether permanent or fluctuating, that adversely affects a child's educational performance but that is not included under the definition of deafness in this section.

Section 300.16 Related Services

(a) As used in this part, the term "related services" means transportation and such developmental, corrective, and other supportive services as are required to assist a child with a disability to benefit from special education, and includes speech pathology and audiology, psychological services, physical and occupational therapy, recreation, including therapeutic recreation, early identification and assessment of disabilities in children, counseling services, including rehabilitation counseling, and medical services for diagnostic evaluation purposes. The term also includes school health services, social work services in schools, and parent counseling and training.

(b) The terms used in this definition are defined as follows:

(1) "Audiology" includes—

(i) Identification of children with hearing loss;

(ii) Determination of the range, nature, and degree of hearing loss, including referral for medical or other professional attention for the habilitation of hearing;

(iii) Provision of habilitative activities, such as language habilitation, auditory training, speech reading (lip-reading), hearing evaluation, and speech conservation;

(iv) Creation and administration of programs for prevention of hearing loss;

(v) Counseling and guidance of pupils, parents, and teachers regarding hearing loss; and

(vi) Determination of the child's need for group and individual amplification, selecting and fitting an appropriate aid, and evaluating the effectiveness of amplification.

(2) "Counseling services" means services provided by qualified social workers, psychologists, guidance counselors, or other qualified personnel.

(3) "Early identification and assessment" means the implementation of a formal plan for identifying a disability as early as possible in a child's life.

(4) "Medical services" means services provided by a licensed physician to determine a child's medically related disability that results in the child's need for special education and related services.

(6) "Parent counseling and training" means assisting parents in understanding the special needs of their child and providing parents with information about child development.

(10) "Rehabilitation counseling services:" means services provided by qualified personnel in individual or group sessions that focus specifically on career development, employment preparation, achieving independence, and integration in the workplace and community of a student with a disability. The term also includes vocational rehabilitation services provided to students with disabilities by vocational rehabilitation programs funded under the Rehabilitation Act of 1973, as amended.

(13) "Speech pathology" includes—

(i) Identification of children with speech or language impairments;

(ii) Diagnosis and appraisal of specific speech or language impairments;

(iii) Referral for medical or other professional attention necessary for the habilitation of speech or language impairments;

(iv) Provision of speech and language services for the habilitation or prevention of communicative impairments; and

(v) Counseling and guidance of parents, children, and teachers regarding speech and language impairments.

(14) "Transportation" includes—

(i) Travel to and from school and between schools;

(ii) Travel in and around school buildings; and

(iii) Specialized equipment (such as special or adapted buses. Iifts, and ramps), if required to provide special transportation for a child with a disability.

[Authority. 20 U.S.C. 1401(a)(17)]

Section 300.17 Special education.

(a)(1) As used in this part, the term "special education" means specially designed instruction, at no cost to the parents, to meet the unique needs of a child with a disability, including—

(i) Instruction conducted in the classroom, in the home, in hospitals and institutions, and in other settings; and

(ii) Instruction in physical education.

(2) The term includes speech pathology, or any other related service, if the service consists of specially designed instruction, at no cost to the parents, to meet the unique needs of a child with a disability, and is considered special education rather than a related service under State standards.

(3) The term also includes vocational education if it consists of specially designed instruction, at no cost to the parents, to meet the unique needs of a child with a disability.

(b) The terms in this definition are defined as follows:

(1) "At no cost" means that all specially designed instruction is provided without charge, but does not preclude incidental fees that are normally charged to nondisabled students or their parents as a part of the regular education program.

[Authority : 20 U.S.C. 1401(a)(16)]

Section 300.18 Transition services.

(a) As used in this part, "transition services" means a coordinated set of activities for a student, designed within an outcome-oriented process, that promotes movement from school to post-school activities, including postsecondary education, vocational training, integrated employment (including supported employment), continuing and adult education, adult services, independent living, or community participation.

(b) The coordinated set of activities described in paragraph (a) of this section must—

(1) Be based on the individual student's needs, taking into account the student's preferences and interests; and

(2) Include needed activities in the areas of—

(i) Instruction;

(ii) Community experiences;

(iii) The development of employment and other post-school adult living objectives; and

(iv) If appropriate, acquisition of daily living skills and functional vocational evaluation.

[Authority: 20 U.S.C. I401(a)(19)]

Section 300.153 Personnel standards.

(a) As used in this part:

(1) "Appropriate professional requirements in the State" means entry level requirements that—

(i) Are based on the highest requirements in the State applicable to the profession or discipline in which a person is providing special education or related services; and

(ii) Establish suitable qualifications for personnel providing special education and related services under this part to children and youth with disabilities who are served by State, local, and private agencies (see section 300.2)

(2) Highest requirements in the state applicable to a specific profession or discipline: means the highest entry-level academic degree needed for any State approved or recognized certification, licensing, registration, or other comparable requirements that apply to that profession or discipline.

[Authority: 20 U.S.C. 1413(a)(14)]

Section 300.220 Child identification.

Each application must include procedures that ensure that all children residing within the jurisdiction of the LEA who have disabilities, regardless of the severity of their disability, and who are in need of special education and related services, are identified, located and evaluated, including a practical method for determining which children are currently receiving needed special education and related services and which children are not currently receiving needed special education and related services.

(Authority: 20 U.S.C. 1414(a)(1)(A)

Note: The LEA is responsible for ensuring that all children with disabilities within its jurisdiction are identified, located and evaluated, including children in all public and private agencies and institutions within that jurisdiction. Collection and use of data are subject to the confidentiality requirements of Section 300.560-300.576.

Section 300.303 Proper functioning of hearing aids.

Each public agency shall ensure that the hearing aids worn by children with hearing impairments including deafness in school are functioning properly.

[Authority: 20 U.S.C. 1412(2)(B)]

Note: The report of the House of Representatives on the 1978 appropriation bill includes the following statement regarding hearing aids:

In its report on the 1976 appropriation bill the Committee expressed concern about the condition of hearing aids worn by children in public schools. A study done at the Committee's direction by the Bureau of Education for the Handicapped reveals that up to one-third of the hearing aids are malfunctioning. Obviously, the Committee expects the Office of Education will ensure that hearing impaired school children are receiving adequate professional assessment, follow-up and services.

[Authority: H.R. Rep. No. 95-381, p. 67 (1977)]

Section 300.308 Assistive Technology

Each public agency shall ensure that assistive technology devices or assistive technology services, or both, as those terms are defined in sections 300.5-300.6 are made available to a child with a disability if required as a part of the child's—

(a) Special education under section 300.17;

(b) Related services under section 300.16; or

(c) Supplementary aids and services under section 300.550(b)(2).

[Authority: 20: U.S.C. 1412(2), (5)(B)]

Appendix: *Analysis of Comments and Changes*

Assistive Technology Device; Assistive Technology Service (Sections 300.5 and 300.6)

Comment: One commenter requested that the proposed definitions of "assistive technology device" and "assistive technology service" be modified to make them as educationally relevant as possible. Another commenter stated that, in the definition of "assistive technology service" [section 300.6(f)], the term "children" should be used in lieu of "individuals." Another commenter suggested that each State be required to include in the State plan its system for providing information and technological assistance for LEAs regarding assistive technology acquisition.

A commenter requested that procedures for determining when a child needs assistive technology be added to the final regulations. Another commenter requested that evaluations be done by personnel qualified to assess the technological needs of children with disabilities. Another commenter was concerned that school personnel would not have the training and knowledge to provide required services.

Discussion: The definitions of "assistive technology device" and "assistive technology service" are taken from sections 602(a)(25) and 602(a)(26) of the Act, and there is no authority to change the substance of those definitions. However, the requirement in section 300.308 limits the provision of assistive technology to educational relevancy— i.e., an assistive technology device or service is only required if it is determined, through the IEP process, to be (1) special education, as defined in section 300.17, (2) a related service, as defined in section 300.16, or (3) supplementary aids and services required to enable a child to be educated in the least restrictive environment. The Secretary believes that the effect of section 300.308 is to limit the provision of assistive technology devices and services to those situations in which they are required in order for a child to receive FAPE.

The Note following "assistive technology service" in the NPRM explained that, except for replacing "child" for "individual," the definition is taken directly from section 602(a)(25) (26) of the Act. The term "individuals" was inad-

vertently included in paragraph (f) of that definition. Therefore, that term is being changed to "children" in these final regulations.

The Secretary believes that while an LEA, at its discretion, might choose to provide technical assistance to LEAs about assistive technology or other provisions required in this part, it would be inappropriate and burdensome to require that a State include a description of a technical assistance system on assistive technology in the State plan.

It is not necessary to add procedures for determining the need for assistive technology services because this determination is made as part of the individual evaluation of each child as required in sections 300.530-300.534. These evaluations must be done by qualified individuals, as specified in section 300.532(a)(3).

In instances where LEA personnel do not have the knowledge to provide assistive technology services, funds under this part may be used to obtain the necessary expertise, and, if appropriate, to train existing school personnel. The Secretary does not believe that further guidance is needed on the matters raised by these commenters.

Changes: In Section 300.6(f), the clause "or are otherwise substantially involved in the major life functions of individuals with disabilities" has been revised to substitute the term "children" for "individuals."

Assistive Technology (Section 300.308)

Comment: A few commenters questioned the Department's authority to require assistive technology devices and services under section 300.308, stating that the only new statutory provisions affecting Part B are the definitions of these terms in 20 U.S.C. 1401 (a)(25) and (a)(26).

Several commenters requested that the provisions on assistive technology devices and services be amended to clarify that the cost of personal or medical devices should be borne by parents or other public agencies and not educational agencies. A few commenters requested that the final regulations clarify that an assistive technology device can be taken home by a child if it is needed to complete a homework assignment; other commenters stated that devices should be used only at school. One commenter suggested that, with respect to a child's need for assistive technology devices and services, the phrase "following evaluation of such needs" be added to proposed section 300.308(a).

Discussion: The Secretary believes that the requirements for assistive technology in this part are fully authorized by law. The report of the House-Committee on Education and Labor on Public Law 101 176 states:

* * * The Committee is aware that since the passage of the Education of the Handicapped Act, advances in the development and use of assistive technology have provided new opportunities for children with many disabilities to participate in educational programs. For many children and youth with disabilities, the provision of assistive technology devices and services will redefine "an appropriate placement in the least restrictive environment" and allow greater independence and productivity * * *.

The Committee bill incorporates definitions for assistive technology service and assistive technology device in order

* * * (2) to increase the awareness of assistive technology as an important component of meeting the special education and related service needs of many students with disabilities, and thus enable time to participate in, and benefit from, educational programs

* * * [House Report No. 101-544, 8-9 (1990).]

The Secretary believes that assistive technology devices and services may be essential to the provision of FAPE to certain children with disabilities. Section 300.308 provides only that these devices and services must be made available if they are required under current provisions of the regulations relating to special education, related services, and supplementary aids and services.

A determination as to whether an assistive technology device or service is required in order for a child to receive FAPE must be made on an individual basis using the evaluation procedures, the procedures for developing IEPs, and the procedures for placement described in these regulations. Similarly a decision as to whether a child may use a device or service in settings other than the child's school (e.g., the child's home or other parts of the community) also must be made on an individual basis.

Under section 300.301, a public agency may use whatever State, local, Federal, and private sources of support are available to provide or pay for services, including assistive technology services or devices. These services and devices must be provided at no cost to the child or parent under section 300.8 and 300.300.

The Secretary does not believe that it is necessary to add the phrase "following evaluation of such needs" because the concept of determining needs based on evaluation is central to these regulations.

Changes: None.

Comment: Several commenters objected to proposed section 300.308(b), regarding the provision of supplementary aids and services for children who are educated in regular classes, because the proposed language implied that assistive technology devices and services under this part must be provided to children who do not receive special education and related services.

Discussion: Under section 300.550(b)(2), "supplementary aids and services" must be provided to children with disabilities who have been determined to be eligible under Part B and are able to be educated in regular classes with the use of those aids and services. Assistive technology can be a form of "supplementary aids and services."

Changes: Section 300.308 has been revised to make it clear that assistive technology devices and services must be provided only if they are required under current regulations as part of a child's special education (section 300.17), related services (section 300.16), or supplementary aids and services [section 300.550(b)(2)].

Source: from Rules and Regulations, *Federal Register* (57)(189), September, 29, 1992, pp. 44794–44852

Appendix I–C

PERTINENT EXCERPTS FROM THE INDIVIDUALS WITH DISABILITIES EDUCATION ACT: EARLY INTERVENTION PROGRAM FOR INFANTS AND TODDLERS WITH DISABILITIES; FINAL RULE

Section 303.7 Children.

As used in this part, *children* means "infants and toddlers with disabilities" as that term is defined in section 303.16.

[Authority: 20 U.S.C. 1472(1)]

Section 303.11 Early Intervention program.

As used in this part, *early intervention program* means the total effort in a State that is directed at meeting the needs of children eligible under this part and their families.

(Authority: 20 U.S.C. 1471-1485)

Section 303.12 Early Intervention services.

(d) *Types of services; definitions.* Following are types of services included under "early intervention services," and, if appropriate, definitions of those services:

(1) *Assistive technology device* means any item, piece of equipment, or product system, whether acquired commercially off the shelf, modified, or customized, that is used to increase, maintain, or improve the functional capabilities of children with disabilities. *Assistive technology service* means a service that directly assists a child with a disability in the selection, acquisition, or use of an assistive technology device. Assistive technology services include—

(i) The evaluation of the needs of a child with a disability, including a functional evaluation of the child in the child's customary environment;

(ii) Purchasing, leasing, or otherwise providing for the acquisition of assistive technology devices by children with disabilities;

(iii) Selecting, designing, fitting, customizing, adapting, applying, maintaining, repairing, or replacing assistive technology devices;

(iv) Coordinating and using other therapies, interventions, or services with assistive technology devices, such as those associated with existing education and rehabilitation plans and programs;

(v) Training or technical assistance for a child with disabilities or, if appropriate, that child's family; and

(vi) Training or technical assistance for professionals (including individuals providing early intervention services) or other individuals who provide services or are otherwise substantially involved in the major life functions of individuals with disabilities.

(2) *Audiology* includes—

(i) Identification of children with auditory impairment, using at risk criteria and appropriate audiologic screening techniques;

(ii) Determination of the range, nature, and degree of hearing loss and communication functions, by use of audiological evaluation procedures;

(iii) Referral for medical and other services necessary for the habilitation or rehabilitation of children with auditory impairment;

(iv) Provision of auditory training, aural rehabilitation, speech reading and listening device orientation and training, and other services;

(v) Provision of services for prevention of hearing loss; and

(vi) Determination of the child's need for individual amplification, including selecting, fitting, and dispensing appropriate listening and vibrotactile devices, and evaluating the effectiveness of those devices.

(e) *Qualified personnel.* Early intervention services must be provided by qualified personnel, including—

(1) Audiologists;

(2) Family therapists;

(3) Nurses;

(4) Nutritionists;

(5) Occupational therapists;

(6) Orientation and mobility specialists;

(7) Pediatricians and other physicians;

(8) Physical therapists

(9) Psychologists;

(10) Social workers;

(11) Special educators; and

(12) Speech and language pathologists.

[Authority: 20 U.S.C. 1401(a)(25), and (a)(26), 1472(2); H.R. REP. No. 198, 102d Cong., 1st Sess. 14 (1991); S. REP. No. 84, 102d Cong., 1st Sess. 21-22 (1991)]

Section 303.16 Infants and toddlers with disabilities.

(a) As used in this part, *infants and toddlers with disabilities* means individuals from birth through age two who need early intervention services because they—

(1) Are experiencing developmental delays, as measured by appropriate diagnostic instruments, in one or more of the following areas:

(i) Cognitive development.

(ii) Physical development, including vision and hearing.

(iii) Communication development.

(iv) Social or emotional development.

(v) Adaptive development; or

(2) Have a diagnosed physical or mental condition that has a high probability of resulting in developmental delay.

(b) The term may also include, at a States discretion, children from birth through age two who are at risk of having substantial developmental delays if early interventions services are not provided.

[Authority: 20 U.S.C. 1472(1)]

Section 303.321 Comprehensive child find system.

(c) *Evaluation and assessment of the child.* The evaluation and assessment of each child must—

(1) Be conducted by personnel trained to utilize *appropriate methods and procedures;*

(2) Be based on informed clinical opinion; and

(3) Include the following:

(i) A review of pertinent records related to the child's current health status and medical history.

(ii) An evaluation of the child's level of functioning in each of the following developmental areas:

(A) Cognitive development.

(B) Physical development, including vision and hearing.

(C) Communication development.

(D) Social or emotional development.

(E) Adaptive development.

(iii) An assessment of the unique needs of the child in terms of each of the developmental areas in paragraph (c)(3)(ii) of this section, including the identification of services appropriate to meet those needs.

Section 303-340 General.

(a) Each system must include policies and procedures regarding individualized family service plans (IFSPs) that meet the requirements of this section and sections 303.341 through 303.346.

(b) As used in this part, *individualized family service plan* and *IFSP* mean a written plan for providing early intervention services to a child eligible under this part and the child's family. The plan must—

(1) Be developed in accordance with sections 303.342 and 303.343;

(2) Be based on the evaluation and assessment described in section 303.322; and

(3) Include the matters specified in section 303.344.

(c) *Lead agency responsibility.* The lead agency shall ensure that an IFSP is developed and implemented for each eligible child, in accordance with the requirements of this part. If there is a dispute between agencies as to who has responsibility for developing or implementing an IFSP, the lead agency shall resolve the dispute or assign responsibility.

(Approved by the Office of Management and Budget under control number 1820-0550)

(Authority: 20 U.S.C. 1477)

Section 303.342 Procedures for IFSP development, review, and evaluation.

(a) *Meeting to develop initial IFSP timelines.* For a child who has been evaluated for the first time and determined to be eligible, a meeting to develop the initial IFSP must be conducted within the 45-day time period in section 303.321(e).

(b) *Periodic review.* (1) A review of the IFSP for a child and the child's family must be conducted every six months, or more frequently if conditions warrant, or if the family requests such a review. The purpose of the periodic review is to determine—

(i) The degree to which progress toward achieving the outcomes is being made; and

(ii) Whether modification or revision of the outcomes or services is necessary.

(2) The review may be carried out by a meeting or by another means that is acceptable to the parents and other participants.

(c) *Annual meeting to evaluate the IFSP.* A meeting must be conducted on at least an annual basis to evaluate the IFSP for a child and the child's family, and, as appropriate, to revise its evaluations conducted under section 303.322(c), and other information available from the ongoing assessment of the child and family, must be used in determining what services are needed and will be provided.

Source: from Rules and Regulations, *Federal Register* (58)145, July 30, 1993, pp. 40958–40989.

Appendix 1–D

CASE LAW

Note: Case law is determined through the rulings of the court. Circuit court and state court decisions are regarded in the region or state that the particular court represents. However, their decisions may serve as the basis for rulings made by the other circuit or state courts. U.S. Supreme Court rulings determine the law of the land. The Office of Civil Rights (OCR) rules on cases which are filed through their office. These rulings also have national implications. The U.S. Department of Education provides further legal interpretation through the Office of Special Education Programs (OSEP). Clarification and interpretation of federal regulations are made through letters written in response to specific inquiries made by state education officials, parents, or other interested parties.

Legal Interpretations Relating to Audiology Services[1]

CASE	INTERPRETATION
Ambient noise levels. Pa. Commw. Ct. 1982. *Silvio v. Commonwealth, Depart. Of Educ.*, 553:577.	District did not have to establish exact ambient noise levels for class room for hearing impaired students because there was sufficient evidence to show that the ambient noise levels were appropriate.
Provision of services within a timely manner. OCR 1988. *Cleveland (OH) Public School District,* 353:307	School district violated 504 when it failed to provide FM systems, individualized speech therapy, and sufficient interpreters in a timely manner.
Insufficient hearing loss. OCR. 1991. *Humboldt (AZ) Unified School District,* 18 IDELR 28.	Lack of evidence to show student's alleged hearing impairment was substantial enough to qualify as a "handicapped person" under 504.
Use of FM system. OSEP 1992. *Letter to Anonymous,* 18 IDELR	Parent may request IEP meeting to consider use of FM system if student has current IEP but IEP does not discuss use of such a system. If student does not have current IEP, parent may request an evaluation to determine if a disability is present, and to discuss use of FM system at time of IEP meeting.
School's role for providing hearing aids. OSEP 1993. *Letter to Seiler,* 20 IDELR 1216.	Declares that a hearing aid is considered a covered device under the definition of "assistive technology device"; therefore, if the hearing aid is required by the student with a disability to receive FAPE, and the hearing aid is specified within the student's IEP as a need, then the district is responsible for providing the hearing aid at no cost to the child or his/her family as per 34 CFR 300.308.
Public agency's role for providing assistive technology. OSEP 1994. *Letter to Gay,* 22 IDELR 373.	When the IEP indicates the requirement of an assistive technology device, such as a hearing aid, as part of the student's special education program, then the responsible public agency must provide the device at no cost to the student or his/her family. If a state's regulations indicate that personal items are to be provided by a student's parents, an additional statement must be included which explains that personal items specified on the student's IEP as necessary for FAPE, would be provided at no cost to parents. When the child attends a state supported school for the deaf, the state's law, regulation, or policy defines whether the student's home school or the school for the deaf pays for the device. The responsible public agency may seek funds from other sources provided they ensure FAPE and there is no cost to the student or his/her family.

(continued)

[1]Summarized from the Individuals with Disabilities Education Law Report

(continued)

CASE	INTERPRETATION
Open classroom/minimal hearing loss. OCR 1994. *Brockton (MA) Public Schools,* 21 IDELR 1076.	Found placement of a student with disabilities, including minimal hearing loss, in an open space resource room was adequate to meet the student's needs. Placement recommendations were made by a team which included initial acceptance by the student's guardian.
Provision of Phonic Ear device. OSEP 1994. *Letter to Anonymous,* 21 IDELR 745.	Regarding parent request for use of Phonic Ear hearing device by student with hearing loss placed by parents at parochial school, OSEP indicated that LEA must ensure genuine opportunity for equitable participation in one of public school's special education programs. However equitable participation does not require district to provide Phonic Ear device as part of its special education and related services. *Comment:* The audiologist along with the IEP team should determine which type of assistive listening device, if any, is most appropriate to meet the educational needs of the individual student. Parents can provide input into the decision, but cannot demand a specific brand or type of equipment.
Hearing loss corrected by a hearing aid. SEA PA 1995. *City of Erie School District,* 22 IDELR 394.	A student whose hearing loss was *corrected by hearing aids,* no longer qualified for special education as hearing impaired. The case found that her hearing loss, because corrected, did not interfere with her performance on an IQ test, and the district did not fail to make necessary accommodations for her hearing loss during the assessment process, and therefore the district's results indicating that she was not gifted were valid.

Other Landmark and Important Case Law Rulings:

Adequate Services and Maximum Potential

Hendrick Hudson School District v. Rowley (1982)
   The first and perhaps most far-reaching ruling regarding the definition of "appropriate" services. The Supreme Court defined "appropriate" as sufficient for educational benefit but not for maximization of the student's potential. In addition, this decision established the school district's right to determine appropriate methodology finding that the provision of a sign language interpreter was not required for this student.

Communication Method

Age v. Bullit County Public Schools, 6th Circuit Court (1982)
   Placement of profoundly deaf children in segregated classroom while being instructed in total communication was an appropriate education.
Silvio v. Commonwealth of Pennsylvania (1982)
   Transfer of child with hearing impairment from private oral school to school using total communication would not impede the child's speaking ability and the association with non-handicapped children would actually improve her communication with others.
Unified School District No. 512, KS (1995)
   The District's plan to serve a student who was hearing impaired in a self-contained classroom using total com-

munication was determined appropriate even though the parents wanted placement in a oral program offered at a private school for deaf students.

Placement/LRE

Letter to Siegel OSEP (1990)
   LRE must include placements options which for students with hearing impairment must include staff members who can interact with the child in his or her mode of communication. The EHA-B (Education for the Handicapped Act-Part B) contains regulations to ensure that children are assessed in their native language or appropriate mode of communication and that individuals providing special education and related services are adequately trained and qualified. OSEP clarified that the placement of a deaf or hearing impaired child should facilitate interaction with language-appropriate peers and staff members who are skilled in the child's mode of communication.
Cobb County Board of Education, GA (1990)
   Placement at a school for the deaf was ordered because the school district's recommended program failed to address the child's need for a total communication environment.
The School District of Philadelphia, PA—OCR (1990)
   The district did not have to provide speech therapy for a hearing impaired child by a certified speech therapist since the teacher of the hearing impaired, by virtue of her coursework in teaching speech to the deaf and district observations of her teaching skill, was sufficiently competent to meet the requirements of Reg. 104.33.

Traverse City Area Public School, MI (1993)

Because student who was deaf had an adequate IEP, continuation of the student's program in total communication at a regular school was determined least restrictive rather than the parent's request for placement at the state school for the deaf.

Dreher ex rel. Dreher v. Amphitheater Unified School District, 9th Circuit Court (1994)

Parents requested reimbursement for speech therapy services at a private school for their profoundly deaf child. The district's program of oral methods and sign language was found to constitute FAPE even though the parents did not choose that option.

Related Services:

Anthony Wayne Local School District, Ohio (1990)

Even though the child (actually two twin sisters) was placed by parents at private, out of district school, the school district the child resided within remained responsible for providing related services at the private school. The district was also ordered to reimburse the parents for tuition to the private school since the district failed to provide the related service (individual and small group instruction) as required by her IEP, thereby denying the child FAPE.

Letter to Dagley, OSEP (1991)

Sign language instruction must be provided to parents (under "parent counseling and training") if IEP team determines instruction for parents is necessary for the child to receive benefit from his education program.

Tugg v. Towey, FL (1994)

The use of interpreters for counseling services for deaf and hearing impaired individuals, including students, was found to be unequal to those provided to the general public. The Florida Department of Health and Rehabilitation Services was ordered to provide mental health services to individuals who were deaf by counselors with sign language skills and an understanding of the mental health needs of the deaf community.

Interpreter Services:

Zobrest v. Catalina Foothills School District, 9th Circuit Court, (1992), U.S. Supreme Court, (1993)

The 9th Circuit Court in 1992 determined that the provision of an interpreter at public expense at a parochial school would violate the Establishment Clause of the U.S. Constitution (dealing with separation of church and state) because the interpreter would be required throughout the school day, for both education and religious instruction.

The U.S. Supreme Court in 1993, however, ruled that the provision of interpreter services to students with disabilities at parochial schools is not barred by the U.S. Constitution as a matter of separation of church and state.

This case only considered whether the Establishment Clause could bar the school district from providing a publicly-paid sign language interpreter on the grounds that it was a religious school. Zobrest did not address the issue of whether private school students are entitled to such services under IDEA.

Cefalu ex re. Cefalu v. East Baton Rouge Parish School Board, LA (1995)

The court ruled that IDEA regulations specifically required the board of education to provide a sign language interpreter to a student in the parochial school his parents had placed him because unlike other special education services, the purpose of the sign language interpreter was to provide the student with assistance most of the time, a service which could not be provided outside of the private school classroom.

Fowler by Fowler v. Unified School District No. 259 KA (1995)

The district was ordered to provide an interpreter at a private, nonsectarian school for the deaf student because there was agreement he needed the service and the district would have had to provide the service if he attended the public school. Because the district had provided services outside of its cluster site to other students, it failed to prove that doing so for this student at a private school would pose an unreasonable burden.

Park City School District, UT (1995)

The district was found to have no obligation to provide a cued speech transliterator for a deaf student in a parochial school since it could provide FAPE within the public school. The ruling indicated that neither IDEA or EDGAR entitled a private school student to services that were essential to maintaining him in the private school placement.

Appendix 1–E

COMPARISON OF SECTION 504, IDEA, AND ADA GUIDELINES FOR EDUCATORS

ISSUES	SECTION 504	IDEA	ADA
TYPE	A Civil Rights Law	An Education Act	A Civil Rights Law
TITLE	The Rehabilitation Act of 1973	The Individuals With Disabilities Education Act (IDEA)	Americans With Disability Act of 1990 (ADA)
RESPONSIBILITY	REGULAR EDUCATION	SPECIAL EDUCATION	PUBLIC AND PRIVATE SCHOOLS
FUNDING	STATE AND LOCAL RESPONSIBILITY (No Federal funding)	STATE, LOCAL, AND FEDERAL IDEA funds cannot be used to serve students eligible only under Section 504	Public and Private responsibility (No Federal funding)
ADMINISTRATOR	SECTION 504 COORDINATOR (Systems with 15 plus employees)	Special Education Director or designee	Suggest to use 504 Coordinator to oversee ADA responsibilities
SERVICE TOOL	ACCOMMODATIONS and/or SERVICES	INDIVIDUALIZED EDUCATION PROGRAM	REASONABLE ACCOMMODATIONS AND LEGAL EMPLOYMENT PRACTICES
PURPOSE	A broad civil rights law which protects the rights of individuals with disabilities in programs and activities that receive Federal financial assistance from the U.S. Department of Education.	A federal funding statute whose purpose is to provide financial aid to states in their efforts to ensure a free appropriate education for students with disabilities	To provide a clear and comprehensive national mandate for the elimination of discrimination against individuals with disabilities.
POPULATION	Identifies student as disabled so long as she/he meets the definition of qualified persons with disabilities; i.e., has a physical or mental impairment which substantially limits a major life activity, has a history of a disability, or is regarded as disabled	Identifies 13 categories of qualifying conditions.	Identifies persons as disabled so long as she/he meets the definition of qualified persons with disabilities; i.e., has a physical or mental impairment which substantially limits a major life activity, or is regarded as disabled by others.

ISSUES	SECTION 504	IDEA	ADA
FREE APPROPRIATE PUBLIC EDUCATION	Both require the provision of a free appropriate public education to eligible students, including individually designed instruction. Requires educational accommodations. "Appropriate" means an education comparable to the education provided to nondisabled students.	Both require the provision of a free appropriate public education to eligible students, including individually designed instruction. Requires the school to provide IEPs. "Appropriate education" means a program designed to provide "educational benefit."	Addresses education in terms of accessibility requirements. Requires appropriate and public entities not to use employment practices that discriminate on the on the basis of a disability.
ELIGIBILITY	A student is eligible so long as she/he meets the definition of qualified person with disabilities, i.e., currently has or has had a physical or mental impairment which substantially limits a major life activity, or is regarded as disabled by others. The student is not required to need special services in order to be protected.	A student is only eligible to receive special education and/or related services if the multidisciplinary team determines that the student has a disability under one of the thirteen qualifying conditions and requires special education services.	A person is eligible so long as she/ he meets the definition of qualified person with disabilities, i.e., currently has or has had a physical or mental impairment which substantially limits a major life activity, or is regarded by others as having a disability. The student is not required to need special education services in order to be protected.
ACCESSIBILITY	Regulations regarding building and program accessibility, requiring that reasonable accommodations be made.	Requires that modifications must be made to provide access to a free appropriate public education.	Requires that public and private programs be accessible to individuals with disabilities.
UNDUE HARDSHIP	Consideration is given for the size of program, extent of accommodation, and cost relative to school budget.	Size of the program and its budget, type of operation, nature and cost of accommodation.	Size of the business and its budget, type of operation, nature and cost of accommodation.
DRUG AND ALCOHOL USE	Current drug use is not considered a disability. An individual who has stopped using drugs and/or alcohol and is undergoing rehabilitation could be protected.	Drug and alcohol use is not covered under IDEA.	Current drug use is not considered a disability. Current alcohol abuse that prevents individuals from performing duties of the job or that constitutes direct threat to property or safety of others is not considered a disability.
CONTAGIOUS DISEASES	Individuals with disabilities excludes any individual with a contagious disease which renders the individual unable.	Could be eligible under the category of "other health impaired."	Permits qualification standard requiring that an individual with a currently contagious disease or infection not pose a direct threat to the health or safety of others.
PROCEDURAL SAFEGUARDS	Both require prior notice to the parent or guardian with respect to identification, evaluation, and placement.		Makes provisions for public notice, hearings, and awarding attorney fees.

(con't.)

(con't.)

ISSUES	SECTION 504	IDEA	ADA
CONSENT	Does not require consent but a district would be wise to do so.	Requires written consent before initial evaluation and placement.	
EVALUATIONS	Evaluation draws on information from a variety of sources in the area of concern; decisions are made by a group knowledgeable about the student, evaluation data, and placement options. Requires parental notice, but not consensus.

Does not require consent, only notice. However, good professional practice indicates informed consent.

Requires periodic reevaluations.

Reevaluation is required before a significant change in placement.

No provision for independent evaluations at school expense. District should consider any such evaluations presented. | A full comprehensive evaluation is required assessing all areas related to the suspected disability. The student is evaluated by a multidisciplinary team. Requires consent before the initial evaluation is conducted.

Requires informed consent before an initial evaluation is conducted.

Requires reevaluations to be conducted at least every 3 years.

A reevaluation is not required before a significant change in placement. However, most students covered by IDEA are also 504 eligible.

Provides for independent educational evaluation. At district expense if parent disagrees with evaluation obtained by school. | All schools should conduct or update their section 504 self-evaluation regarding services, accessibility, practices, and policies to assure discrimination is not occurring to any individual with disabilities. |
| PLACEMENT | When interpreting evaluation data and making placement decisions, both laws require districts to:
• Draw upon information from a variety of sources.
• Ensure that all information is documented and considered.
• Ensure that the placement decision is made by a group of persons, including those who are knowledgeable about the student, the meaning of the evaluation data and placement options.
• Ensure that the student is educated with his/her nondisabled peers to the maximum extent appropriate (least Restrictive Environment—LRE) | | |
| REVIEW | Review periodically. | An IEP review meeting is required before any change in placement. The IEP should be reviewed at least annually. | |

ISSUES	SECTION 504	IDEA	ADA
GRIEVANCE PROCEDURES	Requires districts with more than 15 employees to designate an employee to be responsible for assuring district compliance with Section 504 and provide a grievance procedure for parents, students, and employees.	Does not require a grievance procedure, nor a compliance officer.	Any school district who employs 50 or more shall adopt and publish grievance procedures for resolution of ADA complaints.
DUE PROCESS	Both statues require schools to provide impartial hearings for parents or guardians who disagree with the identification, evaluation, records or placement of student with disabilities.		Due process hearing can be initiated by either party. The court may allow the prevailing party, other than United States, a reasonable attorney's fee.
	Requires that the parent have an opportunity to participate and be represented by counsel. Other details are left to the discretion of the school district. Policy statements should clarify specific details.	Delineates specific requirements.	
EXHAUSTION	Administrative hearing not required prior to OCR involvement or court action.	The parent or guardian should exhaust all administrative hearing before seeking redress in the courts.	An administrative hearing not required prior to OCR involvement or court action.
ENFORCEMENT	Enforced by the U.S. Office for Civil Rights.	Enforced by the U.S. Office of Special Education Programs. Compliance is monitored by the State Department of Education and the Office of Special Education Programs.	Enforced by the U.S. Office of Civil Rights under an agreement with EEOC.
	State Department of Education has no monitoring, complaint resolution or funding involvement.	The State Department of Special Education will resolve complaints under Individuals with Disabilities Education Act.	

(con't.)

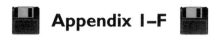

Appendix I–F

FEDERAL MANDATES RELATED TO AUDIOLOGY SERVICES IN THE SCHOOLS

IDEA-PART B (PL 94-142) DEFINITION OF AUDIOLOGY (34CFR300.13[B])

(i)   Identification of children with hearing loss;

(ii) Determination of the range, nature, and degree of hearing loss, including referral for medical or other professional attention for the habilitation of hearing;

(iii) Provision of habilitation activities, such as language habilitation, auditory training, speech reading, (lipreading), hearing evaluation, and speech conservation:

(iv) Creation and administration of programs for prevention of hearing loss;

(v)   Counseling and guidance of pupils, parents, and teachers regarding hearing loss;

(vi) Determination of the child's need for group and individual amplification, selecting and fitting an appropriate aid, and evaluating the effectiveness of amplification. (34 CFR 300.12[b])

IDEA-PART H (PL 99-457) DEFINITION OF AUDIOLOGY (34CFR303.12[d])

(i)   Identification of children with impairments, using at risk criteria and appropriate audiological screening techniques;

(ii) Determination of the range, nature, and degree of hearing loss and communication functions, by use of audiologic evaluation procedures;

(iii) Referral for medical and other services necessary for the habilitation or rehabilitation of children with auditory impairment;

(iv) Provision of auditory training, aural rehabilitation, speech reading and listening device orientation and training, and other services;

(v)   Provision of services for the prevention of hearing loss; and

(vi) Determination of the child's need for individual amplification, including selecting, fitting, and dispensing of appropriate listening and vibrotactile devices, and evaluating the effectiveness of those devices.

IDEA-PART B PROPER FUNCTIONING OF HEARING AIDS (34CFR300.303)

Each public agency shall ensure that the hearing aids worn by children with hearing impairment, including deafness, in school are functioning properly.

IDEA-PART B & PART H: ASSISTIVE TECHNOLOGY (34CFR300.4-6; 34CFR303.12)

Assistive technology devices and services are necessary if a child with a disability requires the device and services in order to receive a free and appropriate education (FAPE); the public agency must ensure that they are made available.

"Assistive technology device" means any item, piece of equipment, or product system, whether acquired commercially off the shelf, modified, or customized, that is used to increase, maintain, or improve the functional capabilities of children with disabilities.

"Assistive technology service" means any service that directly assists a child with a disability in the selection, acquisition, or use of an assistive technology device. The term includes

(a)   The evaluation of the needs of a child with a disability, including a functional evaluation of the child in the child's customary environment;

(b)   Purchasing, leasing, or otherwise providing for the acquisition of assistive technology devices by children with disabilities;

(c)   Selecting, designing, fitting, customizing, adapting, applying, retaining, repairing, or replacing assistive technology devices;

(d)   Coordinating and using other therapies, interventions, or services with assistive technology devices, such as those associated with existing education and rehabilitation plans and programs;

(e)   Training or technical assistance for a child with a disability or, if appropriate, that child's family; and

(f)   Training or technical assistance for professionals (including individuals providing education or rehabilitation services), employers, or other individuals who provide services to, employ, or are otherwise substantially involved in the major life functions of children with disabilities.

DEFINITIONS: IDEA-PART B (34CFR300.7[b])

[2]   "Deaf-blindness" means concomitant hearing and visual impairments, the combination of which causes such severe communication and other developmental and educational problems that they cannot be accommodated in special education programs solely for children with deafness or children with blindness.

[3]   "Deafness" means a hearing impairment that is so severe that the child is impaired in processing linguistic information through hearing, with or without amplification, that adversely affects a child's educational performance.

[4]   "Hearing impairment" means an impairment in hearing, whether permanent or fluctuating, that adversely affects a child's educational performance but that is not included under the definition of deafness in this section.

Appendix 1–G

DEAF STUDENTS EDUCATION SERVICES; POLICY GUIDANCE

4000-01

DEPARTMENT OF EDUCATION

AGENCY: Department of Education

ACTION: Notice of Policy Guidance

SUMMARY: The Department provides additional guidance about Part B of the Individuals with Disabilities Education Act (IDEA) and Section 504 of the Rehabilitation Act of 1973 (Section SW) as they relate to the provision of appropriate education services to students who are deaf. This guidance is issued in response to concerns regarding Departmental policy on the provision of a free appropriate public education (FAPE) to students who are deaf. Many of these concerns were expressed in the report of the Commission on Education of the Deaf. This guidance is intended to furnish State and local education agency personnel with background information and specific steps that will help to ensure that children and youth who are deaf are provided with a free appropriate public education. It also describes procedural safeguards that ensure parents are knowledgeable about their rights and about placement decisions made by public agencies.

FOR FURTHER INFORMATION CONTACT: Jean Peelen or Parma Yarkin, U.S. Department of Education, 400 Maryland Avenue, S.W., Rooms 5046 and 3131, Switzer Building, respectively, Washington, D.C. 20202-2524. Telephone: (202) 205-8637 and (202) 205-8723, respectively. Deaf and hearing impaired individuals may call (202) 205-8449 or (202) 205-8723, respectively, for TDD services.

SUPPLEMENTARY INFORMATION:

Background

In the past twenty-five years, two national panels have concluded that the education of deaf students must be improved in order to meet their unique communication and related needs. The most recent of these panels, the Commission on Education of the Deaf (COED), recommended a number of changes in the way the Federal government supports the education of individuals who are deaf from birth through postsecondary schooling and training. With this notice, the Secretary implements several COED recommendations relating to the provision of appropriate education for elementary and secondary students who are deaf.

The COED's report and its primary finding[1] reflect a fundamental concern within much of the deaf community that students who are deaf have significant obstacles to overcome in order to have access to a free appropriate public education that meets their unique educational needs, particularly their communication and related needs.[2]

The disability of deafness often results in significant and unique educational needs for the individual child. The major barriers to learning associated with deafness relate to language and communication, which, in turn, profoundly affect most aspects of the educational process. For example, acquiring basic English language skills is a tremendous challenge for most students who are deaf. While the Department and others are supporting research activities in the area of language acquisition for children who are deaf, effective methods of instruction that can be implemented in a variety of educational settings are still not available. The reading skills of deaf children reflect perhaps the most momentous and dismal effects of the disability and of the education system's struggle to effectively teach deaf children: hearing impaired students "level off" in their reading comprehension achievement at about the third grade level.[3]

Compounding the manifest educational considerations, the communication nature of the disability is inherently isolating, with considerable effect on the interaction with peers and teachers that make up the educational process. This interaction, for the purpose of transmitting knowledge and developing the child's self-esteem and identity, is dependent upon direct communication. Yet, communication is the area most hampered between a deaf child and his or her hearing peers and teachers. Even the availability of interpreter services in the educational setting may not address deaf children's needs for direct and meaningful communication with peers and teachers.

Because deafness is a low incidence disability, there is not widespread understanding of its educational implications, even among special educators. This lack of knowledge and skills in our education system contributes to the already substantial barriers to deaf students in receiving appropriate educational services.

In light of all these factors, the Secretary believes that it is important to provide additional guidance to State and local education agencies to ensure that the needs of students who are deaf are appropriately identified and met, and that placement decisions for students who are deaf meet the

---

[1]"The present status of education for persons who are deaf in the United States is unsatisfactory. Unacceptably so. This is the primary and inescapable conclusion of the Commission on Education of the Deaf." Commission on Education of the Deaf: *Toward Equality: Education of the Deaf.* (February 1988)

[2]As stated in IDEA, the purpose of the Act is: ". . . to assure that all children with disabilities have available to them . . . a free appropriate public education which emphasizes special education and related services designed to meet their unique needs . . . ." 20 U.S.C. sec. 1400(c). In addition, the Section 504 regulations state: "A recipient [of federal financial assistance] that operates a public elementary or secondary education program shall provide a free appropriate public education to each qualified handicapped person . . ." 34 CFR Section 104.33(a).

[3]Thomas E. Allen, (1981), "Patterns of Academic Achievement Among Hearing Impaired Students: 1974 and 1983," in *Deaf Children in America*, 162–164, Arthur N. Schildroth and Michael A. Karchmer, Eds. San Diego: College-Hill Press .

standards of the applicable statutes and their implementing regulations. It is the purpose of this document to (1) clarify the free appropriate public education provisions of IDEA for children who are deaf, including important factors in the determination of appropriate education for such children and the requirement that education be provided in the least restrictive environment, and (2) clarify the applicability of the procedural safeguards in placement decisions.

Nothing in this notice alters a public agency's obligation to place a student with a disability in a regular classroom if FAPE can be provided in that setting.

The provision of a free appropriate public education based on the unique needs of the child is at the heart of the IDEA. Similarly, the Section 504 regulation at 34 CFR sections104.33-104.36 contains free appropriate public education requirements, which are also applicable to local educational agencies serving children who are deaf. A child is receiving an appropriate education when all of the requirements in the statute and the regulations are met. The Secretary believes that full consideration of the unique needs of a child who is deaf will help to ensure the provision of an appropriate education. For children who are eligible under Part B of the IDEA, this is accomplished through the IEP process. For children determined to be handicapped under Section 504, implementation of an individualized education program developed in accordance with Part B of the IDEA is one means of meeting the free appropriate public education requirements of the Section 504 regulations.

As part of the process of developing an individualized education program (IEP) for a child with disabilities under the IDEA, State and local education agencies must comply with the evaluation and placement regulations at 34 CFR Sections 300.530-300.534. In meeting the individual education needs of children who are deaf under Section 504, LEAs must comply with the evaluation and placement requirements of 34 CFR Section 104.35 of the Section 504 regulation, which contain requirements similar to those of the IDEA. However, the Secretary believes that the unique communication and related needs of many children who are deaf have not been adequately considered in the development of their IEP's. To assist public agencies in carrying out their responsibilities for children who are deaf, the Department provides the following guidance.

The Secretary believes it is important that State and local education agencies, in developing an IEP for a child who is deaf, take into consideration such factors as:

1. **communication needs and the child's and family's preferred mode of communication;**
2. **linguistic needs;**
3. **severity of hearing loss and potential for using residual hearing;**
4. **academic level; and**
5. **social, emotional, and cultural needs, including opportunities for peer interactions and communication.**

In addition, the particular needs of an individual child may require the consideration of additional factors. For example, the nature and severity of some children's needs will require the consideration of curriculum content and method of curriculum delivery in determining how those needs can be met. Including evaluators who are knowledgeable about these specific factors as part of the multidisciplinary team evaluating the student will help ensure that the deaf student's needs are correctly identified.

Under the least restrictive environment (LRE) provision of IDEA, public agencies must establish procedures to ensure that 'to the maximum extent appropriate, children with disabilities, including children in public or private institutions or other care facilities, are educated with children who are not disabled, and that special classes, separate schooling, or other removal of children with disabilities from the regular educational environment occurs only when the nature or severity of the disability is such that education in regular classes with the use of supplementary aids and services cannot be achieved satisfactorily."[4] The section 504 regulation at 34 CFR SECTION 104.34 contains a similar provision.

The Secretary is concerned that the least restrictive environment provisions of the IDEA and Section 504 are being interpreted, incorrectly, to require the placement of some children who are deaf in programs that may not meet the individual student's educational needs. Meeting the unique communication and related needs of a student who is deaf is a fundamental part of providing a free appropriate public education (FAPE) to the child. Any setting, including a regular classroom, that prevents a child who is deaf from receiving an appropriate education that meets his or her needs, including communication needs, is not the LRE for that individual child.

Placement decisions must be based on the child's IEP.[5] Thus, the consideration of LRE as part of the placement decision must always be in the context of the LRE in which appropriate services can be provided. Any setting which does not meet the communication and related needs of a child who is deaf, and therefore does not allow for the provision of FAPE, cannot be considered the LRE for that child. The provision of FAPE is paramount, and the individual placement determination about LRE is to be considered within the context of FAPE.

The Secretary is concerned that some public agencies have misapplied the LRE provision by presuming that placements in or closer to the regular classroom are required for children who are deaf, without taking into consideration the range of communication and related needs that must be addressed in order to provide appropriate services. The Secretary recognizes that the regular classroom is an appropriate placement for some children who are deaf, but for others it is not. The decision as to what placement will provide FAPE for an individual deaf child—which includes a determination as to the LRE in which appropriate services can be made available to the child—must be made only after a full

---

[4] 20 U.S.C. sec. 1412(5)(B).
[5] 20 U.S.C. sec. 1401(18); *see also* 34 CFR section 300.552(a)(2), and 34 CFR section 104.33(b)(2).

and complete IEP has been developed that addresses the full range of the child's needs.

The Secretary believes that consideration of the factors mentioned above will assist placement teams in identifying the needs of children who are deaf and will enable them to place children in the least restrictive environment appropriate to their needs.

The overriding rule regarding placement is that placement decisions must be made on an individual basis.[6] As in previous policy guidance, the Secretary emphasizes that placement decisions may not be based on category of disability, the configuration of the delivery system, the availability of educational or related services, availability of space, or administrative convenience.

States and school districts also are advised that the potential harmful effect of the placement on the deaf child or the quality of services he or she needs must be considered in determining the LRE.

The Secretary recognizes that regular educational settings are appropriate and adaptable to meet the unique needs of particular children who are deaf. For others, a center or special school may be the least restrictive environment in which the child's unique needs can be met. A full range of alternative placements as described at 34 CFR Section 300.551(a) and (b)(1) of the IDEA regulations must be available to the extent necessary to implement each child's IEP. There are cases when the nature of the disability and the individual child's needs dictate a specialized setting that provides structured curriculum or special methods of teaching. Just as placement in the regular educational setting is required when it is appropriate for the unique needs of a child who is deaf, so is removal from the regular educational setting required when the child's needs cannot be met in that setting with the use of supplementary aids and services.

Procedural Safeguards

One important purpose of the procedural safeguards required under Part B and the Section 504 regulations is to ensure that parents are knowledgeable about their rights and about important decisions that public agencies make, such as placement decisions. Under the Section 504 regulations at 34 CFR Section 104.36, a public agency must establish a system of procedural safeguards that includes, among other requirements, notice to parents with respect to placement decisions. Compliance with the Part B procedural safeguards is one means of meeting the requirements of the Section 504 regulations. Under Part B, before a child is initially placed in special education the child's parents must be given written notice and must consent to the placement. The Part B regulations at 34 CFR Section 300.500(a) provide that consent means that parents have been fully informed of all information relevant to the placement decision. The obligation to fully inform parents includes informing the parents that the public agency is required to have a full continuum of placement options available to meet the needs of children with disabilities, including instruction in regular classes, special classes, special schools, home instruction, and instruction in hospitals and institutions. The Part B regulations at 34 CFR §§300.504-300.505 also require that parents must be given written notice a reasonable time before a public agency proposes to initiate or change the identification, evaluation, educational placement or provision of a free appropriate public education to the child. This notice to parents must include a description of the action proposed or refused by the agency, an explanation of why the agency proposes or refuses to take the action, and a description of any options the agency considered and the reasons why those options were rejected. The requirement to provide a description of any option considered includes a description of the types of placements that were actually considered, e.g., special school or regular class, as well as any specific schools that were actually considered and the reasons why these placement options were rejected. Providing this kind of information to parents will enable them to play a more knowledgeable and informed role in the education of their children.

Authority: 20 U.S.C. 1411–1420; 29 U.S.C. 794.

Dated:

Lamar Alexander, *Secretary*

---

[6]34 CFR section 300.552 *Comment. See also* Appendix A to 34 CFR Part 104 at section 24.

Source: From *Federal Register* (57) October 30, 1992, pp. 49274–49276

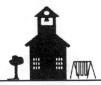

SECTION 2

APPENDIXES

Guidelines

CONTENTS

*Appendixes marked with asterisks (*) are available on an optional computer disk which allows users to customize these forms

Appendix 2–A

COMMUNICATION AND THE ADA
(Effective Communication and Accessibility)

**What is
EFFECTIVE
COMMUNICATION
under ADA?**

- **Taking steps to ensure** that people with communication disabilities
  - Have access to **goods, services, and facilities**
  - Are not excluded, denied services, **segregated or otherwise treated differently** than other people
- **Making information accessible to and useable** by people with communication disabilities

**What is required
to achieve EFFECTIVE
COMMUNICATION
under ADA?**

- **Providing any necessary auxiliary communication aids and services**
  - Unless an undue burden or a fundamental change in the nature of the goods, services, facilities, etc. would result
  - Without a surcharge to the individual
- **Making aurally (via hearing) delivered information available** to persons with hearing and speech impairments (including alarms, nonverbal speech, and computer-generated speech)
- Personally prescribed devices such as hearing aids are **not** required.

**How do you determine
NECESSARY
AUXILIARY
COMMUNICATION
AIDS AND SERVICES?**

- Consideration of:
  - **Expressed preference of the individual with disability**
  - **Level and type of the communication exchange** (complexity, length, and importance of material). For example, interpreter services might not be necessary for a simple business transaction such as buying groceries, but they might be appropriate in lengthy or major transactions such as purchasing a car or provision of legal or medical services.
- **Selection of appropriate aids and services** from available technologies and services (low-tech as well as high-tech) based on facility resources and communication needs (individual's and type of material)

**What are
STRATEGIES
for achieving
EFFECTIVE
COMMUNICATION?**

- **Establishing appropriate attitudes and behaviors:**
  - Assuming that persons with communication disabilities can express themselves if afforded the opportunity, respect, and the necessary assistance to do so
  - Consulting the person with the disability how best to communicate with him or her, and asking about the need for aids and services
  - Traimng staff to communicate more effectively
- **Modifying the communication setting**, for example, reducing noise levels. Improving the communication setting can also reduce the need for assistive devices in some cases.
- **Providing auxiliary aids and services**
- **Responding to auxiliary aids and services requests**
- **Providing materials in accessible formats** (e.g., written transcripts)
- **Keeping written materials simple and direct**
- **Providing visual as well as auditory information**
- **Providing a means for written exchange of information**
- **Informing public of available accommodations**
- **Maintaining devices in good working condition**
- **Consulting a professional** (audiologist, speech-language pathologist)

Source: American Speech-Language-Hearing Association, 10801 Rockville Pike, Rockville, MD 20852. Reprinted by permission.

What are examples of COMMUNICATION (SPEECH AND HEARING) AIDS AND SERVICES?

- **In assembly areas, meetings, conversations:**
  - Assistive listening devices and systems (ALDs), communication boards (word, symbol), qualified interpreters (oral, cued speech, sign language), real-time captioning, written communication exchange and transcripts, computer-assisted note taking, lighting on speaker's face, preferential seating for good listening and viewing position, electrical outlet near accessible seating, videotext displays

- **In telecommunications:**
  - Hearing aid compatible telephones, volume control telephone handsets, amplified telephone mouthpieces (for person with weak voice) (to amplify speech for a hard-of-hearing listener), telecommunication device for the deaf (TDD) or text telephone, facsimile machines (that use visual symbols), computer/modem, interactive computer software with videotext
  - TDD/telephone relay systems

- **In buildings:**
  - Alerting, signaling, warning, and announcement systems using amplified auditory signals, visual signals (flashing, strobe), vibrotactile (touch) devices, videotext displays

- **In prepared (non-live) materials:**
  - Written materials in alternate formats (e.g., symbols, pictures)
  - Aurally-delivered materials in alternate formats (e.g., captioned videotapes, written transcript, sign interpreter)
  - Notification of accessibility options (e.g., alternative formats)

What are COMMUNICATION BARRIERS?

- Factors that hinder or prevent information coming to and/or from a person

- **Visually-related barriers**
  - Inadequate or poor lighting/poor background that interferes with ability to speech-read or see signing
  - Unreadable signage (too small, not in line of vision of people in wheelchairs or of short stature)
  - Lack of visual information (for example, not showing speaker's face)
  - Lack of signage and accessibility symbols

- **Acoustically-related barriers**
  - High noise levels
  - High reverberation levels
  - Lack of aurally-delivered information to supplement visual information (for example, not using amplified auditory as well as visual signals in emergency alarms, partitions that block sound between speaker and listener)

- **Attitudinal and prejudicial barriers**

- **Information complexity** (such as difficult reading level)

What is required for COMMUNICATION ACCESSIBILITY under ADA?

- **Providing TDD and accessible telephone or alternative service**
  - When telephone service is regularly provided to customers/patients on more than just an incidental basis (e.g., hospitals, hotels)
  - When building entry requires aural or voice information exchange (e.g., closed circuit security telephone)

- **Providing means for two-way communication in emergency situations** (e.g., elevator emergency notification system) that does not require hearing or speech for communication exchange

- **Providing closed caption decoders**, upon request, in hospitals that provide televisions, and in places of lodging with televisions in five or more guest rooms

COMMUNICATION ACCESSIBILITY under ADA continued

- **Removing structural communication barriers** in existing buildings when readily achievable (inexpensively and easily removed)

- **Providing alternative service** when barriers are not easily removed (for example, preferential seating area)

- **Following accessibility standards** for new construction/alterations (ADA Accessibility Guidelines, Uniform Federal Accessibility Standard)

What are some READILY ACHIEVABLE STRUCTURAL CARRIER REMOVAL STRATEGIES?

- **Installing sound buffers** to reduce noise and reverberation

- **Installing flashing alarm lights** in restrooms, any general usage areas, hallways, lobbies, and any other common usage areas

- **Integrating visual alarms** into facility alarm systems

- **Removing physical partitions** that block sound or visual information between employees and customers

- **Providing directional signage** with symbols to indicate available services

What is needed for SIGNAGE AND SYMBOLS OF COMMUNICATION ACCESSIBILITY?

- **Symbols** for:
  - **Telephone** accessibility:
    - blue grommet between cord and handset—"hearing aid compatible"
    - telephone handset with radiating soundwaves—"volume control"
  - **TDDs** or text telephones—the international TDD symbol

- **Signage:**
  - **Directional signage** indicating nearest TDD or accessible telephone
  - **Messages for availability of Assistive Listening Devices** (ALDs) in announcements, in key building areas
  - **Messages for communication aids and services** (e.g., interpreters)

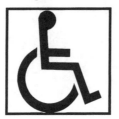

International Symbol of Accessibility

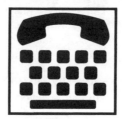

International TDD Symbol

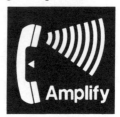

Telephone Handset Amplification Symbol

What types of POLICIES AND PRACTICES NEED TO BE MODIFIED?

- Discriminatory policies such as prohibiting hearing assistance dogs
- Discriminatory eligibility criteria such as restricting access to goods and services unless necessary for the provision of goods and services

What is the best way to ensure COST-EFFECTIVE ADA COMPLIANCE?

- **Perform a facility accessibility audit** that includes identification of communication barriers

- **Determine auxiliary aids and services needs**

- **Develop a plan to remove barriers and acquire assistive devices**

- **Perform ongoing audit and maintenance of accessibility features**

*COST-EFFECTIVE
ADA COMPLIANCE
continued*

- **Modify discriminatory policies, practices, and procedures**
- **Obtain technical assistance and consult** with rehabilitation professionals, disability organizations, consumers, federal agencies as appropriate

The BOTTOM LINE

- **Ask people about their needs, show respect and sensitivity, use what works** (not necessarily what is most expensive), use your resources creatively and effectively.

This document is available in the following formats: large print, audiotape, computer disk, braille, electronic bulletinboard (202-514-6193).

This document provides general information to promote voluntary compliance with the Americans with Disabilities Act (ADA). It was prepared under a grant from the U S. Department of Justice. While the Office on the Americans with Disabilities Act has reviewed its contents, any opinions or interpretations in the document are those of the American Speech-Language-Hearing Association and do not necessarily reflect the views of the Department of Justice. The ADA itself and the Department's ADA regulations should be consulted for further, more specific guidance.

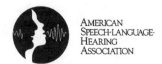

AMERICAN
SPEECH-LANGUAGE-
HEARING
ASSOCIATION

Produced by American Speech-Language-Hearing Association,
10801 Rockville Pike, Rockville, MD 20852,
1-800-638-8255 (V/TDD), 301-897-5700(V); 301-897-0157 (TDD).

Appendix 2–B

GUIDELINES FOR AUDIOLOGY SERVICES IN THE SCHOOLS
Ad Hoc Committee on Service Delivery in the Schools
American Speech-Language-Hearing Association

These guidelines are an official statement of the American-Speech-Language-Hearing Association (ASHA). They provide guidance on the role of the audiologist in school settings, but are not official standards of the Association. These guidelines were prepared by the ASHA Ad Hoc Committee on Service Delivery in the Schools: Frances K. Block, chair; Amie Amiot, ex officio; Cheryl Deconde Johnson; Gina E. Nimmo; Peggy G. Von Almen; Deborah W. White; and Sara Hodge Zeno, Diane L. Eger, 1991–1993 vice president for professional practices, served as monitoring vice president. These guidelines supersede the guidelines titled "Audiology Programs in Educational Settings for Hearing Impaired Children," Asha, May 1976, pages 291–294 and "Audiology Services in the Schools," Asha, May, 1983, pages 53–60.

Contents

Introduction

It has long been recognized that hearing loss affects a child's ability to learn language and achieve academically. Although the effects of hearing loss are variable, depending on several factors, including the nature and degree of the loss, it is essential that children with hearing impairments be provided comprehensive audiological services to reduce the possible negative effects of the loss and to maximize their auditory learning and communication skills. Furthermore, all children can benefit from audiological services through the development of listening skills and the provision of adequate acoustic environments.

Federal legislation continues to refine the responsibilities of public education for children with disabilities (PL 93-112, Rehabilitation Act of 1973, Section 504, 1973; PL 94-142, Education of All Handicapped Act, 1975; PL 99-457, Education of the Handicapped Act Amendments, 1986; PL 100-407, Technology Related Assistance for Individuals with

Disabilities Act, 1988; PL 101–336, Americans with Disabilities Act, 1990; and PL 101–497, Education of the Handicapped Act Amendments, now known as IDEA—Individuals with Disabilities Education Act, 1990). Together these legislative mandates require access to a free and appropriate education (FAPE) for all children with disabilities.

The role of the audiologist in the schools is clearly defined in the Regulations for the Education of All Handicapped Act (PL 94–142), Section 34 CFR 300.13 (b). These regulations were written in 1975 and reauthorized in 1990 without any modification in the definition of audiology. As defined then,

(1) "Audiology" includes:
  (i) Identification of children with hearing loss; (ii) Determination of the range, nature, and degree of hearing loss, including referral for medical or other professional attention for the habilitation of hearing; (iii) Provision of habilitative activities, such as language habilitation, auditory training, speech reading (lipreading), hearing evaluation, and speech conservation; (iv) Creation and administration of programs for prevention of hearing loss; (v) Counseling and guidance of pupils, parents, and teachers regarding hearing loss; and (vi) Determination of the child's need for group and individual amplification, selecting and fitting an appropriate aid, and evaluating the effectiveness of amplification.

The same regulations (34 CFR 300.303) also require that "Each public agency shall insure that the hearing aids worn by deaf and hard of hearing children in school are functioning properly."

Concurrently with the development of these federal mandates, research continues to document the high incidence of hearing loss in school-age children and the negative consequences of all degrees of hearing impairment for psychoeducational and communication development (Berg, 1986; Commission on Education of the Deaf, 1988; Davis, Elfenbein, Schum, & Bentler, 1986; Davis, 1988; Levitt & McGarr, 1988; Matkin, 1986; Wray, Hazleh, & Flexer, 1988). In addition, the importance of the listening environment for children with hearing impairments is now well understood; assistive listening technology has grown; and strategies for selecting, fitting, and evaluating amplification have become more sophisticated (Hawkins, 1988; Levitt, 1985; Musket, 1988).

The foregoing can be summarized as follows:

- Audition is essential to learning for all children; language development and educational achievement are particularly affected when children have unidentified or unmanaged hearing impairments.

Source: From ASHA Desk Reference for Audiology and Speech-Language Pathology, II, pp. 71–82. Copyright 1993 by American Speech-Language-Hearing Association. Available for sale from ASHA Fullfillment Operations (301-897-5700 x218). Reprinted by permission.

- The potential negative impact of mild, fluctuating, and unilateral losses in children is greater than was recognized in the past.
- To ensure optimal use of residual hearing, audiological services must be provided as early in life as possible and be available in the environment in which the child develops and learns. Therefore, certain auditory management services must be delivered in the home and/or the school and be designed to meet the specific needs of the children involved.
- Although private sector audiologists play an important role in the evaluation and management of childhood hearing loss, without provision of direct services in the school environment they cannot be expected to provide the range of services necessary to meet the multifaceted auditory management needs of children with hearing impairments.
- Related and support services are necessary to address the hearing impairments of all but a few of these children. Such services should be sought through appropriate referral and follow-up from other specialists when warranted.
- Audiological services must be provided by personnel who demonstrate the necessary competencies and appropriate American Speech-Language-Hearing Association (ASHA) certification.
- Audiological and educational services delivered must comply with the letter and intent of state and federal mandates.

ASHA addressed the role of the audiologist in the schools in its 1983 position statement "Audiology Services in the Schools." Despite the federal regulations and the ASHA guidelines, there continues to be significant variability in the interpretation of these documents and the provision of services. A recent survey of state departments of education (DeConde-Johnson,1991) substantiated the discrepancy between states and within individual local education agencies in the level of audiology services provided.

The purpose of these guidelines is to provide audiologists and state and local education agencies with recommendations for appropriate cost-effective audiology services in the schools. Information on the following will be provided:

- the characteristics and needs of children with hearing impairments
- the role and function of audiologists in meeting these needs
- the most common delivery models for providing audiology services in the schools, including recommendations for caseload size
- preservice training and certification for audiologists in educational settings

Characteristics and Needs of Children With Hearing Impairments

Although it is well-recognized that hearing is critical to speech-language development, communication, and learning, the complexity of the effects of hearing impairment is not always well understood. A child with hearing impairment suffers both from sensory deprivation and from the effects this deprivation has on communication and learning. Therefore, the effective management of hearing impairment must address medical, communicative, educational, and psychosocial considerations.

Incidence and Types of Hearing Impairment

Although demographic data are difficult to interpret, recent figures suggest that the prevalence of hearing impairment in children from birth to 18 years is as high as 5% (U.S. Department of Health and Human Services, 1991). Berg (1986) and Lundeen (1991) have estimated that among every 1,000 school-age students in the United States, 7 have bilateral and 16 to 19 have unilateral hearing losses that are potentially educationally significant. Included in this number are children with sensorineural hearing losses, as well as children with middle ear infections resulting in conductive hearing losses greater than 25dB. There are many more children who have minimal or fluctuating hearing losses due to otitis media The incidence of hearing loss in special education students is also higher than in the general school population. In addition, there are a significant number of children who have central auditory processing problems. Children with hearing impairments continue to be an underidentified and underserved population. (Berg, 1986; Bess, 1985; Flexer, Wray, & Ireland, 1989; Matkin, 1988).

The most common cause of hearing loss in young children is otitis media, which may result in a conductive hearing impairment. Usually, conductive hearing loss is amenable to medical treatment. Although otitis media is most frequent during the first 3 years of life (Klein, 1988), conductive hearing loss associated with otitis media often continues until the age of 8 to 10 (Stelmachowicz, Davis, Gorga, & Shepard, 1981). Conductive hearing loss is usually not severe in degree, ranging in the slight-to-moderate range. However, it may result in significantly delayed speech, language, and academic skills (Holm & Kunze, 1969; Menyuk, 1986; Needleman, 1977; Teele, Klein, Rosner, & the Greater Boston Otitis Media Study Group, 1984; Zinkus, 1986), because it most often occurs during the early critical learning period.

Sensorineural hearing loss is caused by a variety of illnesses and conditions. It is usually permanent and has a total incidence of at least 10 per 1,000 students. It has been estimated that there are seven times as many students with mild or moderate sensorineural hearing losses as with severe to profound sensorineural hearing losses. Many of these mild to moderate losses are not identified until school entry, and the impact of these losses is often not understood. Sensorineural hearing loss may occur in one or both ears; only recently have the problems caused by unilateral hearing loss been recognized (Bess, 1986). Sensorineural hearing loss can occur at any time, but its prevalence is approximately equal across age groups of children and adolescents. Sensorineural loss in the high frequencies increases dramatically with age and is becoming more common in secondary students because of their exposure to noise (Lass, Woodford, Lundeen, Lundeen, & Everly-Myers, 1986; Montgomery & Fujikawa,

1992; Davis, Shepard, Gorga, Davis, & Stelmachowicz, 1981). The effects of sensorineural loss on language, learning, and psychosocial functioning are usually greater as the degree of hearing loss increases.

When conductive and sensorineural hearing loss are present simultaneously, the resulting loss is called "mixed." In addition to the types of losses mentioned above, many children exhibit central auditory processing problems, the cause and exact nature of which are largely unknown. Children with this type of auditory problem have normal hearing sensitivity but may have deficits in auditory attention, memory, sequencing, and listening when there is background noise.

Hearing loss may occur alone or in combination with other disabilities. The higher incidence of at-risk infants and the presence of other disabilities increase the probability that hearing loss also will occur. Children with language and learning disorders have an increased incidence of hearing loss as well.

Effects of Hearing Impairment

The earlier that hearing impairment occurs in the child's life, the more serious the effects on the child's development. Similarly, the earlier the problem is identified and the intervention begun, the less serious the ultimate impact.

Children with mild or moderate hearing losses are often identified late because they seem to hear and develop socially adequate speech and language. Speech is audible to them, but, depending on the configuration of the hearing loss, parts of words or sentences may not be heard. Therefore, it is often difficult for these children to understand what they hear. A sentence may be audible, but not intelligible. Background noise and distance from the person speaking further impair the child's ability to understand speech.

There are four major ways in which hearing loss affects children:

- It causes delay in the development of receptive and expressive communication skills (speech and language).
- The language deficit causes learning problems that result in reduced academic achievement.
- Communication difficulties often lead to social isolation and poor self concept.
- It may have an impact on vocational choices.

These four problems significantly affect the lives of children. While the magnitude of the educational impact of a hearing loss will vary for each individual child, the language, academic, and psychosocial functioning of children with hearing impairments share several common characteristics, which are summarized below.

- **Vocabulary**
  - ➤ Vocabulary develops more slowly than normal in children with hearing impairments.
  - ➤ Children with hearing impairments learn concrete words (cat, jump, five, red) more easily than abstract ones (before, alter equal to, or jealous). Function words (the, is, are) are also misused frequently.
  - ➤ The gap between the vocabulary of children with normal hearing and those with hearing impairments

widens with age. Children with hearing impairments do not catch up without intervention.
  - ➤ Children with hearing impairments have difficulty understanding the multiple meanings of words.

- **Sentence Structure**
  - ➤ Children with hearing impairments comprehend and produce shorter and more simple sentences than normal.
  - ➤ Children with hearing impairments often misunderstand spoken and written complex sentences (relative clause, passive voice).
  - ➤ Children with hearing impairments often cannot hear word endings, such as "-s" or "-ed," leading to misunderstandings and misuse of tense, pluralization, noun-verb agreement, and possessives.

- **Academic Achievement**
  - ➤ All areas of academic achievement are affected, especially reading and mathematical concepts.
  - ➤ Children with severe to profound hearing losses usually achieve skills no higher than the third or fourth-grade level unless appropriate educational intervention occurs early.
  - ➤ Children with mild to moderate hearing losses, on the average, achieve from 1 to 4 grade levels lower than their peers with normal hearing unless appropriate management occurs.
  - ➤ The gap between children with normal hearing and those with hearing impairments usually widens as they progress through school.
  - ➤ The level of achievement is related to parental involvement and the quantity, quality, and timing of the support services children receive.

- **Psychosocial Functioning**
  - ➤ Children with severe to profound hearing impairments often report feeling isolated, friendless, and unhappy in school, particularly when their socialization with other children with hearing impairments is limited.
  - ➤ These social problems appear to be more prevalent in children with mild or moderate hearing losses than in those with severe to profound impairments.

Service and Program Needs for Children With Hearing Impairments

Minimizing the handicapping effects of hearing impairment depends on early identification and intensive broad-based management of each child. To contribute effectively to this management process, audiologic services within the schools should include the following components:

Prevention. Information concerning methods of prevention, as well as causes and effects, of hearing loss needs to be provided to students, educational staff, and community members on an ongoing basis. This information may be integrated into the school curriculum, as well as take the form of class presentations, parent counseling, professional inservice training, and public information campaigns. The prevention program must be closely tied to efforts aimed toward early identification and intervention.

Identification. An ongoing identification program, which allows for the periodic screening of all children between birth and 21 years of age, must be provided. Each year the identification program should provide screening for all children at specified ages or grade levels; all children referred for or placed in special education programs; all children referred by parents, teachers, and concerned third parties; and all children considered "at-risk" for hearing impairment, including students with a history of exposure to noise. The identification program may include the establishment of at-risk registries, developmental checklists, or pure tone and acoustic immittance screening programs. To be effective, the identification program must develop expedient lines of communication and referral between educators, families, and the medical community. Acoustic immittance screening should be provided for all children who are at risk for middle-ear problems, particularly those under the age of 7. The identification program must be systematic and include complete follow-up procedures. It must be carried out by trained personnel and supervised by an audiologist with demonstrated expertise in this area.

Assessment. Ongoing assessment must be accomplished in order to provide information concerning the nature and extent of hearing impairment and its effect on communicative function, educational performance, and psychosocial well-being. Multidisciplinary and multifaceted assessment to determine amplification, educational, communicative, and psychosocial needs must be completed for all children with hearing loss.

All children who fail screening and all children with known hearing impairments must have an audiologic assessment in order for appropriate treatment to be planned. Children considered for or placed in special education programs; children referred by parents, teachers, and concerned third parties; and children "at-risk" for hearing loss may have either an initial screening or be seen for an audiologic assessment, depending upon the circumstances and available resources. Appropriate audiologic assessment includes, but is not limited to:

- compiling and interpreting available audiometric information
- determining the need for further pre-assessment information, including otologic consultation
- administering, scoring, and interpreting a complete audiologic assessment, which shall include the following, as appropriate:
  - ➤ case history
  - ➤ otoscopic examination
  - ➤ acoustic immittance measurements
  - ➤ pure tone audiometry (air and bone conduction)
  - ➤ speech reception or detection threshold
  - ➤ word recognition (speech discrimination)
  - ➤ word recognition in noise
  - ➤ speech recognition in noise with both auditory and visual inputs
  - ➤ most comfortable loudness level
  - ➤ uncomfortable loudness level
  - ➤ special tests, including auditory brainstem response, otoacoustic emissions, site of lesion, central auditory processing

  - ➤ modified test procedures, including behavior observation, visual reinforcement, and conditioned play audiometry
  - ➤ speechreading
- selecting, administering, scoring, and interpreting tests to determine the benefits of amplification (hearing aids, cochlear implants, and/or FM systems), which shall include the following, as appropriate:
  - ➤ speech audiometry (quiet and noise; auditory and auditory-visual)
  - ➤ functional-gain measurement
  - ➤ real-ear measurement
  - ➤ electroacoustic analysis
  - ➤ listening check and Ling five sound speech test
  - ➤ auditory skill development measurements
- documenting the influence of the hearing loss on communication, learning, psychosocial adjustment, and adaptive behavior
- identifying co-existing factors that may require further evaluation
- referring for assessment and/or treatment, using both school and community resources as appropriate. These may include assessments related to cognitive, academic, visual, and motor skills; emotional status; selection of amplification; and vocational interest and aptitude. In addition, the need for financial assistance in the purchase of a hearing aid should be considered.

Habilitation and Instructional Services. Habilitation and instructional services must be provided for all children identified by a multidisciplinary team as needing such services. Efforts must be made to acquire and interpret information relative to communicative skills, cognitive abilities, motor functioning, social-emotional development, adaptive behavior, health history, and academic status. An Individualized Education Program (IEP) should be tailored to meet the needs of the child and the parents, and should address the academic and support services needed. Educational services may be provided through a number of delivery options, including, but not limited to, home intervention, consultation/collaboration, itinerant instruction, team teaching, resource special education, self-contained special education classes, and residential placement. When determining placements, opportunities for educational and social interaction with other children with hearing impairments, as well as with normal-hearing peers, should be considered.

The habilitative needs of children with hearing impairments encompass many broad and sometimes overlapping areas. Some of the needed services may be provided directly by audiologists, whereas others will be provided by other specialists, such as speech-language pathologists, teachers of the deaf and hard of hearing, psychologists, counselors, social workers, physical therapists, occupational therapists, nurses, or physicians. Some of the most important aspects of habilitation are

- medical treatment, when indicated;
- selection of appropriate amplification (hearing aid, cochlear implant, and/or FM system) at the earliest possible age;

- auditory skill development training;
- training in the use of hearing aids in various settings (including use of amplification in noisy classrooms and social situations);
- structuring a successful learning environment, which includes teacher selection, optimal room acoustics, accessibility to information, and peer and teacher inservices;
- development and remediation of communication, including pragmatic, skills;
- training in the use of visual information to supplement auditory input;
- academic tutoring or specialized instruction;
- counseling; and
- facilitation of transitions between programs, levels, agencies, and vocational settings.

Training in the effective use of hearing is a primary consideration in intervention because such training directly affects the child's success or failure in other areas. Two factors contribute most to the successful use of residual hearing: (a) appropriate amplification that consistently works properly and (b) a favorable acoustic environment. Research indicates that many children who are good candidates for hearing aids still do not wear them (Elfenbein, Bentler, Davis, & Neibuhr, 1988; Kartchmer & Kirwin, 1977; Lipscomb, Von Almen, & Blair, 1992; Davis, Shepard, Stelmachowicz, & Gorga, 1961). Furthermore, children's hearing aids often malfunction. Studies have shown that 50% of the hearing aids worn by children are functioning poorly at any given time (Elfenbein, Bentler, Davis, & Neibuhr, 1988; Gaeth & Lounsbury, 1966; Kemker, McConnell, Logan, & Green, 1979; Potts & Greenwood, 1983; Zink, 1972). These data strongly suggest that programs to monitor hearing aid performance and use which are mandated by PL 94142, 34CFR 300.303, are essential to the effective management of children with hearing impairments.

Children with hearing impairments require a clear signal if they are to understand instructions, class discussions, and other spoken comments. Even when properly functioning hearing aids are worn, the high levels of noise and reverberation that exist in most classrooms reduce their effective use (Anderson, 1989; Crandell, 1991; Crum & Matkin, 1976; FinitzoHieber & Tillman, 1978; Leavitt, 1991). For this reason, noise sources must be eliminated or reduced. Classrooms present a particularly difficult listening situation. Therefore, it is typically necessary to use assistive listening devices that enhance signal-to-noise ratios, in addition to, or instead of, personal hearing aids, to ensure that the child receives the best possible auditory input. The complex interactions between noise, distance from the speaker, acoustic characteristics of the room, and type of amplification make simple recommendations for preferential seating inadequate to ensure good use of hearing in the classroom.

Follow-up and Monitoring. Follow-up services need to be provided as an ongoing and underlying aspect of each component of the hearing identification, conservation, and educational services program. These services include, but are not limited to, teacher consultation, parent and family counseling, monitoring of communicative function, monitoring of educational performance, monitoring of psychosocial needs, and monitoring the performance and effectiveness of individual and group amplification systems, as well as periodic detailed reassessment.

Equipment and Materials. Provision of adequate identification, evaluation, and audiological management services to children with hearing impairments requires access to the following equipment and materials:

- sound-treated test booth
- clinical audiometer with sound field capabilities
- portable acoustic immittance meter
- portable audiometer
- electroacoustic hearing aid analyzer
- otoscope
- sound-level meter
- visual reinforcement audiometry equipment and other instruments necessary for assessing young or difficult-to-test children
- earmold impression materials and modification equipment
- test materials for screening speech and language, evaluating speechreading, and evaluating auditory skills
- test materials for central auditory processing assessment
- loaner or demonstration hearing aids
- FM amplification systems or other assistive listening devices (sound field and personal)
- visual aids for in-service training
- battery testers, hearing aid stethoscopes, and earmold cleaning materials
- auditory, speechreading, speech-language, and communication instructional materials

Technical Assistance and Administrative Support. Although state departments of education have primary responsibility for ensuring that adequate and appropriate services are available within local education agencies, technical assistance for staff and program development should be actively sought from a variety of other sources, including local, state, and national professional organizations; university education and training programs; state departments of health; community speech and hearing centers; private providers of service; and equipment distributors and manufacturers. Such support is critical to maintaining up-to-date services and facilities. In addition, administrative mechanisms should be developed to ensure continuing fiscal support at a level sufficient to properly maintain both the services and the facilities.

Evaluation and Research. Program evaluation must be an ongoing activity to ensure the efficacy of hearing identification, auditory management, educational services, and hearing conservation programs. Ongoing research into the best practices for delivering hearing and educational services is of utmost importance to education agencies and to the children served. In addition, the audiologist must participate in appropriate staff development activities relevant to current educational practices and trends.

Roles and Responsibilities of the Audiologist

Not only are the effects of hearing impairment multifaceted and complex, but identification and audiologic assessment techniques have become increasingly sophisticated.

Unfortunately, the progress and emphasis on management and habilitation have not kept pace with advances in assessment.

In the past audiological services in the schools focused primarily on identification audiometry and pure-tone testing, and the responsibility for providing these services was typically delegated to speech-language pathologists or school nurses. Services usually did not proceed beyond the screening level, and all failures were referred outside the educational setting. Referrals were most often medical, and follow-up was typically limited to that associated with treatment of the medical problem. In the absence of audiologists with educational expertise, the educational, communicative, and psychosocial aspects of hearing impairments may have been neglected.

The responsibility of the audiologist in the schools is finally evolving from a primary focus on identification to that of a consultant, team member, and case manager (Blair, Wilson-Vlotman, & Von Almen, 1989; English, 1991; Flexer, 1990; Flexer, Wray, & Ireland, 1989; Roush, 1991). Schools are beginning to realize the extent of the impact audiologists can have in the assessment and management of children with hearing impairments. Specifically, the audiologist is uniquely qualified to perform the following activities with children:

- provide community leadership to ensure that all infants, toddlers, and youth with impaired hearing are promptly identified, evaluated, and provided with appropriate intervention services
- collaborate with community resources to develop a high-risk registry and follow-up
- develop and supervise a hearing screening program for preschool and school-aged children
- train audiometric technicians or other appropriate personnel to screen for hearing loss
- perform follow-up comprehensive audiological evaluations
- assess central auditory function
- make appropriate referrals for further audiological, communication, educational, psychosocial, or medical assessment
- interpret audiological assessment results to other school personnel
- serve as a member of the educational team in the evaluation, planning, and placement process, to make recommendations regarding placement, related service needs, communication needs, and modification of classroom environments for students with hearing impairments or other auditory problems
- provide in-service training on hearing and hearing impairments and their implication to school personnel, children, and parents
- educate parents, children, and school personnel about hearing loss prevention
- make recommendations about use of hearing aids, cochlear implants, group and classroom amplification, and assistive listening devices

- ensure the proper fit and functioning of hearing aids, cochlear implants, group and class room amplification, and assistive listening devices
- analyze classroom noise and acoustics and make recommendations for improving the listening environment
- manage the use and calibration of audiometric equipment
- collaborate with school, parents, teachers, special support personnel, and relevant community agencies and professionals to ensure delivery of appropriate services
- make recommendations for assistive devices (radio/television, telephone, alerting, convenience) for students with hearing impairment
- provide services, including home programming if appropriate, in the areas of speechreading, listening, communication strategies, use and care of amplification, including cochlear implants, and self-management of hearing needs

Because of the complex and variable nature of hearing impairment and its effects, children with hearing impairments are heterogeneous in nature. It is therefore imperative that individualized intervention plans for all children with hearing impairment be developed and implemented by a multidisciplinary team. In addition, the efforts of that team need to be guided by a complete understanding of the hearing impairment. This knowledge must, in turn, be coordinated with and integrated into ongoing classroom instruction. Unfortunately, most school personnel are unfamiliar with the nature and specific effects of hearing impairment. The audiologist is the only educational team member with comprehensive knowledge about hearing impairments and their consequences. Therefore, audiologists provide an excellent resource for direct service, in-service activities, and public information efforts that can significantly enhance the intervention efforts of the educational team.

Delivery of Audiology Services

The audiologic needs of children with hearing impairments can be addressed through a variety of service delivery models. Implementation of a specific audiology service program will depend on the administrative philosophy of individual state and local school systems and on available resources. However, all states must ensure that local education agencies provide the essential service components necessary to meet state and federal education and civil rights statutes and regulations.

Audiology services may be provided directly by local or intermediate education agencies, may be contracted with private or public entities, or may be a combination of these two delivery models.[1] Factors to consider in the selection of a delivery model include the size and needs of the population to be served, qualifications of available personnel, equipment and facility resources, proximity and timeliness of available services, cost effectiveness, and liability factors.

Whereas the 1980 Ad Hoc Committee on Extension of Audiological Services in the Schools described four delivery models for audiology services in the schools, these four models were essentially combinations of school-based and contracted audiology services.

Substantial coordination, collaboration, and communication among the service provider, the school staff, and the family are critical to the provision of comprehensive services.

Service Delivery Models

School-Based Audiology Services. Audiology services that are school-based are directed or performed by audiologists employed by local or intermediate education agencies or residential programs. Although hearing screening may be delegated to support personnel or volunteers, the audiologist is responsible for developing and supervising hearing identification and prevention programs, including participation with other community agencies for the early identification of hearing impairments. Audiologic assessment is performed by the school audiologist, and results are interpreted and shared directly with others involved in the child's educational program. Necessary referrals outside the school are made with parental consent, and the school audiologist acts as the liaison with physicians and other community professionals. The audiologist in the school is also responsible for the maintenance and calibration of audiological equipment, for recommending and monitoring hearing aids and assistive listening devices, and for evaluating and making recommendations regarding classroom acoustics. Additionally, the audiologist serves as a member of the educational team in the evaluation and Individualized Education Program (IEP) process. Because of the unique perspective the audiologist has as a result of involvement with children throughout their entire education, he or she may serve as the case manager. Along with the teacher of the deaf and hard of hearing and the speech-language pathologist, the audiologist plays an important role in the provision of habilitation services.

Contracted Audiology Services. Audiology services may be provided by school districts through contracts with a variety of sources, including private practitioners, clinics, medical facilities, or public agencies. The contract should specify the exact nature of the services to be provided, the name and credentials of the provider, when and how services will be provided, and the nature of the reporting and consultation requirements. The local or intermediate education agency has the responsibility for ensuring that comprehensive audiology services are delivered to the school population, and may contract for all audiology services or only for those it chooses not to provide directly. Equipment usually belongs to the provider identified in the contract.

Model Selection Considerations

Determination of the most effective service delivery model should be based on considerations related to quality and comprehensiveness of the services, compliance with state and federal regulations, and cost effectiveness. The best alternative for an individual school district may be school-based audiology services, contracted audiology services, or a combination of both. Whatever the delivery model employed, efforts should be made to avoid unnecessary duplication of readily available services and facilities in the community.

School-based audiology services are often more comprehensive and efficient than contracted services, because services are provided directly by audiologists who have constant access to children and well-established daily communication with other educational personnel (Allard & Golden, 1991). Furthermore, audiologists who are employed by schools typically show a greater allegiance and investment by virtue of their employment setting.

Contracted services have the potential to be as effective as school-based services, but care must be taken to ensure that the contracts are not limited in the provision of comprehensive services. Additionally, services, reports, and records must comply with federal, state, and local education agency requirements. It is critical that contractees understand educational policies and procedures, in addition to the educational and communicative implications of a hearing loss in childhood. Staff development activities that pertain to associated educational issues should be included in all contracts. Limited contracts, such as those that provide only for clinical audiologic assessment and leave the school personnel responsible for the interpretation and use of test results in educational planning and remediation efforts, should be avoided.

Another factor in the consideration of a service delivery model is cost effectiveness. The cost of school-based audiology services includes the salaries and fringe benefits of audiology personnel and the purchase or contracting for use of necessary audiologic equipment and materials. The size and nature of the school population will determine the number of staff members and the equipment needed. Contracted services are provided on a fee-for-service basis, which may be calculated in terms of time involved or number of children for whom services are provided. With contracted services, the school is usually not responsible for providing equipment.

When contracted services are used, it is critical that the school's responsibility for assessment, hearing aids, and assistive listening equipment be differentiated from the parent's responsibility. This is necessary to avoid conflict-of-interest situations that arise when the same audiologist fulfills the school contract as well as the private audiology services in a community.

Caseload

To ensure that the identification, auditory management, educational, communication, and psychosocial needs of children with hearing impairments are not neglected, adequate numbers of audiologists must be available to provide services to children. Therefore, fiscal and administrative support must be sufficient to carry out the standards of practice recommended in these guidelines.

A ratio of one full-time audiologist for every 12,000 preschool through secondary students is recommended to provide comprehensive audiologic services. Factors that may reduce this ratio include:

- excessive travel time
- the number of children with hearing impairments
- the number of preschoolers and children with other disabilities

- the number of hearing aids and assistive listening devices in use
- the quantity of special tests provided, including central auditory processing
- the extent of equipment calibration and maintenance responsibilities
- the amount of direct habilitative services
- the extent of supervisory/administrative responsibilities

Preservice Training and Certification

To meet national professional standards established by the American Speech-Language-Hearing Association, audiologists must complete a graduate degree, complete at least 375 hours of supervised clinical practicum, pass a national examination in audiology, and complete a Clinical Fellowship Year under the supervision of a fully certified audiologist. When combined with training and experience in education, these requirements result in the qualifications necessary for audiologists to effectively complement the expertise of other school staff in providing for comprehensive management of children with hearing impairments. In addition to the ASHA certification requirements and as part of graduate training, it is recommended that audiologists who wish to be employed in school settings complete a work experience in a school system under the supervision of a school audiologist and have knowledge and experience in the following areas:

- educational referral procedures and criteria
- multidisciplinary team evaluations, Individualized Educational Plan (IEP) and Individual Family Service Plan (IFSP) development, and placement procedures
- collaborative planning and problem solving with other educational professionals
- interpretation of educational assessments (academic, communication, cognitive, psychosocial, physical)
- legal foundations of regular and special education (current legislation. legal rights, due process)
- sign language systems
- use and modification of instructional materials and media
- development, execution, and supervision of school hearing screening programs
- familiarity with instructional curricula
- acoustic assessment and modifications of classrooms
- record keeping and reporting
- psychoeducational implications of childhood hearing loss
- in-service training and counseling techniques for teachers, parents, and peers
- training and supervision of support personnel
- case management/care coordination with family, school, and community services
- sensitivity to diversity and difficult issues

Summary

The educational needs of children with hearing impairments are the responsibility of local and state education agencies. Comprehensive audiology services to children include prevention, identification, assessment, habilitation and instructional services, supportive in-service and counseling, and follow-up and monitoring services. Audiology programs in schools must be supported by appropriate and adequate equipment and materials, technical assistance, administrative support, and evaluation and research. The needs of children with hearing impairments are diverse. Therefore, a team approach that includes the school audiologist is the only feasible way to ensure that they receive comprehensive services.

Services for children with hearing impairments are greatly enhanced when audiologists are on the educational team. The inclusion of audiologists makes possible the proper interpretation and integration of audiologic data into educational planning for programming. Audiologists bring critical and unique skills and knowledge to the educational setting, thus ensuring the maximal exploitation of residual hearing for auditory learning and communication. Audiology services can be obtained by employing audiologists within the schools or by contracting for their services. Regardless of the service delivery system used, adequate numbers of audiologists must be employed to provide appropriate and comprehensive audiology services to all children.

References

Allard, J., & Golden, F. (1991). Educational audiology: A comparison of service delivery systems utilized by Missouri schools. *Language, Speech and Hearing Services in Schools, 22,* 5–11.

American Speech-Language-Hearing Association. (1983, May). Audiology services in the schools position statement. *Asha, 25,* 53–60.

Anderson, K. (1989). Speech perception and the hard of hearing child. *Educational Audiology Monograph, 1,* 15–30. Berg, F. S. (1986). Characteristics of the target population. In F. Berg, J. C. Blair, S. H. Viehweg, & A. Wilson Vlotman (Eds.), *Educational audiology for the hard of hearing child* (pp. 1–2). New York: Grune and Stratton.

Berg, F., & Fletcher, S. (1970). *The hard of hearing child.* New York: Grune and Stratton.

Bess, F. H. (1985). The minimally hearing impaired child. *Ear and Hearing, 6,* 43–47.

Blair, J., Wilson-Vlotman, A., & Von Almen, P. (1989). Educational audiologist: Practices, problems, directions, and recommendations. *Educational Audiology Monograph, 1,* 1–4.

The Commission on Education of the Deaf. (1988). *Toward equality. Education of the deaf.* Washington, DC: U.S. Government Printing Office.

Craig, H. A. (1965). Sociometric investigation of the self-concept of the deaf child. *American Annals of the Deaf, 110,* 456–478.

Crandall, C. (1991). Effects of classroom acoustics on children with normal hearing; Implications for intervention strategies. *Educational Audiology Monograph, 2,* 18–38.

Crum, M., & Matkin, N. (1976). Room acoustics; The forgotten variable? *Language, Speech and Hearing Services in Schools, 7,* 106–110.

Davis, J. (1974). Performance of young hearing-impaired children on a test of basic concepts. *Journal of Speech and Hearing Disorders, 17,* 342–351.

Davis, J., & Blasdell, R. (1975). Perceptual strategies employed by normal hearing and hearing-impaired children in the comprehension of sentences containing relative. *Journal of Speech and Hearing Research, 18,* 281–295.

Davis, J., Shepard, N., Stelmachowicz, P., & Gorga, M. (1981). Characteristics of hearing-impaired children in the schools: Part I—Demographic data. *Journal of Speech and Hearing Disorders, 46,* 123–129.

Davis, J., Shepard, N., Stelmachowicz, P., & Gorga, M. (1981). Characteristics of hearing-impaired children in the schools: Part II—Psychoeducational data. *Journal of Speech and Hearing Disorders, 46,* 130–137.

Davis, J. M., Elfenbein, J., Schum, R., & Bentler, R. A. (1986). Effects of mild and moderate hearing impairments on language, educational, and psychological behavior of children. *Journal of Speech and Hearing Disorders, 51,* 5362.

Davis, J. M. (1988). Management of the school age child: A psychosocial perspective. In F. H. Bess (Ed.), *Hearing impairment in children* (pp. 401–416). Parkton, MD: York Press.

DeConde-Johnson, C. (1991). The "state" of educational audiology: Survey results and goals for the future. *Educational Audiology Association Monograph, 2,* 74–84.

Eagles, E., Wishik, S., Doerfler, L., Melnick, W., & Levin, H. (1963). Hearing sensitivity and related factors in children. *Laryngoscope,* Special Monograph.

Education of All Handicapped Children. (August 23, 1977). PL 94142 Regulations. *Federal Register, 42*(163).

Elfenbein, J., Bentler, R., Davis, J., & Niebuhr, D. (1988). Status of school children's hearing aids relative to monitoring practices. *Ear and Hearing, 9,* 212–215.

English, K., (1991). Best practices in educational audiology. *Language, Speech, and Hearing Services in Schools, 22,* 283–286.

Finitzo-Hieber, T., & Tillman, T. (1978). Room acoustics effects on monosyllabic word discrimination ability for normal and hearing-impaired children. *Journal of Speech and Hearing Research, 21,* 440–458.

Flexer, C., Wray, D., & Ireland, J. (1989). Preferential seating is NOT enough: Issues in classroom management of hearing impaired students. *Language, Speech, and Hearing Services in Schools, 20,* 11–21.

Flexer, C. (1990, April). Audiological rehabilitation in the schools. *Asha, 32,* pp. 44–45.

Gaeth, J., & Lounsbury, E. (1966). Hearing aids and children in elementary school. *Journal of Speech and Hearing Disorders, 31,* 283–289. Washington, DC: Gallaudet College.

Kemker, F., McConnell, F., Logan, S., & Green, B. (1979). A field study of children's hearing aids in a school environment. *Language, Speech, and Hearing Services in Schools, 10,* 47–53.

Klein, J. (1986). Risk factors for otitis media in children. In J. Kavanagh (Ed.), *Otitis media and child development* (pp. 45–51). Parkton, MD: York Press.

Kodman, F. (1963). Educational status of near deaf children in the classroom. *Journal of Speech and Hearing Disorders, 28,* 297–299.

Lass, N. J., Woodford, C. M., Lundeen, D. J., & Everly-Myers, D. S. (1986). The prevention of noise induced hearing loss in the school-age population: A school educational hearing conservation program. *Journal of Auditory Research, 26,* 247–254.

Levitt, H. (1985). Technology and education of the hearing impaired. In F. Powell, T. Finitzo-Hieber, S. Friel-Patti, & D. Henderson (Eds.), *Education of the hearing impaired child* (pp. 120–129). San Diego: College-Hill Press.

Levitt, H., & McGarr, N. (1988). Speech and language development in hearing impaired children. In F. H. Bess (Ed.), *Hearing impairment in children* (pp. 375–388). Parkton, MD: York Press.

Leavitt, R. (1991). Group amplification systems for students with hearing impairments. *Seminars in Hearing, 12*(4), 380–388.

Ling, D. (1972). Rehabilitation of cases with deafness secondary to otitis media. In A. Glorig and K. Gerwin (Eds.), *Otitis media* (pp. 249–253). Springfield, Ill.: Charles C. Thomas.

Lipscomb, M., Von Almen, P., & Blair, J. (1992). Students as active participants in hearing aid maintenance. *Language, Speech, and Hearing Services in Schools, 23,* 202–213.

Lundeen, C. (1991). Prevalence of hearing impairment among children. *Language, Speech, and Hearing Services in Schools, 22,* 269–271.

Matkin, N. D. (1986). The role of hearing in language development. In J. F. Kavanagh (Ed.), *Otitis media and child development* (pp. 311). Parkton, MD: York Press.

Matkin, N. D. (1988). Re–evaluating our approach to evaluation: Demographics are changing—Are we? In F. H. Bess (Ed.), *Hearing impairment in children* (pp. 101–111). Parkton, MD: York Press.

McClure, W. (1969). Current problems and trends in the education of the deaf. *Deaf American, 18,* 8–14.

Menyuk, P. (1986). Predicting speech and language problems with persistent otitis media. In J. Kavanagh (Ed.), *Otitis media and child development* (pp. 83–96). Parkton, MD: York Press.

Montgomery, J., & Fujikawa, S. (1992). Hearing thresholds of students in the second, eighth, and twelfth grades. *Language, Speech, and Hearing Services in Schools, 23,* 61–63.

Muskett, C. (1988). Assistive listening devices and systems (ALDS) for the hearing impaired student. In R. Roesser & M. P. Downs (Eds.), *Auditory disorders in school children* (pp. 246–259). New York: Thieme Medical Publishers.

Needleman, H. (1977). Effects of hearing loss from early recurrent otitis media on speech and language development. In B. Jaffe (Ed.), *Hearing loss in children* (pp. 640–649). Baltimore: University Park Press.

Peterson, M. (1972). *Achievement of hard of hearing students in regular public schools.* Unpublished doctoral dissertation, Wayne State University.

Potts, P., & Greenwood, J. (1983). Hearing aid monitoring: Are looking and listening enough? *Language, Speech, and Hearing Services in Schools, 14,* 157–163.

Quigley, S., & Thomure, R. (1968). *Some effects of a hearing impairment on school performance.* Champaign, IL: Institute of Research on Exceptional Children, University of Illinois.

Reich, C., Hambleton, D., & Houltron, B. (1977). The integration of hearing-impaired children in regular classrooms. *American Annals of the Deaf, 122,* 534–543.

Ross, M., & Giolas, T. G. (1978). *Auditory management of hearing-impaired children.* Baltimore: University Park Press.

Roush, J. (1991, April). Expanding the audiologist's role. *Asha, 33,* 47–49

Teele, D., Klein, J., Rosner, B., & The Greater Boston Otitis Media Study Group. (1984). Otitis media with effusion during the first three years of life and development of speech and language. *Pediatrics, 74,* 282–287.

U.S. Department of Health and Human Services, Public Health Services (1991). *Healthy people 2000: National health promotion and disease prevention objectives.* DHHS Publication No. 91-50121. Washington, DC: U.S. Government Printing Office, Superintendent of Documents.

Wilcox, J., & Tobin, H. (1974). Linguistic performance of hard-of-hearing and normal-hearing children. *Journal of Speech and Hearing Research, 17,* 286–293.

Wray, D., Hazlett, J., & Flexer, C. (1988). Teaching writing skills to hearing impaired students. *Language, Speech, and Hearing Services in Schools, 19,* 182–190.

Zink, C. (1972). Hearing aids children wear: A longitudinal study of performance. *Volta Review, 74,* 41–51.

Zinkus, P. (1986). Perceptual and academic deficits related to early chronic otitis media. In J. Kavanagh (Ed.), *Otitis media and child development* (pp. 107–116). Parkton, MD: York Press.

Appendix 2–C

AUDIOLOGIC SCREENING OF NEWBORN INFANTS WHO ARE AT RISK FOR HEARING IMPAIRMENT

The following guidelines were developed by the ASHA Committee on Infant Hearing and adopted by the ASHA Legislative Council in November 1988 (LC 28-88). Current and past members of the committee responsible for the development of the guidelines include Deborah Hayes (chair, 1988); Michael Sabo (chair, 1985–87); Fred Bess; Dianne Brackett; Frank Burns: Evelyn Cherow, ex officio: Brad Freidrich; Judith Gravel; Jack Kile; Marcia Kushner; Diane Meyer; Gary Thompson; James Thelin; and Ann Carey, ASHA vice president for professional and governmental affairs (1988–90) and Nancy Becker, vice president for professional and governmental affairs (1985–87).

Background

A Committee on Infant Hearing was established in 1984 by the Legislative Council (LC 27-84). The charge to that committee:

> To gather and synthesize information and policies generated by committees and Boards of ASHA which pertain to special aspects of hearing impairment in infants, models of service delivery to infants, and identification, diagnosis, and management of hearing disorders in infants; to identity and make recommendations on research needs regarding the development of auditory function and dysfunction in infants, prevention of hearing impairment in infants, and the identification, diagnosis, and management of hearing disorders in infants; to provide audiologic consultation to the Joint Committee on Infant Hearing on matters pertinent to prevention, identification, diagnosis, and management of infant hearing.

The initial activity of the committee was to determine procedures that, at the present time, are most appropriate for audiologic screening of infants at risk for hearing impairment. After consideration of the many issues related to infant hearing, the committee concluded that (a) all newborn infants who are at risk for hearing impairment should be identified, (b) infants identified at risk should receive audiologic screening by auditory evoked potentials prior to hospital discharge, and (c) those infants who fail initial audiologic screening or who fail to be screened should enter an audiologic evaluation, follow-up, and management system.

The purpose of this report is to set forth guidelines for the establishment of auditory screening programs for newborn infants who are at risk for hearing impairment.

Guidelines for audiometric evaluation, follow-up, and management of hearing-impaired infants will be considered in forthcoming activities of the Committee on Infant Hearing.

Definitions

Infants at risk: Infants who fall into one or more of the seven risk criteria identified in the 1982 position statement of the Joint Committee on Infant Hearing (1982) are considered at risk for hearing impairment and should receive audiologic screening.[1]
The factors are:

1. A family history of childhood hearing impairment.
2. Congenital perinatal infection (e.g., cytomegalovirus (CMV), rubella, herpes, toxoplasmosis, syphilis).
3. Anatomic malformation involving the head or neck (e.g., dysmorphic appearance including syndronal and nonsyndromal abnormalities, overt or submucous cleft palate, morphologic abnormalities of the pinna).
4. Birthweight less than 1500 grams.
5. Hyperbilirubmemia at level exceeding indications for exchange transfusion.
6. Bacterial menningitis, especially H. influenza.
7. Severe asphyxia which may include infants with Apgar scores of 0–3 who fail to institute spontaneous respiration by 10 minutes and those with hypotonia persisting to two hours of age (Joint Committee on Infant Hearing, 1982).

For a more complete review of these risk criteria and their relation to hearing impairment, see Gerkin (1984).

Hearing impairment: Bilateral conductive and/or sensori-neural deficit in the frequency region important for speech recognition (approximately 1000 through 4000 Hz). Hearing impairment is defined as deficit in auditory sensitivity that interferes with speech recognition and for which intervention strategies are known and available.

---

[1]Investigators have also recommended audiologic screening of infants who manifest other health factors. These factors include: (a) parent consanguinity (Coplan, 1987; Feinmesser & Tell, 1976), (b) severe neonatal sepsis (Feinmesser & Tel, 1976), (c) persistent pulmonary hypertension of the newborn (PPHN; Naulty, Weiss & Herer, 1986; Sell, Gaines, Gluckman, & Williams, 1985), and (d) length of stay in the intensive care nursery and gestational age (Halpern, Hosford-Dunn, & Malachowsky, 1987). Some investigators have also advocated audiologic screening of all infants in neonatal intensive care units (Galambos, Hicks, & Wilson, 1984; Jacobson & Morehouse, 1964). In future risk registries, these additional factors and recommendations may be included. At this time, ASHA recommends, at a minimum, use of the Joint Committee on Infant Hearing 1982 risk criteria pending update of the register.

The impact of childhood hearing impairment on speech and language development and academic achievement is well documented (Allen, 1986: Osberger, 1986). In general hearing-impaired children demonstrate limited speech production skills (Osberger, Robbins, Lybolt, Kent, & Peters, 1986), significantly delayed receptive and expressive language skills (Moeller, Osberger, & Eccarius, 1986; Osberger, Moeller, Eccarius, Robbins, & Johnson, 1986), and reduced academic achievement, especially in language-related areas (Allen, 1986). To minimize these debilitating effects, professionals have urged early identification and habilitation of infants with hearing impairment. Efforts in both the public and private sectors have been undertaken to develop screening, diagnostic, and habilitation programs to meet these goals.

In the public sector, passage of Public Law 99-457, the Education of the Handicapped Amendment of 1986, created (in part) a new discretionary program to address the special needs of handicapped infants and toddlers from birth through 2 years of age and their families. By 1990–91, each state that wants to continue receiving federal financial assistance under the birth through-2 program must have in place a policy to provide early intervention services to all handicapped infants and toddlers. Some components of this program include development of a Child Find system, referral to service providers, research and demonstration projects, and a comprehensive system of personnel development. Provision of services must be by qualified personnel meeting the highest state standards established for employment in each profession or discipline.

In the private sector, representatives from audiology and speech-language pathology, otolaryngology, pediatrics, and nursing have participated in a Joint Committee on Infant Hearing which, over the years, has developed a series of position papers. The most recent position paper (Joint Committee on Infant Hearing, 1982) states that "early detection of hearing impairment in the affected infant is important for medical treatment and subsequent educational intervention to assure development of communication skills." The Joint Committee recommended that infants at risk for hearing impairment be identified and that they receive appropriate evaluation and treatment.

Reliable data on incidence of significant hearing impairment in infants and young children are unavailable (Hotchkiss, 1987; Ries, 1986). National statistics indicate that approximately 3.7 million children are born in the United States each year (Wegman, 1987). Investigators estimate that 7–12% of all newborns are at risk for hearing impairment (Feinmesser & Tell, 1976; Jacobson & Morehouse, 1984; Mahoney & Eichwald, 1987). Moderate to profound hearing impairment is reported present in less than 2% to more than 4% of at-risk infants (Galambos et al., 1984; Jacobson & Morehouse, 1984; Mahoney and Eichwald, 1987; Stein, Ozdamar, Kraus, & Paton, 1983; Hosford-Dunn, Johnson, Simmons, Malachowski, & Low, 1987). Prevalence of milder degrees of hearing impairment in this population is unknown. Retrospective studies have shown that between 50 and 75% of hearing-impaired children were positive for at least one of the Joint Committee's risk criteria (Elssmann, Matkin, & Sabo, 1987; Feinmesser & Tell, 1976; Stein, Clark, & Kraus, 1983).

In addition to infants who are at risk, infants with no known risk factors may have or develop hearing impairment (Feinmesser & Tell, 1976; Simmons, 1980). Prevalence of significant hearing impairment, including mild to moderate hearing impairment, for this population is not well defined.

The dearth of data on the prevalence of hearing impairment in both at-risk newborns and newborns with no known risk factors demonstrates the pressing need for well-controlled studies of the true impairment rate in these populations. Investigations on the prevalence of mild to moderate hearing impairment are especially needed.

Rationale

To prevent or reduce the debilitating effects of childhood hearing impairment, ASHA endorses an aggressive program of early identification and habilitation. Optimally, all newborn infants should receive audiologic screening to identify the majority of infants who require audiologic evaluation, follow-up, and management. At the present time, however, there are no data to indicate that newborn behavioral screening programs are sufficiently sensitive and specific (Durieux-Smith, Picton, Edwards, Goodman, & MacMurray, 1985; Feinmesser & Tell, 1976; Jacobson and Morehouse, 1984), or that evoked potential screening programs can be sufficiently low cost (Mahoney & Eichwald, 1987; Weber, 1987) to warrant mass screening. When cost-effective screening approaches are developed that are sensitive and specific, ASHA recommends evaluation of all newborn infants. In the interim, ASHA recommends audiologic screening of all infants at risk for hearing impairment.

Program Components

A successful program of early identification of hearing impairment in infants includes three components: (a) parent/caregiver education, (b) audiologic screening, and (c) evaluation, follow-up, and management systems.

Parent/caregiver education. Parents/caregivers of all newborns should receive information about normal auditory and speech and language development, and should be informed of the importance of early audiologic evaluation of suspected hearing problems. They should receive information that will enhance their ability both to observe auditory and speech and language development, and to advocate prompt referral for appropriate audiologic evaluation (Elssmann et al., 1987).

Audiologic screening. All newborn infants at risk for hearing impairment by Joint Committee on Infant Hearing criteria (1982) should receive audiologic screening. Screening can occur prior to hospital discharge (Durieux-Smith et al., 1985; Galambos, Hicks, & Wilson, 1982, 1984; Gorga, Reiland, Beauchaine, Worthington, & Jesteadt, 1987; Jacobson & Morehouse, 1984; Stein, Clark, & Kraus, 1983) or may be deferred until age 4 months (Alberti, Hyde, Riko, Corbin, & Fitzhardinge, 1985; Durieux-Smith, Picton, Edwards, MacMurray, & Goodman, 1987; Hyde, Riko, Corbin, Moroso, & Albert, 1984) or even older (Mahoney & Eichwald, 1987). Screening prior to hospital discharge ensures access to all infants who are identified at risk for hearing impairment

(Downs & Sterritt, 1967) and, under appropriate test conditions, does not result in a significantly higher failure rate than deferred screening (Durieux-Smith et al., 1987). Substantial loss to follow-up can occur if screening is deferred (Coplan, 1987; Downs & Sterritt, 1967; Mahoney & Eichwald, 1987; Stein, Clark, & Kraus, 1983). In the absence of systematic nursery-based screening programs, there are data indicating that hearing impairment is typically not identified until age 18 months and older, even for infants at risk for hearing impairment (Elssmann et al., 1987; Stein, Clark, & Kraus, 1983). Further, if screening is deferred until the infant cam be tested with operant conditioning behavioral test procedures, then the goal of identification and habilitation by age 6 months cannot be met for many at-risk infants because developmental age may lag behind chronological age for premature and compromised infants. For these reasons, ASHA recommends audiologic screening prior to hospital discharge.

Screening at-risk newborns (approximately 7–12% of the newborn population) should result in earlier identification and habilitation of approximately 50–75% of hearing-impaired infants (Elssmann et al., 1987; Jacobson & Morehouse, 1984; Mahoney & Eichwald, 1987; Stein, Clark, & Kraus, 1983). It is important to recognize, however, that the remaining 25–50% of hearing-impaired infants will not receive audiologic screening in the newborn nursery and will not, therefore, be identified by these procedures.

Audiologic screening is performed by an audiologist or under the supervision of an audiologist in accordance with current standards (Committee on Audiologic Evaluation, 1987). ASHA recommends that at-risk newborns receive audiologic screening using auditory evoked potential measures prior to discharge from the newborn nursery. At the present time, auditory brainstem response (ABR) provides a reliable and valid estimate of peripheral auditory sensitivity in newborns (Galambos et al., 1982, 1984; Gorga et al., 1987; Jacobson & Morehouse, 1984; Lary, Briassoulis, de Vries, Dubowitz, & Dubowitz, 1985; Schulman-Galambos & Galambos, 1975, 1979).

In addition to technically appropriate application of the ABR test procedure, the audiologic screening includes (a) professional interpretation of test results; (b) parent/caregiver counseling; and (c) when appropriate, guidance into an evaluation, follow-up, and management system.

Evaluation, Follow-up, and Management Systems. Development of programs for identification of hearing impairment in infants is not justified without immediate availability of an appropriate evaluation, follow-up, and management system. Definition of a specific system is outside the scope of this document. At a minimum, the system must include diagnostic and habilitative audiologic services, and general medical and otologic services as recommended by the Joint Committee on Infant Hearing (1982). These services require involvement of an interdisciplinary team.

Protocol for Audiologic Screening of At-Risk Newborn Infants

The recommended process for identification and audiologic screening of at-risk newborn infants is shown in Figure 1.

Population

ASHA recommends that all newborn infants receive evaluation for risk status by Joint Committee on Infant Hearing (1982) criteria prior to discharge from the newborn nursery (well baby nursery for healthy newborns; intensive care nursery for ill or compromised infants). Parents should receive information about expected milestones in auditory and speech-language development and should be informed of the importance of audiologic evaluation of suspected hearing problems. Those infants who have no known risk factors do not receive audiologic screening by ABR prior to discharge. An infant who exhibits abnormal auditory behavior or delayed speech and language development or whose parent/caregiver expresses concern about auditory responsiveness should receive audiologic evaluation.

Procedure

Infants at risk for hearing impairment should receive audiologic screening. The purpose of this screening is to identify those infants whose responses do not meet pass criteria and who therefore should enter an audiologic evaluation, follow-up, and management system.

The recommended procedure is ABR prior to discharge. If the infant is discharged prior to screening, or if ABR screening under audiologic supervision is unavailable, then the parent/caregiver should be informed of the importance of audiologic follow-up for the infant. The infant should be referred to an audiologist for determination of appropriate evaluation, follow-up, and management strategies.

The acoustic stimulus for ABR screening should contain energy in the frequency region important for speech recognition. Clicks are the most commonly used signal for eliciting the ABR (Committee on Audiologic Evaluation, 1987) and contain energy in the speech frequency region (Gorga, Abbas, & Worthington, 1985; Jerger & Mauldin, 1978). Other signals that may be used include tone pips or tone bursts, or clicks in the presence of masking noise.

Pass Criterion

Pass criterion for ABR screening is a response from both ears at intensity levels 40db nHL or less. Infants whose responses meet this criterion should receive audiologic follow-up as necessary for medical evaluation and management and/or developmental evaluation. It is important that parents/caregivers and primary health care providers understand that "pass" on ABR screening does not rule out development of hearing impairment in infancy or early childhood (Nield, Schrier, Ramos, Platzker, & Warburton, 1986). Parents/caregivers and primary health care providers should remain vigilant to the infant's auditory behavior and speech and language development, and should be encouraged to advocate for audiologic evaluation if they are concerned about the infant's communication development.

Infants whose responses meet pass criterion and who are at risk for progressive hearing impairment should receive audiologic monitoring on a periodic basis and probably through the preschool years (Coplan, 1987). Factors that are known at the present time to place an infant at risk for progressive hearing impairment include family history of progressive hearing impairment (Konigsmark & Gorlin, 1976), congenital cytomegalovirus (CMV; Dahle, McCollister, Stagno, Reynolds, & Hoffman, 1979; Stagno et al., 1977), and PPHN (Naulty et al., 1986; Sell et al., 1985).

Refer Criterion/Follow-Up

Infants who do not demonstrate responses at intensity levels 40 dB nHL or less in both ears should enter the audiologic evaluation, follow-up, and management system. Infants who demonstrate responses at 40dB nHL or less from only one ear should receive audiologic monitoring until either (a) both ears meet pass criterion or (b) stable unilateral hearing impairment is confirmed and follow-up and management is initiated.

Comprehensive audiological evaluation may include additional evoked potential evaluation, behavioral testing, and acoustic immittance measures. These infants are also referred for medical evaluation specified by the Joint Committee on Infant Hearing (1982):

1. General physical examination and history including:

   a. Examination of the head and neck,

   b. Otoscopy and otomicroscopy,

   c. Identification of relevant physical abnormalities,

   d. Laboratory tests such as urinalysis and diagnostic tests for perinatal infections.

Habilitation of hearing-impaired infants should be initiated by age 6 months (Joint Committee on Infant Hearing, 1982). Estimates of peripheral sensitivity based on electrophysiologic procedures should be confirmed by behavioral techniques as soon as possible. Efforts to confirm electrophysiologic estimates of peripheral sensitivity may coincide with on-going habitation. In general, precise behavioral estimates of hearing sensitivity can be obtained when the infant can respond to operant conditioning test procedures (approximately 5–6 months developmental age; Thompson & Wilson, 1984). Management decisions made prior to defining the behavioral audiogram may require modification as more precise estimates of hearing sensitivity are obtained.

Summary

The importance of early identification of hearing impairment is well documented. The Joint Committee on Infant Hearing 1982 Position Statement established the goal of identification and habilitation of hearing impaired infants by age 6 months but did not specify the procedure for initial audiologic screening. In these guidelines ASHA specifies the recommended procedure for audiologic screening of infants at risk (for hearing impairment that includes (a) parent/caregiver education; (b) audiologic screening by ABR; and (c) referral to a comprehensive evaluation, follow-up, and management system for those infants who fail initial ABR screening. The procedures recommended in these guidelines are complex and require substantial involvement of a qualified

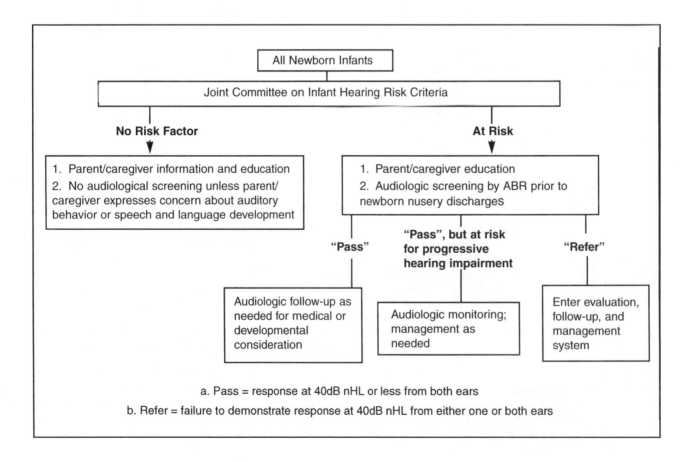

audiologist. Identification programs should be instituted only when all components are available to provide appropriate services to the infant and his/her family. It is hoped that these guidelines will encourage implementation of programs for early identification of hearing impairment in at-risk infants.

References

Alberti, P, Hyde, M, Riko, K, Corbin, H., & Fitzhardinge, P (1985). Issues in early identification of hearing loss. *Laryngoscope, 95*(4), 373–381.

Allen, T. (1986). Patterns of academic achievement among hearing impaired students: 1974 and 1983. In A. Schildroth & M. Karchmer (Eds.), *Deaf children in America* (pp. 161–206). San Diego: College-Hill Press.

Committee on Audiologic Evaluation. Auditory Evoked Potential Measurements Working Group. (1987). *The short latency auditory evoked potentials, a tutorial paper.* Unpublished data.

Coplan, J. (1987). Deafness: Ever heard of it? Delayed recognition of permanent hearing loss. *Pediatrics, 79*(2), 206–213.

Dahle, A., McCollister, F., Stagno, S., Reynolds, D., & Hoffman, H. (1979). Progressive hearing impairment in children with congenital cytomegalovirus infection. *Journal of Speech and Hearing Disorders, 44*(2), 220–229.

Downs, M., & Sterrit, G. (1967). A guide to newborn and infant hearing screening programs. *Archives of Otolaryngology, 85*, 1522.

Durieux-Smith, A., Picton, T., Edwards, C., Goodman, J., & Mac-Murray, B. (1985). The crib-o-gram in the NICU: An evaluation based on brainstem electric response audiometry. *Ear and Hearing, 6*(1), 20–24.

Durieux-Smith, A., Picton, T., Edwards. C., MacMurray, B., & Goodman, J. (1987). Brainstem electric-response audiometry in infants of a neonatal intensive care unit. *Audiology, 26*(3), 284–297.

Elssmann, S., Matkin, N., & Sato, M. (1987). Early identification of congenital sensorineural hearing impairment. *The Hearing Journal, 40*(9), 13–17.

Feinmesser, M., & Tell, L. (1976). Neonatal screening for detection of deafness. *Archives of Otolaryngology, 102*(5), 297–299.

Galambos, R., Hicks, G., & Wilson, M. (1982). Hearing loss in graduates of a tertiary intensive care nursery. *Ear and Hearing, 3*(2), 87–90.

Galambos, R., Hicks, G., & Wilson, M. (1984). The auditory brainstem response reliably predicts hearing loss in graduates of a tertiary intensive care nursery. *Ear and Hearing, 5*(4), 254–260.

Gerkin, K. (1984). The high risk register for deafness. *Asha, 26*(3), 17–23.

Gorga, M., Abbas, P., & Worthington, D. (1985). Stimulus calibration in ABR measurements. In J. Jacobson (Ed.). *The auditory brainstem response* (pp. 49–62). San Diego: College-Hill Press.

Gorga, M., Reiland, J., Beauchaine, K., Worthington, D., & Jesteadt, W. (1987). Auditory brainstem responses from graduates of an intensive care nursery: Normal patterns of response. *Journal of Speech and Hearing Research, 30*(3), 311–318.

Halpern, J., Hosford-Dunn, H., & Malachowski, N. (1987). Four factors that accurately predict hearing loss in "high risk" neonates. *Ear and Hearing, 8*(1), 21–25.

Hosford-Dunn, H., Johnson, S., Simmons, B., Malachowski, N., & Low, K. (1987). Infant hearing screening: Program implementation and validation. *Ear and Hearing, 8*(1), 12–20.

Hotchkiss, D. (1987). Demographic aspects of hearing impairment: Questions and answers. Washington, D.C.: Gallaudet University. Center for Assessment and Demographic Studies.

Hyde, M., Riko, K., Corbin, H., Moroso, M., & Alberti, P. (1984). A neonatal hearing screening research program using brainstem electric response audiometry. *Journal of Otolaryngology, 13*(1), 49–54.

Jacobson, J., & Morehouse, R. (1984). A comparison of auditory brainstem response and behavioral screening in high risk and normal newborn infants. *Ear and Hearing, 5*(4), 247–253.

Jerger, J., & Mauldin, L. (1978). Prediction of sensori-neural hearing level from the brainstem evoked response. *Archives of Otolaryngology, 104*(8), 456–461.

Joint Committee on Infant Hearing. (1982). Position statement. *Asha, 24*(12), 1017–1018.

Konigsmark, B., & Gorlin, R. (1976). *Genetic and metabolic deafness.* Philadelphia, W. B. Saunders Company.

Lary, S., Briassoulis, G., de Vries, L., Dubowitz, L., & Dubowitz, V. (1985). Hearing threshold in preterm and term infants by auditory brainstem response. *Journal of Pediatrics, 107*(4), 593–599.

Mahoney, T., & Eichwald, J. (1987). The ups and "Downs" of high-risk hearing screening: The Utah statewide program. In K. Gerkin, & A. Amochaev (Eds.), *Seminars in Hearing, 8*(2), 155–163.

Moeller, M., Osberger, M., & Eccarius, M. (1986). Receptive language skills. In M. Osberger (Ed.), *Language and learning skills in hearing-impaired students. ASHA Monographs, 23*, 41–53.

Naulty, C., Weiss, I., & Herer, G. (1986). Progressive sensorineural hearing loss in survivors of persistent fetal circulation. *Ear and Hearing, 7*(2), 74–77.

Nield, T., Scbrier, S., Ramos, A., Platzker, A., & Warburton, D. (1986). Unexpected hearing loss in high-risk infants. *Pediatrics, 78*(3), 417–421.

Osberger, M. (Ed.). (1986). Language and learning skills of hearing-impaired students. *ASHA Monographs, 23.*

Osberger, M., Moeller, M., Eccarius, M., Robbins, A., & Johnson, D. (1986). Expressive language skills. In M. Osberger (Ed.). *Language and learning skills of hearing impaired students. ASHA Monographs, 23*, 54–65.

Osberger, M., Robbins, A., Lybolt, J., Kent, R., & Peters, J. (1986). Speech evaluation. In M. Osberger (Ed.). *Language and learning skills of hearing-impaired students. Asha Monographs, 23*, 24–31.

Ries, P. (1986). Characteristics of hearing impaired youth in the general population and of students in special education programs for the hearing-impaired. In A. Schildroth & M. Karchmer (Eds.). *Deaf children in America* (pp. 1–31). San Diego: College-Hill Press.

Schulman-Galambos, C., & Galambos. R. (1975). Brainstem auditory-evoked responses in premature infants. *Journal of Speech and Hearing Research, 18*(3), 456–465.

Schulman-Galambos, C., & Galambos, R. (1979). Brainstem evoked response audiometry in newborn hearing screening. *Archives of Otolaryngology, 105*(2), 86–90.

Sell, E., Gaines, J., Gluckman, C., & Williams, E. (1985). Persistent fetal circulation: Neurodevelopmental outcome. *American Journal of Diseases in Childhood, 139*(1), 25–28.

Simmons, F. B. (1980). Patterns of deafness in newborns. *The Laryngoscope, 90*(3). 448–453.

Stagno, S., Reynolds, D., Amos, C., Dahle, A., McCollister, F., Mohindra, I., Ermocilla, R., & Alford, C. (1977). Auditory and visual defects resulting from symptomatic and subclinical congenital cytomegaloviral toxoplasma infections. *Pediatrics, 59*(5), 669–677.

Stein, L., Clark, S., & Kraus, N. (1983). The hearing-impaired infant: Patterns of identification and habilitation. *Ear and Hearing, 3*(5), 232–236.

Stein, L., Ozdamar, O., Kraus, N., & Paton, J. (1983). Follow-up of infants screened by auditory brainstem response in the neonatal intensive care unit. *Journal of Pediatrics, 103*(9), 447–453.

Thompson, G., & Wilson, W. R. (1984). Clinical application of visual reinforcement audiometry. In T. Mahoney (Ed.), *Seminars in Hearing, 5*(1), 85–99.

Weber, H. (1987). Ten years of searching for the hearing-impaired infant in rural Colorado. In K. Gerkin & A. Amochaev (Eds.). *Seminars in Hearing, 8*(2), 149–154.

Wegman. M. (1987. Annual summary of vital statistics 1986. *Pediatrics, 80*(6), 817–827.

Appendix 2–D

FUNCTIONAL COMMUNICATION MEASURE: HEARING SENSITIVITY[1]

Level 0: Unable to judge.

Level 1: Hearing cannot be used for communication or environmental acoustical awareness.

Level 2: Uses hearing primarily for purposes of environmental acoustical awareness.

Level 3: Limited understanding of spoken language, even when hearing is combined with speechreading and environmental cues.

Level 4: Understands spoken language at normal communication levels only when hearing is combined with speechreading and environmental cues.

Level 5: Understands spoken language at normal conversational levels only if speech is louder than noise.

Level 6: Understands spoken language at normal conversational levels when background noise is as loud as speech.

Level 7: Understands spoken language at normal conversational levels even when background noise is louder than speech.

Note: Levels 1–7 are an initial attempt to reflect a scale of hearing ability influenced by environmental factors (signal–to–noise ratio) and use of contextual cues (speechreading). The levels may not represent equal intervals and could be delineated further to show improvement based on aural rehabilitation efforts. Effects of amplification were not incorporated into the levels so that the clinician can gauge improvement and reflect benefit of amplification fitting and aural rehabilitation.

Source: "Users Guide Phase I, Group I. The American Speech-Language-Hearing Association's National Treatment Outcome Data Collection Project, 1995, FCMS p. 13. Reprinted by permission.

[1]This scale was field tested with adults in health care settings by ASHA in 1995. Reliability and validity testing is still in process.

Appendix 2–E

GUIDELINES FOR IDENTIFICATION AUDIOMETRY

The following revision of the 1974 Guidelines for Identification Audiometry was developed by the Committee on Audiologic Evaluation in compliance with the Committee's charge to periodically review and revise existing ASHA guidelines. The Executive Board of the American Speech Language-Hearing Association (ASHA) approved a draft of this paper for publication in *Asha*, February 1984, for widespread peer review. The present document includes revisions based on members' comments received in response to the February 1984 published draft and was formally adopted by the American Speech-Language-Hearing Association through its Legislative Council in November 1984 (LC 26-84). This revision now replaces the 1974 publication.

Members of the Committee on Audiologic Evaluation included Martin S. Robinette (Chair), Robert H. Brey, J. Michael Dennis, Judy R. Dubno, Earleen Elkins, Sandra Gabriel, Douglas P. Noffsinger, Polly E. Patrick, Gerald R. Popelka, Janet E. Shanks, Michael Valente, and Peggy S. Williams (ex officio). Contributions of Hughlett L. Morris, Vice President for Clinical Affairs, 1982–84, are also acknowledged.

WHEREAS, there has been a charge to the Committee on Audiologic Evaluation to establish guidelines for clinical procedure, and
WHEREAS, guidelines titled "Guidelines for Identification Audiometry" were adopted in LC 21-74, and
WHEREAS, the Committee on Audiological Evaluation has been charged to monitor and, when appropriate, suggest revisions in existing guidelines, and
WHEREAS, information about identification audiometry has changed since 1974, and
WHEREAS, the Committee on Audiologic Evaluation has incorporated in the revised Guidelines for Identification Audiometry solicited comments from individuals involved in conducting identification programs, and
WHEREAS, the entire membership of the Association has had an opportunity to comment on the proposed revised Guidelines (Asha, February 1984), and
WHEREAS, the committee has prepared a final document which incorporates the suggestions of the membership; therefore
RESOLVED, That the revised Guidelines for Identification Audiometry be adopted by the American Speech-Language-Hearing Association; and further
RESOLVED, That notification of the availability of the Guidelines for Identification Audiometry be published in Asha and that the Guidelines be disseminated to appropriate local, state, and federal education officials.

This revised set of "Guidelines for Identification Audiometry," developed by the Committee on Audiologic Evaluation, replaces the original paper of the same title published in 1974.

All ASHA guidelines present a recommended set of procedures based on existing clinical practice and research findings. The spirit of these guidelines is not to mandate a single way of accomplishing the clinical process; rather the intent is to suggest standard procedures that, in the final analysis, will benefit the persons we serve. The intention is to improve interclinician and interclinic comparison of data, thereby allowing for a more effective transfer of information. It is expected that professional members of the Association will recognize the confined scope of guidelines and will use wisdom in relating the usefulness of the guidelines for their specific needs.

The specific purpose of these guidelines is to detail procedures for accomplishing rapid and efficient identification of hearing impairment, particularly for use with young children, As such, these guidelines represent an update of the procedures for identification audiometry for school-age children specified in "Identification Audiometry," *Journal of Speech and Hearing Disorders Monograph Supplement 9* (Darley, 1961). The current need for these guidelines is apparent with the development of increasing numbers of identification audiometry programs administered by state departments of education or health, the development of state mandatory special education statutes, and Medicaid guidelines for Early and Periodic Screening, Diagnosis and Treatment (EPSDT).

For the most part, the philosophy and procedures laid out in these guidelines are based on and supported by published data. ASHA invites data-based input for future modifications of the guidelines.

Scope

A primary goal of identification audiometry using pure-tone air-conduction testing is to identify persons who have hearing impairments that interfere with or that have potential for interfering with communication. The goal of a program using acoustic immittance measurements is the identification of individuals who have middle ear disorders. The program which incorporates both pure-tone testing and acoustic immittance measurements will be the most effective in identifying individuals in need of audiological otological services. The Guidelines for Acoustic Immittance Screening of Middle-Ear Function (ASHA, 1979) describes the procedures recommended for identification of middle ear disorders using acoustic immittance screening measures.

These guidelines are intended for children age 3 years through Grade 3 because early identification of communicative problems in this age group will permit maximum habilitation and avoidance of potential educational problems.

Belkin, Suchman, Bergman, Rosenblatt, and Jacobziner (1964) have reported successful large scale individual pure-tone screening tests with children as young as 3 years of age. In addition, it is this age group which, in our society, is most often involved in the formal educational process through preschools and regular schools. While these guidelines focus on use with young children, they are equally applicable for use with older children and adults. This guideline does not preclude screening below age 3; however, due to unique needs of younger children and infants, a modified screening assessment procedure needs to be utilized.

The guidelines are designed for rapid and efficient identification of hearing impairment. A basic assumption behind the guidelines is that identification audiometry is usually conducted in the relatively poor acoustic environments of schools and offices. Consequently, the procedures recommended are designed to be robust enough to be valid in a wide range of test settings. Naturally, it would be desirable for all identification audiometry to be conducted in acoustic environments that are controlled, but such environments are seldom available.

Identification audiometry is only one component of a hearing conservation program. A well-balanced program will include screening, rescreening, threshold audiometry, referrals for audiologic and medical evaluations, education and habilitation planning, and counseling for parents and teachers. Too often the sole goal is referral for medical evaluation rather than referral for consideration of communicative needs of those who fail screening procedures. Once people have been identified by the program, they should be followed regularly to ensure that their communication and medical needs are met. It is pointless to identify people who have hearing impairments unless there is a concurrent follow-up program to handle their habilitative, educational, and medical needs.

Finally, these guidelines apply only to the use of pure-tone air-conduction screening for the purpose of identifying persons who have hearing impairments that interfere with or have the potential for interfering with communication. Research (Eagles, 1961; Eagles, Wishik, & Doerfler, 1967; Roberts, 1972) demonstrates that pure-tone air-conduction screening is inefficient in identifying many of those who have conductive ear pathology. Thus, if the purpose of an identification audiometry program is also to identify persons with middle-ear pathology, ASHA suggests the inclusion of acoustic immittance screening measurements.

Identification Audiometry

The following recommendations emphasize identification audiometry for children using a manually administered, individual pure-tone air-conduction screening procedure.

Children to Be Screened

Individual limited-frequency screening should be administered annually to children functioning at a developmental level of 3 years through Grade 3 and to any high-risk children including those above Grade 3.[1] The time the program saves by emphasizing the lower grades permits appropriate attention for the high-risk group and focuses the program's efforts during the years when identification of communication problems can lead to intervention that will forestall serious educational, psychological, and social problems. Some school systems may elect to screen routinely after Grade 3 at 3- or 4-year intervals (Darley, 1961). Others may find that a cost/benefit analysis does not justify routine screening beyond Grade 3 (Downs, Doster, & Wever, 1965). To determine the merit of routine screening after Grade 3, more data appear to be necessary.

Procedure

Individual screening. Individual as opposed to group screening is recommended. The Massachusetts Test (Johnston, 1948) is an example of a group pure-tone test that achieved great popularity and is still used in some states. It requires written responses and consequently, like most group screening tests, is limited to children above the second grade. Other limitations of group tests are calibration and maintenance problems of multiple earphones, increased set-up time and excessive time spent in retesting false-positive failures. All these factors combine to increase the total time required for the screening program without increasing accuracy. Many group tests may appear to save time but the time taken to set up, check calibration, score answer sheets, and retest excessive failures may result in no saving of time.

Manual method. A manual versus an automatic method is recommended because it is applicable with children down to 3 years of age. There is no known evidence that a self-recording or other type of automatic method is possible and effective with young children. Certainly, if an effective and more rapid automatic method is developed, its use should be considered.

Signal

Type. Pure-tone signals shall be used. Many different stimuli have been used to screen children and adults for the purpose of identifying persons with hearing impairments. The use of speech materials is not recommended because of the failure of procedures employing those materials to identify individuals with hearing impairment in the frequency range above 500 Hz (Johnson & Newby, 1954).

Test frequencies. When pure-tone testing is used in conjunction with acoustic immittance screening, the test frequencies shall be 1000, 2000, and 4000 Hz. If acoustic immittance screening is not a part of the identification program,

---

[1]Examples of high-risk children are those who (a) repeat a grade; (b) require special education programs; (c) are new to the school system; (d) were absent during a previously scheduled screening exam; (e) failed a threshold test during the previous year; (f) have speech problems, language problems, or obvious difficulty in communication; (g) are suspected of hearing impairment or have a medical problem associated with hearing impairment (children with recurrent or chronic problems such as allergies may require audiometric monitoring); and (h) are involved in coursework which places them at risk for noise exposure (i.e., band, woodworking, and auto mechanics). Additional examples of high-risk children are given in Darley (1961, p. 36).

500 Hz shall be included as a test frequency provided the ambient level does not exceed acceptable levels (ANSI-1977). Research evidence does not support the use of 3000 Hz as an alternative test signal to 4000 Hz (Katt & Sprague, 1981).[2] The interactions between earphones and ears at 6000 Hz (Villchur, 1970) make 6000 Hz a poor choice for inclusion in an identification program.

Screening levels. Screening levels shall be 20 dB HL (re ANSI-1969) at all frequencies tested.[3]

Results

Failure criterion. Failure to respond to the recommended screening levels at any frequency in either ear shall constitute failure.

Mandatory rescreening. All failures should be rescreened preferably within the same session in which they failed. Removing and repositioning the phones, accompanied by careful reinstruction, markedly reduces the number of failures. Wilson and Walton (1974) reported a 52% reduction in failures by rescreening. The rescreening, using the same frequencies, levels, and failure criterion, is an essential procedure for improving the efficiency of a screen program. The time delay for rescreenmg should be as short as feasible, with the maximum delay no greater than 2 weeks.

Disposition of failures. Failures on rescreening should be referred for audiologic evaluation by an audiologist. Some persons, particularly young children, will fail both the screening and rescreening procedures and then yield normal thresholds on an audiologic evaluation. Therefore, a hearing impairment should not be considered identified until verified in an audiologic evaluation. There is no research support for the specification of a priority system for referrals.

The constraints placed on individual programs will determine the referral format, but the hearing conservation program supervisor should be responsible for providing case mamagement necessary to guarantee appropriate referral for audiologic and medical consultation. In addition, the supervisor should sccure educational assistance, if necessary, for students during and after medical therapy or audiologic habilitation. These duties are emphasized because the primary goal of school hearing conservation programs is to reduce the negative effects of communicative problems that are secondary to hearing loss rather than simply to identify children who pass or fail a screening test.

Procedural Considerations

Adherence to the following procedural recommendations should facilitate successful implementation of the ASHA Guidelines for Identification Audiometry.

Personnel

Identification audiometry programs should be conducted or supervised by an audiologist. After appropriate training, support personnel may administer audiometric screenings and rescreenings under the supervision of an audiologist. If properly trained professionals are not involved in supervising an identification audiometry program, an inordinate number of false-positive failures and false-negative passes may occur, thus undermining the validity of the program. Without reservation, the audiologic evaluation should be administered by an audiologist.

Instructions

Instructions are critical in all audiometric procedures, but particular care must be taken in instructing children. Instructions should emphasize the importance of responding "right away even when the beeps sound far away." Groups of children can be instructed at one time. Those waiting for the test profit from watching others being tested. Pantomime may have to accompany verbal instructions for the very young child or the difficult-to-test person, particularly if a conditioned play response is required rather than a hand or verbal response. Careful reinstruction is an important part of the rescreening process. Frequently, children fail because they have misunderstood instructions. This is particularly true of children in the 3- to 6-year age range.

Time

At the third-grade level the entire screening, including earphone placement, occupies less than 1 min. For younger children more time may be necessary. To avoid unnecessary failures with younger children, it is sometimes desirable to present more than one signal per frequency if there is no response. The net effect is a saving of time because the more careful screen process reduces the number of children who fail and require rescreening.

Acoustic Environment

The acoustic environment is an important variable in screening audiometry. Usually school environments are not too noisy for screening at frequencies above 1000 Hz, but sometimes ambient noise will interfere with screening at 1000 Hz and at lower frequencies. The 1000–4000 Hz range was selected for the ASHA guidelines because it is less vulnerable to invalidation by ambient noise and because most significant hearing impairment will include failure in this range.

The allowable octave-band ambient noise levels in the region of the test tone are shown in Table 1. Screening at 500 Hz may be included if the environmental noise in this frequency region is at or below the maximum allowable level. In test environments that have fluctuating noise levels, caution must be used in applying the maximum values shown in this table.

Careful snug placement of the earphones increases attenuation of ambient noise by the earphone cushion assembly.

---

[2]ASHA invites active research on the addition of 3000 Hz to the screening format. Research studies also would be helpful to determine whether 3000 Hz could be substituted for 4000 Hz as a better predictor of subtle communication problems among school-age children.

[3]ASHA is interested in active research concerning screening levels, since there is a great deal of strong feeling expressed concerning the issue, but very little hard data are available.

Table 1

Test frequency	500	1000	2000	4000
Octave-band cutoff	300	600	1200	2400
Frequencies	600	1200	2400	4800
Octave-band levels: Ear covered with earphone mounted in MX-41/AR cushion (ANSI 3.1-1977)	21.5	29.5	34.5	42.0
Plus ASHA screening level re ANSI-1969	20	20	20	20
Resultant maximum ambient noise level allowable for ASHA screening	41.5	49.5	54.5	62

Table 1. Approximate allowable octave-band ambient noise levels (SPL re 20 µPa for threshold measurements at 0 dB HL re ANSI-1969 and for screening at the ASHA-recommended levels re ANSI-1969). In test environments that have fluctuating noise levels, caution must be used in applying the maximum value shown in this table. The committee has used the best information available in the literature to support the levels and is basing its recommendation on these levels until additional information is available.

On the other hand, ASHA does not encourage the use of large sound-attenuating circumaural earphone assemblies (e.g., Auraldomes and Octocups). Below 1000 Hz these devices provide limited improvement in attenuation of ambient noise relative to the attenuation produced by the MX-41 AR cushion (Benson, 1971; Cox, 1955; Webster, 1954). The advantage provided above 1000 Hz is not needed because ambient noise is generally weak above 1000 Hz and the MX-41 AR cushion provides relatively good attenuation of the weak high-frequency ambient noise. Furthermore, the large earphone assemblies are awkward for small children, and they increase test-retest variability in the higher frequencies

Some persons have mistakenly assumed that sound-attenuation headsets eliminate the need for a quiet test environment or, worse, that they substitute for a sound-isolated audiometric test booth. In extremely noisy environments an audiometric test booth is often the only means of providing an environment quiet enough for screening audiometry. The sound-attenuating headsets provide the least benefit in the frequency range where it is needed most.

Audiometric Equipment and Calibration

Audiometers used for screening purposes shall meet the ANSI S36-1969 requirements for either a limited-range or narrow-range audiometer. Audiometers used for audiometric evaluation shall meet the ANSI S3.6-1969 requirements for a wide-range audiometer. Audiometric calibration to ANSI S3.6-1969 specifications should occur regularly, at least once every year, following the initial determination that the

audiometer meets specifications.[4] All the ANSI specifications, not just sound pressure level, should be met. Frequency errors, overshoot, and transient clicks are just a few of the problems that may invalidate a screening test. The sound pressure output of each audiometer should be checked at least every 3 months (preferably more often) in a 6-cc coupler. In addition, a daily listening check should be performed to determine that the audiometer is grossly in calibration and that no defects exist in major components. Efforts should be made to instruct support personnel in the proper handling and operation of audiometric equipment in order to minimize the need for repairs and to improve test accuracy.

Report to Parents

Recommendations for audiologic and medical evaluations will be influenced by the availability of support services. The language used in notices sent to parents about screening or rescreening results should avoid diagnostic conclusions and alarming predictions. The word *fail* probably should be avoided in reporting screening results. Remember that the hearing impairment is not confirmed until the audiometric evaluation is administered. Personal contact would be preferable to sending notices, if possible. Some persons become overly concerned, others express no concern, and still others would like to cooperate but fear the expense that may be involved. If parents believe that their child can "hear," despite what a hearing screening suggests, tact and persuasion will be required to convince them that they may be in error. Careful follow-up is necessary to ensure that recom-

[4]Studies on audiometer calibration suggest that upon receipt, most audiometers may never have been in complete calibration (Eagles & Doefler, 1961; Thomas, Preslar, Summers, & Stewart, 1969; Walton & Williams, 1972). This information underscores the importance of initial calibration of audiometers and indicates that they should be checked to meet ANSI specifications before use in a screening program It has been shown that when specifications are met initially, the audiometers generally remain stable (Walton & Wilson, 1974). Procedures for *Calibration of Pure-Tone Air-Conducted Signals Delivered via Earphones* (1982) may be ordered from ASHA.

mendations are being carried out. A high level of noncompli-amce would indicate the need for evaluating the program's reporting procedures and/or referral recommendations.

Summary

ASHA recommends a manually administered, individual, pure-tone air-conduction screening procedure for identification audiometry. The purpose of this procedure is to identify rapidly and effectively those persons with hearing impairment that interferes with or has the potential for interfering with communication. The procedure is designed to be used with children as young as 3 years old, although it is applicable for use with adults. The pure-tone screening procedure should be part of a program which has, as a second component, acoustic immittance screening for identification of individuals who have middle-ear disorders.

The recommended identification audiometry procedure is: Audiometric screening should be at 20 dB HL (re ANS1-1969) at the frequencies of 1000, 2000, and 4000 Hz if acoustic immittance screening is part of the total identification program. Screening at 20 dB HL at 500 Hz may be included, if acoustic immittance screening is not performed and if the ambient noise level permits testing at that frequency. Failure to respond at the screening level at one or more frequencies in either ear is the criterion for failure. An audiometric rescreening should be administered the same day or no later than within 2 weeks to all persons failing the initial screenmg. An audiologist should administer an audiologic evaluation to persons failing the rescreening. If a hearing impairment is identified by audiometric evaluation, referrals should be made to meet the person's habilitative, education, and medical needs.

Several procedural considerations are vital to implementing successfully the ASHA Guidelines for Identification Audiometry. An audiologist should conduct or supervise an identification audiometry program, although nonprofessional support personnel may be used for the screening procedures after appropriate training. Careful instructions are very important, particularly for young children. Ambient noise levels should not exceed 41.5 dB SPL at 500 Hz, 49.5 dB SPL at 1000 Hz, 54.5 dB SPL at 2000 Hz, and 62 dB SPL at 4000 Hz when measured using a sound level meter with octave-band filters centered on the screening frequencies. Audiometric equipment should initially meet all the ANSI S3.6-1969 specifications and be rechecked at least annually. The sound pressure output at the phones should be checked at least every 3 months, and listening checks for any gross malfunctions should be made daily. Finally, appropriate reporting of screening results should avoid diagnostic conclusions and encourage further evaluation for persons not passing the screening procedures.

Note. When the following Standards referred to in this document are superseded by an approved revision, the revision shall apply:

1. *American National Standard Specification for Audiometers* (53.6-1969);
2. *American National Standard Criteria for Permissible Ambient Noise during Audiometric Testing* (S3.1-1977); and
3. "Guidelines for Acoustic Immittance Screening of Middle-Ear Function" (ASHA, 1979).

References

American National Standard specifications for audiometers (ANSI S3.6-1969). (1970). New York: American National Standards Institute.

American National Standard criteria for background noise in audiometer rooms (ANSI S3.1-1977). (1977). New York: American National Standards institute.

American Speech and Hearing Association. (1975). Guidelines for identification audiometry. *Asha, 17*, 94–99.

American Speech-Language-Hearing Association. (1979). Guidelines for acoustic immittance, screening of middle-ear function. *Asha, 21*, 283–288.

American Speech-Language-Hearing Association, Committee on Audiometric Evaluation. (1982). *Calibration of pure-tone air-conducted signals delivered via earphones.* Rockville, MD: ASHA.

American Speech-Language-Hearing Association. (1984). Draft guidelines for identification audiometry, *Asha, 26*, 47–50.

Belkin, M., Suchman, E., Bergman, M., Rosenblatt, D., & Jacobziner, H. (1964). A demonstration program for conducting hearing tests in day care centers. *Journal of Speech and Hearing Disorders, 20*, 338–338.

Benson, R. (1971). "Auraldomes" for audiometric testing. *National Hearing Aid Journal, 24*, 14–42.

Cox, J. (1955). How quiet must it be to measure normal hearimg? *Noise Control, 1*, 28–29.

Darley, F. (Ed.). (1961). Identification audiometry. *Journal of Speech and Hearing Disorders Monograph Suppl. 9.*

Downs, M., Doster, M., & Wever, M. (1965). Dilemmas in identification audiometry. *Journal of Speech and Hearing Disorders, 30*, 360–364.

Eagles, E. (1961). Hearing levels in children and audiometer performance. *Journal of Speech and Hearing Disorders Monograph Suppl. 9*, 62–62.

Eagles, E., & Doerfler, L. (1961). A study of hearing in children: II. Acoustic environment and audiometer performance. *Transactions of the American Academy of Ophthalmology and Otolaryngology, 65*, 283–296.

Eagles, E., Wishik, S., & Doerfler, L. (1967). Hearing sensitivity and ear disease in children: A prospective study. *Laryngoscope, 274*, 146, 163.

Johnson, K. O., & Newby, H. A. (1954). Experimental study of the efficiency of two group hearing tests. *Archives of Otolaryngology, 60*, 702–710.

Johnston, P. W. (1948). Massachusetts Hearing Test. *Journal of the Acoustical Society of America, 20*, 697-703.

Katt, D., & Sprague, H. (1981). Determining the pure-tone frequencies to be used in identification audiometry. *Journal of Speech and Hearing Disorders, 46*, 433–436.

Roberts, J. (1972). Hearing sensitivity and related medical findings among children in the United States. *Transactions of the American Academy of Ophthalmology and Otolaryngology, 76*, 355–359.

Thomas, W., Preslar, M., Summers, R., & Stewart, J. (1969). Calibration and working condition of 190 audiometers. *Public Health Report, 84*, 311–327.

Villchur, E. (1970). Audiometer-earphone mounting to improve inter-subject and cushion-fit reliability. *Journal of the Acoustical Society of America, 48*, 1387–1396.

Walton, W., & Williams, P. (1972). Stability of routinely serviced portable audiometers. *Language, Speech, and Hearing Services in Schools, 3*, 36–43.

Walton, W., & Wilson, W. (1974). Stability of pure-tone audiometers during periods of heavy use in identification audiometry. *Language, Speech, and Hearing Services in Schools. 5*, 8–12.

Webster, J. (1954) Hearing losses of aircraft repair shop personnel. *Journal of the Acoustical Society of America, 26,* 782–787

Wilson, W., & Walton, W. (1974), Identification audiometry accuracy: Evaluation of a recommended program for school-age children. *Language, Speech, and Hearing Services in Schools, 5,* 132–142.

Additional Sources

Campanelli, P., Krucoff, M., & DiLosa, L. (1964). Hearing screening of school children, *Medical Annals of the District of Columbia, 33,* 309–314.

Jordan, R., & Eagles, E. (1961). The relation of air conduction audiometry to otological abnormalities. *Annals of Otology and Rhinology, 70,* 819–827.

Katz, J. (1978). The effects of conductive hearing loss on auditory function. *Asha, 20,* 879–886.

Kessler, M., & Randolph, K. (1972). The effects of early middle ear disease on the auditory abilities of third grade children. *Journal of the Academy of Rehabilitative Audiology, 12,* 6–20.

Melnick, W., Eagles, E., & Levine, H. (1964). Evaluation of a recommended program of identification audiometry with school age children, *Journal of Speech and Hearing Disorders, 29,* 2–13.

Appendix 2–F

GUIDELINES FOR SCREENING FOR HEARING IMPAIRMENT AND MIDDLE-EAR DISORDERS
Working Group on Acoustic Immittance Measurements and the Committee on Audiologic Evaluation
American Speech-Language-Hearing Association

The Guidelines for Screening for Hearing Impairments and Middle Ear Disorders were developed by the American Speech-Language-Hearing Association (ASHA) Working Group on Acoustic Immittance Measurements and the Committee on Audiologic Evaluation and adopted by the ASHA Legislative Council (LC 22-89) in November 1989. The Working Group members were Robert H. Margolis, chair; Michael G. Block Steven M. Parnes; Ross J. Roeser; Janet E. Shanks; and Richard H. Wilson. The Committee on Audiology Evaluation members included Sandra Gordon-Salant, chair; Evelyn Cherow, current ex officio; John D. Durrant; Thomas E. Fowlkes; Thomas A. Frank Gregg D. Givens; Michael P. Gorga; Carol Kamara, past ex officio; Sharon A. Lesner; and Laura Ann Wilber. The monitoring vice presidents were Gilbert R. Herer, past president, and Teris K. Schery, current vice president for clinical affairs.

Introduction

In 1979, "Guidelines for Acoustic Immittance Screening of Middle-Ear Function" were published in *Asha*. Those guidelines, crafted by the Subcommittee on Impedance Measurement of the Committee on Audiologic Evaluation and approved by Legislative Council in November 1978, presented a procedure for determining pass-fail criteria that could be used to decide upon the need for retest or medical referral of individuals at risk for middle ear disorders. Recognizing the need for additional normative and clinical data, the subcommittee noted that the guidelines "should be considered as interim and subject to revision." The reconstituted subcommittee, now the ASHA Committee on Audiologic Evaluation, Working Group on Acoustic Immittance Measurements, has revised the guidelines with consideration for the following recent developments.

An American standard on aural acoustic immittance instruments has been completed (American National Standards Institute, 1987). This standard has already begun to influence the way aural acoustic immittance measurements are made. Technological advances have improved the instrumentation. Many new instruments provide faster recording speeds, automatically compensate for ear-canal volume, and perform automatic calculations of tympanometric variables that are used as diagnostic indicators. New information on the natural course of otitis media provides important insight into the nature of the conditions that a screening

protocol should detect. Clinical data on screening techniques, including the 1979 ASHA guidelines, are now available and shed new light on the outcomes of such screening strategies.

In 1985, a revised set of "Guidelines for Identification Audiometry" outlined a recommended procedure for audiometric screening for hearing impairment (ASHA, 1985). That document advised that "the pure-tone screening procedure should be part of a program which has, as a second component, acoustic immittance screening for identification of individuals who have middle-ear disorders" (p. 52). ASHA recommends that screening programs include procedures for the detection of all peripheral auditory disorders, not just impairments of auditory sensitivity.

This document supersedes the "Guidelines for Acoustic Immittance Screening of Middle-Ear Function" (ASHA, 1979) and shall be used in conjunction with the "Guidelines for Identification Audiometry" (ASHA, 1985).

Scope

This document provides guidelines for identifying individuals with hearing impairments that potentially interfere with communication and/or individuals with potentially medically significant ear disorders that have been undetected or untreated. Individuals identified by the protocol described herein should, whenever possible, obtain an audiologic evaluation and a medical examination. These guidelines can be used for individuals of all ages who can be tested by behavioral screening audiometry and tympanometry. They are, however, specifically designed for children and young adults (through age 40 years). Other ASHA guidelines address screening procedures for newborn infants (ASHA, 1988).

A thorough understanding of the basic principles of aural acoustic immittance measurement and identification audiometry is essential for competent design and execution of a screening protocol like the one described in these guidelines. A thorough review of acoustic immittance principles is beyond the scope of this document. Several recent reviews are available (Margolis, 1981; Margolis & Shanks, 1985; Shanks, Lilly, Margolis, Wiley, & Wilson, 1988; Van Camp, Margolis, Wilson, Creten, & Shanks, 1986). For a review of the principles of identification audiometry, see ASHA (1985).

Source: From *ASHA Desk Reference for Audiology and Speech-Language Pathology, II*, pp. 85–94. Copyright 1990 by American Speech-Language-Hearing Association. Available for sale from ASHA Fullfillment Operations (301-897-5700 x218). Reprinted by permission.

These guidelines recommend pass-fall criteria that are based, in part, on quantitative measurement of aural acoustic admittance. Where first-generation acoustic immittance instruments provided results in relative ("arbitrary") units and careful calibration was less critical, current instruments present results in physical units. Careful, frequent calibration is essential.

Commercially available acoustic immittance instruments report tympanometric values in various units. Most currently available instruments measure the magnitude of acoustic admittance, which is properly reported in acoustic millimhos (mmho) or as an equivalent volume of air in cubic centimeters (cm^3) or milliliters (ml). However, some manufacturers incorrectly refer to acoustic admittance as "compliance." With a properly calibrated instrument that employs a 226-Hz probe frequency, millimhos, cubic centimeters, and milliliters are equivalent units.

These guidelines are not intended as a recommendation for or against mass screening for middle-ear disorders or hearing loss. The arguments for and against such screening programs are reviewed by Bluestone et al. (1986). Methods for assessing screening programs are discussed by Cadman, Chambers, Feldman, and Sackett (1984). Although this document recommends specific pass-fail criteria, the criteria are not the only acceptable (and perhaps not always the best) choices. It maybe appropriate and beneficial to modify the procedures and pass-fail criteria for specific populations and purposes This document is intended as "guidelines" rather than a protocol that requires strict adherence.

Rationale

Recent studies of the effectiveness of recommended medical referral criteria from tympanometric results have demonstrated that excessive over-referral rates occur when the referral is based on the existence of abnormal tympanometric findings alone (Lous, 1983; Lucker, 1980; Roush & Tait, 1985). Consequently, referral criteria often include provisions for retest after a specified time interval (ASHA, 1979; Harford, Bess, Bluestone, & Klein, 1978) and the use of other screening measures along with tympanometry (Aniansson, 1986; Grimaldi, 1976; Margolis & Heller, 1987; Margolis & Shanks, 1985; Paradise & Smith, 1979; Van Camp, Shanks, & Margolis, 1986). Case history, otoscopic inspection, and audiometric screening frequently produce sufficient evidence of medically significant ear disorders without tympanometric results. To avoid the excessive overreferral rates that characterize screening protocols that are based solely on tympanometry, the screening protocol described in these guidelines includes four sources of data: history, visual inspection, identification audiometry, and tympanometry.

History

It is beyond the scope of a screening program to obtain a complete case history. However, recent occurrence of otalgia (ear pain) or otorrhea (ear discharge) is cause for immediate medical referral. The screening protocol, therefore, includes the acquisition of this information from the most appropriate respondent. It may be obtained at the time of the screening, or it may be requested (especially from parents) in advance of the screening. A request for this information can be included in a letter that explains the purpose of the screening program and requests parental approval for the child to be tested.

Visual Inspection[1]

Visual evidence of ear disease may be evident to the unaided eye or revealed by otoscopy. Although it is not within the purview of this procedure to diagnose ear disease, the inclusion of visual inspection is expected to result in the identification of conditions that require medical attention that are not detected by other components of the screening battery. Because the skill and experience of the individual performing the otoscopic inspection will vary considerably, it is anticipated that more subtle visual evidence of middle-ear disorders will be detected in some screening programs and not in others. Three types of abnormalities should result in an immediate medical referral upon visual detection.

Structural defects of the ear, head, and neck should result in a medical referral. These include a wide variety of conditions such as abnormal position and/or structure of the external ear ranging from complete absence of the pinna and atresia of the ear canal to more subtle abnormalities such as malpositioned pinnae and pre-auricular pits and tags. The presence of visually detectable structural defects may portend the presence of other otologic abnormalities that require medical attention.

Ear-canal abnormalities including inflammation, blood, effusion, excessive cerumen, tumors, or foreign bodies in the ear canal are sufficient cause for a medical referral.

Eardrum abnormalities may be indicative of active middle-ear disorders that require immediate medical attention. Detection of these abnormalities, however, requires more skill and experience in otoscopy than the personnel administering this screening procedure can be expected to possess. In many cases the tympanic membrane is not visible even to an experienced otoscopist. Consequently, only the most obvious eardrum abnormalities are recommended as referral criteria. Obvious perforation, inflammation, or severe retraction of the tympanic membrane are criteria for immediate medical referral. The presence of a pressure-equalization tube indicates that the individual is in the medical treatment/follow-up process. Evaluation of these individuals is, therefore, outside the scope of this screening recommendation.

Identification Audiometry

Although audiometric screening is not adequate for detecting all medically significant otologic disease (Eagles,

---

[1]If any part of this procedure conflicts with state laws governing audiologic or medical practice, it should be modified appropriately.

Wishik, & Doerfler, 1967), identification audiometry is included in this screening protocol for two reasons. First, the existence of hearing loss in association with other abnormal tympanometric results is evidence of a significant medical and communicative disorder. Whereas abnormal tympanometry alone requires a retest to avoid overreferrals associated with transient, self-correcting otitis media, concomitant hearing loss requires immediate follow-up. Second, the inclusion of audiometry in the screening protocol provides the capability to detect sensorineural hearing loss. Consequently, screening audiometry in accordance with the ASHA Guidelines for Identification Audiometry (ASHA, 1985) is included in the screening procedure.

Acoustic Immittance Measurements

In the absence of significant otologic history, visual evidence of middle-ear disorders, and hearing loss, tympanometric abnormalities may result from middle-ear conditions that do not represent medically significant pathology. The transient, self-correcting, secretory otitis media that frequently occurs in children does not often require medical attention (Fiellau-Nikolajsen, 1983; Tos & Poulsen, 1979), and medical referral of these children represents a potentially unacceptable overreferral rate. Tympanometric abnormalities, then, must be interpreted with caution, ensuring referral of conditions requiring medical intervention while avoiding excessive overreferral. The utility of five immittance variables is discussed below, in the context of the four-part screening protocol.

Static admittance (Peak Y) is a measure of the height of the admittance-magnitude tympanogram relative to the tail value.[2] Although the classification of tympanometric shapes has been more commonly employed for determining abnormalities, static admittance can enhance the reliability of the classification of shape. That is, static admittance can be used as an objective criterion for categorizing the shape of a tympanogram. Because the majority of tympanograms recorded with a 226-Hz probe frequency are single-peaked (Van Camp, Creten, Van de Heyning, Decraemer, & Vanpeperstraete, 1983), the classification of tympanometric shapes is based primarily on peak height, that is, static admittance. The distinctions among Type A, Type As, Type Ad, and Type C tympanograms in the Liden-Jerger classification system (Jerger, 1970; Liden, 1969) can be made more reliable within and among clinicians by using an objective criterion. For screening instruments that use a +200 daPa ear-canal vol-

ume correction and 200 daPa/s pump speed, interim norms are presented in Appendix A.[3]

High static admittance is caused by eardrum and ossicular abnormalities. Eardrum abnormalities that cause high static admittance are rarely associated with active disease or hearing loss. Significant ossicular abnormalities are typically associated with large conductive hearing losses. High static admittance, then, in the absence of other signs, is not cause for medical referral. Only low static admittance is employed in these guidelines as a referral criterion.

Equivalent ear-canal volume (Vec) is an estimate of the volume of air in front of the acoustic-immittance probe.[4] It is obtained by measuring the admittance at high positive or high negative ear-canal air pressure. Vec is useful for detecting tympanic membrane perforations accompanied by normal middleear mucosa. When perforations are accompanied by inflammation of the middle ear, Vec may not be abnormally large (Margolis & Shanks, 1985). When measured at an earcanal air pressure of 200 daPa, a Vec value that exceeds the 90% range given in Appendix A, when accompanied by a flat tympanogram, is sufficient cause for immediate medical referral. Although many tympanic membrane perforations do not produce abnormal Vec values, these middle-ear abnormalities will be detected by other tympanometric variables, by pure-tone audiometry, and/or by otoscopy.

Tympanometric width is a quantity that belongs to the class of measurements referred to as tympanometric gradient. Gradient measures are used to describe the shape of the tympanogram in the vicinity of the peak. Measures of this type have been shown to be good indicators of middle-ear effusion (Fiellau-Nikolajsen, 1983; Haughton, 1977; Paradise, Smith, & Bluestone, 1976). Several studies have evaluated the normative distribution characteristics of various gradient measures (de Jonge, 1986; Koebsell & Margolis, 1986; Shanks & Wilson, 1986). On the basis of these results, the gradient measure first described by Liden and his colleagues (Liden, Harford, & Hallen, 1974; Liden, Peterson, & Bjorkman, 1970) appeared to be the procedure of choice. They calculated the pressure interval corresponding to a 50% reduction in peak (static) admittance (the tympanometric width, TW). That measure appeared to be superior to other gradient measures on the basis of (a) normative distribution width in relation to the range of possible values; (b) invariance with pump speed, and (c) low correlation with (and, therefore, supplemental to) static admittance. Gradient measures seem to be sensitive to disease-related mechanical changes in the middle ear that are not always

[2]The ANSI standard on aural acoustic immittance instruments (ANSI S3.39-1987) refers to this quantity as the peak compensated static acoustic admittance.

[3]When other combinations of ear-canal correction and pump speed are employed, normative data must be used that were obtained with such instruments. For example, if an instrument is used that employs a 50 daPa/s pump speed and corrects for ear-canal volume at -250 daPa, the normative values provided by Wiley, Oviatt, and Block (1987, Table 3, p. 165) can be used.

[4]At 226 Hz and standard atmospheric conditions, and with certain constraints on the geometry of the space, the volume of an enclosed quantity of air (in cm^3) is equivalent to its acoustic admittance (in acoustic mmho). When the ear canal is pressurized, the acoustic admittance at the probe tip is a reasonable estimate of the ear canal volume. For example, an acoustic admittance of 0.7 acoustic mmho obtained with an ear-canal air pressure of 400 daPa would indicate an ear-canal volume of 0.7 cm^3. (See Lilly & Shanks, 1981, for a discussion.) When there is a tympanic membrane perforation, the equivalent volume is not always an accurate estimate of the volume in front of the probe. However, an equivalent volume exceeding the normal ranges in Appendix A is strong evidence of perforation.

detected by other tympanometric measures or by otoscopy. Although clinical data are not yet available for tympanometric width, previous studies of patient populations suggest that tympanometric gradient measures are good indicators of middle-ear effusion. Accordingly, the 90% ranges in Appendix A are tentatively recommended as a criterion for medical referral. These values are relevant only to instruments that determine static admittance relative to the admittance at 200 daPa. Gradient measures have been primarily used for the detection of otitis media, which produces abnormally wide tympanograms. Consequently, for the purposes of these guidelines, only abnormally large tympanometric widths will be considered as a criterion for medical referral.

Tympanometric peak pressure (TPP) is an indirect measure of the air pressure in the middle ear. Large, negative intratympanic pressures have been attributed to gas absorption in the middle ear associated with failure of the eustachian tube to open. Negative TPP, then, would be indicative of early stages of otitis media. However, this "ex vacuo" theory has recently been challenged (Buckingham & Ferrer, 1980; Bylander, Ivarsson, Tjernstrom, & Andreasson, 1985; Hergils & Magnuson, 1987). Experimental evidence suggests that gas absorption, by itself, does not account for the large negative pressures observed in some ears. Gas absorption that occurs when the eustachian tube is chronically closed produces pressures that are rarely more negative than -100 daPa (Cantekin, Doyle, Phillips, & Bluestone, 1980; Proud, Odol & Toledo, 1971; Yee & Cantekin, 1986). Mechanisms that have been proposed to account for larger negative intratympanic pressures include alteration of the normal gas absorption rate due to a disturbance in the composition of middle-ear gases (Cantekin et al., 1980), ciliary action of the closed eustachian tube (Hilding, 1944; Murphy, 1979), and sniffing (Falk, 1983; Magnuson, 1981). Positive intratympanic pressures may occur in early stages of acute otitis media (Ostergard & Carter, 1981; Paradise et al., 1976) due to a reduction of middle-ear volume by effusion or by diffusion of gases from the infected tissue into the middle-ear space. In view of the several mechanisms that produce middle-ear pressure and the fact that TPP is an imprecise estimate of the actual middle-ear pressure (Van Camp, Margolis, Wilson, Creten, & Shanks, 1986), it is not surprising that negative TPP associated with an otherwise normal tympanogram is a poor determinant of middle-ear effusion (Fiellau-Nikolajsen, 1983; Haughton, 1977; Paradise at al., 1976). Furthermore, abnormal TPP in the absence of other tympanic membrane abnormalities does not reflect a change in the mechanical properties of the middle ear, only a change in its operating point. For these reasons, and because of the large fluctuations in TPP that have been shown to occur in children who do not develop middle-ear disorders (de Jonge & Cummings, 1985; Lidholdt, 1980), TPP may be judiciously excluded from consideration as a criterion for audiological/medical referral.

Acoustic reflex (AR) measures have been used in screening protocols for middle-ear disorders (ASHA, 1979; Brooks, 1968, 1969, 1974; Harford et al., 1978; McCandless & Thomas, 1974). Although acoustic-reflex thresholds are effective in detecting sensorineural hearing loss in the presence of normal middle-ear function (Popelka, 1981), the efficacy of acoustic-reflex measurements for detecting middle-ear disorders is limited. An absent acoustic reflex may result from (a) a reduction in input to the reflex mechanism due to a middle-ear disorder, (b) a reduction in transmission through the afferent pathway due to sensorineural hearing loss, (c) abnormal function of the efferent portion of the reflex arc due to brainstem or facial nerve disease, or (d) a mechanical disturbance in the middle ear that reduces or eliminates the impedance change that normally results from muscle contraction. Often a combination of these factors operates. In evaluating middle-ear abnormalities, the acoustic-reflex measurement is an indirect index of the status of the middle ear that is more directly assessed with tympanometry. These considerations and their extensive examination of screening programs led several investigators to recommend against the inclusion of acoustic-reflex measurements in screening for middle-ear disorders in children (Cantekin et al., 1980; Renvall, Liden, Jungert, & Nilsson, 1975; Wachtendorf, Lopez, Cooper, Hearn, & Gates, 1984). The use of acoustic-reflex measures contributed to the unacceptably high false positive rates reported in previous assessments of screening protocols (Lous, 1983; Roush & Tait, 1985). AR is not incorporated in the screening protocol described below.

Equipment

The screening protocol requires an otoscope, a pure-tone audiometer, and an acoustic immittance instrument. The audiometer should be calibrated in accordance with the audiometer standard (ANSI S3.6-1969). The acoustic immitance instrument should comply with the ANSI standard on aural acoustic immittance instruments (ANSI S3.39-1987). It should measure acoustic admittance in acoustic millimhos (mmho). Alternatively, acoustic admittance may be expressed in equivalent volume of air in cubic centimeters (cm^3) or milliliters (ml). A number of procedural variables influence the values obtained from tympanograms (see Shanks et al., 1988, for a comprehensive review). The normative admittance data presented in Appendix A pertain to instruments that employ a 226-Hz probe frequency, a pump speed of 200 daPa/s, a positive-to-negative direction of pressure change, and correct for ear-canal volume by subtracting the admittance at 200 daPa from the remaining admittance values. If other measurement parameters are employed, appropriate norms must be used. The data in Appendix A should be considered as interim norms pending a badly needed, large-scale normative study of aural acoustic immittance. Clinical programs may wish to determine their own norms.[5]

Three acoustic immittance measures are used in the screening protocol: static admittance, equivalent ear-canal volume, and tympanometric width. The calculation methods used to

---

[5]The data in Appendix A are placed in an appendix to separate them from the guidelines. Because of the inadequacy of available data, norms are not available that are suitable for inclusion in the guidelines. The normals provided in the Appendix should be considered interim norms for preschool children, school-age children, and adults, until more complete normative data are available.

obtain these measures will substantially influence the values. Static admittance is calculated by subtracting an estimate of the admittance of the ear-canal volume from the peak admittance. The ear-canal volume estimate is obtained from one of the tail values of the tympanogram. Acoustic immittance instruments that automatically calculate static admittance differ in the choice of ear-canal volume correction. Screening instruments typically use the value at +200 daPa whereas clinical instruments often provide a choice.

Equivalent ear-canal volume is obtained from the admittance at the positive or negative tail of the tympanogram. Because of the asymmetry that characterizes most tympanograms, the tail values from the positive pressure side of the tympanogram tend to be greater than those obtained from the negative pressure side. Interim normative values are presented in Appendix A for equivalent ear-canal volume estimated at +200 daPa.

Ideally, tympanometric width (TW) would be calculated automatically by the instrument. When it is not, a template can be constructed that allows graphic determination of normal and abnormal values. Examples of templates for evaluating TW are shown in Appendix B. The method of correcting for ear-canal volume affects TW because the peak value, required in the calculation, is determined after ear-canal correction. The interim normative values for TW in Appendix A pertain to estimates obtained with the 200-daPa ear-canal volume correction.

Personnel

Because screening programs are designed to test large numbers of subjects, the test procedures may be conducted by personnel who are not clinical audiologists. The screening protocol described in these guidelines, however, should be supervised by a clinical audiologist who has training and experience related to the test procedures that comprise the protocol. The personnel who administer the protocol should be sufficiently trained in the procedures to obtain accurate and reliable results.

Recommended Screening Protocol

The recommended screening protocol is based on a four-part procedure consisting of case history, visual inspection, pure-tone audiometry, and tympanometry. Referral criteria are presented in Table 1. The protocol is presented in flow chart format in Figure 1. The flow chart is a representation of the logic used to determine the need for referral. It does not represent the order in which test procedures are administered. With the exception that visual inspection should precede tympanometry, the order of test procedures is unimportant. Each test component, indicated by a numbered box in Figure 1, is described below.

1. A recent, otologic history of otalgia or otorrhea is sufficient cause for immediate medical referral.

2. Visual inspection of the ear may produce sufficient cause for medical referral without the need for further testing. Referral criteria include: structural defect of the ear, head, or neck; inflammation, blood, effusion, excessive cerumen, tumors, or foreign body in the ear canal; or eardrum

appearance consistent with active middle-ear disease. When visual inspection indicates the need for medical referral, tympanometry is not necessary. When visual evidence of middle ear infection is present, or when a pressure-equalization tube is in place, tympanometry should not be performed unless requested by a physician.

3, 4. Audiometric screening should be performed by the method described in the ASHA Guidelines for Identification Audiometry (ASHA, 1985). Those guidelines recommend screening with pure-tone stimuli presented at 20 dB HL (re: ANSI S3.6-1969) with frequencies of 1000, 2000, and 4000 Hz. Failure to respond to any frequency constitutes failure of the audiometric screen. In accordance with the Identification Audiometry Guidelines, failure of the audiometric screen should be confirmed by a rescreen, either on-site or by additional testing at a later date. If the audiometric screen is failed on the second administration, a complete audiologic evaluation should be performed.

5, 6. Low static admittance (Peak Y) associated with an abnormally large volume in front of the probe is evidence of a tympanic membrane perforation and warrants immediate referral. The presence of (Vec) (estimated at 200 daPa) exceeding the 90% range in Appendix A in the presence of a

---

Table 1
Referral Criteria

I. History
   A. Otalgia
   B. Otorrhea

II. Visual Inspection of the Ear
   A. Structural defect of the ear, head, or neck
   B. Ear canal abnormalities
      1. Blood or effusion
      2. Occlusion
      3. Inflammation
      4. Excessive cerumen, tumor, foreign material
   C. Eardrum abnormalities
      1. Abnormal color
      2. Bulging eardrum
      3. Fluid line or bubbles
      4. Perforation
      5. Retraction

III. Identification Audiometry—Fail air conduction screening at 20 dB HL at 1, 2, or 4 kHz in either ear (ASHA, 1985; these criteria may require alteration for various clinical settings and populations).

IV. Tympanometry
   A. Flat tympanogram and equivalent ear canal volume (Vec) outside normal range.
   B. Low static admittance (Peak Y) on two successive occurrences in a 4-6-week interval
   C. Abnormally wide tympanometric width (TW) on two successive occurrences in a 4-6 week interval

Figure 1.

Flow chart for determination of the need for audiologic/medical referral incorporating case history, visual inspection, pure-tone audiometry,and tympanometry. Each numbered box is discussed in the text. The flow chart represents the logic used to determine the need for referral. It does not indicate the order of test procedures.

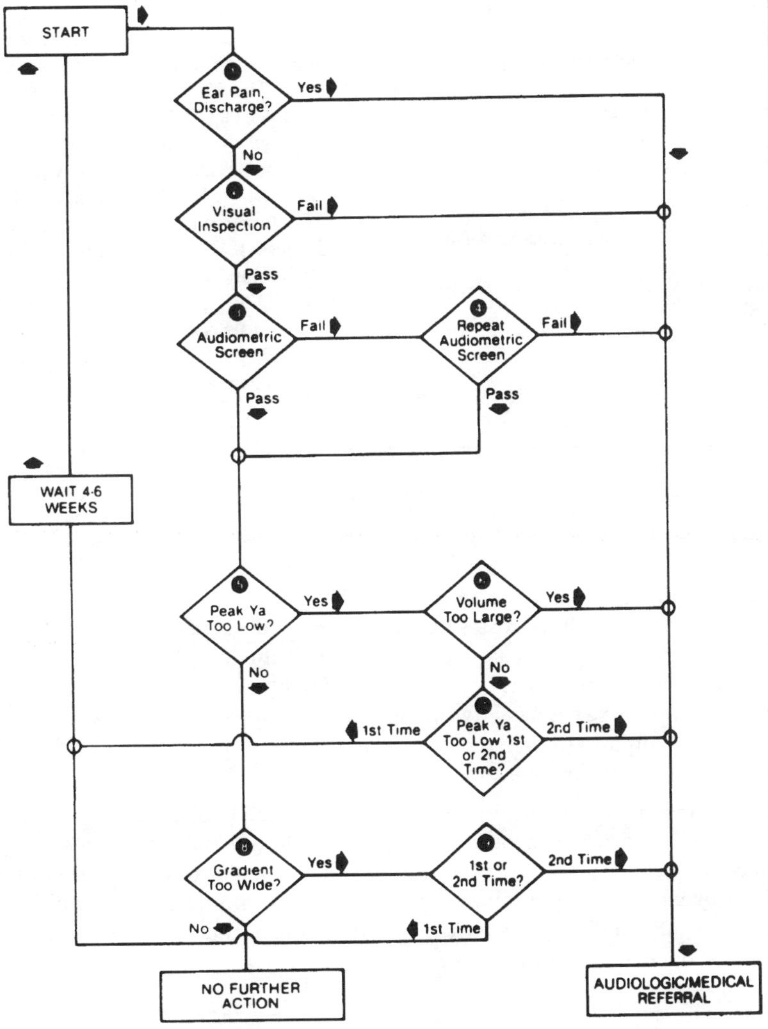

flat tympanogram is evidence of a large volume and should result in a medical referral.

7. Low static admittance (Peak Y) may or may not be associated with significant middle-ear disorders. In the absence of other positive findings, a Peak Y below the 90% range in Appendix A requires observation over an extended period before a medical referral is warranted. Only after two successive abnormal findings over an interval of 4–6 weeks should medical referral be made.

8, 9. An abnormally wide tympanometric width (TW) may occur in the absence of other findings in cases with otitis media. These cases may represent transient secretory otitis media, which does not require medical referral. Like static admittance, abnormal TW in the absence of other signs of middle-ear disorders requires retest after 4–6 weeks, and only then should a medical referral be based on this finding alone.

Audiologic or Medical Referral

Failure of the screen should result in an audiologic evaluation and a medical examination. The nature of the referral may depend on the characteristics of the screening program and the availability of services. For example, the referral may be to a clinic that provides both audiologic and medical services. Alternatively, an audiologic referral may precede the medical referral. If audiologic services are not available, an immediate medical referral should be made on failure of the screening protocol.

Appendix A

Suggested interim norms (means and 90% ranges) for static admittance (Peak Y), equivalent ear-canal volume (Vec), and tympanometric width (TW). The values were extracted from Margolis and Heller (1987) who employed an acoustic immittance screening Instrument (226-Hz probe tone; pump speed –200 daPa/s) that automatically compensated for ear-canal volume by subtracting the admittance at 200 daPa from all values. Normative values for children were obtained from preschool-aged children (3–5 years).

	Peak Y (mmho or cm³)		Vec (cm³)		TW (daPa)	
	Mean	*90% Range*	*Mean*	*90% Range*	*Mean*	*90% Range*
Children	0.5	0.2–0.9	0.7	0.4–1.0	100	60–150
Adults	0.8	0.3–1.4	1.1	0.6–1.5	80	50–110

References

American National Standards Institute. (1970). Specifications for audiometers (ANSI S3.6.-1969). New York: ANSI.

American National Standards Institute. (1988). Specifications for instruments to measure aural acoustic impedance and admittance (aural acoustic immittance) (ANSI S3.39-1987). New York: ANSI.

American Speech-Language-Hearing Association. *(1985)*. Guidelines for identification audiometry. *Asha, 27*, 49–52.

American Speech-Language-Hearing Association. (1979). Guidelines for acoustic immittance screening of middle ear function. *Asha, 21*, 550–558.

Aniansson, G. (1986). Screening diagnosis of secretory otitis media. *Scandinavian Audiology*, Suppl. 26, 65–69.

Bluestone, C.D., Fria, T.J., Arjona, S.K., Casselbrandt, M.L., Schwartz, D.M., Ruben, R.J., Gates, G.A., Downs, M.P., Northern, J.L., Jerger, J.F., Paradise, J.L., Bess, F.H., Kenworthy, O.T., & Rogers, K.D. (1986). Controversies in screening for middle ear disease and hearing loss in children. *Pediatrics, 77*, 57–70.

Brooks, D.N. (1968). An objective method of determining fluid in the middle ear. *International Audiology, 7*, 280–286.

Brooks, D.N. (1969). The use of electro-acoustic bridge in the assessment of middle ear function. *International Audiology, 8*, 563–565.

Appendix B

In the following figures, templates for evaluating tympanometric width are shown for two tympanograms, one recorded from a preschool-aged child (top) and one recorded from an adult (bottom). The shaded regions in each figure represent templates that have widths of 150 daPa (top) and 110 daPa (bottom), the upper limits of the 90% ranges for children and adults, respectively. The template is placed at the ordinate value corresponding to one half of the distance from the peak to the tail value. If the template can be placed at the appropriate admittance value without intersecting the tympanogram, the tympanometric width is outside the normal range. The tympanogram in the upper panel has a tympanometric width of 90 daPa, within the normal range for a preschool-aged child. The tympanogram in the lower panel has a tympanometric width of 165 daPa, an abnormally wide tympanometric width for an adult.

For tympanograms that are automatically corrected for ear-canal volume, the tail value is always zero and the template is placed at the admittance value corresponding to one half of the peak. This is the case for the example in the upper panel. When the tympanogram is not corrected for ear-canal volume (lower panel) the template is placed at the value that lies midway between the peak and the positive tail (if the norms in Appendix A are used). If the negative tail value is used, normative data obtained in that manner must be employed (such as those provided by Shanks & Wilson, 1986).

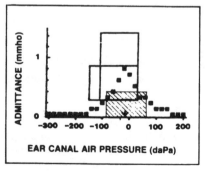

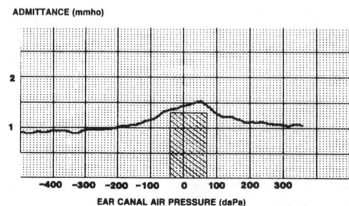

Brooks, D.N. (1974). The role of acoustic impedance bridge in pediatric screening. *Scandinavian Audiology, 3,* 99–104.

Buckingham, R.A., & Ferrer, J. L. (1980). Observations of middle ear pressures: Commentary with movie. *Annals of Otology, Rhinology and Laryngology. 89*(Suppl. 58), 58–61.

Bylander, A.K., Ivarsson, I., Tjernstrom, O., & Andreasson, L. (1985). Middle ear pressure variations during 24 hours in children. *Annals of Otology, Rhinology and Laryngology, 94*(Suppl. 120), 33-35.

Cadman, D., Chambers, L., Feldman, W., & Sackett, D. (1984). Assessing the effectiveness of community screening programs. *Journal of the American Medical Association, 251,* 1580-1585.

Cantekin, E.I., Bluestone, C.D., Fria, T.J., Stool, S.E., Berry, Q.C., & Sabo, D.L. (1980). Identification of otitis media with effusion in children. *Annals of Otology,. Rhinology and Laryngology, 89*(Suppl. 68), 190-195.

Cantekin, E.I., Doyle, W.J., Phillips, D.C., & Bluestone, C.D. (1980). Gas absorption in the middle ear. *Annals of Otology, Rhinology and Laryngology, 89*(Suppl. 68), 71-75.

deJonge, R.R. (1986). Normal tympanometric gradient: A comparison of three methods. *Audiology, 25,* 299-308.

deJonge, R.R., & Cummings, D. (1985). Daily fluctuation in middle-ear pressure. *Asha, 27,* 164.

Eagles, E.I, Wishik, S.M., & Doerfler, L.G. (1967). Hearing sensitivity and ear disease in children: A prospective study. *Laryngoscope,* Monograph Supplement, 1–274.

Falk, B. (1983). Variability of the tympanogram due to eustachian tube closing failure. *Scandinavian Audiology,* Suppl. 17, 11-17.

Fiellau-Nikolajsen, M. (1983). Tympanometry and secretory otitis media. *Acta Otolarynologica,* Suppl. 394, 1-73.

Grimaldi, P. (1976). The value of impedance testing in the diagnosis of middle ear effusion. *Journal of Laryngology and Otology, 90,* 141-152.

Harford, E.R., Bess, F.H, Bluestone, C.D., & Klein, J.O. (1978). *Impedance screening for middle ear disease in children.* New York: Grune & Stratton.

Haughton, P.M. (1977). Validity of tympanometry for middle ear effusions. *Archives of Otolaryngology, 103,* 505-513.

Hergils, L., & Magnuson, B. (1987). Middle-ear pressure under basal conditions. *Archives of Otolaryngology. 113,* 829-832.

Hilding, A.C. (1944). Role of ciliary action in production of pulmonary atelectasis. Vacuum in paranasal sinuses, and on otitis media. *Transactions of the American Academy of Opthalmology and Otolaryugology,* 367-378.

Ivey, R.G. (1975). Tympanometric curves and otosclerosis. *Journal of Speech and Hearing Research, 18,* 554-558.

Jerger, J. (1970). Clinical experience with impedance audiometry. *Archives of Otolaryngology, 92,* 311-324.

Koebsell, K.A., & Margolis, R.H. (1986). Tympanometric gradient measured from normal preschool children. *Audiology, 25,* 149-157.

Liden, (3. (1989). The scope and application of current audiometric tests. *Journal of Laryngology and Otology, 83,* 507-520.

Liden, G., Harford, E., & Hallen, O. (1974). Automatic tympanometry clinical practice. *Audiology, 13,* 126-139.

Liden, G., Peterson, J., & Bjorkman, G. (1970). Tympanometry. *Archives of Otolaryngology, 92,* 248-257.

Lildholdt, T. (1980). Negative middle ear pressure. Variations by season and sex. *Annals of Otology, Rhinology and Laryngology, 89* (Suppl. 68), 67–70.

Lilly, D.J., & Shanks, J.E. (1981). Acoustic immittance of an enclosed volume of air. In G.R., Popelka (Ed.), *Hearing assessment with the acoustic reflex.* New York: Grune & Stratton

Lous, J. (1983). Three impedance screening programs on a cohort of seven-year-old children. *Scandinavian Audiology,* Suppl. 17, 60–64.

Lucker, J.R. (1980). Application of pass-fail criteria to middle ear screening results. *Asha, 22,* 839-840.

Magnuson, B. (1981). Of the origin of the high negative pressure in the middle ear space. *American Journal of Otolaryugology, 2,* 112.

Margolis, R.H. (1981). Fundamentals of acoustic immittance. In G.R. Popelka (Ed.), *Hearing assessment with the acoustic reflex.* (pp. 117-143). New York: Grune & Stratton.

Margolis, R.H. & Heller, J.W. (1 987). Screening tympanometry: Criteria for medical referral. *Audiology, 26,* 197-208.

Margolis, R.H., & Shanks, J.E. (1985). Tympanometry. In J. Katz (Ed.), *Handbook of clinical audiology* (3rd ed., pp. 438–475). Baltimore: Williams & Wilkins.

McCandless, G.A., & Thomas, G.K. (1974). Impedance audiometry as a screening procedure for middle ear disease. *Transactions of The American Academy of Ophthalmology and Otolaryngology, ORL, 78,* 98-102

Murphy, D. (1979). Negative pressure in the middle ear by ciliary propulsion of mucus through the eustachian tube. *Laryngoscope, 89,* 954-961.

Ostergard, C.A, & Carter, D.R. (1981). Positive middle ear pressure shown by tympanometry. *Archives of Otolaryngology, 107,* 353356.

Paradise, J.L., & Smith, C.G. (1979). Impedance screening for preschool children. State of the art. *Annals of Otology, 88,* 56-65.

Paradise, J.L., Smith, C.G., & Bluestone, C.D. (1976). Tympanometric detection of middle ear effusion in infants and young children. *Pediatrics, 58,* 198.210.

Popelka, G.R. (Ed.). (1981). *Hearing assessment with the acoustic reflex.* New York: Grune & Stratton.

Proud, G.O., Odoi, H., & Toledo, P.S. (1971). Bullar pressure changes in eustachian tube dysfunction. *Annals of Otology, Rhinology and Laryngology, 80,* 835-837.

Renvall, U., Liden, G., Jungert, S., & Nilsson, E. (1975). Impedance audiometry In the detection of secretory otitis media. *Scandinavian Audiology, 4,* 119-124.

Roush, J., & Tait, C.A. (1985). Pure-tone and acoustic immittance screening of pre-school aged children: An examination of referral criteria. *Ear and Hearing 6,* 245-250.

Shanks, J.E., & Lilly, D.J. (1981). An evaluation of tympanometric estimates of ear canal volume. *Journal of Speech and Hearing Research, 24,* 557-568.

Shanks, J.E., Lilly, D.J., Margolis, R.H., Wiley, T.L., & Wilson, R.H. (1988). Tympanometry. *Journal of Speech and Hearing Disorders, 53,* 354-377.

Shanks, J.E., & Wilson, R.H. (1986). Effects of direction and rate of ear-canal pressure changes on tympanometric measures. *Journal of Speech and Hearing Research, 29,* 11–19.

Tos, M., & Poulsen, G. (1979). Tympanometry in 2-year-old children. Seasonal influence on frequency of secretory otitis and tubal function. *ORL, 41,* 1-10.

Van Camp, K.J., Creten, W.L., Van de Heyning, P.H., Decraemer, W.F., & Vanpeperstraete, P.M. (1983). A search for the most suitable immittances components and probe tone frequency in tympanometry. *Scandinavian Audiology, 12,* 27-34.

Van Camp, K.J., Margolis, R.H., Wilson, R.H., Creten, W.L., & Shanks, J.E. (1986). Principles of tympanometry. *ASHA Monographs, 24.*

Van Camp; K.J., Shanks, J.E., & Margolis, R.H. (1986). Simulation of pathological high impedance tympanograms. *Journal of Speech and Hearing Research, 29,* 505-514.

Wachtendorf, C.A., Lopez, L.L, Cooper, J.C., Hearn, E.M., & Gates, G.A. (1984). The efficacy of school screening for otitis media. In D.J. Lim, C.D. Bluestone, J.O. Klein, & J.D. Nelson (Eds.), *Recent advances in otitis media with effusion* (pp. 242-246). Philadelphia: B.C. Becker.

Wiley, T.L., Oviatt, D.L., & Block, M.G. (1987). Acoustic immittance measures in normal ears. *Journal of Speech and Hearing Research, 30,* 161-170.

Yee, A.L., & Cantekin, E.I. (1986). Effect of changes in systemic oxygen tension on middle ear gas exchange. *Annals of Otology Rhinology and Laryngology, 95,* 369-372.

Appendix 2–G

GUIDELINES FOR THE AUDIOLOGIC ASSESSMENT OF CHILDREN FROM BIRTH THROUGH 36 MONTHS OF AGE

The Guidelines for the Audiologic Assessment of Children From Birth Through 36 Months of Age were developed by the American Speech-Language-Hearing Association (ASHA) Committee on Infant Hearing and adopted by the ASHA Legislative Council (LC 25–90) in November 1990. Current and past members of the committee responsible for the development of the guidelines include Jack E. Kile, chair; Fred Bess; Evelyn Cherow, ex officio; Janet Coscarelli; Judith S. Gravel; O. T. Kenworthy; Marcia R. Kushner; Noel D. Matkin; James W. Thelin; and Barbara Cone Wesson. Ann L. Carey, vice president for professional and governmental affairs (1988–90), was the monitoring vice president.

Scope

In accordance with the recommendations of the "Guidelines for Audiologic Screening of Newborn Infants Who Are at Risk for Hearing Impairment" (*Asha*, 1989), the ASHA Committee on Infant Hearing has developed "Guidelines for the Audiologic Assessment of Children From Birth Through 36 Months of Age." The committee has specifically limited the scope of this document to assessment. Guidelines relative to identification and management will be addressed in forthcoming documents from other committees of ASHA.

In developing these guidelines, the ASHA Committee on Infant Hearing recognizes the complex and multidimensional nature of hearing and its development. The committee further recognizes the growing number of infants with multiple developmental disabilities and the resulting challenge of accurately delineating their hearing status. Therefore, the committee recommends the use of multiple nonduplicative procedures that sample various dimensions of auditory function (e.g., responses to threshold and suprathreshold stimuli). Yet the committee remains mindful of the need for cost containment in healthcare delivery (Administration on Developmental Disabilities, 1988; Kurent, 1989; U.S. General Accounting Office, 1985). Accordingly, the committee acknowledges that the type and number of procedures administered to any child should be dictated as much by the reliability and completeness of the results as by any specified assessment protocol (Turner, Frazer, & Shepard, 1984).

This document should be regarded as guidelines for practice, not standards. The committee recognizes that each individual case presents unique characteristics that may influence the approach to the evaluation. Nevertheless, the committee has provided specific procedural recommendations that are supported by research evidence and cumulative clinical experience. The committee encourages further study of these guidelines to evaluate the efficacy of the procedures and protocols recommended.

Background

Early and comprehensive assessment of hearing status is critical to the provision of appropriate, individualized intervention strategies for children[1] Pursuant to the screening guidelines (ASHA, 1989) and the Joint Committee on Infant Hearing Position Statement (1982), the present report sets forth guidelines for the audiologic evaluation of children who are either identified through screening programs or referred directly to audiologists for hearing assessment.

The mandate for developing these guidelines is derived from several sources. Public Law 99-57, a discretionary program to address the special needs of handicapped children from birth through 2 years of age, emphasizes the need for appropriate assessments and for personnel qualified to provide these procedures. Second, ASHA's Legislative Council (LC 27-84) charges the Committee on Infant Hearing to gather and synthesize policies that pertain to identification, diagnosis, and management of hearing disorders in infants. Third, research on the impact of hearing impairment on speech-language, social, and cognitive development as well as subsequent academic achievement supports the need for early identification and rehabilitation of children with hearing impairment. (See Davis, 1988, for a review).

ASHA (1989) guidelines for screening newborn infants recommend audiologic assessment for high-risk infants who fail audiologic screening by auditory brainstem response (ABR) procedures. Furthermore, those guidelines recommend that any child (regardless of risk or screening status) "who exhibits abnormal auditory behavior or delayed speech and language development, or whose parent/caregiver expresses concern about auditory responsiveness should receive audiologic evaluation" (*Asha*, 1989, p. 91). The underlying principle is that once a child is suspected of having hearing impairment, then a comprehensive assessment must be completed in a timely fashion in order

Source: From *ASHA Desk Reference for Audiology and Speech-Language Pathology, II,* pp. 41–49. Copyright 1993 by American Speech-Language-Hearing Association. Available for sale from ASHA Fullfillment Operations (301-897-5700 x218). Reprinted by permission.

Reference this material as follows: American Speech-Language-Hearing Association. (1991). Guidelines for the audiological assessment of children from birth through 36 months of age. *Asha, 33*(Suppl. 5), 37–43.

[1]For the purposes of these guidelines, the generic terms child and children will be used throughout the document.

to initiate medical referrals, aural rehabilitation, and educational management.

Behavioral assessment of hearing sensitivity in children has been complicated by developmental and maturational limitations. Thus, early behavioral assessment techniques relied on observation of reflexive responses and/or state changes in the presence of an auditory stimulus (Downs & Sterritt, 1967; Eisenberg, 1976; Friedrich, 1985; Thompson & Weber, 1974). Behavioral Observation Audiometry (BOA) techniques, even with normal-hearing children, often are confounded by nonspecific responses to sound, false positive responses, or differential responses depending on stimulus spectrum, observer bias, and widely variable threshold values (Bench, Collyer, Mentz, & Wilson, 1976; Northern & Downs, 1984; Weber, 1969; Wilson & Thompson, 1984).[2] Published age-related response levels for various stimuli (pure tones, white noise, speech) have been used for judging normal versus abnormal auditory responses (Northern & Downs, 1984). The validity of this approach has not been supported by research that focused on *unconditioned* auditory responses involving large samples of normal-hearing and hearing-impaired children.

In contrast, research by Moore, Thompson, Wilson, and their colleagues (Moore, Thompson, & Thompson, 1975; Moore, Thompson, & Wilson, 1977; Primus & Thompson, 1985; Thompson, 1985; Thompson & Folsom, 1981; 1984; Thompson & Wilson, 1984; Thompson, Wilson, & Moore, 1979; Wilson, 1978; Wilson & Thompson, 1984) has demonstrated that it is possible to elicit reliable *conditioned* auditory responses from children using an operant, visually reinforced behavioral response technique. Normally developing children as young as 5 months of age may be trained to produce a motor response contingent upon the presence of an auditory stimulus (Wilson & Thompson, 1984). The behavior, usually a head turn, is reinforced by an appealing visual display. These researchers, as well as others, have demonstrated that frequency-specific thresholds may be obtained from infants, allowing the accurate evaluation of hearing sensitivity regardless of type, degree, or configuration of impairment (Bernstein & Gravel, 1990; Diefendorf, 1988; Gravel 1989; Nozza & Wilson, 1984; Wilson & Thompson, 1984).

Auditory evoked potential measurements, especially the ABR, can provide estimates of threshold sensitivity. The use of the ABR has an important role in both identification and assessment protocols, particularly with children too young or too disabled to be reliably assessed using conditioned behavioral techniques (Stein & Kraus, 1989). The ABR elicited by air-conducted clicks provides an estimate of sensitivity in high-frequency regions (Coats & Martin, 1977; Jerger & Mauldin, 1978; Yamada, Kodera, & Yagi, 1979; Yamada, Yagi, Yamame, & Suzuki, 1975). ABR tests employing frequency-specific stimuli such as tone-pips (Gorga, Worthing-

ton, Reiland, Beauchaine, & Goldgar, 1985; Hyde, 1985; Stapells, Picton, Perez-Abalo, Read, & Smith, 1985) further extend the application of ABR tests for defining the degree and configuration of hearing impairment. The use of bone-conducted stimuli (Mauldin & Jerger, 1979; Stapells & Ruben, 1989; Yang, Rupert, & Moushegian, 1987; Ysunza & Cone-Wesson, 1987) may serve to define the type of loss.

Other audiologic procedures are being developed and researched, such as electrocochleography (Cullen, Berlin, Gondra, & Adams, 1976), middle and late auditory evoked potentials (Krause, Reed, Smith, Stein, & Cartee, 1985; Kurtzberg, 1989; McRandle, Smith, & Goldstein, 1974; Mendel, Adkinson, & Harker, 1977; Mendelson & Salamy, 1981), and, most recently, otoacoustic emissions (Kemp, 1978; Kemp, Ryan, & Bray, 1990; Norton & Widen, 1990), which may also contribute to the assessment of auditory function in children. However, further research is needed to define their clinical application.

Acoustic immittance measures (tympanometry and acoustic reflex thresholds) are an integral part of the audiologic assessment of children. Both tympanometry and acoustic reflex threshold measurements contribute to the description of middle ear status. Acoustic reflex threshold determination provides additional information relevant to hearing status (Northern, 1988).

There remain undefined parameters for the examination of tympanometric configuration and acoustic reflex measurements in young infants (McMillan, Bennett, Marchant, & Shurin, 1985; Sprague, Wiley, & Goldstein, 1985). Recognition of these limitations, however, should not preclude the routine use of acoustic immittance measures in the pediatric test battery. Rather, thoughtful interpretation of test results should be made *in combination with* other clinical findings. In young infants, the interpretation of acoustic reflex findings may be compromised when only the 220/226 Hz probe tone is used. The use of a higher probe tone frequency (e.g., 660/678 Hz), may provide a more valid indication of middle ear status and peripheral auditory integrity for this group of children (ASHA, 1988; Bennett & Weatherby, 1982; Himmelfarb, Popelka, & Shannon, 1979; Marchant et al., 1986; Margolis, 1978 Margolis & Popelka, 1975; Weatherby & Bennett, 1980).

In summary, the committee recommends a comprehensive audiologic assessment of children from available behaviorial, electrophysiologic, and acoustic immittance measures. Responses should be replicable and either there should be agreement among measures or assessment should be continued until consensus is reached. The use of *any test alone* for assessing children's hearing sensitivity is discouraged (Friedrich, 1985; Gravel, Kurtzberg, Stapells, Vaughan, & Wallace, 1989). Corroboration of test results through case history, parent report, and observations of behavior are crucial to assess functional use of hearing. Effective diagnosis

[2]In pediatric evaluation, the terms threshold and minimal response level (MRL, Matkin, 1977) have been used to define the lowest intensity level at which an infant responds to an auditory stimulus. The Committee recommends that if the value was acquired using standard or modified up down audiometric procedures (ASHA Guidelines for Manual Pure Tone Audiometry) and represents a point on the psychometric function (that is, 50% or 71%), then the term threshold is appropriate. Threshold is not an absolute value but rather represents a criterion level that accounts for motivation, attention, and the specifics of the response task. However, if the value represents on y the lowest level at which a behavioral response was obtained from a child, then the torn MRL is appropriate, regardless of the evaluation technique employed. With maturation and auditory stimulation, the lowest intensity level at which a threshold or MRL is obtained may improve during subsequent evaluation.

and management also includes involvement of the parent/ caregiver at all stages of assessment and intervention to enable families to be active participants rather than passive recipients (Cherow, 1985; Dunst, Trivette, & Deal, 1988; Education of the Handicapped Act Amendments of 1986). Ultimately, the goal is to define precisely the type, degree, and configuration of the hearing impairment for each ear. The need for such precision should not preclude initiation of intervention, including the selection and fitting of amplification (hearing aids and FM systems) and other assistive devices. Accordingly, ongoing assessment is viewed as an integral part of the management process. Further, it should be recognized that single-point assessment does not adequately address the issue of progressive hearing loss. In cases where progressive hearing loss may be suspected, routine reevaluation in conjunction with otologic management is essential.

Definitions

ASSESSMENT. An in-depth examination of auditory function utilizing behavioral, electrophysiologic, and acoustic immittance measures to determine the degree, configuration, type, and symmetry of any auditory impairment or to determine that the child does not have hearing impairment that could impede normal communication development. Assessment facilitates medical referral/treatment, aural rehabilitation, and education planning.

BEHAVIORAL ASSESSMENT. An examination of hearing function using procedures in which the child provides overt, reliable responses to a variety of auditory stimuli for which the spectra and signal intensity are known. These procedures include visual reinforcement audiometry (VRA), visual or tangible reinforced operant conditioning audiometry (VROCA, TROCA), and conditioned play audiometry (CPA). All behavioral measurements of auditory sensitivity must be completed in a test environment meeting standards for background noise levels (ANSI, 1977). Signals need to be calibrated in accordance with current national standards, when applicable. When national standards do not exist, as is the case with sound field audiometry, signal calibration may be referenced to other published standards, to published data, or to values established by the clinic performing the audiologic tests. Appropriate sound field calibration is particularly critical in the behavioral audiologic assessment of children who cannot be tested under earphones. (Morgan, Dirks, & Bower, 1979; Rochlin, 1990; Walker, Dillon, & Byrne, 1984).

ELECTROPHYSIOLOGIC ASSESSMENT. For the purpose of these guidelines, electrophysiologic assessment refers to the measurement of evoked potentials to auditory stimuli (AEP). The most widely used AEP is the auditory brainstem response (ABR). At this time, the ABR is considered the AEP of choice for audiologic evaluation using established normative data for latency by age (ASHA, 1987). Consistent with other measurements of auditory sensitivity, all AEP measurements must be completed in a test environment meeting standards for background noise levels (ANSI S3.1-1977).

ACOUSTIC IMMITTANCE ASSESSMENT. Acoustic immittance refers to the measurement of middle ear function by tympanometry and the determination of acoustic reflex thresholds using tonal stimuli and noise bands.

HEARING IMPAIRMENT. Unilateral or bilateral conductive and/or sensorineural deficit in the frequency range most important for speech recognition (500–4,000 Hz). Based largely on adult, pure-tone normative values, various classifications of hearing impairment have been published (Clark, 1981). However, research and clinical experience with children suggests that any classification of hearing loss by degree may not adequately indicate the adverse impact of hearing impairment on development (Kenworthy, Bess, Stahlman, & Lindstrom, 1988).

TARGET POPULATION. The following children should be referred for audiologic evaluation:

➤ any child who failed a newborn hearing screening;
➤ any child who is suspected by a parent/primary caregiver, educator, or primary care physician of having hearing loss;
➤ any child "who exhibits abnormal auditory behavior or delayed speech and language development" (ASHA Guidelines, 1989, p. 91);
➤ any child not previously screened who is identified as at high risk for hearing loss based on the Joint Committee on Infant Hearing Position Statement (1982) or any subsequent revisions (Joint Committee on Infant Hearing 1990 Position Statement, 1991, Suppl. 5, p. 3).

Procedures

Several guiding principles were of paramount importance in compiling the recommendations for appropriate assessment procedures. These principles include (a) individualized timely assessment protocol, (b) use of frequency-specific stimuli, (c) ear-specific assessment and (d) determination of middle ear status by bone conduction and acoustic immittance measurements.

Individualized, Timely Assessment Protocol

Children undergo rapid sensory, motor, and cognitive development. Thus, it is essential that assessment tools be chosen that are appropriate for the neurodevelopmental state of the young child. Although a thorough assessment of the hearing impairment may not be completed at one point in time, prolonged delays between assessments should be avoided. Although serial evaluations yield the best information upon which to base management decisions, the diagnosis and remediation of any existing hearing loss should not be delayed because of an inability to reliably complete any particular test.

Use of Frequency-Specific Stimuli

Acoustic stimuli used for assessment should provide frequency-specific[3] information regarding auditory sensitivity. Therefore, responses to pure tones, FM tones, or narrow bands of

---

[3]Bandwidth should be considered when using narrow band noise stimuli for behavioral assessment (Orchik & Mosher, 1975; Orchik & Rintelmann, 1978; Stephens & Rintelmann, 1978) and when using brief duration tones for electrophysiologic assessment (Gorga, Abbas, & Worthington, 1985; Stapells et al., 1985). Frequency specificity may be compromised if the stimulus bandwidth is not sufficiently narrow, thereby possibly contributing to an inaccurate determination of audiometric configuration.

noise should be obtained in behavioral testing of children regardless of the response levels obtained to broadband signals (e.g., speech, music, or environmental sound). Because high-frequency spectral energy (above 1,000 Hz) is critical to speech perception, audiologic assessment of children should always include test stimuli that allow the clinician to evaluate hearing sensitivity within the high-frequency range. The Committee suggests that at a minimum, thresholds be obtained at 500 Hz and 2,000 Hz to allow for the selection of appropriate amplification (Matkin, 1987).

Frequency-specific stimuli are also recommended for ABR assessment. The use of click stimuli alone is not sufficient for the estimation of audiometric configuration (Eggermont, 1982; Stapells et al., 1985; Stapells, 1989). Thus, it is recommended that frequency-specific stimuli be used when comprehensive ABR testing is undertaken (Hyde, 1985; Stapells, et al, 1985; Stapells, 1989). ABR thresholds for clicks generally correlate well with pure-tone thresholds in the high-frequency range (Coats & Martin, 1977; Jerger & Mauldin, 1978; Yamada, Yagi Yamane, & Suzuki, 1975; Yamada, Kodera, & Yagi, 1979). The ABR thresholds for low-frequency stimuli (Gorga et al., 1985), and low-frequency stimuli in notched noise (Hyde, 1985; Picton, Ouellette, Hamel, & Smith, 1979; Stockard, Stockard, & Coen, 1983;) can be used to estimate thresholds for the low-frequency region. Derived band analysis of ABR responses may also be used for this purpose (Don & Eggermont, 1978; Don, Eggermont, & Brackmann, 1979; Parker & Thornton, 1978a, 1978b). ABR test protocols should be chosen to estimate threshold in both the high and low-frequency range.

Ear-Specific Assessment

Ear-specific assessment is the goal for both behavioral and electrophysiologic procedures because a unilateral hearing loss, even in the presence of a normal-hearing ear, may place a child at significant developmental and/or educational risk (Bess, 1982; Bess, Klee, & Culbertson, 1986; Oyler, Oyler, & Matkin, 1988). Therefore, determining hearing sensitivity for each ear is important for establishing supportive evidence for medical/surgical diagnosis and treatment, selecting appropriate amplification, establishing baseline function, and monitoring auditory status when progressive or fluctuating hearing loss is suspected. Effective masking of the non-test ear should be utilized as necessary.

Determination of Middle Ear Status by Bone Conduction and Acoustic Immittance Measurements

When air-conduction thresholds obtained by either behavioral or electrophysiologic methods are found to be elevated, estimates of bone conduction sensitivity should be completed. In contrast, acoustic immittance should be accomplished during each test session in order to assist in the determination of middle ear status. Findings from acoustic immittance alone are not sufficient for middle ear assessment, but they provide valuable information when considered in conjunction with other audiologic results.

Protocols

Assessment Protocol for Children Chronologically/Developmentally Birth Through 4 Months of Age (Age Adjusted for Prematurity)

At these very young ages, or for very compromised children (severely developmentally delayed or multiply impaired), the suggested methods for the comprehensive assessment of auditory function are the ABR (using click and low-frequency stimuli) and acoustic immittance in combination with case history, parent/caregiver report, and behavioral observation of the infant's responses to a variety of auditory stimuli. The behavioral observation is intended for corroboration of parent/caregiver report of the child's auditory behavior rather than for threshold estimation.

ELECTROPHYSIOLOGIC ASSESSMENT. ABR threshold and latency-intensity function should be measured for air conducted clicks and/or tones for each ear. At a minimum, responses to clicks and low-frequency stimuli should be obtained to provide an estimate of audiometric configuration. When air-conducted ABR is elevated, an ABR to bone-conducted stimuli should be considered when equipment, normative data, and expertise are available (Mauldin & Jerger, 1979; Stapells, 1989; Stapells & Ruben, 1989; Yang, Rupert, & Moushegian, 1987; Ysunza & Cone-Wesson, 1987).

ACOUSTIC IMMITTANCE ASSESSMENT. Tympanograms and acoustic reflexes should be assessed for both ears. The use of a probe frequency higher than 220/226 Hz for obtaining acoustic reflexes in this age range should be considered.

BEHAVIORAL ASSESSMENT. At present, reliable procedures for the behavioral assessment of hearing in this age population are not clinically available. However, this should not preclude the clinician's consideration of behavioral methods now being researched and developed (Olsho, Koch, Halpin, & Carter, 1987).

Assessment Protocol for Children Who Are Chronologically/Developmentally 5–24 Months of Age (Age Adjusted for Prematurity)

Behavioral techniques, in combination with acoustic immittance measures, are often sufficient for the comprehensive assessment of hearing for children in this age range. ABR is recommended when the validity or adequacy of behavioral test results are limited or the neurologic integrity of the auditory pathways to the level of the brainstem is in question.

BEHAVIORAL ASSESSMENT. Visual reinforcement audiometry (VRA) should be employed to assess hearing sensitivity for speech and frequency-specific stimuli. The VRA test results should include indicators of the child's response reliability. Minimally, both high- and low-frequency signals should be used, preferably at octave frequencies from 500–4,000 Hz. Ear-specific threshold information is preferable to sound field findings. Nevertheless, it is often useful to initiate VRA in the sound field or by bone conduction because the response behavior is more easily established. Word recognition measures should be applied at suprathreshold levels as early as possible, while recognizing the child's language limitations (see Assessment Protocol for Young Children). If air conduction results are elevated, unmasked bone conduction thresholds, at a minimum, should be obtained.

ACOUSTIC IMMITTANCE ASSESSMENT. Tympanograms and acoustic reflex thresholds should be assessed in both ears. Additional acoustic reflex measurements using broadband noise stimuli may provide useful information about auditory status (Jerger, Burney, Mauldin, & Crump, 1974; Jerger, Hayes, Anthony, & Mauldin, 1978; Margolis & Fox, 1977; Neimeyer & Sesterhenn, 1974; Popelka, Margolis, & Wiley, 1976; Silman & Gelfand, 1978; 1981; see comments regarding probe-tone frequency in *Assessment Protocol for Children Through 4 Months of Age*.)

ELECTROPHYSIOLOGIC ASSESSMENT. When behavioral findings are incomplete or inconclusive or are judged as unreliable, an ABR to air-conducted clicks and/or tones is recommended. If air-conducted ABR threshold estimates are elevated, bone-conducted measures should be considered when equipment, normative data, and expertise are available (Mauldin & Jerger, 1979; Stapells, 1989; Stapells & Ruben, 1989; Yang, Rupert, & Moushegian, 1987; Ysunza & Cone-Wesson, 1987). The same testing protocol described above for neonates and infants through 4 months of age applies.

Assessment Protocol for Children Who Are Chronologically/Developmentally 25–36 Months of Age

Behavioral techniques, in combination with acoustic immittance measures, are generally sufficient for the comprehensive assessment of hearing for children in this age range. ABR is recommended when the validity or adequacy of behavioral test results are limited or the neurologic integrity of the auditory pathways to the level of the brainstem is in question.

BEHAVIORAL ASSESSMENT. Conditioned play audiometry (CPA), tangible or visually reinforced operant conditioning audiometry (TROCA, VROCA), or visual reinforcement audiometry (VRA) should be employed, depending on the child's ability to perform the necessary task. Frequency-specific thresholds should be determined at octave frequencies 500–4,000 Hz (at a minimum). Thresholds should be determined for each ear by air conduction. Bone conduction thresholds should be determined when air-conducted thresholds are elevated. A threshold for speech using a closed set (picture-point, object-point, or repetition) response task should also be obtained. A formal assessment of word recognition ability using standardized tests such as Word Intelligibility by Picture Identification—WIPI; (Ross & Lerman, 1971), the Northwestern University Children's Perception of Speech—NU-CHIPS (Elliot & Katz, 1980) and the Pediatric Speech Intelligibility Test—PS (Jerger & Jerger, 1984) is recommended whenever appropriate. When the use of a standardized test is not possible, an attempt should be made to informally assess word recognition using objects or body parts within the child's demonstrated receptive vocabulary (Matkin,

1979; Olsen & Matkin, 1979). In the latter case, results should be reported descriptively and not quantitatively, as such tests are nonstandardized measures of word recognition ability.

ACOUSTIC IMMITTANCE ASSESSMENT. See *Assessment Protocol for Children Who Are Chronologically/Developmentally 5–24 Months of Age.*

ELECTROPHYSIOLOGIC ASSESSMENT. See *Assessment Protocol for Children Who Are Chronologically/Developmentally 5–24 Months of Age.*

Personnel and Scope of the Assessment

Audiologic assessment is performed by an ASHA-certified audiologist who is responsible for the administration and interpretation of behavioral, electrophysiologic, and acoustic immittance measures. Audiologic assessment includes provision of input regarding audiologic follow-up and management including candidacy for use, fitting, and dispensing of amplification and/or alternative communication devices. Audiologic assessment also includes professional interpretation of case history and test results, parent/caregiver counseling, and, when appropriate, referral to allied professionals such as the primary care physician, medical specialist, speech-language pathologist, or psychologist. Where programs addressing the special needs of children with hearing impairment are in place, the audiologist and parent/caregiver are mandated members of the multidisciplinary team and participate in decisions regarding child and family needs (PL 99–57). Where no such programs are in place, guidance should be provided regarding available education and intervention options, so that the parent/caregiver can make informed decisions.

References

Administration on Developmental Disabilities. (1988). *Mapping the future for children with special needs: PL 99–457.* Iowa City: University of Iowa.

American National Standards Institute. (1977). *American national standard for permissible ambient noise during audiometric testing.* (ANS31.-1977) New York ANSI.

American Speech-Language-Hearing Association. (1987). *The short latency auditory evoked potentials.* Rockville MD: ASHA Committee on Audiologic Evaluation, Auditory Evoked Potential Measurements Working Group.

American Speech-Language-Hearing Association. (1988). Tutorial on tympanometry. ASHA working group on aural acoustic-immittance, measurements committee on audiologic evaluation. *Journal of Speech and Hearing Disorders, 53,* 354–377.

American Speech-Language-Hearing Association. (1989). Guidelines for audiologic screening of newborn infants who are at risk for hearing impairment. *Asha, 31*(3), 89–92.

Bench, J., Collyer. Y., Mentz, L., & Wilson, I. (1976). Studies in infant behavioral audiometry. I. Neonates. *Audiology, 15,* 85–105.

Bennett, M., & Weatherby, L. (1982). Newborn acoustic reflexes to noise and puretone signals. *Journal of Speech and Hearing Research, 25,* 383–387.

Bernstein, R., & Gravel, J. (1991). A method for determining hearing sensitivity in infants: The interweaving staircase procedure (ISP). *Journal of the American Academy of Audiology, 1,* 138–145.

Bess, F. (1982). Children with unilateral hearing loss. *Journal of the Academy of Rehabilitative Audiology, 15*, 131–143.

Bess, F., Klee, T., & Culbertson, J. (1988). Identification, assessment and management of children with unilateral sensorineural hearing loss. *Ear and Hearing, 7*, 43–51.

Cherow, E. (Ed.). (1985). *Hearing-impaired children with developmental disabilities: An interdisciplinary foundation for service*. Washington. DC: Gallaudet University Press.

Clark, J. (1981). Uses and abuses of hearing loss classification. *Asha, 23*, 493–500.

Coats, A., & Martin, J. (1977). Human auditory nerve action potentials and brainstem evoked responses. *Archives of Otolaryngology, 103*, 605–622.

Cullen, J., Berlin, C., Gondra, M., & Adams, M. (1978). Electrocochleography in children: A retrospective study. *Acta Otolaryngologica, 102*, 482–490.

Davis, J. (1988). Management of the school age child: A psychological perspective, In F. Bess (Ed.), *Hearing impairment in children* (pp. 401–416). Parkton, MD: York Press.

Diefendorf, A. (1988). Pediatric audiology. In J. Lass, L. McReynolds, J. Northern, & D. Yoder (Eds.), *Handbook of speech-language pathology and audiology* (pp. 1315–1338). Toronto: B. C. Decker.

Don, M., & Eggermont, J. (1978). Analysis of the click evoked brainstem potentials in man using high-pass noise masking. *Journal of the Acoustical Society of America, 63*, 1084–1092.

Don, M., Eggermont, J., & Brackmann, D. (1979). Reconstruction of the audiogram using brainstem responses and high pass noise masking. *Annals of Otology, Rhinology and Laryngology, Suppl. 57*, 1–20.

Downs, M. P., & Sterritt, G. M. (1987). Guide to newborn and infant hearing screening programs. *Archives of Otolaryngology, 85*, 15–22.

Dunst, C., Trivette, C., & Deal, C. (1988). Help giver and family functioning. In *Enabling and empowering families* (pp. 35–45). Cambridge, MA: Bookline Books.

Education of the Handicapped Act Amendments of 1986, Public Law 99-457, 34 CFR Part 303, Part H. *Federal Register, 54*(119), 119, 26306–26348, June 22, 1989.

Eggermont, J. J., & Salamy, A. (1988). Electrophysiologic techniques in audiology and otology: Development of ABR parameters in a preterm and a term born population. *Ear and Hearing, 9*(5), 283–289.

Eisenberg, R. (1976). *Auditory competence in early life*. Baltimore, MD: University Park Press.

Elliot, L., & Katz, D. (1980). *Northwestern University Children's Perception Speech (NU Chips)*. St. Louis: Auditec.

Friedrich, B. W. (1985). The state of the art in audiologic evaluation and management. In E. Cherow, N. Matkin, and R. J. Trybus (Eds.), *Hearing-impaired children and youth with developmental disabilities: An interdisciplinary foundation for service* (pp. 122–152). Washington, DC: Gallaudet University Press.

Gorga, M., Worthington, D., Reiland, J., Beauchaine, K., & Goldgar, D. (1985). Some comparisons between auditory brainstem response thresholds, latencies, and the pure tone audiogram. *Ear and Hearing, 6*, 105–109.

Gorga M., Abbas, P., & Worthington, D. (1985). Stimulus calibration and ABR measurements. In J. Jacobson (Ed.), *Auditory brainstem response* (pp. 49–62). San Diego: College-Hill Press.

Gravel J. (1989). Behavioral assessment of auditory function. In J. Gravel (Ed.), *Assessing auditory system integrity in high-risk infants and young children* (pp. 216–228). *Seminars in Hearing, 10*(3).

Gravel, J., Kurtzberg, D., Stapells, D., Vaughan, H., & Wallace, I. (1989). Case studies. In J. Gravel (Ed.), *Assessing auditory system integrity in high-risk infants and young children*. (pp. 272–286). *Seminars in Hearing, 10*(3). New York: Thieme Medical Publishers.

Himelfarb, M., Popelka. G., & Shannon, E. (1979). Tympanometry in normal neonates. *Journal of Speech and Hearing Research, 22*, 179–191.

Hyde, M. L. (1985). Frequency specific BERA in infants. *Journal of Otolaryngology, 14* (Supplement), 19–27.

Jerger, J., Burney, P., Mauldun, L., & Crump, B. (1974). Predicting hearing loss from the acoustic reflex. *Journal of Speech and Hearing Disorders, 39*, 11–22.

Jerger, J., Hayes, D., Anthony, L., & Mauldin, L. (1978). Factors influencing prediction of hearing loss from the acoustic reflex. *Monographs of Contemporary Audiology, 1*, 1–20.

Jerger, J., & Mauldin, L. (1978). Prediction of sensorineural hearing level from the brainstem evoked response. *Archives of Otolaryngology, 104*, 456–461.

Jerger, S., & Jerger, J. (1984). *Pediatric Speech Intelligibility Test - PSI* St. Louis: Auditec.

Joint Committee on Infant Hearing. (1982). Position statement. *Asha, 24*, 1017–1018.

Joint Committee on Infant Hearing. (1991). 1990 Position Statement. *Asha, 33*(Suppl. 5), 3–6.

Kemp, D. (1978). Stimulated acoustic emission from the human auditory system. *Journal of the Acoustical Society of America, 64*, 1386–1391.

Kemp, D., Ryan, S., & Bray, P. (1991). A guide to the effective use of otoacoustic emissions. *Ear and Hearing, 11*, 93–105.

Kenworthy, O.T., Bess, F., Stahlman, M., & Lindstrom, D. (1987). Hearing, speech and language outcome in infants with extreme immaturity. *American Journal of Otology, 8*, 419–425.

Kraus, N., Reed, N., Smith, O., Stein, L., & Cartee, M. (1985). Auditory middle latency responses in children: Effects of age and diagnostic category. *Electroencephalography and Clinical Neurophysiology, 62*, 343–351.

Kurent, H. (1989). Future trends in health care. *Asha, 31*(12), 40–42.

Kurtzberg, D. (1989). Cortical event-related potential assessment of auditory system integrity. In J. Gravel (Ed.), *Assessing auditory system integrity in high-risk infants and young children* (pp. 252–261). *Seminars in Hearing, 10*(3).

Marchart, D., McMillan, P., Shurin, P., Johnson, C., Turcgyk, V., Feinstein, J., & Panek, D. (1986). Objective diagnosis of otitis media in early infancy by tympanometry and ipsilateral acoustic reflex thresholds. *Journal of Pediatrics, 102*, 590–595.

Margolis, R. H. (1978). Tympanometry in infants. State of the art. In E. R. Harford, F. H. Bess, C.D. Bluestone, and J. O. Klein (Eds.), *Impedance screening for middle ear diseases in children* (pp. 41–56). New York: Grune & Stratton.

Margolis, R. H. & Fox, C. M. (1977). A comparison of three methods for predicting hearing loss from the acoustic reflex. *Journal of Speech and Hearing Research, 20*, 241–253.

Margolis, R. H., & Popelka, G. R. (1975). Static and dynamic acoustic impedance measurements in infant ears. *Journal of Speech and Hearing Research, 18*, 435–443.

Matkin, N. (1977). Assessment of hearing sensitivity during the preschool years. In F. Bess (Ed.), *Childhood deafness* (p. 138). New York: Grune & Stratton.

Matkin, N. (1979). The audiologic examination of young children at risk. *Ear, Nose, and Throat Journal, 58*, 29–38.

Matkin, N. (1987). Hearing instruments for children: Premises for selecting and fitting. *Hearing Instruments, 38*(9), 14–16.

Mauldin, L., & Jerger, J. (1979). Auditory brain stem evoked responses to bone-conducted signals. *Archives of Otolaryngology, 105*, 656–661.

McMillan, P., Bennett, M., Marchant, C., & Shurin, P. (1985). Ipsilateral and contralateral acoustic reflexes in neonates. *Ear and Hearing, 6*, 320–324.

McRandle, D., Smith, M., & Goldstein R. (1974). Early averaged electroencephalic responses to clicks in neonates. *Annals of Otology, Rhinology, and Laryngology, 83*, 695-702.

Mendel M., Adkinson, I., & Harker, L. (1977). Middle components of the auditory evoked potentials in infants. *Annals of Otology, Rhinology, and Laryngology, 86*, 293–299.

Mendelson, R., & Salamy, A. (1981). Maturational effects on the middle components of the averaged electroencephalic response. *Journal of Speech and Hearing Research, 24*, 104–144.

Moore, J. M., Thompson, G., & Thompson, M. (1975). Auditory localization of infants as a function of reinforcement conditions. *Journal of Speech and Hearing Disorders, 40*, 29–34.

Moore, J., Thompson, G., & Wilson. W. (1977). Visual reinforcement of head-turn responses in infants under 12 months of age. *Journal of Speech and Hearing Disorders, 42*, 328–333.

Morgan, D., Dirks, D., & Bower, D. (1979). Suggested threshold sound pressure levels for frequency modulate warble tones in the sound field. *Journal of Speech and Hearing Disorders, 44*, 37–54.

Neimeyer, W., & Sesterhenn, G. (1974). Calculating the hearing threshold from the stapedius reflex threshold for different sound stimuli. *Audiology, 13*, 421–427.

Northern, J. L. (1988). Recent developments in acoustic immittance measurements with children. In F. H. Bess (Ed.), *Hearing impairment in children*. Parkton, MD: York Press.

Northern, J. L., & Downs, M. P. (1984). *Hearing in children* (3rd ed.) Baltimore, MD: Williams & Wilkins.

Norton, S., & Widen, J. (1990). Evoked otoacoustic emissions in normal hearing infants and children: Emerging data and issues. *Ear and Hearing, 11*, 121–127.

Nozza, R., & Wilson, W. R. (1984). Masked and unmasked pure tone thresholds of infants and adults: Development of auditory frequency selectivity and sensitivity. *Journal of Speech and Hearing Research, 27*(4), 613–622.

Olsen, W., & Matkin, N. (1979). Speech audiometry. In W. Rintelmann (Ed.), *Hearing assessment*. Baltimore, MD: University Park Press.

Olsho, L., Koch, E., Halpin, C., & Carter, E. (1987). An observer-based psychoacoustic procedure for use with young infants. *Developmental Psychology, 23*, 627–640.

Orchik, D., & Mosher, N. (1975). Narrow band noise audiometry: The effect of filter slope. *Journal of the American Audiology Society, 1*, 50–53.

Orchik, D., & Rintelmann, W. R. (1978). Comparison of pure-tone, warble-tone, and narrow-band noise thresholds of young normal hearing children. *Journal of the American Audiology Society, 3*, 214–220.

Oyler, R., Oyler, A., & Matkin, N. (1988). Demographics and educational impact. *Language, Speech, and Hearing Services in Schools, 19*, 201–209.

Parker, D., & Thornton, A. (1978a). Derived cochlear nerve and brainstem evoked responses of the human auditory system. *Scandinavian Audiology, 7*, 1–8.

Parker, D., & Thornton, A. (1978b). Frequency specific components of the cochlear nerve and brainstem evoked responses of the human auditory system. *Scandinavian Audiology, 7*, 53–60.

Picton, T., Ouellette, J., Hamel, G., & Smith, A. (1979). Brainstem evoked potentials to tone-pipe in notched noise. *Journal of Otolaryngology, 8*, 289–314.

Popelka, G., Margolis, R., & Wiley, T. (1976). The effect of activating signal bandwidth on acoustic-reflex thresholds. *Journal of the Acoustical Society of America, 59*, 153–159.

Primus, M., & Thompson, G. (1985). Response strength of young children in operant audiometry. *Journal of Speech and Hearing Research, 28*, 539–547.

Rochlin, G. (1990). *Status of sound field audiometry among audiologists in the United States*. Paper presented at the annual meeting of the American Academy of Audiology, New Orleans.

Ross, M., & Lerman, J. (1971). *Word Intelligibility by Picture Identification-WIPI*. St. Louis: Auditec.

Silman, S., & Gelfand, S. (1978). Prediction of hearing levels from acoustic reflex thresholds in persons with high-frequency hearing losses. *Journal of Speech and Hearing Research, 22*, 697–707.

Silman, S., & Gelfand, S. (1981). The relationship between magnitude of hearing loss and acoustic reflex threshold levels. *Journal of Speech and Hearing Disorders, 46*, 312–316.

Sprague, B., Wiley, T., & Goldstein, R. (1985). Tympanometric and acoustic-reflex studies in neonates. *Journal of Speech and Hearing Research, 28*, 265–272.

Stapells, D. (1989). Auditory brainstem response assessment of infants. In J. Gravel (Ed.), *Assessing auditory system integrity in high-risk infants and children* (pp. 229–251). *Seminars in Hearing, 10*(3).

Stapells, D., Picton, T., Perez-Abalo, M., Read, D., & Smith, A. (1985). Frequency specificity in evoked potential audiometry. In J. T. Jacobson (Ed.), *Auditory brainstem response* (pp. 147–177). San Diego, CA: College-Hill Press.

Stapells, D., & Ruben, R. (1989). Auditory brainstem responses to bone-conducted tones in infants. *Annals of Otology, Rhinology and Laryngology, 98*, 941–949.

Stein, L., & Kraus, N. (1985). Auditory brainstem response measures with multiply handicapped children and adults. In J. T. Jacobson (Ed.), *Auditory brainstem response* (pp. 337–348). San Diego, CA: College-Hill Press.

Stephens, M., & Rintelmann, W. (1978). The influence of audiometric configuration on pure-tone, warble-tone and narrow band noise thresholds of adults with sensorneural hearing losses. *Journal of the American Audiology Society, 3*, 221–226.

Stockard, J. E., Stockard, J. J., & Coen, R. (1983). Auditory brain stem response variability in infants. *Ear and Hearing, 4*, 11–23.

Thompson, G. T. (1985). Reinforced and nonreinforced head-turn responses of infants as a function of stimulus bandwidth. *Ear and Hearing, 6*, 125–129.

Thompson, G. & Folsom, R. (1981). Hearing assessment of at risk infants. *Clinical Pediatrics, 20*, 257–261.

Thompson, G. T., & Folsom, R. C. (1984). A comparison of two conditioning procedures in the use of visual reinforcement audiometry (VRA). *Journal of Speech and Hearing Disorders, 49*, 241–245.

Thompson, G. T., & Weber, B. A. (1974). Responses of infants and young children to behavior observation audiometry (BOA). *Journal of Speech and Hearing Disorders, 39*, 140–147.

Thompson, G. T., Wilson, W. R., & Moore, J. M. (1979). Clinical application of visual reinforcement audiometry (VRA) to low-functioning children. *Journal of Speech and Hearing Disorders, 44*, 80–90.

Thompson, G., & Wilson, W. (1984). Clinical application of visual reinforcement audiometry. *Seminars in Hearing, 5*, 85–99.

Turner, R., Frazer, G., & Shepard, N. (1984). Formulating and evaluating audiological test protocols. *Ear and Hearing, 5*, 321–330.

U.S. General Accounting Office. (1985). *Constraining national health care expenditures; Achieving quality care at an affordable cost.* GAO/HRD 85–105. Gaithersburg, MD: Author.

Walker, G., Dillon, H., & Byrne, D. (1984). Sound field audiometry: Recommended stimuli and procedures. *Ear and Hearing, 5*, 13–21.

Weatherby, L., & Bennett, M. (1980). The neonatal acoustic reflex. *Scandinavian Audiology, 9*,193–110.

Weber, B. A. (1969). Validation of observer judgments in behavior observation audiometry. *Journal of Speech and Hearing Disorders, 34*, 350–354.

Wilson, W. R. (1978). Behavioral assessment of auditory function in infants. In F. D. Minifie & L. L. Lloyd (Eds.), *Communicative and cognitive abilities—early behavioral assessment*. Baltimore, MD: University Park Press.

Wilson, W. R., & Thompson, G. (1984). Behavioral audiometry. In J. Jerger (Ed.), *Pediatric audiology* (pp. 1–44). San Diego, CA: College-Hill Press.

Yamada, O., Kodera, K., & Yagi, T. (1979). Cochlear processes affecting wave latency of the auditory evoked brainstem response. *Scandinavian Audiology, 8*, 67–70.

Yamada, O., Yagi, T., Yamane, H., & Suzuki, J. (1975). Clinical evaluation of the auditory evoked brain stem response. *Auris-Nasus-Larynx, 2,* 97–105.

Yang, E. Y., Rupert, A. L., & Moushegian, G. (1987). A developmental study of bone conduction auditory brainstem response in infants. *Ear and Hearing, 8,* 244–251.

Ysunza, A., & Cone-Wesson, B. (1987). Bone conduction masking for brainstem auditory evoked-potentials (BAEP) in pediatric audiological evaluations. Validation of the test. *International Journal of Pediatric Otorhinolaryngology, 12,* 291–302.

Appendix 2–H

AMPLIFICATION AS A REMEDIATION TECHNIQUE FOR CHILDREN WITH NORMAL PERIPHERAL HEARING

This report was prepared by the American Speech-Language-Hearing Association (ASHA) Committee on Amplification for the Hearing Impaired. Present and past committee members responsible for this report include Thomas S. Rees, current chair; Walt Smoski, past chair; G. Jean Boggess; Evelyn Cherow, ex officio; Alice E. Holmes; Barbara J. Moore-Brown; Polly E. Patrick; Valenta G. Ward-Gravely; Linda Van Dyke; and Peter Ivory. Teris K. Schery, 1988–1990 vice president for clinical affairs, was monitoring vice president. The ASHA Executive Board accepted the report in August 1990 for publication in Asha (EB 116–90).

The use of various amplification devices for populations other than those with hearing disorders—that is, for persons with normal peripheral hearing—has been reported as a therapeutic tool in recent years. This type of habilitation/rehabilitation has been suggested for use primarily with children in educational and clinical settings as a remedial technique for those with phonological disorders, central auditory processing disorders (CAPD), and language/learning disabilities. The goals of such intervention include increasing attention span, reducing distractibility, improving signal-to-noise ratio, and increasing sound (phonological) awareness and discrimination. This application is apparently based on the premise that the development of these skills affects children's speech sound production, language processing, and academic achievement. The committee is responding to questions and concerns that have been raised regarding the efficacy of this practice and potential detrimental effects on hearing. The limited literature addressing the use of amplification with children who have normal peripheral hearing is reviewed in this report. Finally, concerns about clinical practice and recommendations for further research needs are offered.

Review of the Literature

Amplification for the purpose of increasing the intensity level of stimulus presentation in order to improve response accuracy has been reported to be effective in several studies. During the development and evaluation of the Northwestern University Children's Perception of Speech Test (NU-CHIPS), Elliot and Katz (1980) reported that normal-hearing 3-year-olds required increased intensity levels during stimulus presentation to reach criterion on a picture-naming task. In a subsequent study, normal-hearing 6- and 10-year-olds required higher intensity levels than adults to identify Consonant-Vowel (CV) syllables (Elliot, Longinotti, Clifton, & Meyer, 1981). A higher stimulus presentation level also was reported to be necessary for children with articulation disorders to achieve more accurate productions when compared to those without articulation disorders (Clifton & Elliot, 1982).

Intervention programs for children with articulation or phonological disorders have included ongoing or intermittent use of amplification devices. Shriberg (1983) recommended the use of "augmented input" as an integral component in articulation programs for children. Hodson and Paden (1983) described a 2-minute period of auditory bombardment with amplification at the beginning and end of each session in the treatment of phonological disabilities. Stimulus words targeting specific phonemes were read to children using a "low level of amplification." Hodson and Paden stated that children with phonological disorders benefited from a program including emphasis by intense presentation of sounds and sound sequences. Amplification was felt to direct the child's attention to the target and to be more successful than other methods for improving the production of sounds. The authors emphasized the use of "low level amplification" and stated that "caution must be taken to keep the level minimal . . . in order to avoid any possible damage to the child's hearing mechanism" (p. 50).

FM assistive listening devices also have been used as a possible intervention strategy for children with central auditory processing disorders. Stach, Loiselle, and Jerger (1987) reported on 25 such children who were given a trial period with FM systems set to minimal gain, 11 of whom were subsequently fit with the devices. The parents and teachers of these children stated that they observed improved academic and behavioral performance. Stach, Loiselle, Jerger, Mintz, and Taylor (1987) also reported on a single case study of a 7-year-old who was fit with an FM device. Improved academic achievement and modification of behavior were noted by parents and teachers.

The use of low-power FM wireless systems for children with learning disabilities has been described in two reports by a manufacturer. The first involved using FM systems with learning-disabled children from 6- to 12-years of age for 30 minutes to 2 hours per day for 3–6 weeks (Loose, 1984). Teachers reported that the students appeared to show increases in attention, productivity, and accuracy. The second manufacturer's report involved 40 normal hearing 5-10-year-olds who were judged to have attention problems

Source: From *ASHA Desk Reference for Audiology and Speech-Language Pathology, II,* pp. 127–130. Copyright 1991 by American Speech-Language-Hearing Association. Available for sale from ASHA Fullfillment Operations (301-897-5700 x218). Reprinted by permission.

Reference this material as follows:

American Speech-Language-Hearing Association (1991). Amplification as a Remediation Technique for Children With Normal Peripheral Hearing. *Asha, 33*(Suppl. 3), 22–24.

(Blake, Torpey, & Wertz, 1986). Twenty of the children used auditory trainers during instructional periods for 24 weeks, and the other 20 served as a control group. Pre- and post-intervention observations for target behaviors were made for both groups. Statistical analyses were not reported; however, preliminary findings indicated that 95% of the experimental group demonstrated improved attending behavior (e.g., increased eye contact with teacher, increased rate and appropriateness of response, increased ability to follow directions, and increased awareness of verbal cues, body position, and body control). In addition, decreased body movement and reduction in extraneous verbalizations and distractibility were also noted.

Shapiro and Mistal (1985) reported on the use of high-frequency amplification in reading- and spelling-disabled children. Four reading-disordered children, 2 with normal hearing and 2 with hearing loss at 6,000 Hz and 8,000 Hz, were fit with an in-the-ear (ITE) hearing aid in the right ear. Use of amplification reportedly enhanced only the frequencies between 2,500 Hz and 6,000 Hz, although no functional or real ear measurements were reported. The authors reported an improvement in the areas of auditory memory, articulation of complex words, and intelligibility of phonetically balanced words. A subsequent study (Shapiro & Mistal, 1986) evaluated the long-term effects of high-frequency amplification. Fourteen normal-hearing students referred for reading/spelling delays were divided into 2 groups: 7 were fit with high-frequency ITEs, and 7 served as a matched control group. After 13 months of use, testing of the unamplified group did not show any group differences in spelling, reading progress, or speech discrimination; however, the amplified group showed an enhancement in speech discrimination in noise over the unaided condition. The amount of gain provided by the ITEs was not specified.

Project MARRS (Mainstream Amplification Resource Room Study) (Sarff, Ray, & Bagwell, 1981; Ray, Sarff, & Glassford, 1984) was the first study to report the use of sound field amplification for children with academic achievement deficits. Fourth-, fifth-, and sixth-grade classes in four schools were equipped with an FM teacher transmitter and two speakers that provided amplified speech at intensity levels of approximately 10 dB above the ambient noise level. Target students were selected using the following criteria: each student had a minimal hearing loss (15 dB to 35 dB HL), had academic deficits of 6 months or more, and had average intellectual potential. Half of the target students were placed in amplified classrooms; the other half were placed in unamplified classrooms and received supplemental instruction from a resource room teacher. The target students were not identified for the teachers. Typical use of the sound systems was 3 hours per day. Students received 1, 2, or 3 years of treatment. The results indicated that target students in amplified classrooms demonstrated significantly improved Scholastic Reading Achievement scores, and this increase was equal to or greater than that of the target students who received resource room instruction. Additionally, regarding the MARRS project, Ray (1987) stated that, "questionnaire data obtained from administrators, teachers, and students indicated the intervention is helpful to teachers and to non-handicapped students as well as those with mild hearing losses" (p. 14).

Flexer (1989) reported results obtained from another school system utilizing 47 sound field amplification systems in regular classrooms. The educators had found that 43% of primary-level students failed a 15 dB HL hearing screening considered to be educationally significant. After 3 years of use, results indicated that even though pupil count had increased in the school, the number of students receiving special services had decreased from 945 at the beginning of the study to 850 after amplifying the classrooms. In general, higher scores were obtained on the Iowa Test of Basic Skills for students in amplified classrooms in kindergarten through third grade. Teachers reported improved on-task behavior, improved use of voices, use of longer utterances, and increased confidence when using the microphone.

Although this review has focused on children with normal peripheral hearing, the use of assistive listening devices with normal-hearing head-injured adult clients was addressed by Casterline, Flexer, & DePompei (1989). They reported decreases in distracting behaviors and increased attention.

Concerns Related to Current Practices

The current literature leaves several questions unanswered regarding safety and efficacy in the use of amplification devices on children with normal peripheral hearing. Several concerns arise related to this practice.

RESEARCH DESIGN. Although the literature cited has suggested benefit with the use of amplification in individuals with normal peripheral hearing, conclusions were based primarily on anecdotal reports in nonrefereed publications and without specific empirical data to support the investigators' conclusions.

Specific data regarding the gain provided, the acoustic environments in which amplification was used, the cumulative wearing time, and the method of selection and fitting were not reported and are essential. Research is needed in controlled settings to eliminate extraneous factors that have threatened the internal validity of previous findings. In addition, information about the involvement of audiologists in the methodology described is absent in the current literature.

POTENTIAL FOR NOISE-INDUCED HEARING LOSS. Risk management practices dictate that caution be exercised in the fitting of any amplification device because of the potential for noise-induced hearing loss. The potential for damage to the normal auditory mechanism through exposure to intense sounds is well-documented. The Occupational Safety and Health Administration (U.S. Department of Labor, 1983) warns that adults who are exposed to noise levels at or above 85 dBA for an 8 hour time-weighted average are at risk for noise-induced hearing loss. As the intensity of the sound increases, the acceptable exposure time decreases dramatically. For example, the maximum allowable exposure levels for occupational noise are 90 dBA for 8 hours, 110 dBA for 30 min., and 125 dBA for less than 4 min.

It is not uncommon for personal hearing aids and amplification systems to produce 135 to 145 dB SPL at the tympanic membrane. More conservative levels are advisable with children, who have been reported to be at greater risk for incurring noise-induced hearing loss than adults (Humes, 1988; Mills, 1975). Although many amplification devices are marketed as mild gain instruments, the actual peak output of these instruments may vary depending on such factors as input level, distance from the microphone, and receiver coupling. Because younger children have smaller ear canal volumes, the sound pressure level (SPL) at the tympanic membrane may be even higher than in adults (Jirsa & Norris, 1978). Only real ear measurements with the device on the child can assure that excessive SPLs are not being produced.

SELECTION AND MONITORING PROCEDURES. Currently, there are no uniform procedures for the selection and fitting of amplification devices other than personal hearing aids. Procedures need to be developed that include the real ear measurement of SPL delivered to the ear and measurement of discomfort levels. Traditional coupler gain or functional gain measurements are not appropriate with children who have no peripheral hearing loss. Consumer protection and the qualifications of professionals responsible for recommending amplification devices on persons with normal peripheral hearing need to be addressed. Close monitoring of the electroacoustic properties of these devices and of the thresholds of the children wearing them is essential. Selection and monitoring of these devices are the responsibilities of a licensed or certified audiologist (ASHA, 1984).

Summary and Recommendations

The use of amplification devices including FM systems, auditory trainers, personal amplification devices, and other assistive listening devices with normal-hearing children who have disorders of articulation, auditory processing, language, and learning has been reported. This practice raises three areas of concern: efficacy, consumer safety, and professional liability. Well-designed research is needed to evaluate the efficacy of using amplification with normal-hearing individuals. These studies should be carefully controlled for factors that would influence the validity of the research. The issue of potential damage to the auditory mechanism should be considered when fitting any amplification device. Instruments that improve the signal-to-noise ratio may be an alternative when treating normal-hearing children with special needs. Finally, whenever personal hearing aids or assistive listening devices are being utilized, a certified or licensed audiologist should be involved as a member of the research or clinical team. This committee urges collaborative research among audiologists, speech-language pathologists, and educators to evaluate the efficacy, safety, and associated risk management when using amplification as a remediation technique for children with normal peripheral hearing.

References

American Speech-Language-Hearing Association. (1984). Guidelines for graduate training in amplification. *Asha, 26*(5), 43.

Blake, R., Torpey, C., & Wertz, P. (1986). Preliminary findings: Effect of FM auditory trainers on attending behaviors of learning disabled children. *Telex Communications.*

Casterline, C., Flexer, C., & DePompei R. (1989). Use of assistive listening devices with head injured survivors. Paper presented at the meeting of the American Speech-Language-Hearing-Association, St. Louis, MO.

Clifton, L., & Elliot, L. (1982). CV identification thresholds for speech-language-learning disordered listeners. *Journal of the Acoustical Society of America, 71*, 857.

Elliot, L., & Katz, J. (1980). *The Northwestern University Children's Perception of Speech Test: NU-CHIPS.* St. Louis: Auditec.

Elliot, L., Longinotti C., Clifton, L., & Meyer, D. (1981). Detection and identification thresholds for consonant vowel syllables. *Perception and Psychophysics, 30*, 411–416.

Flexer, C. (1989). Turn on sound: An odyssey of sound field amplification. *Educational Audiology Association Newsletter, 5*, 6.

Hodson, B., & Paden, E. (1983). *Targeting intelligible speech.* San Diego: College-Hill Press.

Humes, L. E. (1978). Can children's hearing be more readily damaged by noise? *Journal of Childhood Communication Disorders, 2*, 49–55.

Jirsa, R. E., & Norris, T. W. (1978). Relationship of acoustic gain to aided threshold improvement. *Journal of Speech and Hearing Disorders, 43*, 384–352.

Loose, F. (1984). Learning disabled students use FM wireless systems. *Telex Communications.*

Mills, J. H. (1975). Noise and children: A review of literature. *Journal of Acoustical Society of America, 58*, 767–779.

Ray, H. (1987, Spring). Put a microphone on the teacher: A simple solution for the difficult problem of mild hearing loss. *The Clinical Connection*, 14–15.

Ray, H., Sarff, L. S., & Glassford, J. E. (1984, Summer/Fall). Sound field amplification: An innovative educational intervention for mainstreamed learning disabled students. *The Directive Teacher*, 18–20.

Sarff, L., Ray, H., & Bagwell, C. (1981). Why not amplification in every classroom? *Hearing Aid Journal, 34*(10), 11, 47–52.

Shapiro, A. H., & Mistal, G. (1985). ITE-aid auditory training for reading- and spelling-disabled children. Clinical case studies. *The Hearing Journal, 38*(2), 26–31.

Shapiro, A. H., & Mistal, G. (1986). ITE-aid auditory training for reading- and spelling-disabled children: A longitudinal study of match groups. *The Hearing Journal, 39*(2), 14–16.

Shriberg, L. (1983). Natural phonologic process approach. In W. Perkins (Ed.), *Phonologic-articulatory disorders* (pp. 3–9). New York: Theime-Stratton.

Stach, B. A., Loiselle, L. H., & Jerger, J. F. (1987, November). FM systems used by children with central auditory processing disorders. Paper presented at the annual convention of the American Speech-Language-Hearing Association, New Orleans, LA.

Stach, B. A., Loiselle, L. H., Jerger, J. F., Mintz, S. L, & Taylor, C. D. (1987). Clinical experience with personal FM assistive listening devices. *The Hearing Journal, 40*(5), 24–30.

U.S. Department of Labor, Occupational Safely and Health Administration. (1983). Occupational Noise Exposure, Hearing Conservation Amendment, Final Rule. *Federal Register, 48*(46), 9738–9785.

Appendix 2–I

GUIDELINES FOR FITTING AND MONITORING FM SYSTEMS

Ad Hoc Committee on FM Systems and Auditory Train-ers American Speech-Language-Hearing Association

The Guidelines for Fitting and Monitoring FM Systems were developed by the American Speech-Language-Hearing Association (ASHA) Ad Hoc Committee on FM Systems and Auditory Train-ers and adopted by the ASHA Legislative Council (LC 27-93) in November 1993. Members of the committee include Ruth A. Bent-ler, chair; Evelyn Cherow, ex officio; Joseph J. Curry; David B. Hawkins; Sherrin L. T. Massie; Jean Lovrinic, Vice President for Governmental and Social Policies, monitoring vice president; and Kimberly Parker-Bright. These guidelines are an official statement of the American Speech-Language-Hearing Association. They pro-vide guidance on use of specific practice procedures but are not offi-cial standards of the Association.

Introduction

Frequency modulated (FM) systems/auditory trainers[1] have been standard equipment for children with hearing loss in educational settings for many years. The improvement of the signal-to-noise ratio in noisy and reverberant environments has been recognized as the primary advantage of FM use (Ross, 1992). Technological advances have widened the application of these devices. Use of FM systems has been reported for children and adults with hearing loss, as well as for persons with normal hearing who exhibit disorders of articulation, auditory processing and learning, and language (ASHA, 1991d; Bess, Klee, & Culbertson, 1986; Blake, Field, Foster, Platt, & Wertz, 1991; Cargill & Flexer, 1989; Loose, 1984; Pfeffer, 1992; Ross, 1992; Smith, McConnell, Walter, & Miller, 1985), although these guidelines do not address those latter applications. The availability and use of FM systems have increased as a result of Public Law 101–336, the Ameri-cans with Disabilities Act, and PL 101–476, the Individual with Disabilities Education Act (IDEA) and Section 504 of the Rehabilitation Act of 1973. All of these mandate access to technology for persons with hearing/communication deficits in order to reduce communication barriers.

The FM system has been shown to present approximately 15–20 dB greater intensity of the speech signal than back-ground noise at the ear of the listener (Hawkins, 1984). The increase in the signal-to-noise ratio is needed to maximize auditory capabilities (especially speech understanding), lan-guage learning, and the resultant academic success for chil-dren (Ross & Giolas, 1971; Ross, Giolas, & Carver, 1973).

Achieving the most effective use of residual hearing may best be accomplished when an FM system is considered early in the process of fitting amplification. In fact, consider-ation of the FM system as the primary amplification system rather than as a supplemental system has been suggested (Madell, 1992a, b; Maxon & Smaldino, 1991). Reported addi-tional benefits of an improved signal-to-noise ratio include increased attention span, reduced distractibility, and increased sound awareness/discrimination (Blake et al., 1991; Caster-line, Flexer, & DePompei, 1989; Flexer, 1989; Stach, Loiselle, & Jerger, 1987).

Although FM systems are of potential benefit for many listeners in a variety of settings and applications, certain cautions/issues need to be considered:

1. Little regulatory consumer protection has been mandat-ed because most states do not classify these devices as hearing aids.
2. FM systems are available commercially, and many are purchased without consultation with an audiologist.
3. The American National Standards Institute has not yet issued a standard for performance measurements of FM systems.
4. No guidelines are currently available for the selection, evaluation, and fitting of FM systems for persons with hearing loss or for use by persons with normal hearing.
5. Researchers have raised concerns regarding specific problems related to electroacoustic performance factors, for example, variability, nonlinearity, lack of stability, coupling and maintenance (Hawkins & Schum, 1985; Thibodeau, 1990; Thibodeau & Saucedo, 1991).
6. Candidacy, effectiveness of fit, cost and lifestyles, needs and aesthetics are important concerns and must be con-sidered on an individual basis.

By addressing these issues as well as the benefits and lim-itations of FM systems, the audiologist facilitates their suc-cessful use.

Scope

This paper provides guidelines for fitting and monitoring of personal and self-contained FM systems for children and adults with hearing loss.[2] Included are preselection and

---

Source: From *ASHA Desk Reference for Audiology and Speech-Language Pathology, II,* pp. 107–120. Copyright 1994 by American Speech-Language-Hearing Association. Available for sale from ASHA Fullfillment Operations (301-897-5700 x218). Reprinted by permission.

Reference this material as: American Speech-LanguageHearing Association. (1994, March). Guidelines for fitting and monitoring FM systems. *Asha, 36* (Suppl. 12), pp. l-9.

[1]FM systems are also called auditory trainers. Traditionally the term *auditory trainer* has been used to refer to hard-wired, FM, infrared, or any amplification system other than a personal hearing aid. Because of the ambiguous nature of the term, only *FM systems* will be used in this guidelines paper.

[2]Currently, one ear-level FM system is available. That system could be classified as a self-contained FM system, and the basic protocol out-lined herein can be used. These guidelines were not intended to address selection, evaluation, fitting, and monitoring of sound-field systems.

management considerations for the use of FM systems, as well as recommended procedures for performance measurements. The appropriate personnel responsible for selecting, fitting, and monitoring are defined. The committee acknowledges the complexity and the continuing evolution of FM technology. In that it is not possible to consider every configuration of design and implementation, these guidelines are intentionally limited in scope. They supersede that portion of the Position Statement: Definitions and Competencies of Aural Rehabilitation, III., C., Evaluation of Personal and Group Amplification and Other Sensory Aids (ASHA, 1984).

Personnel

The audiologist is the professional who is uniquely qualified to select, evaluate, fit, and dispense FM systems. Section IIA of the ASHA Code of Ethics (ASHA, 1992) states that "Individuals shall engage in the provision of clinical services only when they hold the appropriate Certificate of Clinical Competence or when they are in the certification process and are supervised by an individual who holds the appropriate Certificate of Clinical Competence." IIB of the Code of Ethics further states that "Individuals shall engage in only those aspects of the profession that are within the scope of their competence, considering their level of education, training, and experience." In an "Issues in Ethics" statement (ASHA, 1991a) it was further clarified that "Services relating to evaluating, selecting, fitting, or dispensing hearing aids and other amplification devices shall be provided only by individuals who hold the CCC-A" (A.5). Daily monitoring checks by other personnel (including speech-language pathologists, teachers, etc.) are appropriate after such personnel have received instruction in monitoring techniques from a certified audiologist.

Preferred Practice Patterns for Professions of Speech-Language Pathology and Audiology (ASHA, 1993a), specifically 9.0 (Aural Rehabilitation), 10.0 (Product Dispensing), 11.0 (Product Repair/Modification), 25.0 (Hearing Aid Assessment), and 25.1 (Assistive Listening System/Device Selection), are consistent with these guidelines.

Other ASHA policies and reports have addressed the appropriateness of the audiologist as the professional qualified to select, evaluate, and fit amplification devices. They include Amplification as a Remediation Technique for Children With Normal Peripheral Hearing (ASHA, 1991b), The Use of FM Amplification Instruments for Infants and Preschool Children With Hearing Impairment (ASHA, 1991d), Scope of Practice: Speech-Language Pathology and Audiology (ASHA, 1990), Guidelines for Graduate Education in Amplification (ASHA, 1991c), and Guidelines for Audiology Services in the Schools (ASHA, 1993b). Federal regulations 34 FR Chapter II § 300.13 (Federal Register, 1992a) and 34 FR Chapter III § 303.12 (Federal Register, 1992b) further define and support the audiologist's role in the evaluation and habilitation of the population aged 0–21.

Preselection Considerations

Before selecting an FM system for personal use, it is necessary to assess the present level of receptive (auditory com-

munication) function and to identify other factors related to device use. Implicit in the preliminary stages is determining whether to use a personal FM system (coupled to one's own hearing aids) or a self-contained FM system (coupled directly to the ear). If a personal FM system is being considered, hearing aids should be chosen with appropriate coupling capabilities and flexibility to maximally interface with the FM system. For instance, the hearing aids should have strong telecoils, and direct audio input may be desirable as well. In addition, hearing aid switch options (such as M/T/MT) must be carefully considered so as to provide flexibility in listening arrangements. Alternatively, if a self-contained system is going to be used, appropriate decisions should be made relative to the necessary gain and output requirements for that listener.

Other factors to be considered in the preselection process include

- the person's ability to wear, adjust, and manage the device;
- support available in the educational setting (e.g., in-service to teachers, classmates);
- acceptance of the device;
- appropriate situations and/or settings for use;
- time schedule for use;
- compatibility with personal hearing aids and other audio sources as well as options for coupling;
- individual device characteristics and accessories;
- external source interference (e.g., pagers, radio stations, computers, etc.);
- cost and accessibility;
- legislative mandates.

Assessments may include, but are not limited to, audiological evaluations, observations of auditory performance in representative settings, consultations with the user or others knowledgeable of the user's performance, questionnaires and scales, hands-on demonstration, and a trial period.

The issue of potential damage to the auditory mechanism should be considered when fitting any assistive listening device. This is of special concern when considering the fitting of an FM system to a person with normal hearing or mild fluctuating hearing loss.

Management

I. Orientation

The subject's (and family's) ability to accept and use an FM system depends upon several factors, including but not limited to (a) a hands-on demonstration of the FM system and its types and components, and (b) the training of personnel (e.g., speech-language pathologists, teachers) in its appropriate use and troubleshooting.

A hands-on demonstration session provides the user and family an opportunity to assess the components of the FM system(s) as they relate to specific needs. This session serves to establish the user/family's role in (re)habilitation.

The audiologist is responsible for the training of individual(s) responsible for the use and maintenance of the FM system. As part of this training, the audiologist should ensure that the modes of use (i.e., FM only/FM plus environment/environment only) are understood by the user and family as well as the support personnel.

Trial periods and return policies vary by manufacturer and by state and local laws. Applicable policies should be investigated and discussed with the user and family. Research on the trial use of FM systems in the home with parents and toddlers (Benoit, 1989) and with college students (Flexer, Wray, Black, & Millin, 1987) suggests that acceptance and compliance may depend on the user's knowledge of how the system works in relation to the hearing loss and the perception that the benefits outweigh the risks. In light of this, the audiologist may choose to make available loaner and/or rental equipment.

2. Monitoring

A. Daily. It is well documented that malfunctions of FM systems occur in normal-use situations (Bess, Sinclair, & Riggs, 1984; Hoverstein, 1981; Maxon & Brackett, 1981). Daily monitoring is required to determine if the device is functioning properly. This daily check can be performed by the user, parent, teacher, speech-language pathologist, or any one who has received appropriate training by the audiologist.

Generally, a daily check consists of visual inspection of the device and its coupling, followed by listening to the sound quality of the device. In a sense, the user monitors sound quality continuously and may well detect such problems as intermittent function or a condition that "doesn't sound normal." However, an individual with normal hearing also should perform a listening check. This ensures detection of more subtle problems that the user may not identify. If possible, the listening check should be performed in the room/location where it will be used so that any interference will be detected.

The user or other appropriate individuals should have accessory supplies available to remedy routine problems as they occur. These supplies typically include such items as spare microphones, button receivers, boots, batteries, cords, and neckloops.

If a malfunction persists or otherwise cannot be identified and remedied through the daily check procedure, the audiologist should be notified.

B. Comprehensive Monitoring. Periodic monitoring by the audiologist may include on-site tests, such as electroacoustic analysis, probe microphone measurements, and troubleshooting measures. These procedures may be performed at any time, that is, whenever an unresolved problem is identified during the daily check. In any case, such procedures should be implemented at least once a year. With children it is advisable to monitor on a more frequent basis (at least semiannually).

At this writing, there is no electroacoustic measurement standard procedure for FM systems. However, many manufacturers make these measurements and provide the results with their devices. Therefore, until a measurement standard procedure is available, devices should be evaluated at least according to the measurement procedures used by the manufacturer, which are typically those of ANSI S3.22 (1987) Specifications of Hearing Aid Characteristics. Measurements such as full-on gain, SSPL90, harmonic distortion,

and so forth, should be obtained and should be compared to the manufacturer's values. Both the FM and environmental microphone(s) should be evaluated separately, with care taken to properly position the FM microphone transmitter in relation to the test signal source.

C. Audiologic Re-Evaluation. Periodic evaluations of hearing and performance with the FM device are necessary to monitor stability of hearing, appropriate device settings, function, and degree of benefit. These evaluations should be performed at least annually for adults and semiannually when the device is worn by a child.

These assessments may include, but are not limited to, audiologic evaluations, coupler and real ear performance measurements, assessments of speech recognition, consultations, observations of performance in normal-use settings, questionnaires, and subjective scales of performance benefit.

Performance Measurements

In spite of the widespread use of FM systems in educational and other environments, little attention has been directed toward specific methods of measurements and fitting. Often the typical methods used with personal hearing aids have been used. These approaches may be appropriate in some aspects, but they have distinct limitations. Although there are no validated procedures for measurement and fitting of FM systems, several recent approaches have been proposed and can form the basis for a guideline for clinical assessment of these devices.

Types of Performance Measurements. There are two basic reasons for obtaining performance measurements with an FM system: (a) adjustment of control settings (e.g., SSPL90, tone controls) on the FM system to achieve the desired output, gain, and frequency response, and (b) assessment of speech recognition ability with the FM system.

Two methods will be described that allow adjustment of the control settings. One involves adjusting the FM system's electroacoustic characteristics in a 2cm^3 coupler, and the other uses real-ear measurements with a probe-microphone unit. Speech recognition ability can be assessed with the FM system and compared to performance with hearing aids by using specific sound-field arrangements and appropriate signal-to-noise ratios. After several general principles are discussed, each of these approaches will be described below and a recommended approach provided.

General Principles in Assessment of FM Systems. Although FM systems are amplification devices similar to hearing aids, there are some distinct differences that need to be taken into account in developing measurement strategies. First, and perhaps most important, the input level of speech to the FM microphone is more intense than to the hearing aid microphone. With the FM microphone appropriately located 6–8 inches from the talker's mouth, the overall level of speech is approximately 80–85 dB SPL (Cornelisse, Gagne & Seewald, 1991; Hawkins, 1984; Lewis, 1991; Lewis, Feigin, Karasek & Stelmachowicz, 1991). This is 10–20 dB more intense than the typically assumed 60–70 dB SPL input to the microphone of the personal hearing aid 1–2 meters from the talker. This fact has important implications in the assessment and fitting of FM systems. If output measurements are being made to adjust and fit FM systems, then typical input levels should be used. This is particularly important given that most FM microphone transmitters employ some type of input compression. The gain and output of the FM system may be quite different if lower-level signals, which are not representative of the speech input to the FM microphone, are used in the measurement procedure.

A second issue relates to the increased complexity of the FM systems compared with hearing aids. Many FM systems have several microphone input possibilities. These include lapel, lavalier, boom, and conference microphones for the transmitter and ear-level or body-worn microphones at the receiver. There may be one or two environmental microphones, and they may be omnidirectional or directional. It is important that each input channel in the FM system to be evaluated and that the microphones be positioned in the proper manner. Input levels may need to be altered for different microphone types and locations.

In a similar vein, the FM system may have more than one volume control wheel (VCW). Some units have one VCW for the FM signal and one for the environmental microphone(s). On personal FM systems, there will be one VCW for the FM system and one for the personal hearing aid. In addition, there may be a VCW on the FM microphone transmitter. It is important that careful thought be given to the setting of these VCWs, as certain combinations can produce undesired results (Hawkins & Schum, 1985; Hawkins & Van Tasell, 1982; Lewis, 1991, 1992).

Finally, modifications must be made in some testing procedures to account for the way certain systems are physically arranged on the user. For instance, if a personal FM system with a neck loop is to be evaluated in a 2-cm^3 coupler, then the hearing aid (attached to the coupler) and neck loop must be located appropriately on a person (preferably the user) if the measurements are to be valid.

Electroacoustic Measures in a 2-cm^3 Coupler for Fitting and Adjustment of FM Systems. Measurements of the FM system in a 2-cm^3 coupler can be used to adjust the FM system for appropriate amplification characteristics for an individual user. The use of 2-cm^3 coupler measurements to achieve this purpose has been described in detail by Lewis et al. (1991) and Seewald and Moodie (1992). In this approach one important assumption must be made: the personal hearing aids are functioning properly and have been adjusted to meet the client's amplification needs. If this assumption can be made or verified, then the task becomes one of adjusting the FM system so that it performs similarly to the hearing aid, given the differences in input levels described earlier.[3,4] The following brief outline gives an overview of the approach for such adjustments and is a modified version of that proposed by Seewald and Moodie (1992) and discussed by Lewis et al. (1991). For complete details, see Insert 1.

I. Determine that the user's personal hearing aids are functioning properly and have been set appropriately.

2. Measure critical electroacoustic characteristics on the personal hearing aid: (a) SSPL90, (b) output of the hearing aid with a 65 dB SPL input at user VCW position and control settings. The measures of maximum output and output for typical inputs will serve as targets for the adjustment of the FM system.

3. Place the microphone of the FM system in the calibrated test position. Couple the external receiver of the FM system to the 2-cm^3 coupler appropriately. Obtain an SSPL90 curve and adjust the maximum output control on the FM system until the SSPL90 curve most closely matches that obtained with the hearing aid alone in #2 above.

4. Using an 80 dB SPL input to the FM microphone, adjust the FM VCW and tone control(s) until the 2-cm^3 coupler output levels most closely match those obtained for the hearing aid alone in #2 above. Note that output is being matched, not gain. The gain of the FM system will be less than that of the hearing aid, because of input levels. (If a personal FM system is being used, leave the hearing aid VCW at the user setting and adjust only the FM VCW until the closest match is obtained.) When the closest match has been achieved, harmonic distortion measurements should be obtained and a careful listening check performed to verify that the adjusted control settings on the FM system produce a clear and undistorted speech signal.

If a self-contained FM system is being used, the environmental microphone(s) portion of the FM system should be assessed using the same input levels as were used above with the hearing aids alone. The SSPL90 measured in the environmental-microphone mode may be different from that measured in the FM-only mode. As a result, the audiologist should recheck the FM-only SSPL90 if the control has been adjusted during the environmental microphone assessment. For many FM systems there is only one VCW on the FM receiver that affects the level of both the FM signal and the environmental microphone(s). Under these circumstances, a decision will have to be made regarding which input mode will be adjusted. The decision can be modified in cases through the use of a control that affects the level of the FM signal relative to the environmental microphone signal. For some systems, there are VCWs for both the FM and the environmental microphone(s); in these cases the two can be adjusted independently. The reader is referred to Lewis (1993) and Lewis et al. (1991) for a discussion of the issue of how to conceptualize the adjustment of the FM signal relative to the environmental microphone signal.

Real-Ear Measurements for Fitting and Adjustment of FM Systems. Two approaches have been used to fit and adjust FM systems using assessment of real-ear performance: functional gain or aided sound-field thresholds, and probe-microphone measurements. While behavioral measurements of real-ear performance such as functional gain have been recommended by some investigators (Madell, 1992b; Turner & Holte, 1985; Van Tasell, Mallinger, & Crump,

---

[3]For self-contained FM systems that use earbuds or walkman-type headsets, probe microphone measures may be preferred because those receivers cannot be coupled adequately to the 2-cm^3 coupler.

[4]It is important to use the same type of signal (such as pure tones or speech-weighted noise) when making measurements on the hearing aid and FM system for comparison purposes.

1986), several distinct limitations of this approach have been described recently (Lewis et al., 1991; Seewald & Moodie, 1992). The major problem with the functional gain approach is that the input levels to the FM microphone at the aided threshold will typically be quite low during the measurement procedure. These lower input levels will not be representative of the talker's voice entering the FM microphone during actual use of the FM system. These input level differences, combined with the fact that most FM microphone-transmitters incorporate input compression, make the aided sound field threshold values difficult to interpret. While the threshold values would represent the lowest intensity signal that the user could detect with the FM system, they would lead to an overestimate of both the amount of gain of the FM signal under normal use conditions and the sensation level at which speech would be present (Lewis et al., 1991; Seewald, Hudson, Gagne, & Zelisko, 1992; Seewald & Moodie, 1992).

The limitations of behavioral testing, along with the inability to assess the maximum output of the FM system with threshold measurements, have led to an increasing emphasis on the use of probe-microphone measurements. Using this approach, the real-ear gain/frequency response and maximum output can be assessed with realistic input levels. Details on various approaches can be found in Hawkins (1987), Lewis et al. (1991), Mueller, Hawkins, and Northern (1992), and Seewald and Moodie (1992).

One approach to probe-microphone measurements is similar to that described above for 2-cm^3 coupler measurements. The task is to match the real-ear output of the FM system using appropriate input levels to the real-ear output of the user's personal hearing aid. Again, the assumption must be made that the personal hearing aid is functioning acceptably. A second approach is to determine what amplification characteristics are desirable and adjust the FM system to best match that goal, regardless of the performance of the personal hearing aid. If this latter approach is used, then a procedure that specifies goals for real-ear maximum output and aided output levels for speech is needed. One such procedure is the Desired Sensation Level (DSL) approach described by Seewald, Zelisko, Ramji, and Jamieson (1991).

An example of how probe-microphone measurements can be made with FM systems is briefly outlined below (see Insert 2 for a detailed description).

1. The FM microphone is placed in the calibrated spot in front of the sound-field loudspeaker of the probe-microphone system (exactly how this is accomplished may depend on the particular probe-microphone system being used) or next to the controlling microphone of the probe system (Hawkins, 1987).
2. The probe-microphone tube is placed in the ear canal of the client and the FM receiver is set to receive only the FM signal. A real-ear SSPL90 curve, or Real Ear Saturation Response (RESR) is obtained. (NOTE: Care should be exercised in making this measurement so as to prevent exces-

sive output levels in the ear and to avoid discomfort; for the first RESR measurements, the output control should be set to the minimum position.) The output control is adjusted until the desired RESR is obtained (see Hawkins, 1992, for more details), which could be either the RESR of the personal hearing aid or an independently generated target value. An alternative to directly measuring the RESR has been outlined by Sullivan (1987) and described further by Hawkins (1992, 1993).

3. Using an 80 dB SPL input to the FM microphone, adjust the FM VCW and tone control(s) until the desired output levels in the ear canal are obtained. If a personal FM system is used, the hearing aid VCW should be set to the typical use position, and the FM VCW should be adjusted for the desired output levels.
4. If an environmental microphone(s) is present, turn off the FM microphone and obtain an RESR measurement through the environmental microphone mode. (If an adjustment to the SSPL90 control is necessary, the FM-only measurement should be repeated to determine if it is still appropriate.) Repeat #3 using 65 dB SPL input. As described earlier, if only one VCW exists on the FM receiver and it controls both the level of the FM signal and the environmental microphone(s), then a decision must be made as to where the single setting will be. If separate VCWs are present for the FM signal and environmental microphone(s), then the environmental microphone VCW can be adjusted to appropriate level relative to the FM signal (see Lewis, 1993, and Lewis et al., 1991, for more discussion of this issue).

Speech Recognition Testing With FM Systems. It is often necessary and/or desirable to assess the speech recognition ability of a user with an FM system. It may also be important to compare such performance with that obtained using a personal hearing aid(s). Lewis et al. (1991) have described a procedure for making assessments of speech recognition ability with FM systems and hearing aids in a sound booth. A brief outline of this procedure follows (see Insert 3 for a detailed description).

1. For the hearing aid assessment, speech recognition is assessed with a speech signal of 55 dB HL and in a background noise of 50 dB HL, yielding a S/N ratio of +5 dB, a value typical of many elementary school classrooms (Crandell & Smaldino, 1993; Finitzo-Hieber, 1988; Markides, 1986). Assuming the sound field has been calibrated for a 45-degree azimuth, the intensity of the speech would be 68 dB SPL, a level that should be typical of the input to the hearing aid microphone.[5] A measure of speech recognition is obtained with an age- and language-appropriate test.
2. To assess performance with the FM system, the user is removed from the sound booth and placed next to the audiologist at the audiometer. The FM microphone is

---

[5]Instead of using the plus and minus 45-degree azimuth loudspeaker arrangement, the audiologist may prefer that speech originate from 0 degrees and noise from 180 degrees. This would eliminate the possibility of a head shadow effect for either the speech or noise in the case of monaural fitting. If the 0/180 arrangement is used and the sound field is calibrated with the appropriate 17 dB reference, then the speech signal can be presented at 50 dB HL (67 dB SPL) and the noise at 45 dB HL (62 dB SPL).

placed in the calibrated spot in the sound field where the user was earlier seated. The noise remains at 50 dB HL, but the speech signal is increased to 70 dB HL (83 dB SPL). This 15 dB increase in speech intensity (from 55 to 70 dB HL) is equivalent to the increase in SPL that occurs at the FM microphone (Hawkins, 1984). A speech recognition score is now obtained under these conditions. The effective S/N ratio at the FM microphone is +20 dB and represents the actual situation that would exist at the FM microphone.

It should be noted that the above testing arrangement addresses speech recognition performance in the FM-only mode, that is, the environmental microphone(s) are not active. If the performance of the FM system's environmental microphones are to be assessed without the FM signal present, then the measurement should be made under the hearing aid-only protocol. Assessment of the FM system with the FM signal and environmental microphone(s) requires a different arrangement. The physical arrangement for the hearing aid-only assessment is used with two important exceptions (see Insert 3, Figure 3–C, for more details). The user wears the FM receiver with the FM and environmental microphone(s) active. The FM microphone is located at a position in front of the loudspeaker that produces a speech input of 83 dB SPL to the FM microphone. A potential problem may exist with this physical arrangement, as the high-frequency input to the FM microphone can be reduced at this close location in front of the loudspeaker (Lewis et al., 1991).

Conclusion. These guidelines were developed to provide direction to audiologists in the selection and fitting of FM systems. The committee recognizes the complexity of the technology (including microphone and coupling strategies) and the many unresolved issues of measurement (including input stimulus type and level). These guidelines should be viewed as a reflection of the current understanding of these issues. Future technology and research will mandate consideration of alternate approaches and tools.

References

American National Standards Institute. (1987). Specifications of hearing aid characteristics (ANSI §3.22). New York: ANSI.

American Speech-Language-Hearing Association. (1984). Definition of and competencies for aural rehabilitation. Rockville, MD: ASHA.

American Speech-Language-Hearing Association. (1990, April). Scope of practice, speech-language pathology and audiology. *Asha* (Suppl. 2), pp. 1–2.

American Speech-Language-Hearing Association. (1991a, December). Issues in ethics. *Asha*, p. 51.

American Speech-Language-Hearing Association. (1991b, January). Amplification as a remediation technique for children with normal peripheral hearing. *Asha* (Suppl. 3), pp. 22–24.

American Speech-Language-Hearing Association. (1991c, March). Guidelines for graduate education in amplification. *Asha* (Suppl. 5), pp. 35–36.

American Speech-Language-Hearing Association. (1991d, March). The use of FM amplification instruments for infants and preschool children with hearing impairment. *Asha* (Suppl. 5), pp. 1–2.

American Speech-Language-Hearing Association. (1992, March). Code of ethics. *Asha* (Suppl. 9), pp. 1–2.

American Speech-Language-Hearing Association. (1993a, March). Preferred practice patterns for the professions of speech-language pathology and audiology. *Asha* (Suppl. 11).

American Speech-Language-Hearing Association. (1993b, March). Guidelines for audiology services in the schools. *Asha* (Suppl. 10), pp. 24–32.

Benoit, R. (1989). Home use of the FM amplification systems during the early childhood years. *Hearing Instruments, 40,* 8–12.

Bess, F., Klee, T., & Culbertson, J. (1986). Identification, assessment and management of children with unilateral sensorineural hearing loss. *Ear and Hearing, 7(1),* 43–51.

Bess, F., Sinclair, J., & Riggs, D. (1984). Group amplification in schools for the hearing impaired. *Ear and Hearing, 5,* 138–143.

Blake, R., Field, B., Foster, C., Platt, F., & Wertz, P. (1991). Effect of FM auditory trainers on attending behaviors of learning-disabled children. *Language, Speech, and Hearing Services in the Schools, 22,* 111–114.

Cargill, S., & Flexer, C. (1989). Issues in fitting FM units to children with unilateral hearing losses; Two case studies [Monograph]. *Journal of the Educational Audiology Association, 1(1),* 30–47.

Casterline, C., Flexer, C., & DePompei, R. (1989). *Use of assistive listening devices with head injured survivors.* Paper presented at the meeting of the American Speech-Language-Hearing Association, St. Louis, MO.

Cornelisse, L.E., Gagne, J.P., & Seewald, R.C. (1991). Long term average speech spectrum at the chest level microphone location. *Canadian Journal of Speech-Language Pathology and Audiology, 15(3),* 7–12.

Crandell, C., & Smaldino, J. (in press). The importance of room acoustics. In R. Tyler (Ed.), *Assistive listening devices.*

Federal Register. (1992a). 34 FR Chapter II § 300.16, Vol. 57, No. 189, p. 44303.

Federal Register. (1992b). 34 FR Chapter III § 303.12, Vol. 57, No. 85, p. 18993.

Finitzo-Hieber, T. (1988). Classroom acoustics. In R. Roeser (Ed.), *Auditory disorders in school children* (2nd ed., pp. 221–233). New York: Thieme-Stratton.

Flexer, C. (1989). Turn on sound: An odyssey of sound field amplification. *Educational Audiology Association Newsletter, 5,* 6.

Flexer, C., Wray, D., Black, T., & Millin, J. (1987). Amplification devices: Evaluating classroom effectiveness for moderately hearing-impaired college students. *Volta Review, 89(7),* 347–57.

Hawkins, D. (1984). Comparisons of speech recognition in noise by mildly to moderately hearing-impaired children using hearing aids and FM systems. *Journal of Speech and Hearing Disorders, 49(4),* 409–418.

Hawkins, D. (1987). Assessment of FM systems with probe tube microphone system. *Ear and Hearing, 8(5),* 301–303.

Hawkins, D. (1992). Selecting SSPL90 using probe-microphone measurements. In H. Mueller, D. Hawkins, & J. Northern (Eds.), *Probe microphone measurements: Hearing aid selection and assessment* (pp. 145–158). San Diego, CA: Singular Publishing Group.

Hawkins, D.B. (1993). Assessment of hearing aid maximum output. *American Journal of Audiology, 2(1),* 36–37.

Hawkins, D., & Schum, D. (1985). Some effects of FM-system coupling on hearing aid characteristics. *Journal of Speech and Hearing Disorders, 50(2),* 132–141.

Hawkins, D., & Van Tasell, D. (1982). Electroacoustic characteristics of personal FM systems. *Journal of Speech and Hearing Disorders, 47(4),* 335–362.

Hoverstein, G.H. (1981). A public school audiology program: Amplification maintenance, auditory management, and inservice education. In F.H. Bess, B.A. Freeman, & J.S. Sinclair (Eds.), *Amplification in education* (pp. 224–247). Washington, DC: A.G. Bell Publishers.

Lewis, D. (1991). FM systems and assistive devices: Selection and evaluation, In J.A. Feigin & P.G. Stelmachowicz (Eds.), *Pediatric amplification: Proceedings of the 1991 National Conference* (pp. 115-138). Omaha, NE.

Lewis, D.E. (1992). FM systems. *Ear and Hearing, 13*(5), 290–293.

Lewis, D. (in press). Assistive devices for classroom listening: FM systems. *American Journal of Audiology.*

Lewis, D., Feigin, J., Karasek, A., & Stelmachowicz, P. (1991). Evaluation and assessment of FM systems. *Ear and Hearing, 12*(4), 268–280.

Loose, F. (1984). *Learning disabled students use FM wireless systems.* Rochester, MN: Telex Communications.

Madell, J.R. (1992a). FM systems as a primary amplification for children with profound hearing loss. *Ear and Hearing, 13*(2), 102–107.

Madell, J.R. (1992b). FM systems for children birth to age 5. In M. Ross (Ed.), *FM auditory training systems: Characteristics, selection, and use* (pp. 15–174). Timonium, MD: York Press.

Markides, A. (1986). Speech levels and speech-to-noise ratios. *British Journal of Audiology, 20,* 115–120.

Maxon, A.B., & Brackett, D. (1981). Mainstreaming hearing-impaired children. *Audio Journal for Continuing Education, 6,* 10.

Maxon, A.B., & Smaldino, J. (1991). Hearing aid management in children. In C. Flexer (Ed.), *Current audiologic issues in educational management of children with hearing loss.* New York: Seminars in Hearing.

Mueller, H.G., Hawkins, D.B., & Northern, J. (1992). Probe microphone measurements: Hearing aid selection and assessment. San Diego, CA: Singular Publishing Group.

Pfeffer, E.B. (1992). Alternate uses for FM systems. In M. Ross (Ed.), *FM auditory training systems: Characteristics, selection, and use* (pp. 211–224). Timonium, MD: York Press.

Ross, M. (Ed.). (1992). *FM auditory training systems: Characteristics, selection and use.* Timonium, MD: York Press.

Ross, M., & Giolas, T. (1971). Effect of three classroom listening conditions on speech intelligibility. *American Annals of the Deaf, 116,* 580–584.

Ross, M., Giolas, T., & Carver, D. (1973). Effect of three classroom listening conditions on speech intelligibility. A replication in part. *Language, Speech, Hearing Services in Schools, 4,* 72–76.

Seewald, R., Hudson, S., Gagne, J., & Zelisko, D. (1992). Comparison of two methods for estimating the sensation level of amplified speech. *Ear and Hearing, 13*(3), 142–149.

Seewald, R., & Moodie, K. (1992). Electroacoustic considerations. In M. Ross (Ed.), *FM auditory training systems: Characteristics, selection, and use* (pp. 75–102). Timonium, MD: York Press.

Seewald, R., Zelisko, D., Ramji, K., & Jamieson, D. (1991). *DSL 3.0 user's manual.* London, Ontario, Canada: University of Western Ontario.

Smith, D., McConnell, J., Walter, T., & Miller, S. (1985). Effect of using an auditory trainer on the attentional, language, and social behaviors of autistic children. *Journal of Autism Developmental Disorders, 15,* 285–302.

Stach, B.A., Loiselle, L.H., & Jerger, J.F. (1987). FM systems used by children with central processing disorders. Paper presented at the annual convention of the American Speech-Language-Hearing Association, New Orleans, LA.

Sullivan, R. (1987). Aided SSPL90 response in the real ear: A safe estimate. *Hearing Instruments, 38,* 36.

Thibodeau, L. (1990). Electroacoustic performance of direct-input hearing aids with FM amplification systems. *Language, Speech and Hearing Services in the Schools, 21,* 49–56.

Thibodeau, L., & Saucedo, K. (1991). Consistency of electroacoustic characteristics across components of FM systems. *Journal of Speech and Hearing Research, 34*(4), 628–635.

Turner, C., & Holte, L. (1985). Evaluation of FM amplification systems. *Hearing Instruments, 36,* 6–12, 56.

Van Tasell, D., Mallinger, C., & Crump, E. (1986). Functional gain and speech recognition with two types of FM amplification. *Language Speech and Hearing Services in Schools, 17,* 28–37.

Insert 1—Outline for FM System Adjustment Using 2 cm³ Coupler Measurements

1. Verify through coupler measurements and/or probe-microphone measurements that the client's hearing aid is functioning properly and has been fitted appropriately for the hearing loss.
2. Obtain 2 cm³ measurements on the client's personal hearing aid.
   a. Obtain an SSPL90 curve using a 90 dB SPL swept pure tone with the hearing aid VCW full-on.
   b. Adjust the hearing aid VCW to the use position. Using a 65 dB SPL input, obtain an output (not gain) curve in the 2 cm³ coupler.
3. Set up the FM system for 2 cm³ coupler measurements (See Figure 1–A).
   a. Place the FM microphone in the calibrated test position.
   b. With the FM receiver outside the test box, set the receiver for FM-only reception. Attach the button or behind-the-ear (BTE) receiver to the HA-2 2 cm³ coupler. Maintain a minimum distance of 2 ft between the FM transmitter and receiver.
   c. If a personal FM system is used, connect the FM receiver to the personal hearing aid (also located outside the test box) via the coupling method that the client will use (direct audio input, neck loop, or silhouette). If a neck loop is used, the hearing aid should be placed on the client (or other person of similar size, if possible, if the client is not available) and the earhook connected to the HA-2 2 cm³ coupler (or individual earmold connected to the HA-1 2 cm³ coupler) which is held next to the client's ear (see Figure 1–B).
4. Adjust the FM system SSPL90 to match the personal hearing aid SSPL90.
   a. Turn the FM receiver VCW full-on (also turn the personal hearing aid VCW full-on if a personal FM system is being evaluated) and obtain an SSPL90 curve with a 90 dB SPL pure-tone sweep.
   b. Adjust the FM systems SSPL90 control until the SSPL90 curve most closely matches that of the personal hearing aid (#2 above).

5. Adjust the FM system output and frequency response to match the personal hearing aid.
   a. Using an 80 dB SPL input delivered to the FM microphone in the test box, adjust the FM receiver VCW and tone control(s) until the 2 cm³ coupler output (not gain) most closely matches the output obtained with the personal hearing aid (#2b above).
   b. With a personal FM system, leave the hearing aid VCW and tone control(s) at the user setting and adjust only the FM receiver VCW and tone control(s) to obtain the closest match to the personal hearing aid alone response (#2b above).
6. Measure the maximum output and frequency response of the environmental microphone(s) if a self-contained FM system is being used.
   a. Turn the FM VCW to full-on, measure the SSPL90, and adjust as necessary. If the SSPL90 control is changed, measure the FM-only SSPL90 again and determine if readjustment is needed.
   b. Measure the output using a 65 dB SPL input. If only one VCW exists on the FM receiver and it controls both the level of the FM signal and the environmental microphone(s), then a decision must be made as to where the single setting will be. If separate VCWs are present for the FM signal and environmental microphone(s), then the environmental microphone VCW can be adjusted to an appropriate level relative to the FM signal (see Lewis et al., 1991, and Lewis, 1993, for more discussion of this issue). If matching desired output values for the FM-only mode and environmental microphone mode leads to different control settings, priority should be given to matching the FM-only targets.
7. Measure harmonic distortion to verify acceptable values.
8. Perform a complete listening check to assure acceptable clarity and low distortion.

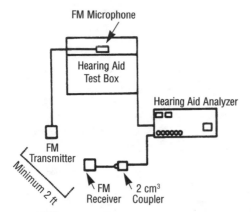

Figure 1-A. Physical arrangement for 2 cm³ coupler measurements FM systems when measuring FM transmission mode only. The FM receiver may be attached to the HA-2 2 cm³ coupler via an external button receiver, BTE receiver, or via a personal hearing aid if direct audio input or a silhouette inductor is utilized. (Adapted from Thibodeau, 1992).

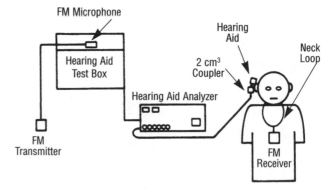

Figure 1-B. Physical arrangement for 2 cm³ coupler measurements of the FM system connected to a personal hearing aid via a neck loop. The hearing aid is set to the "T" position and the environmental microphone(s), if present, on the FM system are deactivated if possible.

Insert 2—Outline for FM System Adjustment Using Probe-Microphone Measurements

1. Determine a set of target real-ear maximum output and frequency response values through either
   a. using existing real-ear measurements obtained from an appropriately fit personal hearing aid OR
   b. a published amplification selection scheme, e.g. DSL (Seewald et al., 1991)
2. Prepare the test environment for probe-microphone measurements.
   a. The placement of the FM microphone in the sound field will depend on the specific probe-microphone system. See Figure 2–A for a possible arrangement if the probe system uses an off-line (or stored) equalization method. During equalization, the reference microphone is placed at the location of the FM microphone. During the measurements the reference microphone is disabled. If the system uses a controlling microphone for on-line equalization, it can be located near the FM microphone, as shown in Figure 2B. (Note: In this latter arrangement, if the reference microphone is near the ear, then feedback may be a problem in higher gain instruments.)
   b. Place the probe tube in the ear canal at an appropriate location, connect the FM system (set to FM only) to the client via the coupling method that will be used.
3. Adjust the FM system maximum output to the desired position.
   a. Set the maximum output control to the minimum position.
   b. Set the FM VCW to the highest level before feedback (and the client's hearing aid VCW to the highest possible use position if it is a personal FM system). Obtain a measure of the Real Ear Saturation Response (RESR) by introducing a 90 dB SPL swept tonal signal and measuring the output in the ear canal. (NOTE: Extreme care should be exercised in making this measurement so as to prevent excessive output and/or discomfort; the output control should be set to the minimum

position for the first measurement.) An alternative to directly measuring the RESR has been outlined by Sullivan (1987) and described further by Hawkins (1992, 1993).
   c. Adjust the output control until the RESR most closely matches the personal hearing aid RESR or the desired RESR targets.
4. Adjust the FM system real-ear output and frequency response for the FM signal to match the personal hearing aid values or the desired real-ear values.
   a. Using an 80 dB SPL signal delivered to the FM microphone, adjust the FM receiver VCW and tone control(s) until the desired real-ear values are most closely matched.
   b. With a personal FM system, leave the hearing aid VCW and tone control(s) at the user setting and adjust only the FM receiver VCW and tone control(s) to obtain the closest match.
5. Measure the real-ear maximum output and frequency response of the environmental microphone(s) if a self-contained FM system is being used.
   a. Turn off the FM microphone and place the user in the sound field as for probe-microphone measurements with a personal hearing aid.
   b. Adjust the FM VCW to just below feedback, measure the RESR, and adjust as necessary. If the SSPL90 control is changed, measure the FM-only RESR again and determine if readjustment is needed.
   c. Measure the real-ear output using a 65 dB SPL signal. If matching desired output values for the FM-only mode and environmental microphone mode leads to different control settings, priority should be given to matching the FM-only targets.
6. Remove the FM system from the user and measure harmonic distortion in a 2 cm^3 coupler to verify acceptable values.
7. Perform a complete listening check to assure acceptable clarity and low distortion.

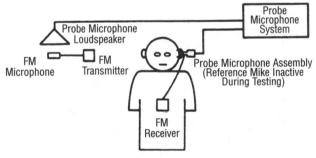

Figure 2-A. Physical arrangement for probe-microphone evaluation of FM system for the FM-only mode when the probe-microphone system uses an off-line (or stored) equalization method. During the equalization procedure the reference phone is active and located next to the FM microphone. During the actual probe measurements the reference microphone is disabled.

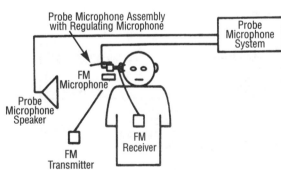

Figure 2-B. Physical arrangement for probe-microphone evaluation of FM system for the FM-only mode when the probe-microphone system uses a controlling microphone for on-line equalization.

Insert 3—Speech Recognition Measures With FM Systems and Personal Hearing Aid(s)

1. Select a speech recognition test that is appropriate for the age and language of the client.
2. Place the hearing aid(s) on the client and set up the arrangement shown in Figure 3–A.
   a. Speech is at 55 dB HL (68 dB SPL) and noise at 50 dB HL (63 dB SPL), producing a S/N ratio of +5 dB. The loudspeakers are located at plus and minus 45 degree azimuths.
   b. Obtain a speech recognition score.
3. Place the FM receiver set to FM-only on the client and set up the arrangement shown in Figure 3–B.
   a. Speech is 70 dB HL (83 dB SPL) and noise is 50 dB HL (63 dB SPL), producing a S/N ratio of +20 dB at the FM microphone. The loudspeakers are located at plus and minus 45 degrees azimuth. With directional microphones, point the microphone at the loudspeaker producing the speech signal.
   b. Obtain a speech recognition score.
4. If a speech recognition measure is desired for FM system with environmental microphone(s) active, set up the arrangement shown in Figure 3–C.
   a. Speech is 55 dB HL (68 dB SPL) at the client's location and noise is 50 dB HL (63 dB SPL), producing a S/N ratio of +5 dB at the environmental microphone(s).
   b. The FM microphone is positioned in front of the speech loudspeaker at a location designed to produce 83 dB SPL speech input to the FM microphone.

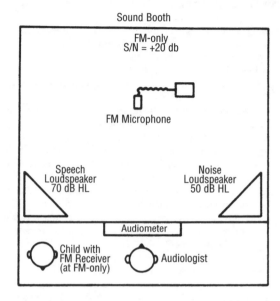

Figure 3-B. Physical arrangement in sound booth for speech recognition testing of FM system set to FM-only for comparison purposes to hearing aid(s) only.

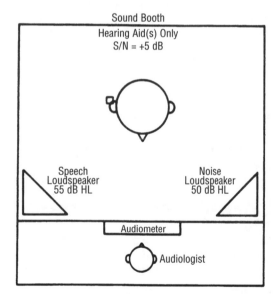

Figure 3-A. Physical arrangement in sound booth for speech recognition testing of hearing aid(s) only for comparison purposes to FM system. (Modified from Lewis et al., 1991)

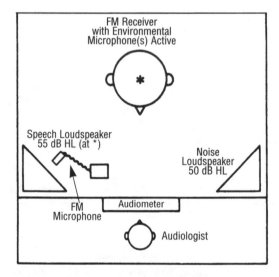

Figure 3-C. Physical arrangement in sound booth for speech recognition testing of FM system with environmental microphone(s) active. (See Lewis et al., 1991, for potential difficulties in high-frequency input to the FM microphone using this arrangement.)

Appendix 2–J

THE USE OF FM AMPLIFICATION INSTRUMENTS FOR INFANTS AND PRESCHOOL CHILDREN WITH HEARING IMPAIRMENT

Committee on Amplification for the Hearing Impaired
American Speech-Language-Hearing Association

The following position statement was adopted by the American Speech-Language-Hearing Association (ASHA) Legislative Council (LC 17-90) in November 1990. Members of ASHA's Committee on Amplification for the Hearing Impaired responsible for the development of this position statement include Thomas S. Rees, chair; G. Jean Boggess; Evelyn Cherow, ex officio; Alice E. Holmes; Barbara J. Moore-Brown; Polly E. Patrick; and Valenta G. Ward-Gravely, with the guidance of Teris K. Schery, 1988–90 vice president for clinical affairs.

Position Statement

It is the position of the American Speech-Language-Hearing Association that it is incumbent on audiologists to provide optimum amplification to young children with hearing impairment during the early years of their lives—the most critical period for speech and language development. Appropriate audiological management for these children must include selection and fitting of suitable amplification for all listening environments. Personal hearing aids may be appropriate for some communication situations, but the use of FM amplification may be necessary in other listening contexts to ensure optimal use of residual hearing.

Background

The importance of early identification and appropriate audiologic management of children with hearing impairment is well known. In order to achieve optimal use of residual hearing for the development of speech and language, a consistent and nondistorted auditory signal is necessary. The major goal in fitting amplification is to improve the signal-to-noise ratio (S/N) in order to increase the understanding of speech.

Unfortunately, the ability of personal amplification (i.e., a hearing aid) to provide an optimal speech signal to the hearing-impaired child is compromised by acoustic conditions commonly encountered in various listening environments. Speaker-to-listener distance, background noise, and reverberant room characteristics combine, resulting in a deterioration in speech recognition ability in hearing-impaired listeners regardless of age.

Very young children experience language under a variety of acoustic conditions. Typically, an infant or toddler receives close, one-to-one attention from the parent or caregiver with abundant opportunities for communicative interaction. Exposure to incidental speech that occurs naturally in the home is also critical for normal speech and language development. This incidental speech and language development does not necessarily occur in quiet nor with the infant nearby. In addition, with the rise in the use of day-care facilities, infants and toddlers may frequently encounter listening environments less suitable than the ideal, one-to-one situation. Similar acoustic conditions are known to be completely unsuitable for school-aged children with hearing impairments.

FM amplification systems have been designed to provide a solution for deleterious acoustic circumstances that listeners with hearing impairment encounter at home, in the classroom, or in many other common listening environments. The significant advantage of FM amplification over personal hearing aids has been documented for school-aged children with hearing impairments. In principle, FM listening allows a constant distance of approximately 6–8 inches to be maintained between the speaker's lips and the FM transmitter microphone. Thus, a greatly enhanced S/N is provided regardless of the distance between the child and the speaker or the acoustic environment.

In the past, FM systems have been used separately from the personal hearing aid and primarily in a formal classroom environment. Technological improvements currently allow the FM system to be coupled to the child's personal hearing aids. This provides the advantages of FM transmission while, in theory, maintaining the electroacoustic characteristics of the child's own hearing aid. These systems are also well suited for use in less structured environments.

Public Law 99-457 expands identification and education of disabled infants and toddlers, including those with hearing impairments. Appropriate audiological management for these children must include selection and fitting of suitable amplification for all listening environments. Personal hearing aids may be appropriate for some communication situations, but the use of FM amplification may be necessary in others. It is incumbent on professionals providing services to young children with hearing impairment to provide optimum amplification during the early years of life—the most critical period for speech and language development.

Appendix 2–K

ACOUSTICS IN EDUCATIONAL SETTINGS

Subcommittee on Acoustics in Educational Settings, Bioacoustics Standards & Noise Standards Committee

This position statement and these guidelines were developed by the American Speech-Language-Hearing Association (ASHA) Subcommittee on Acoustics in Educational Settings of the Bioacoustics Standards and Noise Standards Committee and approved by the ASHA Legislative Council (LC 9-94) in November 1994. Subcommittee members include Robert Burkard, chair; Daniel Ostergren, subcommittee chair; Carl Crandell; Noel Matkin; Wayne Olsen; Joseph Smaldino; Maureen Thompson, ex officio; Jo Williams, past ex officio; and Tanya Gallagher, 1992-1994 vice president for research and technology.

Position Statement

It is the position of the American Speech-Language-Hearing Association (ASHA) that all students (children and adults) be provided with appropriate acoustical environments in educational settings, to include classrooms, assembly areas, and communication-related treatment rooms. Acoustical characteristics of classrooms are of particular concern because inaccurate perception of speech in these environments is known to affect a student's attention, behavior, speech perception, and learning. If additional factors exist, such as hearing loss (even a minimal loss), learning disability, possible central auditory processing deficit, developmental delays, and/or English as a second language, a poor acoustic environment may be a primary determinant of academic success. Achieving appropriate classroom acoustics is particularly important considering the emphasis of the Americans with Disabilities Act of 1990 (Public Law 101-336) on removing barriers and improving accessibility of educational facilities.

Background

The acoustical properties of educational settings could be considered the "forgotten variables" in ensuring students' academic success, particularly for those students with unique communication or educational needs (Crum & Matkin, 1976). Factors that affect the acoustical properties of a room include the intensity and spectral/temporal characteristics of competing noise and the reverberation characteristics of the enclosure. (An additional factor is the distance between the student and the teacher; however, this is not an acoustic characteristic of the listening environment itself and shall be discussed separately.) Though researchers have well documented the deleterious effects of excessive levels of classroom noise and reverberation on

speech-recognition ability and educational/social development (Bess & Tharpe, 1986; Blair, Peterson, & Viehweg, 1985; Crandell & Bess, 1986; Crandell, 1992, 1993; Davis, Elfenbein, Schum, & Bentler, 1986; Finitzo-Hieber, 1988; Finitzo-Hieber & Tillman, 1978; Leavitt & Flexer, 1991; Ross, 1978; Ross & Giolas, 1971; Shepard, Davis, Gorga, & Stelmachowicz, 1981; Smaldino & Flexer, 1991), studies of the acoustical conditions in classrooms consistently reveal environments that exhibit excessive levels of noise and reverberation (Bess & McConnell, 1981; Crandell, 1993; Crandell & Bess, 1986, 1987; Crum, 1974; Finitzo-Hieber, 1988; Finitzo-Hieber & Tillman, 1978; McCroskey & Devens, 1975; Niemoeller, 1968; Olsen, 1977, 1981, 1988).

The term noise (or variations—background noise, classroom noise, etc.) refers to any auditory disturbance that interferes with what a listener wants to hear (Finitzo-Hieber, 1988). The source(s) of the noise may or may not be within the classroom itself, though noise generated in the classroom (such as students talking, desks/chairs sliding on noncarpeted flooring, and shuffling books and papers) is typically the most detrimental to the child, because this form of noise is spectrally similar in frequency to the desired signal (the teacher's voice). Sanders (1965) measured noise levels in 47 occupied and unoccupied classrooms in 15 buildings and noted mean occupied noise levels ranging from 52 dB(B) in classrooms for students with hearing loss to 60 dB(B) in kindergarten classrooms. Other studies have reported similar occupied noise levels (Crandell, 1992; Crandell & Smaldino, 1994; Nober & Nober, 1975; Paul 1967).

Externally generated noise from sources such as hallway traffic and heating/ventilation/air conditioning (HVAC) operation, or noise emanating from large assembly areas such as gymnasiums or cafeterias, is also present in the classroom. Mean unoccupied noise levels are typically reported to range from 45 to 60 dB(A). See Crandell and Smaldino (1992) for a review.

Whether internally or externally generated, the presence of high noise levels has led to relatively poor signal-to-noise ratios (SNRs) being measured in the classroom setting. Depending on grade level and programming, reported SNRs have ranged from +5 to –7 dB (Blair, 1977; Finitzo-Hieber, 1988; Markides, 1986; Paul, 1967; Sanders, 1965). Such values are discouraging; several investigators have noted that students with normal hearing require a +6 dB SNR for optimum communication efficiency (see Crandell, 1992). Indeed, the presence of even a minimal hearing loss (pure tone average of 15–30 dB HL) compromises speech recognition ability by 13% at +6 SNR and by 33% at –6 SNR when compared to peers with normal hearing (Crandell, 1993).

The presence of a poor SNR is not the only variable that negatively affects speech recognition in the classroom. Interference caused by reverberation, or reflected sound energy, occurs as well. Reverberation time (T) is the time differential between the cessation of vibration of the sound source and a measured decay of 60 dB. The amount of reverberation present in an enclosure increases linearly with room volume and is inversely related to the amount of sound-absorbing material present; low frequencies are typically absorbed less efficiently. (See Benarek, 1955; Borrild, 1983; or Knudsen & Harris, 1978, for specific measurement procedures for reverberation.) The degradation of speech recognition by reverberation occurs through the masking of direct sound energy by the temporally delayed reflected energy (Bolt & MacDonald, 1949; Houtgast, 1981; Kurtovic, 1975; Lochner & Burger, 1964; Nabalek & Pickett, 1974a, b). Because vowel (low frequency) sounds are more intense than consonant (high-frequency) sounds, reflected vowel phonemes tend to mask consonant information, particularly word-final consonants. Several researchers have noted that noise and reverberation combine synergistically to degrade speech recognition in classroom settings (Crandell & Bess, 1986; Crum, 1974; Nabalek, 1981; Nabalek & Pickett, 1974a, b). This effect is caused by (a) reflected noise energy causing an increase in ambient noise level and (b) integration of background noise with reflected and delayed speech energy, which makes the resulting noise more uniform both temporally and spectrally.

The measured range of reverberation for unoccupied classrooms has been shown to range from 0.4 to 1.2 seconds (Bradley, 1986; Crandell, 1992; Finitzo-Hieber, 1988; Kodaras, 1960; McCroskey & Devens, 1975; Olsen, 1988; Ross, 1978). Given that Ts longer than 0.4 seconds appear to degrade speech recognition for many listeners (Crandell & Bess, 1986; 1987a; Crum, 1974; Finitzo-Hieber & Tillman, 1978; Niemoeller, 1968; Olsen, 1977, 1981), the above-noted Ts appear to be much too long for effective speech recognition

Guidelines

In consideration of the data regarding the acoustical properties of classrooms and other learning environments, and to ensure that all students (particularly those students with specific communication/educational needs) be provided with appropriate acoustical environments in educational settings, ASHA recommends the following guidelines for acoustics in educational settings. These guidelines should be considered when adding to, remodeling, or building new schools:

1. Unoccupied classroom noise levels should not exceed 30 dB(A) or a Noise Criteria (NC) 20 dB curve (Beranek, 1954; Borrild, 1978; Crandell, 1992; Crandell & Smaldino, 1994; Fourcin et al., 1980; Gengel, 1971; Finitzo-Hieber, 1988; Finitzo-Hieber & Tillmam, 1978; Niemoeller, 1968; Olsen, 1988). This recommendation is made in order to maintain appropriate SNRs (see recommendation #2) in the classroom. Noise levels in classrooms/treatment rooms should be compared with NC curves, as this procedure provides additional information regarding the spectral characteristics of the noise;

2. SNRs at the student's ear should exceed a minimum of +15 dB (Beranek, 1954; Borrild, 1978; Crandell, 1992; Crandell & Smaldino, 1994; Fourcin et al., 1980; Gengel, 1971; Finitzo-Hieber, 1988; Finitzo-Hieber & Tillman, 1978; Niemoeller, 1968; Olsen, 1988). This guideline is based on findings that the speech recognition of listeners with hearing loss tends to remain relatively constant at SNRs in excess of +15 dB but deteriorates at poorer SNRs;

3. Reverberation times should not exceed 0.4 seconds (Crandell & Bess, 1986; Crandell, 1992; Crum, 1974; Finitzo-Hieber & Tillman, 1978; Niemoeller, 1968; Olsen, 1988). A T of 0.4 seconds is recommended based on the findings that speech recognition by listeners with hearing loss shows significant deterioration at higher Ts. It is also recommended that, whenever possible, reverberation levels be measured at a wide range of discrete frequencies, rather than at 500, 1000, and 2000 Hz only. This procedure provides additional information regarding the spectral characteristics of the reflected energy

Considerations Regarding Implementation of Guidelines #2

The above guidelines represent idealized goals for classroom acoustics and it is recognized that instrumentation/technical constraints may make it difficult to determine if a given classroom or other educational setting achieves these acoustical characteristics. In problematic situations, it may be advisable to consult with professionals in the area of acoustical measurement and analysis. Generally, however, taking steps to improve the acoustical properties of the enclosure may help to provide an adequate, if not optimal, listening environment.

A number of investigators (Crandell, 1993; Finitzo-Hieber, 1988; Nabalek & Nabalek, 1985; Olsen, 1978) have provided a discussion of methods by which background noise and reverberation may be minimized and the desired signal maximized. These include locating classrooms—particularly those intended for instruction of students with hearing loss or other educational considerations—away from external noise sources, such as adjacent traffic or construction areas, HVAC equipment, or playground areas. Effective landscaping, such as the placement of trees, shrubs, and earthen banks, may be helpful in reducing noise from these sources. Locating rooms away from busy hallways and other large group areas, such as gymnasiums and cafeterias, is critical as well. Internal acoustical treatments, such as heavy carpeting, thick curtains, and acoustical wall and ceiling panels, help reduce both unwanted classroom noise and room reverberation, particularly when applied to hard, parallel surfaces.

Though room location and acoustical treatment are critical to providing an optimal listening/learning environment, additional communication benefit may be realized by ensuring that the student receives optimal acoustic cuing from the teacher via manipulation of the distance between the student and teacher. This variable, although not an acoustical property of the room itself, clearly has an impact on both the SNR and the ratio of reverberant- to direct-sound energy at the listener's ear.

Minimizing speaker-to-listener distance helps place the listener in the direct sound field of the speaker. This simply means that the signal from the speaker reaches the listener with little or no interference from energy reflected off room surfaces. As the distance between speaker and listener increases, there is a decrease in the intensity of the speaker's voice, with a corresponding decrease in the ratio of direct to reverberant sound. Eventually, the distance between speaker and listener reaches a point at which the intensity of the direct sound is equal to the intensity of the reverberant sound. This distance is defined as the critical distance of an enclosure (Puetz, 1971). Several investigators have reported that speech recognition scores decrease as speaker-to-listener distance increases, until the critical distance is reached (Crandell & Bess, 1986; Crandell, 1991; Klem, 1971; Niemoeller, 1981; Puetz, 1971). At listening distances exceeding the critical distance, recognition ability tends to remain essentially constant. It is therefore advisable to minimize speaker-to-listener distances whenever possible. Restructuring the classroom by favoring small-group instruction over the more traditional lecture presentation may help place the student within the direct sound field (Crandell, 1993). It is crucial to note that as the amount of room reverberation increases, critical distance decreases. It may be tempting to ignore the acoustical characteristics of the room and simply provide "preferential seating" for those students with unique educational needs, but this approach provides benefit only if acoustical improvements are made to the room as well.

Given the possible impracticality of seating all students within the direct sound field, an artificial method to reduce the distance between student and teacher, such as using an assistive listening system, is an appropriate additional consideration. These devices include systems that transmit the teacher's voice from a microphone to a receiver on the child and are coupled to the child's ear (e.g., FM, infrared, and induction systems), as well as the free-field FM amplification system. The free-field system delivers low-level amplification (i.e., 10 dB) of the teacher's voice throughout the classroom via loudspeaker(s), thereby equalizing or enhancing the SNR throughout the classroom. Several investigators have reported improved speech recognition for both students with normal hearing and students with hearing loss using free-field amplification systems (e.g., Berg, 1987; Crandell & Bess, 1987; Crandell & Smaldino, 1994; Flexer, 1989; Flexer, Millen, & Brown, 1990; Ray, Sarff, & Glassford, 1984; Sarff, 1981; Sarff Ray, & Bagwell, 1981). Discussions concerning the proper utilization of amplification systems in the classroom environment are provided in additional ASHA guidelines (ASHA, 1991a, b). The reader is directed also to Bess and Sinclair (1985), Hawkins (1988), and Ross, Brackett, and Maxon (1991).

Summary

The Americans with Disabilities Act (enacted July 26, 1990) has brought into focus the need for removing barriers and improving accessibility of all buildings and facilities. It is clear that the definition of barrier must be expanded to include not only structural features that limit physical accessibility, but also acoustical barriers that limit access to communication and information. Acoustical interference caused by inappropriate levels of background noise and reverberation presents a barrier to learning and communication in educational settings and school-sponsored extracurricular activities, particularly for students with hearing loss or other language/learning concerns.

ASHA has provided these guidelines and acoustical improvement strategies in order to assist communication related professionals, teachers, school officials, architects, contractors, state education agencies, and others in developing the best possible learning environment for all students. Additional research on both the acoustical characteristics of learning environments and the communication requirements of learners is encouraged.

References

American Speech-Language-Hearing Association Committee on Amplification for the Hearing Impaired. (1991, January). Amplification as a remediation technique for children with normal hearing. *Asha* (Suppl. 3), pp. 22–24.

American Speech-Language-Hearing Association Committee on Amplification for the Hearing Impaired. (1991, March). The use of FM amplification instrument for infants and preschool children with hearing impairment. *Asha* (Suppl. 5), pp. 1–2.

Beranek, L. (1954). *Acoustics*. New York: McGraw-Hill.

Berg, F. (1987). *Facilitating classroom listening*. Boston: College-Hill.

Bess, F., & McConnell, F. (1981). *Audiology, education and the hearing-impaired child*. St. Louis: CV Mosby.

Bess, F., & Sinclair, S. (1985). Amplification systems used in education. In J. Katz (Ed.), *Handbook of clinical audiology* (pp. 970–985). Baltimore: Williams & Wilkins.

Bess, F., & Tharpe, A. (1986). An introduction to unilateral sensorineural hearing loss in children. *Ear and Hearing, 7*, 313.

Blair, J. (1977). Effects of amplification, speechreading, and classroom environment on reception of speech. *Volta Review, 79*, 443–449.

Blair, J., Peterson, M., & Viehweg, S. (1985). The effects of mild hearing loss on academic performance of young school-age children. *Volta Review, 87*, 87–93.

Bolt, R., & MacDonald, A. (1949). Theory of speech masking by reverberation. *Journal of the Acoustical Society of America, 21*, 577–580.

Borrild, K. (1978). Classroom acoustics. In M. Ross & T. Giolas (Eds.), *Auditory management of hearing impaired children* (pp. 145–179). Baltimore: University Park.

Bradley, J. (1986). Speech intelligibility studies in classrooms. *Journal of the Acoustical Society of America, 80*, 846–854.

Crandelt C. (1991). Classroom acoustics for normal-hearing children: Implications for rehabilitation. *Educational Audiology Monograph, 2*, 18–38.

Crandell, C. (1992). Classroom acoustics for hearing-impaired children. *Journal of the Acoustical Society of America, 92*, 2470.

Crandell, C. (1993). Noise effects on the speech recognition of children with minimal hearing loss. *Ear & Hearing, 14*, 210–216.

Crandell, C., & Bess, F. (1986, October). Speech recognition of children in a "typical" classroom setting. *Asha*, p. 82.

Crandell C., & Bess, F. (1987, October). Sound-field amplification in the classroom setting. *Asha*, p. 87.

Crandell, C. & Smaldino, J. (1994). Room acoustics. In R. Tyler & D. Schum (Eds.), *Assistive devices for the hearing impaired*. Needham Heights, MA: Allyn & Bacon.

Crum, D. (1974). *The effects of noise, reverberation, and speaker-to-listener distance on speech understanding.* Unpublished doctoral dissertation, Northwestern University, Evanston, IL.

Crum, D. & Matkin, N. (1976). Room acoustics: The forgotten variable? *Language, Speech, and Hearing Services in Schools, 7*(2), 106–110.

Davis, J., Elfenbein, J., Schum, R., & Bentler, R. (1986). Effects of mild and moderate hearing impairments on language, educational, and psychosocial behavior of children. *Journal of Speech and Hearing Disorders, 51*, 53

Finitzo-Hieber, T. (1988). Classroom acoustics. In R. Roeser (Ed.), *Auditory disorders in school children* (2nd ed.) (pp. 221–223). New York: Thieme-Stratton.

Finitzo-Hieber, T., & Tillman, T. (1978). Room acoustics effects on monosyllabic word discrimination ability for normal and hearing-impaired children. *Journal of Speech and Hearing Research, 21*, 440–458.

Flexer, C. (1989). Turn on sound: An odyssey of sound amplification. *Educational Audiology Newsletter, 5*, 6–7.

Flexer, C., Millen, J., & Brown, L. (1990). Children with developmental disabilities: The effects of sound field amplification in word identification. *Language, Speech, and Hearing Services in Schools, 21*, 177–182.

Fourcin, A., Joy, D., Kennedy, M., Knight, J., Knowles, S., Knox, E., Martin, M., Mort, J., Penton, J., Poole, D., Powell C., & Watson, T. (1980). Design of educational facilities for deaf children. *British Journal of Audiology, 3*(Suppl. 3), 124.

Gengel, R. (1971). Acceptable signal-to-noise ratios for aided speech discrimination by the hearing impaired. *Journal of Auditory Research, 11*, 219–222.

Hawkins, D. (1988). Options in classroom amplification systems. In F. Bess (Ed.), *Hearing impairment in children* (pp. 253–265). Parkton, MD: York Press.

Houtgast, T. (1981). The effect of ambient noise on speech intelligibility in classrooms. *Applied Acoustics, 14*, 15–25.

Klein, W. (1971). Articulation loss of consonants as a criterion for speech transmission in a room. *Journal of the Audio Engineering Society, 19*, 920–922.

Knudson, V., & Harris, C. (1978). *Acoustical designing in architecture.* American Institute of Physics—Acoustical Society of America.

Kodaras, M. (1960). Reverberation times of typical elementary school settings. *Noise Control, 6*, 17–19.

Kurtovic, H. (1975). The influence of reflected sound upon speech intelligibility. *Acoustica, 33*, 32–39.

Leavitt, R., & Flexer, C. (1991). Speech degradation as measured by the Rapid Speech Transmission Index (RASTI). *Ear and Hearing, 12*, 115–118.

Lochner, J., & Burger, J. (1964). The influence of reflections in auditorium acoustics. *Journal of Sound and Vibration, 4*, 426–454.

Markides, A. (1986). Speech levels and speech-to-noise ratios. *British Journal of Audiology, 20*, 115–120.

McCroskey, F., & Devens, J. (1975). Acoustic characteristics of public school classrooms constructed between 1890 and 1960. *Proceedings of NoisExpo, National Noise and Vibration Control Conference* (pp. 101–103). Bay Village, OH: Acoustical Publications.

Nabelek, A. (1981). Temporal distortions and noise considerations. In G. Studebaker & F. Bess (Eds.), *Vanderbilt hearing aid report: State of the art research needs* (pp. 51–59). Upper Darby: Monographs in Contemporary Audiology.

Nabelek, A., & Nabelek, I. (1985). Room acoustics and speech perception. In J. Katz (Ed.), *Handbook of clinical audiology* (3rd ed.) (pp. 834–846). Baltimore: Williams & Wilkins.

Nabelek, A., & Pickett, J. (1974a). Monaural and binaural speech perception through hearing aids under noise and reverberation with normal and hearing impaired listeners. *Journal of Speech and Hearing Research, 17*, 724–739.

Nabelek, A., & Pickett, J. (1974b). Reception of consonants in a classroom as affected by monaural and binaural listening, noise, reverberation, and hearing aids. *Journal of the Acoustical Society of America, 56*, 628–639.

Neimoeller, A. (1968). Acoustical design of classrooms for the deaf. *American Annals of the Deaf, 113*, 1040–1045.

Neimoeller, A. (1981). Physical concepts of speech communication in classrooms for the deaf. In F. Bess, B. Freeman, & J. Sinclair (Eds), *Amplification in education* (pp. 164–179). Washington, DC: Alexander Graham Bell Association for the Deaf.

Nober, L., & Nober, E. (1975). Auditory discrimination of learning disabled children in quiet and classroom noise. *Journal of Learning Disabilities, 8*, 656–773.

Olsen, W. (1977). Acoustics and amplification in classrooms for the hearing impaired. In F. H. Bess (Ed.), *Childhood deafness: Causation, assessment and management* (pp. 251–266). New York: Grune & Stratton.

Olsen, W. (1981). The effects of noise and reverberation on speech intelligibility. In F. H. Bess, B. A. Freeman, & J. S. Sinclair (Eds.), *Amplification in education* (pp. 151–163). Washington, DC: Alexander Graham Bell Association for the Deaf.

Olsen, W. (1988). Classroom acoustics for hearing-impaired children. In F. H. Bess (Ed.), *Hearing impairment in children.* Parkton, MD: York Press.

Paul, R. (1967). *An investigation of the effectiveness of hearing aid amplfcation in regular and special classrooms under instructional conditions.* Unpublished doctoral dissertation, Wayne State University, Detroit, MI.

Peutz, V. (1971). Articulation loss of consonants as a criterion for speech transmission in a room. *Journal of the Audio Engineering Society, 19*, 915–919.

Ray, H., Sarff, L. S., & Glassford, F. E. (1984). Sound field amplification: An innovative educational intervention for mainstreamed learning disabled students. *Directive Teacher, 18*–20.

Ross, M. (1978). Classroom acoustics and speech intelligibility. In J. Katz (Ed.), *Handbook of clinical audiology* (pp. 469–478). Baltimore: Williams & Wilkins.

Ross, M., Brackett, D., & Maxon, A. (1991). *Assessment and management of mainstreamed hearing-impaired children: Principles and practices.* Austin, TX: Pro-Ed.

Ross, M., & Giolas, T. (1971, December) Effects of three classroom listening conditions on speech intelligibility. *American Annals of the Deaf, 116*, 580–584.

Sanders, D. (1965). Noise conditions in normal school classrooms. *Exceptional Child, 31*, 344–353.

Sarff, L. S. (1981). An innovative use of free field amplification in regular classrooms. In R. Roeser & M. Downs (Eds.), *Auditory disorders in school children* (pp. 263–272). New York: Thieme-Stratton.

Sarff L. S., Ray, H. R., & Bagwell, C. (1981). Why not amplification in every classroom? *Hearing Aid Journal, 11*, 44–52.

Shepard, N., Davis, J., Gorga, M., & Stelmachowicz, P. (1981). Characteristics of hearing-impaired children in the public schools: Part I—Demographic data. *Journal of Speech and Hearing Disorders, 46*, 123–129.

Smaldino, J., & Flexer, C. (1991, June). *Improving listening in the classroom.* Paper presented at the 1991 Academy of Rehabilitative Audiology Annual Meeting, Breckenridge, CO.

Appendix 2–L

TECHNICAL REPORT ON SERVICE PROVISION UNDER IDEA, PART H, TO CHILDREN WHO ARE DEAF AND HARD OF HEARING, AGES BIRTH TO 36 MONTHS

Joint Committee of ASHA and the Council on Education of the Deaf

The following report was prepared by the Joint Committee of the American Speech-Language-Hearing Association (ASHA) and the Council on Education of the Deaf (CED) to provide all represented organizations with information regarding the provision of services mandated under the Individuals with Disabilities Education Act—Part H, as amended (IDEA—Part H). Specifically, this document pertains to children who are deaf and hard of hearing ages birth to 36 months who are eligible for services under the Individuals with Disabilities Education Act— Part H, as amended (IDEA—Part H). The report was approved in August 1993 by the ASHA Executive Board (EB 110-93) and by the CED Board in December 1993.

Present and past committee members responsible for the development of this technical report include Stephen J. Boney, ASHA chair (1990-1992); Antonia Brancia Maxon, ASHA chair (1986-1989); Linda Seestedt-Stanford,ASHA chair (1993); Harold Meyers, CED chair (1991); Jean Moog, CED chair (1986-1990); Evelyn Cherow, ASHA ex officio; Gerry Bateman; Bert Bell; Stan Brooks; Kathleen Christensen; Diane Golden; Winfield McCord; Marilyn Sass-Lehrer; and Harriet Alexander-Whiting. The monitoring officers included Ann L. Carey, 1992 ASHA president; Diane L. Eger, past vice president for professional practices (1991-93) and Crystal S. Cooper, vice president for professional practices (1994).

Definitions

Key terms used throughout this statement are defined as follows:

Individual Family Service Plan (IFSP): A written plan for providing early intervention services for a child and the child's family. This should be developed jointly by the family and appropriate qualified personnel involved in the provision of early identification/intervention services. The purpose of this plan is described in the Individuals with Disabilities Education Act—Part H, as amended (IDEA—Part H).

Birth to 36-month-old child with hearing loss: A child 0–36 months of age with hearing levels what deviate from audiometric normal. This includes hearing loss of any degree (mild to profound), type, laterality (ear), or age of onset of hearing loss. The terms *deaf* and *hard-of-hearing* are used throughout this document and cover the range of hearing loss.

Multidisciplinary team: involvement of two or more disciplines or professions to provide integrated and coordinated services that include evaluation and assessment activities and development of an IFSP. The professionals on the team should meet the highest educational standards set for their profession and in their respective state in addition to having expertise with deaf and hard of hearing youngsters and their families.

Mode of Communication: Primary sensory modality through which an individual with hearing loss receives and produces language. This includes oral/aural, visual/gestural, sign communication, cued speech, and combinations thereof.

Sensory devices: Any device that is used to improve, augment, or supplement communication. Such devices could include personal hearing aids, wireless FM systems, cochlear implants, vibrotactile units, or other assistive listening devices.

Background

Children who are deaf or hard of hearing and their families/caregivers constitute a unique group whose needs differ from those of other families. The variables that set children with hearing loss apart from those with other disabilities are related to the lack of full access to communication. This can have long-term effects on the child's cognitive, speech, language, and social-emotional development, as well as affect the family system. Early identification, assessment, and management should (a) be conducted by professionals who have the qualifications to meet the needs of children who are deaf or hard of hearing, particularly infants, toddlers, and their families; (b) be designed to meet the unique needs of the child and family; and (c) include families in an active, collaborative role with professionals in the planning and provision of early intervention services.

Roles, Knowledge, and Experience

The descriptions of knowledge and experience given below are provided with the understanding that the individuals with Disabilities Education Act—Part H, as amended (IDEA—Part H) requires a team approach and a strong family focus in the development and implementation of the IFSP.

1.0 Role: Participation as a member of a multidisciplinary team

Proficient In:

1.1 Involving families as equal partners on the multidisciplinary team

1.2 Recognizing expertise and roles of members of the multidisciplinary team

1.3 Sharing and consulting in joint goal setting and planning with all members of the team

Knowledge and Experience Needed:

1a. Skill in involving families as equal partners of the multidisciplinary team

1b. Knowledge of first language acquisition and the effects of hearing loss

1c. Knowledge of hearing loss and/or other conditions and their effect on early development of cognition, communication, speech, motor, adaptive and social-emotional development

1d. Knowledge of how a child who is deaf or hard of hearing and/or has special needs affects relationships within the family and community

1e. Knowledge that assessment and management is a dynamic, ongoing process requiring a variety of skills and techniques

1f. Skill in sharing, consulting, joint goal setting and planning with all members of the team

1g. Skill in using appropriate counseling strategies

1h. Knowledge of the various roles of members on the multidisciplinary team

1i. Skill in integrating and implementing the knowledge and recommendations of other team members

1j. Knowledge of resources available for deaf and hard of hearing children and their families including local, state, and national organizations

1k. Knowledge of range of services appropriate to meet the individual needs of the child and family

1l. Knowledge of Deaf culture and issues of cultural diversity as they affect children who are deaf or hard of hearing and their families

1m. Skill in summarizing and integrating assessment information into an educational report and program plan

2.0 Role: Working with Families

Proficient In:

2.1 Facilitating parent/caregiver/professional collaboration

2.2 Recognizing family strengths and challenges and incorporating these in the IFSP

2.3 Providing information to families, in a sensitive manner, regarding financial and emotional support

2.4 Providing families with information pertaining to federal, state, and local legislation for children who are deaf or hard of hearing

Knowledge and Skills Needed:

2a. Sensitivity to cultural diversity and socioeconomic issues

2b. Knowledge and understanding of the child's current level of development and needs and those of the family

2c. Knowledge and understanding of Deaf culture and heritage

2d. Knowledge of federal state, and local legislation/regulations regarding service provision for 036-month-old children who are deaf or hard of hearing

2e. Familiarity with federal, state, and local funding sources for services for 0-36-month-old children who are deaf or hard of hearing

2f. Knowledge of child advocacy agencies and other community service agencies

2g. Knowledge of the range of educational and other related services (e.g., occupational therapy, physical therapy, etc.) available for the child and family

2h. Knowledge of legal rights and due process procedures available for families and children

2i. Knowledge of the range of language and communication options available for the child and family (e.g., American Sign Language, cued speech, simultaneous communication, aural/oral)

2j. Ability to involve adults who are deaf or hard of hearing and families of children who are deaf and hard of hearing as resources for children with hearing loss and their families

3.0 Role: Assessment and diagnosis of hearing loss in 0-36-month-old children

Proficient In:

3.1 Conducting appropriate audiological assessments of 0-36-month-old children according to established guidelines (ASHA, 1991; ASHA, 1989)*

Knowledge and Experience Needed:

3a. Certification and licensure (where applicable) in audiology

3b. Knowledge of pre- and postnatal development of the auditory system and audition

3c. Knowledge of behavioral and electrophysiological techniques for assessing infants and toddlers

3d. Skill in performing and interpreting audiological assessments of infants and toddlers

4.0 Role: Assessment of communication competence of 0-36-month-old children with hearing loss

Proficient In:

4.1 Administering the appropriate formal and informal communication assessments of 0-36-month-old children

---

* For more specific information regarding audiological assessment techniques, see Joint Committee on Infant Hearing Draft Position Statement (1994); Diefendorf (1988); Gravel (1989); Martin (1987); Northern & Downs (1991); and Wilson and Thompson (1984).

with hearing loss using the child's mode of communication and primary language

Knowledge and Skills Needed:

4a. Certification and/or licensure in speech-language pathology with expertise in working with deaf and hard of hearing infants or education of the deaf and hard of hearing

4b. Knowledge of communication development including both visual/gestural and aural/oral

4c. Knowledge of assessment tools appropriate for 0-36-month-old children with hearing loss

4d. Knowledge of techniques for acquiring communication data through observation and interaction

4e. Skill in working with 0-36-month-old children who are deaf or hard of hearing

4f. Skill in assessing parent/caregiver and child communication interactions

4g. Skill in interpreting results with respect to the hearing loss

5.0 Role: Assessment of cognitive, motor, and social skills of 0-36-month-old children with hearing loss**

Proficient In:

5.1 Administering formal, and informal developmental assessments with tools appropriate for 0-36-month-old children who are deaf or hard of hearing using the child's mode of communication and primary language

Knowledge and Skills Needed:

5a. Certification and licensure (where appropriate) in respective areas specific to psychology, occupational therapy, physical therapy, and social work

5b. Knowledge of the development of cognitive, motor, and social skills

5c. Knowledge of the appropriate tools to use with a 0-36-month-old child with hearing loss

5d. Skill in adapting to the needs of the individual child

5e. Ability to incorporate information about hearing loss to modify assessment procedures

5f. Skill in interpreting the above evaluation results with respect to the hearing loss.

6.0 Role: Otological evaluation of the 0-36-month-old child with hearing loss

Proficient In:

6.1 Providing otological information with respect to risk factors, craniofacial anomalies, and syndromes associated with hearing loss

6.2 Conducting routine otological evaluations to rule out and treat conditions amenable to medical or surgical treatment

6.3 Conducting otological evaluations to provide medical clearance for selection and fitting of amplification

Knowledge and Skills Needed:

6a. Certification and licensure in medicine with a specialty in otolaryngology or otology

6b. Knowledge of infant/child development

6c. Knowledge of risk factors for hearing loss

6d. Knowledge of medical genetics related to hearing loss

6e. Knowledge of common etiologies of hearing loss in infants and young children

6f. Knowledge of the possible effects of sequelae of chronic otitis media on language and academic achievement

6g. Experience with the pediatric population

6h. Skill in working with families

7.0 Role: Developing and Implementing the Individual Family Service Plan

Proficient In:

7.1 Establishing family-professional collaboration and partnership

7.2 Coordinating/participating in assessment and identification of services to child and family with multidisciplinary team including the family

7.3 Communicating proficiently in the child and family's mode of communication and primary language

Knowledge and Skills Needed:

7a. Demonstrated understanding of the diversity of family's structure, roles, values and beliefs, and coping styles

7b. Demonstrated understanding of the racial, ethnic, and cultural diversity of the family

7c. Demonstrated understanding of the significance of the family-centered approach

7d. Coordinate/participate in family-directed assessment of the family's resources, priorities, and concerns related to the developmental needs of the child within the family context

7e. Coordinate/participate in comprehensive assessment of the child including relevant professionals and family participation

7f. Communicate results of assessment(s) with family input and participation

7g. Coordinate/participate in identification and provision of recommended services to family and child

7h. Coordinate/participate in IFSP meetings in which family is encouraged to be an active participant

---

** For more specific information regarding assessment techniques see, Brackett (1990); Geers and Moog (1987), Moeller, Osenberger, and Morford (1987); and Moeller, Coufal, and Hixon (1990); Spencer, P, Bodner-Johnson, B, and Gutfreund, M. (1992), Schuyler and Rushmer (1987).

7i. Communicate family rights regarding services and confidentiality issues

7j. Knowledge of legislation related to the provision of services to families with children birth to 36 months

7k. Coordinate/participate in development of expected outcomes for child and family with family participation

8.0 Role: Provision of sensory devices (the use of the term sensory device is specified in the Definitions section of this document)

Proficient In:

8.1 Selecting and fitting the appropriate sensory devices when appropriate

8.2 Evaluating the effectiveness of the sensory devices

8.3 Respecting the child's and families' values regarding the use of sensory devices

Knowledge and Skills Needed:

8a. Certification and licensure (where applicable) in audiology

8b. Knowledge of the various types of sensory devices

8c. Knowledge of the appropriate application of the various types of sensory devices

8d. Knowledge of assessment techniques appropriate for the 0-36-month-old child

8e. Skill in working with the 0-36-month-old child and family members

9.0 Role: Management of sensory devices

Proficient In:

9.1 Observing and evaluating the ongoing benefits of sensory devices

9.2 Troubleshooting of sensory devices

9.3 Care and maintenance of sensory devices

Knowledge and Skills Needed:

9a. Knowledge of the characteristics of sensory devices

9b. Knowledge of troubleshooting techniques for sensory devices

9c. Knowledge of room acoustics, including the effects of noise, reverberation, and distance on speech recognition and environmental modifications to improve room acoustics (ASHA, 1984b)

9d. Knowledge of functional benefit of the sensory device

9e. Skill in troubleshooting and electroacoustic evaluation of the sensory device in compliance with existing or proposed standards

9f. Skill in implementing the use of sensory devices

9g. Skill in working with families and teaching them to appropriately monitor the various sensory devices

10.0 Role: Maximizing Auditory Potential

Proficient In:

10.1 Determining a child's potential use of residual hearing

10.2 Determining the benefit afforded a child by the sensory device

10.3 Determining the effects of different listening conditions on the use of residual hearing

10.4 Determining the auditory areas in which skills can be improved

10.5 Developing and implementing an appropriate management program to address those areas

10.6 Respecting the families' values and choices regarding the use of residual hearing

Knowledge and Skills Needed:

10a. Those persons who provide aural rehabilitation services should meet competencies as oulined in Defnition and Competencies for Aural Rehabilitation (ASHA, 1984b)

10b. Knowledge of the sequence of auditory development and skill in integrating those processes into training

10c. Knowledge of the potential effects of a child's hearing loss on the use of residual hearing

10d. Knowledge of potential effects of sensory devices on the use of residual hearing

10e. Knowledge of the effects of room acoustics on the use of residual hearing

10f. Knowledge of integrating auditory and visual information for speech perception

10g. Skill in interpreting aided test results with respect to acoustic cues of speech

11.0 Role: Facilitating Communication Development

Proficient In:

11.1 Providing intervention in the child's primary language and mode of communication

11.2 Determining the child's strengths with respect to communication

11.3 Facilitating family understanding of language and communication options and assisting the family in selecting an appropriate approach for their child

11.4 Implementing a language/communication approach that is appropriate for the child and supported by the family

11.5 Implementing an appropriate communication intervention program for the child and the family

11.6 Facilitating access to adult and peer communication in the child's primary language and communication mode

11.7 Using the communication modality and primary language of the child and/or family

Knowledge and Skills Needed:

11a. Knowledge of language acquisition

11b. Knowledge of the potential effects of hearing loss on language acquisition

11c. Skill in determining the potential effects of hearing loss for the particular child

11d. Knowledge of various language/communication approaches appropriate for individuals who are deaf and hard of hearing

11e. Skill in separating the effects of hearing loss from those language differences not related to hearing

11f. Skill in facilitating caretaker/parent and child interactions

11g. Skill in the techniques for facilitating spoken and sign language acquisition for children 0-36-month-old children who are deaf and hard of hearing

12.0 Role: Facilitating cognitive development

Proficient In:

12.1 Assisting families to develop ways to foster cognitive development of 0-36-month-old children who are deaf and hard of hearing

Knowledge and Skills Needed:

12a. Knowledge of normal cognitive development

12b. Knowledge of the possible effects of hearing loss on language acquisition

12c. Knowledge of the difference between and the interaction of cognition and language

12d. Skill in separating the effects of language problems related to hearing loss from those related to cognitive problems

Summary and Conclusions

Since positive family-child relationships are initially established during the first 3 years, it is imperative that service providers focus their efforts on the family unit, as well as on the child. The Individuals with Disabilities Education Act—Part H, as amended (IDEA—Part H) supports this concept and has mandated development of an IFSP for each infant and toddler and his or her family eligible for early intervention services.

The confirmed diagnosis of hearing loss for a child may have long-term effects on the family. Usually children who are deaf or hard of hearing are born into families with normal-hearing parents and siblings who have limited knowledge of the implications of hearing loss. In addition, parents may go through stages of grieving after learning that their child is deaf or hard of hearing (Luterman, 1979; Moses, 1985). Early experiences with adults who are deaf or hard of hearing, parents who have deaf or hard of hearing children and other support services are essential.

The effects of hearing loss on communication may interfere with parent-child interaction, especially when the primary communication system of the child and family are different.

The following areas are those in which a family may benefit from consultation, information, and education:

1. Immediate and easy access to a professional who can help them understand the hearing loss and its potential effects, both long and short term

2. Immediate and ongoing access to deaf and hard of hearing adults and children and their families

3. Immediate and ongoing access to professionals who can help facilitate the development of effective parent-child interaction

4. Immediate and easy access to a professional who can provide information, education and emotional support to families

5. Ongoing access to broad-based informational programs that enable families to become more familiar with hearing loss, assessment, sensory devices, communication techniques, management, educational options, and deaf community resources

Professionals providing services to families of children who are deaf and hard of hearing can facilitate parents' and caregivers' acquisition of knowledge regarding their child's short- and long-term needs by working with families to do the following:

1. Plan and implement assessment and management as early as possible

2. Develop an IFSP that will enable the family to assist the child in reaching his/her full potential

3. Understand the potential effects of hearing loss in the context of the individual abilities and differences

4. Foster knowledge of legal rights as provided by federal legislation/regulations (the Individuals with Disabilities Education Act—Part H, as amended (IDEA—Part H); Americans with Disabilities Act; Technology Assistance Act) and state legislation

5. Identify potential funding sources at the federal, state, and local levels to assist with assessment and management of individuals who are deaf and hard of hearing

6. Provide information regarding procedures for accessing programs offered by governmental and private agencies

7. Understand the family/caregiver's crucial role in developing an appropriate family service plan and becoming their child's primary advocate

References

American Speech-Language-Hearing Association. (1984a, May). Definition and competencies for aural rehabilitation. *Asha, 26,* 37–41.

American Speech-Language Hearing Association. (1984b, May). Guidelines for graduate training in amplification. *Asha, 26,* 46.

American Speech-Language-Hearing Association. (1989, March). Audiologic screening of newborn infants who are at risk for hearing impairment. *Asha, 31,* 89–92.

American Speech-Language-Hearing Association. (1991, March). Guidelines for the audiologic assessment of children from birth through thirty-six months of age. *Asha, 33*(Suppl. 5), 37–43.

Bess, F. (Ed.). (1988). *Hearing impairment in children.* Parkton, MD: York Press.

Brackett, D. (1990). Communication assessment. In M. Ross, D. Brackett, & A.B. Maxon (Eds.), *Assessment and management of hearing-impaired children: Principles and practices.* Austin, TX: Pro-Ed.

Diefendorf A. (1988). Behavioral evaluation of hearing impaired children. In F. Bess (Ed.), *Hearing impairment in children* (pp. 133–151). Parkton, MD: York Press.

Early intervention program for infants and toddlers with handicaps; final regulations. (1989). *Federal Register, 54*(119); 26306–26348.

Geers, A., & Moog, J. (1987). Predicting spoken language acquisition of profoundly hearing-impaired children. *JSHD, 52,* 84–94.

Gravel, J. (1989). Assessing auditory system integrity in high risk infants and young children. *Seminars in Hearing,* 10.

Joint Committee on Infant Hearing. (1994). *1994 draft position statement.* (Publication pending final review).

Luterman, D. (1979). *Counseling parents of hearing-impaired children,* Boston, MA: Little, Brown and Company.

Martin, F. (Ed.). (1987). *Hearing disorders in children.* Austin, TX: Pro-Ed.

Moeller, M., Osberger, M.J., & Mortord, J. (1987). Speech-language assessment and intervention with preschool hearing-impaired children. In J. Alpiner & P. McCarthy (Eds.), *Rehabilitative audiology; Children and adults* (pp. 163–187). Baltimore, MD: Williams and Wilkins.

Appendix 2–M

MINIMUM COMPETENCIES FOR EDUCATIONAL AUDIOLOGISTS

I. The educational audiologist should demonstrate competency for providing services to individuals birth through 21 years of age and their families in the following areas:

A. Identification audiometry, including pure tone audiometric screening, immittance measures, and newborn screening criteria.

B. Threshold audiometric evaluation for pure tone air and bone conduction, speech reception and word recognition testing, immittance measurements, otoscopy, special tests including interpretation of electrophysiological measures, differential diagnosis of auditory disorders, and diagnosis of central auditory processing disorders.

C. Medical and educational referral and follow-up procedures and criteria.

D. Audiological assessment of individuals using procedures appropriate to their receptive and expressive language skills, cognitive abilities, and behavioral functioning.

E. Evaluation of the need for and selection of hearing aids, FM systems, cochlear implants, vibrotactile devices, and other hearing assistance technology. This includes making earmold impressions and modifications.

F. The structure of the learning environment, including classroom acoustics and implications for learning.

G. General child development and management.

H. Written and verbal interpretation of auditory assessment results and implications appropriate for the intended audience, such as parents, teachers, physicians, and other professionals.

I. IFSP/IEP planning process and procedures:
1. Interpretation of auditory assessment results and their implications on psychosocial, communicative, cognitive, physical, academic, and vocational development.
2. Educational options for individuals who are deaf or hard of hearing including appropriate intensity of services and vocational and work-study programming as part of multidisciplinary team process.
3. Legal issues and procedures, especially the legal rights of and due process for students, parents, teachers, administrators, and school boards, including the implications of the Americans with Disability Act, the Individual with Disabilities Education Act, and Section 504 of the Vocational Rehabilitation Act of 1974.

J. Consultation and collaboration with classroom teachers and other professionals regarding the relationship of hearing and hearing loss to the development of academic and psychosocial skills:
1. Ensure support for enhancing the development of auditory functioning and communication skills.

2. Recommend appropriate modifications of instructional curricula and academic methods, materials, and facilities.

K. Participation in team management of communication treatment for individuals who are deaf or hard of hearing or who have difficulties processing speech/language through the auditory system. These procedures should integrate the following:
1. Orientation to, and the use and maintenance of, appropriate amplification instrumentation and other hearing assistance technologies.
2. Auditory skills development.
3. Speech skills development including phonology, voice, and rhythm.
4. Visual communication including speechreading and manual communication.
5. Language development (expressive and receptive oral, signed, and/or written language).
6. Selection and use of appropriate instructional materials and media.
7. Structuring of learning environments including acoustic modifications.
8. Case management/care coordination with family, school, medical, and community services.
9. Facilitation of transitions between levels, schools, programs, agencies, etc.

L. Knowledge of communication systems and language used by individuals who are deaf and hard of hearing.

M. Counseling for the family and individual who is deaf or hard of hearing, including emotional support, information about hearing loss and its implications, and interaction strategies to maximize communication and psychosocial development.

N. Selection and maintenance of audiological equipment.

O. Maintenance of records including screening, referral, follow-up, assessment, IFSP/IEP planning, and services.

P. Implementation of a hearing conservation program.

Q. Awareness of cerumen management concerns and techniques.

R. Implementation of inservice training for staff and support personnel.

S. Train and supervise paraprofessionals.

T. Sensitivity to family systems, diversity, and cultures, including Deaf culture.

U. Knowledge of school systems, multidisciplinary teams, and community and professional resources.

V. Effective interpersonal and communication skills.

II. The educational audiologist should have an internship/practicum in a school setting under the supervision of an educational audiologist. A preferred internship would be a full-time experience lasting approximately six weeks.

Source: "Minimum competencies for educational audiologists" by Educational Audiology Association, 1994, *Educational Audiology Association Newsletter, 11*(4), p. 7. Reprinted by permission.

Appendix 2–N

AMPLIFICATION FOR INFANTS AND CHILDREN WITH HEARING LOSS
The Pediatric Working Group
Conference on Amplification for Children With Auditory Deficits

In October 1994, Vanderbilt University, Bill Wilkerson Center, and the Academy of Dispensing Audiologists cosponsored a conference designed to address various contemporary issues associated with hearing aids in children. The proceedings of this conference, "Amplification for Children With Auditory Deficits" (Bess, Gravel, & Tharpe, 1996) is available through the Bill Wilkerson Center Press, Nashville, Tennessee. Following the conference, a small working group was assembled from the conference faculty to develop a Position Statement on amplification for infants and children with hearing loss. The members of the committee who prepared the following statement include: Fred H. Bess, Chair, Vanderbilt University School of Medicine/Bill Wilkerson Center, Nashville, Tennessee; Patricia A. Chase, Vanderbilt University School of Medicine, Nashville, Tennessee; Judith S. Gravel, Albert Einstein College of Medicine, Bronx, New York; Richard C. Seewald, The University of Western Ontario, London-Ontario, Canada; Patricia G. Stelmachowicz, Boys Town National Research Hospital, Omaha, Nebraska; Anne Marie Tharpe, Louisiana State University Medical Center, New Orleans, Louisiana; and Andrea Hedley-Williams, Bill Wilkerson Center, Nashville, Tennessee.

Introduction

The timely fitting of appropriate amplification to infants and children with hearing loss is one of the more important responsibilities of the pediatric audiologist. Although the importance of providing an audible signal for the development and maintenance of aural/oral communication for formal and informal learning is undisputed, the methods used to select and evaluate personal amplification for infants and children with hearing loss vary widely among facilities. Few audiologists use any systematic approach for selecting and fitting amplification for young children and many do not use current technologies in the fitting process (Hedley-Williams, Tharpe, & Bess, 1996). Because of the improvement in early identification of hearing loss in children (Bess & Paradise, 1994; Stein, 1995), continued changes in technology, and a new array of amplification options available for application to infants and children, there is a critical need for a systematic, quantifiable, and evidence-based approach to providing amplification for the pediatric population. The goal is to ensure that children will receive full-time and consistent audibility of the speech signal at safe and comfortable listening levels.

The audiologist is the professional singularly qualified to select and fit all forms of amplification for children, including personal hearing aids, FM systems, and other assistive listening devices. To perform this function capably, an audiologist must have experience with the assessment and management of infants and children with hearing loss and the commensurate knowledge and test equipment necessary for use with current pediatric hearing assessment methods and hearing aid selection and evaluation procedures. Facilities that lack the expertise or equipment should establish consortial arrangements with those that do.

This statement sets forth guidelines and recommendations associated with the fitting of personal amplification to infants and children with hearing loss. The approach stresses an objective, timely strategy and discourages the traditional comparative approach. We envision the provision of appropriate, reliable, and undistorted amplification as a four-stage process involving assessment, selection, verification, and validation. We herein present a discussion on need, audiologic assessment, preselection of the physical characteristics of hearing aids, selection and verification of the electroacoustic characteristics of hearing aids, and validation of aided auditory function. Because the focus of this position statement is on the fitting process, the topics of counseling and follow-up are discussed but not treated in detail. Readers are referred elsewhere for comprehensive coverage of these important topics (Brackett, 1996; Diefendorf, Reitz, Escobar, & Wynne, 1996; Edwards, 1996). Finally, we include a question/answer section regarding issues frequently raised by pediatric audiologists.

Criteria for Provision of Personal Amplification

A child needs hearing aids when there is a significant, permanent, bilateral peripheral hearing loss. Some children with variable and/or unilateral losses may also need hearing aids. There are no empirical studies that delineate the specific degree of hearing loss at which need for amplification begins. However, if one considers the acoustic spectrum of speech at normal conversational levels in the 1000–4000 Hz range, hearing thresholds of 25 dB HL or greater can be assumed to impede a child's ability to perceive the acoustic features of speech necessary for optimum aural/oral language development. Hence, thresholds equal to or poorer than 25 dB HL would indicate candidacy for amplification in some form. For children with unilateral hearing loss, rising or high frequency hearing loss above 2000 Hz, and/or milder degrees of hearing loss (<25 dB HL), need should be based on the audiogram plus additional information including cognitive function, the exis-

Source: "Amplification for infants and children with hearing loss" by The Pediatric Working Group of the Conference on Amplification for Children with Auditory Deficits, 1996, *American Journal of Audiology* 5(1), pp. 53–68. Reprinted by permission.

Suggested reference: The Pediatric Working Group of the Conference on Amplification for Children With Auditory Deficits. (1996). Amplification for infants and children with hearing loss. *American Journal of Audiology, 5*(1), 53–68.

tence of other disabilities, and the child's performance within the home and classroom environment.

The Audiologic Assessment

The efficacy of the hearing aid fitting is predicated on the validity of the audiologic assessment. The ultimate goal of the audiometric evaluation is to obtain ear- and frequency-specific threshold data from the child at the earliest opportunity.

When testing very young children, however, complete audiologic data are seldom obtained. In the absence of a complete audiogram, and even with one, consistencies among several audiometric measures—behavioral findings, click-evoked and/or tone evoked ABR threshold recordings, aural acoustic immittance measures (reflexes and tympanometry), evoked otoacoustic emissions, and bone-conduction responses (behavioral and/or ABR)—are essential.

For children with a developmental age at or under 6 months, behavioral responses should be confirmed with ABR threshold assessment. When behavioral results are unreliable, such as in the case of children with multiple disabilities, behavioral and ABR assessments should be completed and the findings for both measures should be examined for agreement. However, in the absence of reliable behavioral thresholds, hearing aid fitting should proceed based on frequency-specific ABR results unless neurologic status contraindicates such action.

It is not sufficient to base binaural hearing aid fitting only on soundfield thresholds, nor is it acceptable to fit hearing aids to infants and young children based solely on a click-ABR threshold. In both such cases, critical information is lacking that could affect the efficacy of the fit, or in the worst-case scenario, be detrimental to the child's performance. With regard to soundfield audiometric assessment, it is inadvisable to assume that both ears have equal hearing loss or hearing loss of the same configuration based on behavioral soundfield results alone. Therefore, it is preferable to obtain thresholds using earphones. Insert earphones are recommended because the child's real-ear-to-coupler difference (RECD) (described in the Selection and Verification Section) can then be used to convert threshold measures to real-ear SPL. Other behavioral measures such as speech detection and speech recognition may be useful in determining amplification need. The click-ABR provides insufficient information regarding both the degree and configuration of hearing loss—information that is critical for use with today's prescriptive selection and evaluation procedures. At a minimum, click and 500-Hz tone ABR thresholds should be obtained in order to reflect low- and high-frequency hearing sensitivity (ASHA, 1991). Finally, auditory behaviors should be consistent with parental reports of auditory function as well as more formal, systematic observations of behavioral responses to calibrated acoustic stimuli.

Preselection—Physical Characteristics

Even at a very young age, consideration should be given to the availability of appropriate coupling options on hearing aids, so that the child will have maximum flexibility for accessing the various forms of current assistive device technology. Consequently, hearing aids for most children should include the following features: Direct Audio Input (DAI), telecoil (T), and microphone-telecoil (M-T) switching options. Hearing aids used with young children also require more flexibility in electroacoustic parameters (e.g., tone, gain, output limiting) than for adults, as well as more safety-related features such as battery and volume controls that are tamper resistant.

The physical fit of the hearing aids (in most cases worn behind the pinnae) and the earmolds is important for both comfort and retention. Color of the hearing aids and earmolds needs to be considered across ages, and size of the hearing aids is an especially important cosmetic concern for older children. Earmolds should be constructed of a soft material.

While consideration needs to be given to the aforementioned physical factors, the ultimate goal is the consistency and integrity of the amplified signal that the child receives. Providing the best possible amplified speech signal should not be compromised for cosmetic purposes, particularly in the early years of life when speech-language learning is occurring at a rapid pace.

Binaural amplification should always be provided to young children unless there is a clear contraindication. Even if there is audiometric asymmetry between ears as evidenced by pure tones or speech perception, hearing aids should be fitted binaurally until it is apparent from behavioral evidence that a hearing aid fitted to the poorer ear is detrimental to performance.

In general, behind-the-ear (BTE) hearing aids are the style of choice for most children. However, for children with profound hearing loss, body aids or FM systems may be more appropriate because of acoustic feedback problems limiting sufficient gain to provide full audibility of the speech signal in BTE arrangements. Other circumstances that may indicate the need for body-worn amplification include children with restricted motor capacities and those confined by a head restraint. In-the-ear (ITE) hearing aids may be considered appropriate when ear growth has stabilized—at about 8-10 years of age—as long as the flexibility and options available are not markedly restricted by concha and ear-canal size.

Selection and Verification of Electroacoustic Characteristics

The use of a systematic approach when selecting the electroacoustic characteristics of hearing aids for children is considered of utmost importance. Sound pressure levels measured in infants' and young children's ears typically exceed adult values (Bratt, 1980; Feigin, Kopun, Stelmachowicz, & Gorga, 1989; Nelson Barlow, Auslander, Rines, & Stelmachowicz, 1988) and external ear resonance characteristics vary as a function of age (Bender, 1989; Kruger, 1987; Kruger & Ruben, 1987). In addition, children may be unable to provide subjective feedback regarding their hearing aid fittings (i.e., comfortable and uncomfortable listening levels). Therefore, probe microphone measurements of real-ear hearing aid performance should be obtained with children whenever possible (Stelmachowicz & Seewald,

1991). If probe measures are used, target values for frequency/gain and frequency/output limiting characteristics should be selected via a systematic approach that seeks to optimize the audibility of speech (e.g., Byrne & Dillon, 1986; Byrne, Parkinson, & Newall, 1991; McCandless & Lyregaard, 1983; Schwartz, Lyregaard, & Lundh, 1988; Seewald, 1992; see Appendix A for details). For selecting maximum hearing aid output, similar approaches exist (e.g., McCandless & Lyregaard, 1983; Seewald, 1992; Skinner, 1988; see Appendix A for details). Many of these prescriptive approaches were developed for adults and may not be appropriate for children in the process of developing speech and language without some modification. However, such approaches do provide a starting point after which modifications can be made in the verification and validation stages of the process. Some procedures for calculating target gain and output limiting characteristics for children are available in computer-assisted formats (Seewald, Ramji, Sinclair, Moodie, & Jamieson, 1993) although such values can also be calculated manually (Moodie, Seewald, & Sinclair, 1994; see Appendix A for details).

Once the preselected hearing aid frequency-gain and output characteristics have been determined theoretically, verification of the selected electroacoustic parameters should be completed. Because large variability in RECDs are expected in young children, custom earmolds should be available at the time hearing aid performance is verified. Prior to the direct evaluation of the hearing aid on the child, the hearing aid gain and maximum output characteristics should be preset in a hearing aid test box using published or preferably measured RECD values (Feigin et al., 1989; Seewald et al., 1993; see Appendix A, Table 7).

Probe microphone measurements are preferable for use in the verification stage. When probe microphone measures of real-ear hearing aid performance are not possible, however, real-ear hearing aid performance can be predicted by applying average RECD values to coupler measures. Average RECD values from adults, however, are not appropriate for use with children due to the differences in adult and child ear-canal characteristics (Bentler & Pavlovic, 1989; Hawkins, Cooper, & Thompson, 1990). Thus, transforms designed for use with infants and children should be used to predict hearing aid performance (Moodie et al., 1994; Seewald, Sinclair, & Moodie, 1994; Sinclair et al., 1994). Examples of how to use age-appropriate correction factors for determining target gain and maximum output values for children are shown in Appendix A: Worksheets 1 and 2. No facility should fit hearing aids to children if it lacks the equipment for electroacoustic evaluation.

Verification of Output Limiting

The primary purposes of output limiting are to protect the child from loudness discomfort and to avoid potential damage to the ear from amplified sound. Setting the output-limiting characteristics of hearing aids for children is considered of equal, if not greater, importance as other amplification selection considerations. To this end, the audiologist must know what output levels exist in the ear canal of the child. Coupler-based SSPL targets are insufficient for use with infants and young children in particular unless RECDs are applied (Seewald, 1991; Snik & Stollman, 1995). Recommended options for determining output-limiting levels include direct measurement of the real-ear saturation response (RESR) for each ear or the use of measured or average age-related RECD values added to the tabled response (see Appendix A, Table 7B for HA-2/RECD values). It is recommended that swept pure tones or swept warble tones should be used when measuring hearing aid output (Revit, 1991; Seewald, & Hawkins, 1990; Stelmachowicz, 1991; Stelmachowicz, Lewis, Seewald, & Hawkins, 1990).

Clearly, these approaches are predicated on the availability of frequency-specific threshold data. Thus, in cases where full audiometric information is not available, the clinician must make a "best estimate" of the residual hearing across the frequency range important for speech. The use of formulae may necessitate some extrapolation and interpolation of audiometric information from limited audiometric data, taking into account additional clinical and/or familial information that may be available. In such cases, continued observation and assessment of the child are mandatory.

Although none of the threshold-based selection procedures is guaranteed to ensure that a child will not experience loudness discomfort or that output levels are safe, the use of a systematic objective approach that incorporates age-dependent variables into the computations is preferred. Finally, frequency-specific loudness discomfort levels should be obtained when children are old enough to provide reliable responses (Gagné, Seewald, Zelisko, & Hudson, 1991; Kawell, Kopun, & Stelmachowicz, 1988; Macpherson, Elfenbein, Schum, & Bentler, 1991; Stuart, Durieux-Smith, & Stenstrom, 1991).

Verification of Gain/Frequency Response

The hearing aid should be adjusted to approximate the previously determined target gain values for each ear. Aided soundfield threshold measurements are not the preferred procedure for verifying the frequency-gain characteristics of hearing aids in children for several reasons: (a) prolonged cooperation from the child is required, (b) time needed for such testing can be excessive, (c) frequency resolution is poor, and (d) test-retest reliability is frequently poor (Seewald, Moodie, Sinclair, & Cornelisse, 1996). In addition, misleading information may be obtained in cases of severe to profound hearing loss, minimal/mild loss, or when nonlinear signal processing is used (Macrae, 1982; Schwartz & Larson, 1977; Seewald, Hudson, Gagné, & Zelisko, 1992; Snik, van den Borne, Brokx, & Hoekstra, 1995; Stelmachowicz & Lewis, 1988).

Gain should be verified using probe-microphone measures or 2cc coupler and RECD (individually measured or age-related average) values. A 60-dB SPL input using swept pure tones or speech-weighted noise should be used with linear hearing aid systems (Stelmachowicz, 1991; Stelmachowicz et al., 1990). When using nonlinear instruments with children, audiologists should be using advanced verification technology such as the use of multiple signal levels and types to obtain a family of response characteristics (Revit, 1994).

Validation of Aided Auditory Function

Once the prescriptive procedure is complete and the settings of the hearing aids have been verified, the validation process begins. Validation of aided auditory function is a critical, yet often overlooked, component of the pediatric amplification provision process. The purpose of validating aided auditory function is to demonstrate the benefits/limitations of a child's aided listening abilities for perceiving the speech of others as well as his or her own speech. Validation is accomplished, over time, using information derived through the aural habilitation process, as well as the direct measurement of the child's aided auditory performance.

With input provided by parents, teachers, and speech-language pathologists, the pediatric audiologist determines whether the ultimate goals of the hearing aid fitting process have been achieved. These goals are that the speech signal is audible, comfortable, and clear, and that the child is resistant to noise interference in the vast majority of communication environments in which formal and informal learning takes place. Measurements of aided performance quantify the child's auditory abilities at the time of the initial hearing aid fitting, and, as importantly, serve as a baseline for monitoring the child's incorporation of audible speech cues into his or her communication repertoire. Examples of measures of aided auditory performance include aided soundfield responses to various stimuli, including speech measures (see Appendix B, Table I for examples of speech materials to be used with children). Other functional performance measures include the SIFTER (Anderson, 1989), the Pre-School SIFTER (Anderson & Matkin, in development), and the Meaningful Auditory Integration Scale (MAIS; Robbins, Renshaw, & Berry, 1991). Measures of aided performance are not to be used for the purpose of changing hearing aid settings unless there is an obvious behavioral indicator to the contrary. These include loudness tolerance problems or an inability to perceive particular speech cues that should be audible in the aided condition. It is recommended that performance measures be obtained in a binaural presentation mode unless one's intent is to document asymmetry in aided auditory performance.

It is stressed that the contributions provided by all members of the habilitation team promote an atmosphere of mutual cooperation and respect that ultimately results in more effective management for the child with hearing impairment (Edwards, 1996).

Informational Counseling and Follow-Up

In order to ensure that hearing aids will be used successfully, proper counseling, monitoring, and follow-up are essential. Hearing aid orientation programs should include all family members who will be assisting the child with the hearing aid and any professionals working directly with the child and his or her family (e.g., teachers and therapists). The need for parents, teachers, and therapists to receive inservice training on the routine troubleshooting of the child's hearing instruments and the child's performance using amplification cannot be overemphasized. When appropriate, children should be assisted in understanding the details of their hearing loss; instructed in the use, care, and monitoring of their personal hearing aids; and given information on communication strategies under different listening conditions (Edwards, 1996; Elfenbein, 1994; Seewald & Ross, 1988).

It is recommended that young children be seen by an audiologist every 3 months during the first 2 years of using amplification; thereafter children should be seen at least every 6 months if there are no concerns. Reasons for more aggressive monitoring include fluctuating and/or progressive hearing loss (Tharpe, 1996). The follow-up examinations should include audiometric evaluation, electroacoustic evaluation and listening checks of the hearing aid(s), and re-evaluation of the RECD and other probe-microphone measures as appropriate. In addition, the RECD should be measured whenever earmolds are replaced.

Functional measures, as discussed above, should be obtained on a periodic basis to document the development of auditory skills. These measures should include input from family, educators, and other interested professionals regarding communication and educational abilities, and social and behavioral development (Diefendorf et al., 1996). Finally, the audiologist should routinely assess the acoustic conditions in which children use amplification and offer suggestions on ways to optimize the listening environments (Crandell, 1993).

Questions and Answers

The following section has been developed to provide information about questions commonly asked by audiologists working with the pediatric population.

1. *Can an FM system be used in lieu of traditional hearing aids for an infant or young child?*
    Theoretically, an FM system (in the FM mode of operation) should provide an improved signal-to-noise (S/N) ratio for any user. A number of investigators have suggested that use of FM systems as primary amplification can be advantageous for children with severe to profound hearing loss (Benoit, 1989; Brackett, 1992; Kramlinger, 1985; Madell, 1992). In addition, Moeller, Donaghy, Beauchaine, Lewis, and Stelmachowicz (1996) monitored language acquisition in a small group of young children with mild to moderate hearing loss fitted with FM systems in the home setting over a 2-year period. In this study, practical problems such as system bulkiness, signal interference, multiple talkers, the need for extensive parent/caregiver training, and the complications associated with inappropriate mode of operation (e.g., FM transmission of irrelevant conversations and communication at great distances) limited and/or complicated FM system use in many situations. At the end of the 2-year study, the parents reported that they preferred to use the FM system as an assistive device rather than as primary amplification. Although manufacturers have attempted to address some of these practical problems with recent technological advances (e.g., BTE FM systems, voice-activated microphones), currently no single system can be expected to solve all of these problems. If an FM system is recommended for a young child, the practi-

cal issues cited above should be considered in the context of the child's degree of hearing loss, environment, and family structure.

2. What assistive devices, if any, are appropriate for young children?

Assistive devices are often overlooked in the management of young children with hearing loss. Assistive devices can help ensure safety, foster independence, and maintain privacy for older children with hearing loss. FM systems can be used as assistive devices even for very young children in situations where noise, reverberation, and/or distance are a concern. Normal-hearing children learn the meaning of various environmental sounds in an incidental fashion. If a child cannot be expected to hear environmental sounds such as the telephone, doorbell, smoke alarm, or alarm clock when he or she is unaided, the use of appropriate alerting devices should be considered. There will be many situations (e.g., bath time, sleeping) when hearing aids will not be worn, yet the children with hearing loss should be able to identify and respond to familiar environmental and alerting signals. Normal-hearing children begin to attend to television programs by 2–4 years of age. A TV amplifier can provide access to television for children with varying degrees of hearing loss. In addition, for children with severe to profound hearing loss, closed captioning can be introduced at this early age to foster preliteracy skills, such as print awareness. Children with normal hearing are often introduced to the concept of telephone conversations shortly after their first birthday; something as simple as a telephone amplifier may enable the child with hearing loss to talk to friends, grandparents, or other relatives. Children with more severe hearing loss may require a telephone device for the deaf (TDD). TDDs can be can be used once the child can read and write. See Compton (1989) for a more thorough discussion of assistive devices in general and Lewis (1991) for a discussion of the application of these devices with young children.

3. Is there a minimum age at which hearing aids should be fitted? And what factors need to be considered when fitting hearing aids to children under 6 months of age?

If the clinical picture clearly suggests that a permanent, educationally significant hearing loss exists and the family is motivated to proceed with habilitation, then the child is a candidate for amplification regardless of age. Consider, for example, a child who is screened at birth because of a family history of hearing loss (two older siblings with severe bilateral sensorineural hearing loss). If the ABR shows elevated click-evoked and/or tone-burst thresholds, an absence of otoacoustic emissions, and normal middle ear function, there is little reason to delay the hearing aid fitting once the infant is awake sufficient lengths of time to introduce the device effectively. If the clinical picture is less straightforward, then additional testing is warranted before the hearing aid fitting. Under 6 months of age, a successful hearing-aid fitting can often be compromised by practical issues. The complicating factors include: parental acceptance of the hearing loss, ear canal and concha size, financial considerations, additional handicapping condi-

tions or health concerns, conductive component to the hearing loss, problems with retention of the earmold/hearing aid, and acoustic feedback. Some of these problems can be circumvented by the use of loaner hearing aids, body-worn hearing aids, specialized devices to assist with device retention (kiddie tone hooks, double-sided tape, headbands, bonnets, Huggie Aids™) and feedback control via use of a remote microphone. In cases where the hearing aid fitting must be delayed, it is still important to proceed with counseling, parent education, and habilitative services.

4. What about a young child with a conductive hearing loss or a conductive overlay?

In these cases, the first goal is to determine if the hearing loss is entirely conductive or mixed in nature. If it is entirely conductive and cannot be treated medically or surgically (e.g., congenital ossicular anomalies), then it should be viewed in the same way as a sensorineural hearing loss. An air-conduction hearing aid, if it can be used, is preferable to a bone-conduction aid. Bone-conducted amplification is limited by several factors, including low fidelity, the complexity and number of components, the difficulty of keeping the bone vibrator against the mastoid, and, in some cases, malformation of the skull.

If the hearing loss is caused by otitis media, then the child should be followed closely in lieu of amplification. In cases where the conductive component is substantial, ossicular anomalies and/or a cholesteatoma should be ruled out by the managing physician.

When a child has a mixed hearing loss, a bone-conduction hearing aid may or may not be appropriate, depending on the degree and configuration of the sensorineural component and the reason for the conductive component. (Again, air-conduction hearing aid fittings are most appropriate.) In these cases, it is important to work closely with the managing physician.

When a conductive component exists, concern for overamplification is minimized, since the SPL actually reaching the cochlea will be reduced by the amount of the conductive component.

5. How should children with progressive or fluctuating hearing loss be managed?

Progressive hearing loss is known to be associated with certain etiologies (e.g., cytomegalovirus, branchio-oto-renal syndrome, Stickler syndrome, family history of progressive hearing loss). In addition, it has been reported that as many as 21% of children with sensorineural hearing loss showed evidence of fluctuating and/or progressive hearing loss that is not related to middle ear disease (Brookhouser, Worthington, & Kelly, 1994). Accordingly, parents, caregivers, and teachers should be counseled to be aggressive if changes in auditory awareness are suspected in a young child. Obviously, in some cases (e.g., fistula), early medical intervention may halt or actually reverse the progression of hearing loss. When progressive or fluctuating hearing loss has been identified, close follow-up by both the audiologist and the managing otolaryngologist is essential, and a referral to a geneticist may be warranted. Professional counseling should be considered for older children with progressive hearing loss to help them cope with potential changes in their communication abilities. Hearing aids should have flexible frequency response and maximum output characteristics. It may be necessary to recommend more than one volume control setting and/or changes in the internal settings as hearing changes. In some instances, programmable or multi-memory hearing aids may be the best choice.

6. *What about amplification for young children with minimal hearing loss, unilateral hearing loss, rising or unusual configuration, or hearing loss only above 2000 Hz?*
   Minimal, unilateral, rising, and high-frequency hearing losses are not often identified at an early age (Bess & Tharpe, 1986; Mace, Wallace, Whan, & Stelmachowicz, 1991). When identified, however, they pose a special challenge for the pediatric audiologist. These losses should be monitored closely for progression, and middle-ear problems should be treated aggressively. Parents, caregivers, and teachers should be counseled to watch for changes in auditory awareness. Safety issues should be discussed for children with unilateral hearing loss, and the topic of hearing protection should be addressed. Hearing aids and other assistive devices should be considered on a case-by-case basis. Factors such as speech and language development, additional handicapping conditions, academic performance, and communication needs should be considered in conjunction with the audiological data when making decisions about amplification.

7. *What additional factors need to be considered when fitting hearing aids/assistive devices to children with multiple handicapping conditions?*
   Estimates suggest that as many as 30% of children with permanent sensorineural hearing loss have at least one additional handicapping condition (Karchmer, 1985). For many of these children, the accurate determination of hearing status may be difficult. Developmental delays often preclude behavioral audiological testing, and neurological problems often complicate the interpretation of ABR measures. In cases where the existence of educationally significant hearing loss can be established, however, a multidisciplinary approach is mandatory. Parents, physicians, audiologists, teachers, speech-language pathologists, physical and/or occupational therapists, and social workers need to be involved in the decision to proceed with amplification. Because these children often have atypical early life experiences, a primary goal should be to meet the needs of both the child and his or her family. It is important to recognize that for many of these children, hearing per se may not be a priority for the family. In many cases, it may be appropriate to delay the hearing aid fitting or to use some type of assistive device instead of conventional amplification. (A child on a ventilator, for example, may benefit from a hearing aid with a remote microphone).

When a decision is made to proceed with amplification, it is essential to evaluate its impact in relation to the child's physical challenges, environment, and communication needs.

Future Directions

The selection and evaluation of properly fitted and functioning hearing aids for children with hearing loss is one of the major challenges facing today's pediatric audiologist. This challenge is compounded by a continued decrease in the average age of identification of hearing loss in children, as well as the ever-changing technology in hearing aids and the associated instrumentation used in the selection and evaluation of hearing aids. Hence, it is critical for the pediatric audiologist to stay abreast of the trends, practices, and technologies used in the hearing assessment and hearing aid fitting of very young children. To this end, the Pediatric Working Group recognizes the need for systematic research and encourages controlled studies in all areas of pediatric amplification. Examples of important directions for future research include:

➤ Develop/validate audiometric assessment protocols for fitting amplification in infants.
➤ Examine the relationship between aided performance and auditory/communicative function.
➤ Develop additional psychoacoustic data from children with hearing loss, and consider the implications of such data on amplification selection and evaluation.
➤ Validate various prescriptive procedures for this population.
➤ Evaluate current technologies designed to enhance signal-to-noise ratio.
➤ Develop procedures and guidelines for fitting advanced technology hearing aids to children.
➤ Determine the efficacy of amplification for children with minimal hearing loss, unilateral hearing loss, or unusual audiometric configurations.
➤ Develop better models for predicting performance and establishing safety and efficacy.

Acknowledgments

We are grateful to Arthur Boothroyd, whose comprehensive and critical review strongly influenced the final version of this statement.

Supported in part by Project #MCI-TN 217 from the Maternal and Child Health Bureau (Title V, Social Security Act), Health Resource and Services Administration, Department of Health and Human Services.

References

American Speech-Language-Hearing Association. (1991, March). Guidelines for the audiologic assessment of children from birth through 36 months of age. *Asha, 33*(Suppl. 5), 37–43.
Anderson, K. (1989). *Screening Instrument for Targeting Education Risk* (SIFTER). Austin, TX: Pro-Ed.
Anderson, K., & Matkin, N. D. (in development). Preschool S.I.F.T.E.R. Screening Instrument for Targeting Educational Risk in Preschool Children (age 3-kindergarten).
Benoit, R. (1989). Home use of FM amplification systems during the early childhood years. *Hearing Instruments, 40*(3), 8–12.
Bentler, R. A. (1989). External ear resonance characteristics in children. *Journal of Speech and Hearing Disorders, 54*, 264–268.

Bentler, R. A., & Pavlovic, C. V. (1989). Transfer functions and correction factors used in hearing aid evaluation and research. *Ear and Hearing, 10*, 58–63.

Bess, F. H., Gravel, J. S., & Tharpe, A. M. (Eds.). (1996). *Amplification for children with auditory deficits.* Nashville, TN: Bill Wilkerson Center Press.

Bess, F. H., & Paradise, J. L. (1994). Universal screening for infant hearing impairment: A reply. *Pediatrics, 94*(6), 959–963.

Bess, F. H., & Tharpe, A. M. (1986). Case history data on unilaterally hearing-impaired children. *Ear and Hearing, 7*(1), 14–19.

Brackett, D. (1992). Effects of early FM use on speech perception. In M. Ross (Ed.), *FM auditory training systems—Characteristics, selection and use.* Timonium, MD: York Press.

Brackett, D. (1996). Developing auditory capabilities in children with severe and profound hearing loss. In F. H. Bess, J. S. Gravel, & A. M. Tharpe (Eds.), *Amplification for children with auditory deficits.* Nashville, TN: Bill Wilkerson Center Press.

Bratt, G. W. (1980). *Hearing and receiver output in occluded ear canals in children.* Unpublished doctoral dissertation. Nashville, TN: Vanderbilt University.

Brookhouser, P., Worthington, D., & Kelly, W. (1994). Fluctuating and/or progressive sensorineural hearing loss in children. *Laryngoscope, 104*, 958–964.

Byrne, D., & Dillon, H. (1986). The National Acoustic Laboratories' (NAL) new procedure for selecting the gain and frequency response of a hearing aid. *Ear and Hearing, 7*, 257–265.

Byrne, D., Parkinson, A., & Newall, P. (1991). Modified hearing aid selection procedure to severe-profound hearing losses. In G. Studebaker, F. Bess, & L. Beck (Eds.), *The Vanderbilt Hearing-Aid Report 11.* Parkton, MD: York Press.

Compton, C. (1989). *Assistive devices: Doorways to independence.* Washington, DC: Gallaudet University.

Crandell, C. C. (1993). Speech recognition in noise by children with minimal degrees of sensorineural hearing loss. *Ear and Hearing, 14*, 210–216.

Diefendorf, A. O., Reitz, P. S., Escobar, M. W., & Wynne, M. K. (1996). Initiating early amplification: Tips for success. In F. H. Bess, J. S. Gravel, & A. M. Tharpe (Eds.), *Amplification for children with auditory deficits.* Nashville, TN: Bill Wilkerson Center Press.

Edwards, C. (1996). Auditory intervention for children with milder auditory deficits. In F. H. Bess, J. S. Gravel, & A. M. Tharpe (Eds.), *Amplification for children with auditory deficits.* Nashville, TN: Bill Wilkerson Center Press.

Elfenbein, J. (1994). Monitoring preschoolers' hearing aids: Issues in program design and implementation. *American Journal of Audiology, 3*(2), 65–70.

Feigin, J. A., Kopun, J. G., Stelmachowicz, P. G., & Gorga, M. P. (1989). Probe-tube microphone measures of ear canal sound pressure levels in infants and children. *Ear and Hearing, 10*(4), 254–258.

Gagné, J.-P., Seewald, R. C., Zelisko, D. L., & Hudson, S. P. (1991). Procedure for defining the auditory area of hearing-impaired adolescents with a severe/profound hearing loss II: Loudness discomfort levels. *Journal of Speech-Language Pathology and Audiology, 15*(4), 27–32.

Hawkins, D. B., Cooper, W. A., & Thompson, D. J. (1990). Comparison among SPL's in real ears, 2CM³ and 6CM³ couplers *Journal of the American Academy of Audiology, 1*, 154–161.

Hedley-Williams, A., Tharpe, A. M., & Bess, F. H. (1996). Fitting hearing aids in children: A survey of practice procedures. In F. H. Bess, J. S. Gravel, & A. M. Tharpe (Eds.), *Amplification for children with auditory deficits.* Nashville, TN: Bill Wilkerson Center Press.

Karchmer, M. A. (1985). A demographic perspective. In E. Cherow (Ed.), *Hearing impaired children and youth with developmental disabilities.* Washington DC: Gallaudet Press, 37–56.

Kawell, M. E., Kopun, J. G., & Stelmachowicz, P. G. (1988). Loudness discomfort levels in children. *Ear and Hearing, 9*(33), 133–136

Kramlinger, M. (1985). How I helped my children communicate: Adapting an auditory trainer for everyday use. *Exceptional Parent, 15*, 19–25.

Kruger, B. (1987). An update on the external ear resonance in infants and young children. *Ear and Hearing, 8*(16), 333–336.

Kruger, B., & Ruben, A. J. (1987). The acoustic properties of the infant ear. *Acta Oto-Laryngologica* (Stockholm) *103*, 578–585.

Lewis, D. (1991). FM systems and assistive devices: Selection and evaluation. In J. A. Feigin & P. G. Stelmachowicz (Eds.), *Pediatric amplifcation: Proceedings of the 1991 National Conference.* Omaha, NE: Boys Town National Research Hospital.

Mace, A. L., Wallace, K. L., Whan, M. A., & Stelmachowicz, P. G. (1991). Relevant factors in the identification of hearing loss. *Ear and Hearing, 12*, 287–293.

Macpherson, B. J., Elfenbein, J. L., Schum, R. L., & Bentler, R. (1991). Thresholds of discomfort in young children. *Ear and Hearing, 12*(3), 184–190.

Macrae, J. (1982). Invalid aided thresholds. *Hearing Instruments 33*(9), 20, 22.

Madell, J. R. (1992). FM systems for children birth to age five. In M. Ross (Ed.), *FM auditory training systems—Characteristics, selection and use.* Timonium, MD, York Press.

McCandless, G., & Lyregaard, P. (1983). Prescription of gain/output (POGO) for hearing aids. *Hearing Instruments 34*, 16–21.

Moeller, M. P., Donagby, K., Beauchaine, K, Lewis, D. E., & Stelmachowicz, P. G. (1996). Longitudinal study of FM system use in non-academic settings: Effects on language development. *Ear and Hearing, 17*, 28–41.

Moodie, K S., Seewald, R. C., & Sinclair, S. T. (1994). Procedure for predicting real-ear hearing aid performance in young children. *American Journal of Audiology, 3*(1), 23–31.

Nelson Barlow, N., Auslander, M.-C., Rines, D., & Stelmachowicz, P. G. (1988). Probe-tube microphone measures in hearing-impaired children and adults. *Ear and Hearing, 9*, 243–247.

Revit, L. J. (1991). New tests for signal-processing and multichannel hearing instruments. *Hearing Journal, 44*, 20–23.

Revit, L. J. (1994). Using coupler tests in the fitting of hearing aids. In M. Valente (Ed.), *Strafegies for selecting and verifying hearing aid fittings.* New York: Thieme Medical Publishers.

Robbins, A. M., Renshaw, J. T., & Berry, S. W. (1991). Evaluating meaningful auditory integration in profoundly hearing impaired children. *American Journal of Otology, 12*, 144–150.

Schwartz, D. M., & Larson, V. D. (1977). A comparison of three hearing aid evaluation procedures for young children. *Archives of Otolaryngology, 103*, 401–406.

Schwartz, D., Lyregaard, P., & Lundh, P. (1988). Hearing aid selection for severe-to-profound hearing loss. *Hearing Journal, 41*, 13–17.

Seewald, R. C. (1991). Hearing aid output limiting considerations for children. In J. Feigin & P. G. Stelmachowicz (Eds.), *Pediatric amplification: Proceedings of the 1991 National Conference.* Omaha, NE: Boys Town National Research Hospital.

Seewald, R. C. (1992). The desired sensation level method for fitting children: Version 3.0. *The Hearing Journal, 45*(4), 36–41.

Seewald, R. C., Hudson, S. P., Gagné, J.-P., & Zelisko, D. L. (1992). Comparison of two procedures for estimating the sensation level of amplified speech. *Ear and Hearing, 13*(3), 142–149.

Seewald, R. C., Moodie, K. S., Sinclair, S. T., & Cornelisse, L. E. (1996). Traditional and theoretical approaches to selecting amplification for infants and young children. In F. H. Bess, J. S. Gravel, & A. M. Tharpe (Eds.), *Amplification for children with auditory deficits.* Nashville, TN: Bill Wilkerson Center Press.

Seewald, R. C., Ramji, K. V., Sinclair, S. T., Moodie, K S., & Jamieson, D. G. (1993). *Computer-assisted implementation of the desired sensation level method for electroacoustic selection and fitting in children: User's manual.* London, ON: University of Western Ontario.

Seewald, R., & Ross, M. (1988). Amplification for young hearing-impaired children. In M. Pollack (Ed.), *Amplification for the hearing impaired.* New York: Grune & Stratton.

Seewald, R. C. Sinclair, S. T., & Moodie, K. S. (1994). Predictive accuracy of a procedure for electroacoustic fitting in young children. Presented at the XXII International Congress of Audiology, July 1994, Halifax.

Sinclair, S. T., Beauchaine, K. L., Moodie, K. S., Feigin, J. A., Seewald, R. C., & Stelmachowicz, P. G. (1994). Repeatability of a real-ear to coupler difference measurement as a function of age. Presented at the American Academy of Audiology Sixth Annual Convention, April 1994, Richmond.

Skinner, M. (1988). *Hearing aid evaluation.* Englewood Cliffs, NJ: Prentice Hall.

Snik, A. F. M., & Stollman, M. H. P. (1995). Measured and calculated insertion gains in young children. *British Journal of Audiology, 29,* 7–11.

Snik, A. F. M., van den Borne, S., Brokx, J. P. L., & Hoekstra, C. (1995). Hearing aid fitting in profoundly hearing impaired children; comparison of prescription rules. *Scandinavian Audiology.*

Stein, L. K (1995). On the real age of identification of congenital hearing loss. *Audiology Today, 7*(1), 10–11.

Stelmachowicz, P. G. (1991). Clinical issues related to hearing aid maximum output. In G. A. Studebaker, F. H. Bess, & L. B. Beck (Eds.), *The Vanderbilt/VA hearing aid report* (pp. 141–148). Parkton: York Press.

Stelmachowicz, P. G., & Lewis, D. E. (1988). Some theoretical considerations concerning the relation between functional gain and insertion gain. *Journal of Speech and Hearing Research, 31,* 491–496.

Stelmachowicz, P. G., Lewis, D. E., Seewald, R. C., & Hawkins, D. B. (1990). Complex vs. pure-tone stimuli in the evaluation of hearing aid characteristics. *Journal of Speech and Hearing Research, 33,* 380–385.

Stelmachowicz, P. G., & Seewald, R. C. (1991). Probe-tube microphone measures in children. *Seminars in Hearing, 12,* 62–72.

Stuart, A., Durieux-Smith, A., & Stenstrom, R. (1991). Probe-tube microphone measures of loudness discomfort levels in children. *Ear and Hearing, 12,* 140–143.

Tharpe, A. M. (1996). Special considerations for children with fluctuating/progressive hearing loss. In F. H. Bess, J. S. Gravel, & A. M. Tharpe (Eds.), *Amplification for children with auditory deficits.* Nashville, TN: Bill Wilkerson Center Press.

Received May 8, 1995
Accepted July 12, 1995

Contact author: Fred H. Bess, PhD, Vanderbilt University, Division of Hearing and Speech Sciences, Nashville, TN 37232-8700

Key Words: infants, amplification, children, assistive devices, research

Appendix A

Procedures for Calculating Target Gain and Output Limiting Characteristics for Children

A.1. Prescription of Gain and Output (POGO)

POGO was introduced in 1983 by McCandless and Lyregaard. It is based on the following assumptions: (a) frequency-gain response and maximum output limiting are essential characteristics in a basic prescriptive fitting, and (b) a valid prescriptive fitting can be derived based on audiometric information obtained with pure-tone or other stationary signals that will ensure an amplified signal that is audible and delivered at a comfortable listening level.

Required insertion gain is calculated using the formula in Table 1.

POGO II was introduced in 1987 to prescribe the additional gain required for individuals with severe to profound hearing losses. Therefore, *for losses greater than 65 dB*, the formula shown in Table 2 is used.

Reserve Gain

The POGO formula includes a 10-dB reserve gain

Conductive and/or Mixed Hearing Losses

The POGO formula does not provide recommendations regarding the gain requirements of those with conductive or mixed hearing loss.

Maximum Output Calculations

The calculation of hearing aid maximum output characteristics requires the measurement of UCLs at .5, 1, and 2 kHz, and is made using the equation shown in Table 3.

Defining 2cc Coupler Criteria

Table 4 provides transformation values to convert the pre-scribed insertion gain for ITE or BTE hearing aids to 2cc coupler gain. The values shown in this table are subtracted from the POGO desired insertion gain values. To assist in the selection of hearing aids from manufacturer's published specification books, one must add the desired reserve gain across frequencies.

A.2. National Acoustic Laboratories (NAL) Procedure

The first version of the NAL procedure was introduced in 1976 (Byrne & Tonnison). The rationale of this procedure is to amplify all frequency bands of speech to MCL. In 1986, Byrne and Dillon published a revised version of the NAL procedure (NAL-R). In the revised version, the prescribed real-ear gain is dependent on both degree of hearing loss and slope of hearing thresholds across frequencies. In 1991, the NAL-R procedure was further modified to provide more overall gain for individuals with severe to profound hearing losses. The calculation of X has been modified (see line 1, Table 5) to provide more overall gain for mean thresholds over 60 dB HL. In addition, when the threshold at 2 kHz is 95 dB HL or greater, more gain is prescribed in the low frequencies and less gain in the high frequencies.

Required insertion gain is calculated as a function of frequency using the formulas shown in Table 5.

Reserve Gain

The NAL formula includes a 15-dB reserve gain to be added to the desired insertion gain values.

Conductive and/or Mixed Hearing Losses

For these individuals, additional gain is needed at each frequency, equal to one-fourth of the difference between air- and bone-conduction thresholds.

A.3. Desired Sensation Level (DSL) Method

The general rationale of the DSL method is to use a systematic procedure to provide children with hearing loss with an amplified speech signal that is audible, comfortable, and undistorted across the broadest relevant frequency range possible. This method applies age-appropriate individual or average values for relevant acoustic characteristics that are known to vary as a function of age—specifically, external ear resonance characteristics and real-ear to 2cc coupler differences (RECD). A computer-assisted implementation of the DSL method is available.

TABLE 1. POGO formula for calculating required insertion gain.

Frequency (Hz)	Insertion Gain (dB) Formula
250	1/2 HTL - 10
500	1/2 HTL - 5
1000	1/2 HTL
2000	1/2 HTL
3000	1/2 HTL
4000	1/2 HTL

TABLE 2. POGO II formula for losses greater than 65 dB.

Frequency (Hz)	Insertion Gain (dB) Formula
250	1/2 HL + 1/2 (HL-65) - 10
500	1/2 HL + 1/2 (HL-65) - 5
1000	1/2 HL + 1/2 (HL-65)
2000	1/2 HL + 1/2 (HL-65)
3000	1/2 HL + 1/2 (HL-65)
4000	1/2 HL + 1/2 (HL-65)

TABLE 3. Formula for maximum power output (MPO) calculations (in dB SPL re: 2cc coupler).

$$MPO = \left(\frac{UCL_{500} + UCL_{1000} + UCL_{2000}}{3} \right) + 4$$

TABLE 4. Correction values (in dB) to be subtracted from the POGO insertion gain values to estimate the corresponding 2cc coupler gain as a function of frequency.

	Frequency (Hz)					
	250	500	1000	2000	3000	4000
ITE	3	1	2	-6	-6	5
BTE	3	1	0	-2	-11	-9

TABLE 5. NAL-R formulas for calculating required real-ear gain (REG) as a function of frequency modified for severe/profound hearing losses.

1. Calculate $X_{dB} = 0.05 \times (HTL_{500} + HTL_{1000} + HTL_{2000}$ up to 180 dB) + 0.116 $\times$ combined HTL in excess of 180 dB.

2. Calculate the prescribed real-ear gain (REG) at each frequency:

$$REG_{250} \text{ (dB)} = X + 0.31\ HTL_{250} - 17 \qquad REG_{2000} \text{ (dB)} = X + 0.31\ HTL_{2000} - 1$$
$$REG_{500} \text{ (dB)} = X + 0.31\ HTL_{500} - 8 \qquad REG_{3000} \text{ (dB)} = X + 0.31\ HTL_{3000} - 2$$
$$REG_{750} \text{ (dB)} = X + 0.31\ HTL_{750} - 3 \qquad REG_{4000} \text{ (dB)} = X + 0.31\ HTL_{4000} - 2$$
$$REG_{1000} \text{ (dB)} = X + 0.31\ HTL_{1000} + 1 \qquad REG_{6000} \text{ (dB)} = X + 0.31\ HTL_{6000} - 2$$
$$REG_{1500} \text{ (dB)} = X + 0.31\ HTL_{1500} + 1$$

3. When the 2000-Hz HTL is 95 dB or greater, add the following gain (dB) values.

HTL 2 kHz	250	500	750	1000	1500	2000	3000	4000	6000
95	4	3	1	0	-1	-2	-2	-2	-2
100	6	4	2	0	-2	-3	-3	-3	-3
105	8	5	2	0	-3	-5	-5	-5	-5
110	11	7	3	0	-3	-6	-6	-6	-6
115	13	8	4	0	-4	-8	-8	-8	-8
120	15	9	4	0	-5	-9	-9	-9	-9

Frequency (Hz) column headers

TABLE 6. The desired real-ear aided response values (in dB gain)[a] as a function of threshold (dB HL) and audiometric frequency for the DSL Method.

Threshold (dB HL)	250	500	750	1000	1500	2000	3000	4000	6000
0	1	2	3	1	4	11	14	13	6
5	1	2	3	2	5	12	16	15	8
10	1	3	4	4	7	15	18	18	10
15	2	4	5	6	10	17	21	20	13
20	3	5	7	9	12	20	24	23	16
25	5	7	9	12	15	23	27	26	19
30	7	9	11	15	18	26	30	30	23
35	10	12	14	18	22	29	34	33	27
40	13	15	17	21	25	32	38	37	31
45	17	18	20	25	29	36	41	40	35
50	20	21	24	28	32	40	45	44	39
55	24	25	28	32	36	43	49	48	43
60	28	28	31	36	40	47	53	52	47
65	32	32	35	39	44	50	57	55	51
70	36	36	39	43	48	54	60	59	55
75	41	40	42	47	51	57	64	63	59
80	44	43	46	50	55	61	67	66	62
85	48	47	50	54	58	64	71	70	66
90	52	50	53	57	62	67	74	73	69
95	55	54	56	60	65	70	76	76	71
100	58	57	59	62	67	72	79	79	73
105	—	60	62	65	70	75	81	81	—
110	—	62	64	67	72	77	83	85	—

Frequency (Hz) column headers

[a]The values presented in this table assume a real-ear unaided response (REUR) approximating published average adult values (Shaw & Vaillencourt, 1985). Furthermore, if audiometric data have been collected using 3A insert earphones (in dB HL), the above values assume an average adult real-ear to coupler difference.

Desired Real-Ear Aided Response Values (in dB gain) as a Function of Threshold (dB HL)

The real-ear aided response values, in dB gain, required to amplify the long-term speech spectrum to the desired sensation levels as a function of threshold (dB HL) and audiometric frequency are shown in Table 6.

Estimated real-ear to 2cc coupler difference (RECD) values as a function of age are shown in Table 7. These age-appropriate estimated RECD values can be used when individual RECD measures cannot be obtained. The use of these values to derive corresponding 2cc coupler targets enables hearing aid electroacoustic response shaping to occur in the hearing aid test chamber.

The DSL Unamplified Long-Term Average Speech Spectrum

The DSL unamplified speech spectrum attempts to strike a compromise between the average speech levels of potential conversational partners and the average speech levels of a child's own speech productions at the ear-level position. The overall level of the DSL long-term average speech spectrum (LTASS) is 70 dB SPL. The DSL unamplified LTASS levels are shown in Table 8 as a function of frequency.

Reserve Gain

The DSL method currently applies 12 dB of reserve gain.

Conductive and/or Mixed Hearing Losses

The DSL method does not currently provide recommendations regarding additional gain requirements for individuals with conductive or mixed hearing loss.

Desired Real-Ear Maximum Sound-Pressure Level (SPL) Values (in dB) as a Function of Threshold (dB HL)

The desired real-ear maximum SPL values as a function of threshold (dB HL) and audiometric frequency are shown in Table 9.

Defining 2cc Coupler Criteria

The DSL worksheets on pages 65 and 66 provide information on how to calculate 2cc coupler gain criteria for the purposes of electroacoustic selection and fitting.

A.4. References

POGO

McCandless, G. A. (1994). Overview and rationale of threshold-based hearing aid selection procedures. In M. Valente (Ed.), *Strategies for selecting and verifying hearing aid fittings.* New York: Thieme Medical Publishers.

McCandless G. A., & Lyregaard P. E. (1983). Prescription of gain

TABLE 7. Estimated real-ear to 2cc coupler difference (RECD) transformations as a function of age and audiometric frequency.

A. HA-1 coupler

	\multicolumn{9}{c}{Frequency (Hz)}								
	250	500	750	1000	1500	2000	3000	4000	6000
0–12 months	5.4	9.8	10.0	13.0	14.4	14.5	18.5	21.6	22.4
13–24 months	7.3	10.2	9.9	12.6	13.7	14.2	16.1	18.5	15.5
25–48 months	4.0	8.5	8.7	11.8	13.2	13.2	15.5	16.2	15.4
49–60 months	2.8	8.0	8.5	9.8	11.9	12.7	14.0	15.0	14.8
>60 months[a]	2.2	4.6	4.3	6.3	7.7	8.8	11.2	13.1	13.7

B. HA-2 coupler

	\multicolumn{9}{c}{Frequency (Hz)}								
	250	500	750	1000	1500	2000	3000	4000	6000
0–12 months	5.5	9.7	9.6	11.9	11.6	10.5	16.2	19.4	17.8
13–24 months	7.4	10.1	9.5	11.5	10.9	10.2	13.8	16.3	10.9
25–48 months	4.1	8.4	8.3	10.7	10.4	9.2	13.2	14.0	10.8
49–60 months	2.9	7.9	8.1	8.7	9.1	8.7	11.7	12.8	10.2
>60 months	2.3	4.5	3.9	5.2	4.9	4.8	8.9	10.9	9.1

[a]Values for individuals > 60 months were derived by Seewald, Ramji, Sinclair, Moodie, and Jamieson (1993), at The University of Western Ontario. Values for individuals < 60 months were derived by applying age group data reported by Feigin, Kopun, Stelmachowicz, and Gorga (1989) to the values of Seewald and colleagues. HA-2 coupler values were derived by applying an HA-1 to HA-2 coupler transformation (Seewald et al., 1993) to the HA-1 coupler values.

TABLE 8. The one-third octave band levels (dB SPL) of the University of Western Ontario long-term average speech spectrum for hearing aid fitting in children.

	\multicolumn{9}{c}{Frequency (Hz)}								
	250	500	750	1000	1500	2000	3000	4000	6000
dB SPL	62.8	64.3	60.1	56.4	52.1	51.0	45.0	42.3	42.1

TABLE 9. The desired real-ear maximum sound-pressure level (SPL) values (in dB)[a] as a function of threshold (dB HL) and audiometric frequency for the DSL Method.

Threshold (dB HL)	Frequency (Hz)								
	250	500	750	1000	1500	2000	3000	4000	6000
0	94	102	101	99	99	100	100	98	97
5	94	102	101	99	99	101	100	99	97
10	94	102	101	100	100	102	101	100	98
15	95	103	102	101	100	103	102	101	98
20	95	103	102	101	101	104	103	102	99
25	96	104	103	103	102	105	105	103	100
30	97	105	104	104	104	106	106	104	101
35	99	106	106	105	105	108	108	106	103
40	100	107	107	107	107	110	110	108	105
45	102	109	109	109	109	112	112	109	106
50	104	111	110	110	111	114	114	111	108
55	106	113	112	112	113	116	116	113	111
60	109	115	114	114	115	118	118	115	113
65	111	117	117	117	117	120	120	118	115
70	114	119	119	119	119	122	123	120	117
75	117	121	121	121	121	124	125	122	120
80	120	123	123	123	123	126	127	124	122
85	123	126	125	125	125	128	129	126	124
90	126	128	127	127	127	130	130	128	125
95	129	130	129	129	129	131	132	130	127
100	132	131	131	130	131	133	133	132	128
105	—	133	132	131	132	134	135	133	—
110	—	134	134	133	133	135	136	135	—

[a]See note at end of Table 6.

and output (POGO) for hearing aids. *Hearing Instruments, 3,* 16–21.

Schwartz, D., Lyregaard, P. E., & Lundh, P. (1988). Hearing aid selection for severe-to-profound hearing loss. *Hearing Journal, 41*(2), 13–17.

NAL

Battaglia, D., Dillon, H., & Byrne, D. (1991). *HASP: Version 2 user's manual.* Chatswood, Australia: The National Acoustics Laboratories.

Byrne, D., & Dillon, H. (1986). The National Acoustic Laboratories' (NAL) research for hearing aid gain and frequency response selection strategies. In G. A. Studebaker & I. Hochberg (Eds.), *Acoustical factors affecting hearing aid performance* (2nd ed.). Boston, MA: Allyn and Bacon.

Byrne, D., Parkinson, A., & Newall, P. (1991). Modified hearing aid selection procedure for severe-profound hearing losses. In G. Studebaker, F. Bess, & L. Beck (Eds.), *The Vanderbilt Hearing-Aid Report II.* Parkton, MD: York Press.

Byrne, D., & Tonisson, W. (1976). Selecting the gain of hearing aids for persons with sensorineural hearing impairments. *Scandinavian Audiology, 5,* 51–59.

DSL

Feigin, J. A., Kopun, J. G., Stelmachowicz, P. G., & Gorga, M. P. (1989). Probe-tube microphone measures of ear-canal sound pressure levels in infants and children. *Ear and Hearing, 10*(4), 254–258.

Seewald, R. C. (1992). The desired sensation level method for fitting children: Version 3.0. *Hearing Journal, 45*(4), 36–41.

Seewald, R. C., Ramji, K. V., Sinclair, S. T., Moodie, K. S., & Jamieson, D. G. (1993). *Computer-assisted implementation of the desired sensation level method for electroacoustic selection and fitting in children: User's manual.* London, ON: University of Western Ontario.

Seewald, R. C., Ross, M., & Spiro, M. K. (1985). Selecting amplification characteristics for young hearing-impaired children. *Ear and Hearing, 6*(1), 48–53.

Shaw, E. A., & Vaillancourt, M. M. (1985). Transformation of sound-pressure level from the free field to the eardrum presented in numerical form. *Journal of the Acoustical Society of America, 78*(3), 1120–1123.

Worksheet #1: Calculating target 2cc coupler gain values as a function of frequency.

	250	500	750	1000	1500	2000	3000	4000	6000
Threshold (dB HL)									
Desired real-ear aided response									
RECD values									
Mic Effects[a]									
Target coupler gain (row 2-3-4)									
Measured coupler gain									
Difference (row 5-6)									

[a]*Mic Location Effect values* as a function of hearing aid type and audiometric frequency.

	Frequency (Hz)								
	250	500	750	1000	1500	2000	3000	4000	6000
BTE	0.5	1.2	0.9	0.3	2.5	4.1	2.8	3.7	1.6
ITE	0.5	1.8	2.0	1.5	-0.3	3.8	3.3	4.3	0.4
ITC	0.3	0	0.4	1.2	-1.9	2.1	3.5	6.4	-1.8
BODY AID	3.0	4.0	2.0	0	-4	-4	0	0	0

1. Enter the individual's hearing threshold measures as a function of frequency.

2. Using Table 6, determine the desired real-ear aided response as a function of frequency and hearing threshold level. For example, if the audiometric threshold at 250 Hz is 30 dB HL, the desired real-ear aided response (in gain) is 7 dB.

3. Enter the individual's measured RECD values. If measured values cannot be obtained, use estimated age-appropriate RECD values as a function of frequency from Table 7(A) for ITE fittings and Table 7(B) for BTE fittings.

4. Enter the appropriate mic location effect values as a function of hearing aid style.

5. To determine the target 2cc coupler gain values across frequencies, subtract the RECD and mic location effect values from the desired real-ear aided response values (row 2–3–4).

6. Using the frequency-specific University of Western Ontario (UWO) LTASS values from Table 8 as a guideline for test signal input levels, adjust the electroacoustic characteristics of the hearing aid in the hearing aid test chamber to approximate the target 2cc coupler values as a function of frequency. For example, using a 50-dB stimulus level, adjust the volume control wheel to approximate the target 2cc gain at 2000 Hz. Using a 65-dB stimulus level, adjust the hearing aid tone control to approximate the target 2cc gain at 500 Hz. (Note: for linear and output compression hearing aids, set maximum output characteristics before setting the hearing aid gain/frequency response characteristics).

Worksheet #2: Calculating target saturation SPL (SSPL) values as a function of frequency.

	250	500	750	1000	1500	2000	3000	4000	6000
Threshold (dB HL)									
Desired real-ear maximum SPL									
RECD values									
Target coupler SSPL (row 2–3)									
Measured coupler SSPL									
Difference (row 3–4)									

1. Enter the individual's hearing threshold measures as a function of frequency.

2. Using Table 9, determine the desired real-ear maximum SPL (dB) as a function of frequency and hearing threshold level. For example, if the audiometric threshold at 250 Hz is 30 dB HL, the desired maximum SPL (dB) is 97.

3. Enter the individual's measured RECD values. If measured values cannot be obtained, use estimated age-appropriate RECD values as a function of frequency from Table 7.

4. To determine the target SSPL values across frequencies, subtract the RECD values from the desired real-ear maximum SPL values (row 2–3).

5. With the hearing aid volume control wheel adjusted to a full-on position, place the hearing aid in the hearing aid test chamber. Using a 90-dB stimulus level, look for the primary peak in the hearing aid response. Adjust the hearing aid maximum output control so that it does not exceed the target coupler SSPL value for that frequency.

6. Using a 90-dB pure-tone stimulus level, enter the measured coupler SSPL values as a function of frequency.

7. Determine the difference between the target and measured SSPL values.

8. Once the hearing aid maximum output characteristics have been adjusted to approximate the 2cc target values, the frequency gain characteristics should be quickly re-evaluated to ensure that adjustments are not necessary. In addition, if the hearing aid being fitted is a compression instrument, an evaluation of the compression characteristics at user's settings should be conducted.

Appendix B

Common Speech Recognition Materials Used With Children

TABLE 1 (page 1 of 2). Common speech recognition materials used with children. Children's lists.

Test name	Investigator(s)	Material	Number of Lists	Items Per List	Response Format	Response Task	Age Range	Degree of HL
1. PBK-50	Haskins (1949)	Monosyllables	4	50	Open set	Verbal	6-9 years	Mild to moderate
2. Word Intelligibility by Picture Identifica-Identification (WIPI)	Ross & Lerman (1970)	Monosyllables	4	25	Closed set (6 picture matrix)	Psycho-motor	3-6 years	Mild to severe
3. Sound Effects Recognition Test (SERT)	Finitzo-Hieber, Gerlin, Matkin, Cherow-Skalka (1980)	Environmental Sounds	3	10	Closed set (4 picture matrix)	Psycho-motor	≥3 years	Severe to profound
4. Spondee Recognition Test	Erber (1974)	Spondees	1	25	Closed set	Written	8-16 years	Severe to profound
5. Six Sound Test	Ling (1978); Ling (1989)	Vowels /u/, /a/, /I/, /ʃ/, /s/, /m/	1	6	Open set	Psycho-motor	Infant/ children	Moderate to profound
6. Glendonald Auditory Screening Procedure (GASP)	Erber (1982)	Phonemes Words Sentences	1 1 1	10 12 10	Closed Set	Psycho-motor and verbal	6–13 years	Moderate to profound
7. Childrens Perception of Speech (NUCHIPS)	Katz & Elliott (1978)	Monosyllables	4 (ran-domiza-tions)	50	Closed set	Psycho-motor	≥3 years	Mild to moderate
8. Discrimination by the Identification of Pictures (DIP)	Siegenthaler & Haspiel (1966)	Monosyllables	3	48	Closed set (2 picture matrix)	Psycho-motor	3-8 years	Mild to severe
9. BKB Sentences	Bench, Koval, & Bamford (1979)	Sentences	21 11	16 16	Open set	Verbal	8-15 years	Mild to moderate
10. Auditory Numbers Test (ANT)	Erber (1980)	Numbers	1	5	Closed set	Psycho-mothor	3-8 years	Severe to profound
11. Pediatric Speech Intelligibility Test (PSI)	Jerger, Lewis, Hawkins, & Jerger (1980)	Monosyllables Sentences	1 2	20 10	Closed set	Verbal	3-10 years	Mild to moderate
12. Hoosier Auditory Visual Enhancement Test (HAVE)	Renshaw, Robbins, Miyamoto, Osberger, & Pope (1988)	Monosyllables	1	40	Closed set	Verbal/Sign	≥2 years	Mild to profound
13. Minimal Pairs Test	Robbins, Renshaw, Miyamoto, Osberger, & Pope (1988)	Monosyllables	2	80	Closed set	Psycho-motor	≥5 years	Mild to profound
14. Imitative tests of Speech Pattern Contrast Perception (IMSPAC)	Boothroyd (1996)	Syllables	4 (plus random-izations)	40	Auditors: Closed set	Child: Imitation	≥3 years	Mild to profound
15. Three Interval Force Choice Test of Speech Pattern Contrast Perception (THRIFT)	Boothroyd (in press)	Syllables	1 (plus random-izations)	54 or 108	Choose odd one of 3	Pointing, button-press, or verbal	≥7 years	Mild to profound
16. Arthur Boothroyd Lists (AB lists)	Boothroyd (1968)	Phonemes in CVC words	15	30 pho-nemes	Open set	Verbal/ written	≥4 years	Mild to profound

TABLE 1 (page 2 of 2). Common speech recognition materials used with children. Adult lists.

Test name	Investigator(s)	Material	Number of Lists	Items Per List	Response Format	Response Task	Age Range	Degree of HL
1. Northwestern University Auditory Test No. 6 (NU-6)	Tillman & Carhart (1966)	Monosyllables	4	50	Open set	Verbal/ written	≥9 years	Mild to moderate
2. Central Institute for the Deaf W-22 (CID W-22)	Hirsh et al. (1952)	Monosyllables	20	50	Open set	Verbal/ written	≥7 years	Mild to moderate
3. Nonsense Syllable Test (NST)	Levitt & Resnick (1978)	Syllables	16 (7 subtests within a list)	62	Closed set	Written	≥6 years	Mild to moderate

References (Appendix B)

Bench, J., Koval, A., & Bamford, J. (1979). The BKB (Bamford-Koval-Bench) sentence lists for partially-hearing children. *British Journal of Audiology, 13*, 108–112.

Boothroyd, A. (1968). Developments of speech audiometry. *Sound, 2*, 3–10.

Boothroyd, A. (1996). Speech perception and production in hearing-impaired children. In F. H. Bess, J. S. Gravel, & A. M. Tharpe (Eds.) *Amplification for children with auditory deficits.* Nashville, TN: Bill Wilkerson Center Press.

Boothroyd, A. (in press). Speech perception tests and hearing-impaired children. In G. Plant & C. E. Spens (Eds.), *Speech communication and profound deafness.* London: Whurr Publishers.

Erber, N. P. (1974). Pure-tone thresholds and word-recognition abilities of hearing-impaired children. *Journal of Speech and Hearing Research, 17*, 194–202.

Erber, N. P. (1980). Use of the auditory numbers test to evaluate speech perception abilities of hearing-impaired children. *Journal of Speech and Hearing Disorders, 45*, 527–532.

Erber, N. P. (1982). *Auditory training.* Washington, DC: Alexander Graham Bell Association for the Deaf.

Finitzo-Hieber, T., Gerlin, I. J., Matkin, N. D., & Cherow-Skalka, E. (1980). A sound effects recognition test for the pediatric evaluation. *Ear and Hearing, 1*, 271–276.

Haskins, H. A. (1949). A phonetically balanced test of speech discrimination for children. Master's thesis. Northwestern University: Evanston, IL.

Hirsh, I. J., Davis, H., Silverman, S. R., Reynolds, E. G., Eldert, E., & Bensen, R. W. (1952). Development of materials for speech audiometry. *Journal of Speech and Hearing Disorders, 17*, 321–337.

Jerger, S., Lewis, S., Hawkins, J., & Jerger, J. (1980). Pediatric speech intelligibility test. I. Generation of test materials. *International Journal of Pediatric Otorhinolaryngology, 2*, 217–230.

Katz, D. R., & Elliott, L. L. (1978). Development of a new children's speech discrimination test. Paper presented at the convention of the American Speech-Language-Hearing Association, November 18–21, Chicago.

Levitt, H., & Resnick, S. B. (1978). Speech reception by the hearing impaired: Methods of testing and the development of new tests. *Scandinavian Audiology, 6*(Suppl.), 107–130.

Ling, D. (1978). Auditory coding and reading—An analysis of training procedures for hearing impaired children. In M. Ross & T. G. Giolas (Eds.), *Auditory management of hearing-impaired children* (pp. 181–218). Baltimore, MD: University Park Press.

Ling, D. (1989). *Foundations of spoken language for hearing-impaired children.* Washington, DC: Alexander Graham Bell Association for the Deaf.

Renshaw, J., Robbins, A. M., Miyamoto, R., Osberger, M. J., & Pope, M. (1988). *Hoosier Auditory Visual Enhancement Test (HAVE).* Indiana University School of Medicine, Department of Otolaryngology–Head and Neck Surgery, Indianapolis, IN.

Robbins, A. M., Renshaw, J., Miyamoto, R., Osberger, M. J., & Pope, M. (1988). *Minimal Pairs Test.* Indiana University School of Medicine, Department of Otolaryngology–Head and Neck Surgery, Indianapolis, IN.

Ross, M., & Lerman, J. (1970). A picture identification test for hearing impaired children. *Journal of Speech and Hearing Research, 13*, 44–53.

Siegenthaler, B., & Haspiel, G. (1966). Development of two standardized measures of hearing for speech by children. (Project No. OE-5-10-003). Washington, DC: U.S. Department of Health, Education and Welfare.

Tillman, T. W., & Carhart, R. (1966). An expanded test for speech discrimination utilizing CNC monosyllabic words. Northwestern University Auditory Test No. 6. Technical Report No. SAM-TR-66-55, USAF School of Aerospace Medicine, Brooks Air Force Base, TX.

Appendix 2–O

POSITION STATEMENT AND GUIDELINES OF THE CONSENSUS PANEL ON SUPPORT PERSONNEL IN AUDIOLOGY

This policy paper was developed by the Consensus Panel on Support Personnel in Audiology whose members come from the following professional organizations that represent audiologists: Academy of Dispensing Audiologists (ADA), American Academy of Audiology (AAA), American Speech-Language-Hearing Association (ASHA), Educational Audiology Association (EAA), Military Audiology Association (MAA), and the National Hearing Conservation Association (NHCA). Audiologists who served as organizational representatives to the panel included Donald Bender (AAA) and Evelyn Cherow (ASHA), co–chairs; James McDonald and Meredy Hase (ADA); Albert deChiccis and Cheryl DeConde Johnson (AAA); Chris Halpin and Deborah Price (ASHA); Peggy Benson (EAA); James Jerome (MAA); and Lloyd Bowling and Richard Danielson (NHCA).

I. Introduction

The consensus panel recognizes that federal and state health care and education reform initiatives, changing U.S. demographics, and the broadening scope of practice of audiologists (ASHA, 1996; Educational Testing Service, 1995; AAA, 1993) have affected the delivery of audiology services. Audiologists are using support personnel in audiology service delivery systems to ensure both the accessibility and the highest quality of audiology care while addressing productivity and cost–benefit concerns. In an analysis of state licensure laws (Larson & Lynch, 1995), ASHA found that in the 45 states that regulate one or both professions of audiology and speech–language pathology, 30 recognize support personnel. Not all of these states actually regulate support personnel; 22 states have promulgated rules regulating support personnel in all work settings and 5 were in process of creating these rules. This position statement and guidelines do not supersede federal legislation and regulation requirements, any existing state licensure laws, or affect the interpretation or implementation of such laws. The document may serve, however, as a guide for the development of new laws or, at the appropriate time, for revising existing licensure laws.

II. Position Statement

It is the position of the following organizations represented on the Consensus Panel on Support Personnel in Audiology (Academy of Dispensing Audiologists, American Academy of Audiology, Educational Audiology Association, Military Audiology Association, and National Hearing Conservation Association) that support personnel may assist audiologists in delivery of services. The roles and tasks of audiology support personnel will be assigned **only** by supervising audiologists. Supervising audiologists will provide appropriate training that is competency-based and specific to job performance. Supervision will be comprehensive, periodic, and documented. The supervising audiologist maintains the legal and ethical responsibilities for all assigned audiology activities provided by support personnel. The needs of the consumer of audiology services and protection of that consumer will always be paramount (ASHA, 1996; ASHA, 1994; AAA, 1996; NHCA, 1995). Audiologists are uniquely educated and specialize in the diagnosis and rehabilitation of hearing and related disorders. As such, audiologists are the appropriate, qualified professionals to hire, supervise, and train audiology support personnel.

III. Guidelines

A. Definitions

SUPPORT PERSONNEL: People who, after appropriate training, perform tasks that are prescribed, directed, and supervised by an audiologist.
SUPERVISING AUDIOLOGIST: An audiologist who has attained license (where applicable) or certification credentials and who has been practicing for at least one year after meeting these requirements.

B. Qualifications for Support Personnel

1. Have a high school degree or equivalent.
2. Have communication and interpersonal skills necessary for the tasks assigned.
3. Have a basic understanding of the needs of the population being served.
4. Have met training requirements and have competency–based skills necessary to the performance of specific assigned tasks.
5. Have any additional qualifications established by the supervising audiologist to meet the specific needs of the audiology program and the population being served.

C. Training

Training for support personnel should be well-defined and specific to the assigned task(s). The supervising audiologist will ensure that the scope and intensity of training encompass all of the activities assigned to the support personnel. Training should be competency-based and provided through a variety of formal and informal instructional methods. Audiologists should provide support personnel with information on roles and functions. Continuing opportunities should be provided to ensure that practices are current and that skills are maintained. The supervising audiologist will maintain written documentation of training activities.

D. Role

Audiology support personnel may engage in only those tasks that are planned, delegated, and supervised by the audiologist. The specific roles of audiology support personnel will be influenced by the particular needs of the audiologist and must be determined by the audiologist responsible for the support personnel's training and supervision.

Audiology support personnel will **not engage independently** in the following activities. **This list provides examples and is not intended to be all-inclusive.**

➤ Interpreting observations or data into diagnostic statement of clinical management strategies or procedures.
➤ Determining case selection.
➤ Performing habilitative or rehabilitative tasks that require in-process clinical judgments.
➤ Transmitting clinical information, either verbally or in writing, to anyone without the approval of the supervising audiologist.
➤ Composing clinical reports except for progress notes to be reviewed by the audiologist and held in the patient's/client's records.
➤ Referring a patient/client to other professionals or agencies.
➤ Referring to him– or herself either orally or in writing with a title other than one determined by the supervising audiologist.
➤ Signing any formal documents (e.g., treatment plans, reimbursement forms, or reports).
➤ Discharging a patient/client from services.
➤ Communicating with the patient/client, family, or others regarding any aspect of patient/client status or service without the specific consent of the supervising audiologist.

E. Supervision

Supervising audiologists will have the primary role in all administrative actions related to audiology support personnel, such as hiring, training, determining competency, and conducting performance evaluations. In addition, the supervising audiologist maintains final approval of all directives given by administrators and other professionals regarding audiology tasks.

Supervising audiologists will assign specific tasks to the support person. Such tasks **must not** 1) require the exercise of professional judgment, 2) entail interpretation of results (with the exception of hearing screening), or 3) encompass the development or modification of treatment plans.

The amount and type of supervision required should be based on skills and experience of the support person, the needs of patients/clients served, the service-delivery setting, the tasks assigned, and other factors. For example, more intense supervision will be required during orientation of a new support person; initiation of a new program, task, or equipment; or a change in patient/client status.

The number of support personnel supervised by a given audiologist must be consistent with the delivery of appropriate, quality service. It is the responsibility of the individual supervisor to protect the interests of patients/clients in a manner consistent with state licensure requirements, where applicable, and the Code of Ethics of that audiologist's respective professional organization.

References

American Academy of Audiology. (1993). Audiology: Scope of practice. *Audiology Today, 5*(1), 16–17.

American Academy of Audiology. (1996). *Code of ethics.* McLean, VA: Author.

American Speech-Language-Hearing Association. (1994). Code of ethics. *Asha, 36*(Suppl. 13), 1–2.

American Speech–Language–Hearing Association. (1996). Scope of practice in audiology. *Asha, 38*(Suppl. 16), 12–14.

Educational Testing Service. (1995). *The practice of audiology: A study of clinical activities and knowledge areas for the certified audiologist.* Rockville, MD: American Speech-Language-Hearing Association.

Larson, S., & Lynch, C. (1995). *Report: State regulation of audiology and speech—anguage pathology support personnel.* Rockville, MD: American Speech-Language-Hearing Association. Unpublished manuscript.

National Hearing Conservation Association. (1995). *Code of ethics.* Milwaukee, WI: Author.

Source: "Position statement and guidelines of the consensus panel on support personnel in audiology" by Consensus Panel on Support Personnel in Audiology, 1997. Reprinted by permission.

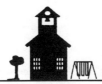

SECTION 3

APPENDIXES

Screening

CONTENTS

*Appendixes with asterisks (*) are available on an optional computer disk which allows users to customize these forms.

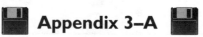 **Appendix 3–A**

BEHAVIORS FREQUENTLY EXHIBITED BY A CHILD WITH A HEARING LOSS

1. Has poor attention.
2. Frequently requests repetition.
3. Frowns or strains when listening.
4. Is easily fatigued.
5. Rarely participates in class discussions.
6. Cannot localize sounds.
7. Gives inappropriate answers to simple questions.
8. May be isolated.
9. Is overly dependent on visual cues.
10. Has low tolerance for frustration.
11. Often speaks too loudly.
12. Has poor reading skills.
13. Tends to do better in math than in reading.
14. Has poor spoken or written language.
15. Has frequent misarticulations in speech.
16. Has harsh, breathy, nasal, or monotone voice quality.
17. Has inappropriate pitch, rhythm, stress, and inflection in speech.
18. Has history of frequent earaches or ear discharge.
19. Is a mouth breather or has other nasal symptoms.
20. Complains of ringing, buzzing, or other noises in the head.

Source: Adapted from "Teacher tips for identifying a possible hearing impaired child" by V. Berry, 1988, in R.J. Roeser & M.P. Downs (Eds.), *Auditory disorders in school children,* p. 339. Copyright 1988, by Thieme Medical Publishers, Inc.

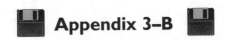 **Appendix 3–B**

HISTORY OF EAR AND HEARING PROBLEMS

Children who have had many ear infections and periods of hearing loss are more likely to have language, vocabulary and listening difficulties when they start school. We would like to identify these students so that we are more aware of their possible hearing problems and can be alert for present or developing learning problems.

Parent or guardian, please answer the following questions:

Child's Name: _____   **Birthdate:** _____

	NO	YES
1. Did your child have *any* ear problems before the age of 1?	____	____
2. Has your child ever had a draining ear?	____	____
3. Approximately how many ear problems has your child had in his/her life? 0–2 _____ 3–5 _____ 6–10 _____ 10 or more _____		
4. Does your child tend to have 4 or more ear problems each year?	____	____
5. Has your child had an ear problem in the last 6 months?	____	____
6. Has your child ever had an ear problem that lasted 3 months or longer? (with or without medication)	____	____
7. Has anyone related to the child had many ear problems? (parents, brothers or sisters, cousins)	____	____
8. Has your child ever been seen by an Ear Doctor (Otologist)? If yes, what doctor _____ Month/Year of last visit? _____	____	____
9. Has your child ever had tubes placed in his/her eardrums? If yes, how many times? _____ At what age(s)? _____	____	____
10. Does your child have any permanent hearing loss that you know about? (For example: deaf in one ear, can't hear high-pitched sounds) Please describe:	____	____

EAR PROBLEM = ear infection, earaches, draining ears, medicine taken for ears, doctor noticed fluid behind eardrum, hole in eardrum, etc.

Source: From "Hearing Conservation in the Public Schools Revisited" by K. Anderson, 1991, *Seminars in Hearing, 12*(4), p. 360. Copyright 1991 by Thieme Medical Publishers, Inc. Reprinted by permission.

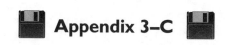

Appendix 3–C

HEARING QUESTIONNAIRE

NAME: _____ DOB: _____

SCHOOL: _____ GRADE: _____

FORM COMPLETED BY: _____ DATE COMPLETED: _____

1. Does this child have an identified heaing loss?   ___ YES ___ NO
2. If not, do you feel this child has a hearing problem?   ___ YES ___ NO
3. Does this child startle to loud sound?   ___ YES ___ NO
4. Does this child turn to sound?   ___ YES ___ NO
   If not, is it due to a motor problem?   ___ YES ___ NO
5. Does this child respond to his/her name?   ___ YES ___ NO
6. Give an example of how this child responds to sound in his/her environment:

   _____

   _____
7. Has this child had recent ear or upper respiratory infections? ___ YES ___ NO
8. What is this child's developmental age? _____
9. Does this child's motor development interfere with his/her ability to respond
   to sound?   ___ YES ___ NO
10. Do you feel this child's hearing has changed in the past year? ___ YES ___ NO

RETURN THIS FORM TO YOUR EDUCATIONAL AUDIOLOGIST:

_____

_____

_____

Source: "Hearing questionnaire" by the Colorado Educational Audiology Group. Reprinted by permission.

Appendix 3–D

FISHER'S AUDITORY PROBLEMS CHECKLIST

Student Name _____ District/Building _____

Date _____ Grade_____ Observer _____ Position _____

Please place a check mark before each item that is considered to be a concern by the observer:

___ 1. Has a history of hearing loss.

___ 2. Has a history of ear infection(s).

___ 3. Does not pay attention (listen) to instruction 50% or more of the time.

___ 4. Does not listen carefully to directions - often necessary to repeat instructions.

___ 5. Says "Huh?" and "What?" at least five or more times per day.

___ 6. Cannot attend to auditory stimuli for more than a few seconds.

___ 7. Has a short attention span.
(if this item is checked, _____ 0-2 minutes _____ 5-15 minutes
also check the most
appropriate time frame.) _____ 2-5 minutes _____ 15-30 minutes

___ 8. Daydreams - attention drifts - not with it at times.

___ 9. Is easily distracted by background sound(s).

___ 10. Has difficulty with phonics.

___ 11. Experiences problems with sound discrimination.

___ 12. Forgets what is said in a few minutes.

___ 13. Does not remember simple routine things from day to day.

___ 14. Displays problems recalling what was heard last week, month, year.

___ 15. Has difficulty recalling a sequence that has been heard.

___ 16. Experiences difficulty following auditory directions.

___ 17. Frequently misunderstands what is said.

___ 18. Does not comprehend many words - verbal concepts for age/grade level.

___ 19. Learns poorly through the auditory channel.

___ 20. Has a language problem (morphology, syntax, vocabulary, phonology).

___ 21. Has an articulation (phonology) problem.

___ 22. Cannot always relate what is heard to what is seen.

___ 23. Lacks motivation to learn.

___ 24. Displays slow or delayed response to verbal stimuli.

___ 25. Demonstrates below average performance in one or more academic area(s).

Scoring: Four percent credit for each numbered item not checked.

Number of items not checked _____ x 4 = _____.

Normative data - grade score from reverse side _____.

Source: "Fisher's auditory problems checklist" by L.I. Fisher, 1985. Copyright 1985 by Lee I. Fisher. Reprinted by permission.

Fisher's Auditory Problems Checklist includes
the following components of auditory processing:

Association	Localization
Attention	Long Term Memory
Attention Span	Motivation
Auditory-Visual Integration	Performance
Closure	Recognition
Comprehension	Sensitivity
Discrimination	Sequential Memory
Figure-Ground	Short Term Memory
Identification	Speech-Language Problems

NORMATIVE DATA FOR FISHER'S AUDITORY PROBLEMS CHECKLIST

GROUP	APPROXIMATE AGE RANGE	MEAN
Kindergarten	(Age 0 - 5.11)	92.0%
First	(Age 6.0 - 6.11)	89.9%
Second	(Age 7.0 - 7.11)	87.0%
Third	(Age 8.0 - 8.11)	85.6%
Fourth	(Age 9.0 - 9.11)	85.9%
Fifth	(Age 10.0 - 10.11)	87.4%
Sixth	(Age 11.0 - 11.11)	80.0%
Total Group (N=280)		86.8%
Cut-Off Score Suggesting Need For Further Evaluation		72.0%
One SD Below Group Mean		68.6%
Two SD Below Group Mean		50.4%

Fisher, Lee I., Learning Disabilities and Auditory Processing.

In VanHattum, Rolland J. (Ed.), "*Administration of Speech-Language Services In The Schools*", College Hill Press, 1985, pp. 231-292.

Additional Copies of this form are available in pads of 100 each from
The Educational Audiology Association 1-800-460-7322
4319 Ehrlich Road, Tampa, FL 33624

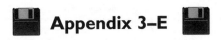

Appendix 3-E

PARENT NOTIFICATION/HISTORY FORM

NAME OF PROGRAM

Dear Parent,

Hearing is important to your child's ability to learn and to progress satisfactorily at school. For this reason, your school will be checking your child's hearing on __(DATE)__. This hearing screening is a very simple procedure and will take only a few minutes. If you do *not* want your child to participate in the screening, please let your child's teacher know prior to the screening date.

In order for us to be aware of factors that might affect your child's performance on the hearing screening, please answer the questions below and return this form to your child's teacher before the screening date.

If your child is absent or has difficulty with the hearing screening test, we will recheck him/her in 2–3 weeks and will notify you if there is a continued concern. If you have any questions about the hearing screening or wish to talk with me, please contact me at (INSERT PHONE NUMBER).

Sincerely,

Educational Audiologist

RETURN THIS TO YOUR CHILD'S TEACHER PRIOR TO _____(DATE)_____

CHILD'S NAME: _____   GRADE: _____

TEACHER: _____   SCHOOL: _____

Has your child had ear pain at any time during the past month?   _____ YES _____ NO

Has your child had drainage from the ears during the past month? _____ YES _____ NO

Appendix 3–F

SCREENING INSTRUMENT FOR TARGETING EDUCATIONAL RISK (S.I.F.T.E.R.)

S.I.F.T.E.R.

SCREENING INSTRUMENT FOR TARGETING EDUCATIONAL RISK

by Karen L. Anderson, Ed.S., CCC-A

STUDENT _____ TEACHER _____ GRADE _____

DATE COMPLETED _____ SCHOOL _____ DISTRICT _____

The above child is suspect for hearing problems which may or may not be affecting his/her school performance. This rating scale has been designed to sift out students who are educationally at risk possibly as a result of hearing problems.

Based on your knowledge from observations of this student, circle the number best representing his/her behavior. After answering the questions, please record any comments about the student in the space provided on the reverse side.

#	Question	High		Mid		Low	Category
1.	What is your estimate of the student's class standing in comparison of that of his/her classmates?	UPPER 5	4	MIDDLE 3	2	LOWER 1	ACADEMICS
2.	How does the student's achievement compare to your estimation of her/his potential?	EQUAL 5	4	LOWER 3	2	MUCH LOWER 1	
3.	What is the student's reading level, reading ability group or reading readiness group in the classroom (e.g., a student with average reading ability performs in the middle group)?	UPPER 5	4	MIDDLE 3	2	LOWER 1	
4.	How distractible is the student in comparison to his/her classmates?	NOT VERY 5	4	AVERAGE 3	2	VERY 1	ATTENTION
5.	What is the student's attention span in comparison to that of his/her classmates?	LONGER 5	4	AVERAGE 3	2	SHORTER 1	
6.	How often does the student hesitate or become confused when responding to oral directions (e.g., "Turn to page . . .")?	NEVER 5	4	OCCASIONALLY 3	2	FREQUENTLY 1	
7.	How does the student's comprehension compare to the average understanding ability of her/his classmates?	ABOVE 5	4	AVERAGE 3	2	BELOW 1	COMMUNICATION
8.	How does the student's vocabulary and word usage skills compare with those of other students in his/her age group?	ABOVE 5	4	AVERAGE 3	2	BELOW 1	
9.	How proficient is the student at telling a story or relating happenings from home when compared to classmates?	ABOVE 5	4	AVERAGE 3	2	BELOW 1	
10.	How often does the student volunteer information to class discussions or in answer to teacher questions?	FREQUENTLY 5	4	OCCASIONALLY 3	2	NEVER 1	CLASS PARTICIPATION
11.	With what frequency does the student complete his/her class and homework assignments within the time allocated?	ALWAYS 5	4	USUALLY 3	2	SELDOM 1	
12.	After instruction, does the student have difficulty starting to work (looks at other students working or asks for help)?	NEVER 5	4	OCCASIONALLY 3	2	FREQUENTLY 1	
13.	Does the student demonstrate any behaviors that seem unusual or inappropriate when compared to other students?	NEVER 5	4	OCCASIONALLY 3	2	FREQUENTLY 1	SCHOOL BEHAVIOR
14.	Does the student become frustrated easily, sometimes to the point of losing emotional control?	NEVER 5	4	OCCASIONALLY 3	2	FREQUENTLY 1	
15.	In general, how would you rank the student's relationship with peers (ability to get along with others)?	GOOD 5	4	AVERAGE 3	2	POOR 1	

Additional copies of this form are available in pads of 100 each from
The Educational Audiology Association
4319 Ehrlich Road, Tampa, FL 33624
ISBN 0-8134-2845-9

Source: "Screening instrument for targeting educational risk" by K. Anderson, 1989. Copyright 1989 by Karen Anderson. Reprinted by permission.

TEACHER COMMENTS

Has this child repeated a grade, had frequent absences or experienced health problems (including ear infections and colds)? Has the student received, or is he/she now receiving, special support services? Does the child have any other health problems that may be pertinent to his/her educational functioning?

The S.I.F.T.E.R. is a SCREENING TOOL ONLY

Any student failing this screening in a content area as determined on the scoring grid below should be considered for further assessment, depending on his/her individual needs as per school district criteria. For example, failing in the Academics area suggests an educational assessment, in the Communication area a speech-language assessment, and in the School Behavior area an assessment by a psychologist or a social worker. Failing in the Attention and/or Class Participation area in combination with other areas may suggest an evaluation by an educational audiologist. Children placed in the marginal area are at risk for failing and should be monitored or considered for assessment depending upon additional information.

SCORING

Sum the responses to the three questions in each content area and record in the appropriate box on the reverse side and under Total Score below. Place an **X** on the number that corresponds most closely with the content area score (e.g., if a teacher circled 3, 4 and 2 for the questions in the Academics area, an **X** would be placed on the number 9 across from the Academics content area). Connect the **X**'s to make a profile.

CONTENT AREA	TOTAL SCORE	PASS						MARGINAL		FAIL				
ACADEMICS		15	14	13	12	11	10	9	8	7	6	5	4	3
ATTENTION		15	14	13	12	11	10	9	8	7	6	5	4	3
COMMUNICATION		15		14	13		12	11	10	9	8	7	6	5	4	3
CLASS PARTICIPATION		15	14	13	12	11	10	9	8	7	6	5	4	3
SOCIAL BEHAVIOR		15	14	13	12	11	10	9	8	7	6	5	4	3

Appendix 3–G

SCREENING INSTRUMENT FOR TARGETING EDUCATIONAL RISK IN PRESCHOOL CHILDREN (AGE 3–KINDERGARTEN) (PRESCHOOL S.I.F.T.E.R.)

PRESCHOOL S.I.F.T.E.R.

**Screening Instrument for Targeting Educational Risk
in Preschool Children (age 3-Kindergarten)**
by Karen L. Anderson, Ed.S. & Noel Matkin, Ph.D.

Child ———————————————— Teacher ——————————— Age ————————

Date Completed ____/____/____ School ———————————————— District ——————

The above child is suspect for hearing problems which may affect his/her ability to listen, pay attention, develop language, follow teacher instruction and learn normally. This rating scale has been designed to sift out children who are at risk for educational delay and who may need further evaluation. Based on your knowledge of this child, circle the number that best represents his/her behavior. If the child is a member of a class that has students with special needs, comparisons should be made to normal learning classmates or normal developmental milestones. Please share additional comments about the child on the reverse side of this form.

PRE-ACADEMICS

1. How well does the child understand basic concepts when compared to classmates (e.g., colors, shapes, etc.)? — ABOVE 5 AVERAGE 4 3 2 BELOW 1

2. How often is the child able to follow two-part directions? — ALWAYS 5 FREQUENTLY 3 2 SELDOM 1

3. How well does the child participate in group activities when compared to classmates (e.g., calendar, sharing)? — ABOVE 5 AVERAGE 4 2 BELOW 1

ATTENTION

4. How distractible is the child in comparison to his/her classmates during large group activities? — SELDOM 4 OCCASION 2 FREQUENT 1

5. What is the child's attention span in comparison to classmates? — LONGER 5 AVERAGE 3 2 SHORTER 1

6. How well does the child pay attention during a small group activity or time? — ABOVE 5 AVERAGE 4 3 2 BELOW 1

COMMUNICATION

7. How does the child's vocabulary and word usage skills compare to classmates? — ABOVE 5 AVERAGE 4 3 2 BELOW 1

8. How proficient is the child at relating an event when compared to classmates? — ABOVE 5 AVERAGE 4 3 2 BELOW 1

9. How does the child's overall speech intelligibility compare to classmates (i.e., production of speech sounds)? — ABOVE 5 AVERAGE 4 3 2 BELOW 1

CLASS PARTICIPATION

10. How often does the child answer questions appropriately (verbal or signed)? — ALMOST ALWAYS 5 FREQUENTLY 4 3 2 SELDOM 1

11. How often does the child volunteer information during group discussions? — ALMOST ALWAYS 5 FREQUENTLY 4 3 2 SELDOM 1

12. How often does the child participate with classmates in group activities or group play? — ALMOST ALWAYS 5 FREQUENTLY 4 3 2 SELDOM 1

SOCIAL BEHAVIOR

13. Does the child play in socially acceptable ways (i.e., turn taking, sharing)? — ALMOST ALWAYS 5 FREQUENTLY 4 3 2 SELDOM 1

14. How proficient is the child at using verbal language or sign language to communicate effectively with classmates (e.g., asking to play with another child's toy)? — ABOVE 5 AVERAGE 4 3 2 BELOW 1

15. How often does the child become frustrated, sometimes to the point of losing emotional control? — NEVER 5 SELDOM 4 3 FREQUENTLY 2 1

Source: "Screening instrument for targeting educational risk in preschool children (age 3–kindergarten)" by K. Anderson and N. Matkin, 1996. Copyright 1996 by Karen Anderson & Noel Matkin. Reprinted by permission.

TEACHER COMMENTS: (frequent absences, health problems, other problems or handicaps in addition to hearing?)

The Preschool S.I.F.T.E.R. is a SCREENING TOOL ONLY. The primary goal of the Preschool S.I.F.T.E.R. is to identify those children who are at-risk for developmental or educational problems due to hearing problems and who merit further observation and investigation. Analysis has revealed that two factors, expressive communication and socially appropriate behavior, discriminate children who are normal from those who are at-risk. The greater the degree of hearing problem, the greater the impact on these two factors and the higher the validity of this screening measure. If a child is found to be at-risk then the examiner is encouraged to calculate the total score in each of the five content areas. Analysis of the content area score may assist in developing a profile of the child's strengths and special needs. The profile may prove beneficial in determining appropriate areas for evaluation and developing an individual program for the child.

SCORING

There are two steps to the scoring process. First, enter scores for each of the indicated questions in the spaces provided and sum the total of the 6 questions for the expressive communication factor and then the 4 questions for the socially appropriate behavior factor. If the child's scores fall into the At-Risk category for either or both of these factors, then sum the 3 questions in each content area to develop a profile of the child's strengths and potential areas of need.

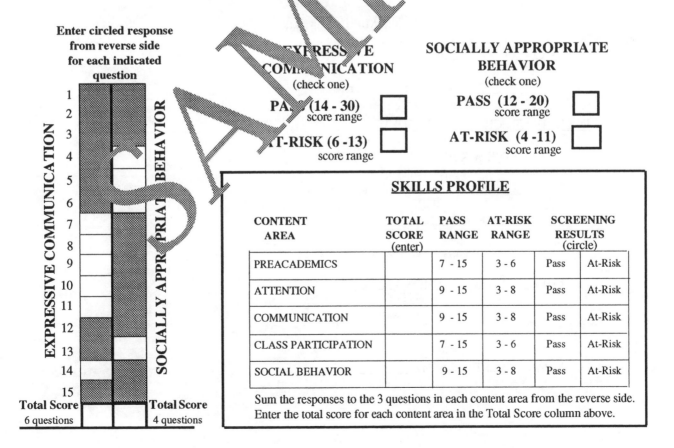

Enter circled response from reverse side for each indicated question

EXPRESSIVE COMMUNICATION

SOCIALLY APPROPRIATE BEHAVIOR

EXPRESSIVE COMMUNICATION (check one)

PASS (14 - 30) score range ☐

AT-RISK (6 - 13) score range ☐

SOCIALLY APPROPRIATE BEHAVIOR (check one)

PASS (12 - 20) score range ☐

AT-RISK (4 - 11) score range ☐

Total Score 6 questions

Total Score 4 questions

SKILLS PROFILE

CONTENT AREA	TOTAL SCORE (enter)	PASS RANGE	AT-RISK RANGE	SCREENING RESULTS (circle)	
PREACADEMICS		7 - 15	3 - 6	Pass	At-Risk
ATTENTION		9 - 15	3 - 8	Pass	At-Risk
COMMUNICATION		9 - 15	3 - 8	Pass	At-Risk
CLASS PARTICIPATION		7 - 15	3 - 6	Pass	At-Risk
SOCIAL BEHAVIOR		9 - 15	3 - 8	Pass	At-Risk

Sum the responses to the 3 questions in each content area from the reverse side. Enter the total score for each content area in the Total Score column above.

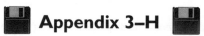 **Appendix 3–H**

INDIVIDUAL AND CLASS HEARING SCREENING FORMS

NAME OF PROGRAM
HEARING SCREENING RESULTS

Please File Completed Form in Medical Section of Student's Permanent Folder

Student: _____   School: _____

Teacher: _____   Grade: _____

<u>INITIAL SCREENING RESULTS</u>   DATE: _____

    PURE-TONE SCREENING:

        _____ Pass - Normal Hearing   _____ Rescreen

    IMMITTANCE SCREENING:

        _____ Pass - Normal Middle Ear Function   _____ Rescreen

    OTOACOUSTIC EMISSIONS SCREENING

        _____ Pass - Normal Hearing   _____ Rescreen

<u>FOLLOW-UP SCREENING RESULTS</u>   DATE: _____

    PURE-TONE SCREENING:

        _____ Pass - Normal Hearing   _____ Refer

    IMMITTANCE SCREENING:

        _____ Pass - Normal Middle Ear Function   _____ Refer

    OTOACOUSTIC EMISSIONS SCREENING

        _____ Pass - Normal Hearing   _____ Refer

DATE PARENT LETTER SENT:_____

NAME OF PROGRAM

CLASS HEARING SCREENING RESULTS

SCHOOL: _____

TEACHER: _____ GRADE: _____

NAME	Screening Date: _____		Rescreening Date: _____	
	PURE TONE	IMMITTANCE	PURE TONES	IMMITTANCE
	R___ L___	R___ L___	R___ L___	R___ L___
	R___ L___	R___ L___	R___ L___	R___ L___
	R___ L___	R___ L___	R___ L___	R___ L___
	R___ L___	R___ L___	R___ L___	R___ L___
	R___ L___	R___ L___	R___ L___	R___ L___
	R___ L___	R___ L___	R___ L___	R___ L___
	R___ L___	R___ L___	R___ L___	R___ L___
	R___ L___	R___ L___	R___ L___	R___ L___
	R___ L___	R___ L___	R___ L___	R___ L___
	R___ L___	R___ L___	R___ L___	R___ L___
	R___ L___	R___ L___	R___ L___	R___ L___

KEY: + = Pass   R = Refer

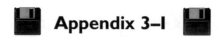

Appendix 3–I

HEARING RESCREENING FORM

NAME OF PROGRAM

HEARING RESCREENING LIST

SCHOOL: _____   DATE: _____

NAME	TCHR GRADE	Screening			Rescreening			FOLLOW-UP
		PT	IMMIT	VSL INSP	PT	IMMIT	VSL INSP	

Screening Codes: **A** = Absent **N** = Normal **R** = Rescreen **AR** = Audiological Referral **MR** = Medical Referral
Follow-Up Codes: **SN** = Sensorineural **COND** = Conductive **MXD** = Mixed **NL** = Normal on later tests
MI = Mild **MOD** = Moderate **SEV** = Severe **PROF** = Profound **HF** = High Frequency
UNI = Unilateral **RT** = Right **LF** = Left **DR** = Under doctor's care **HA** = Hearing Aid
WD = Withdrew from school **NR** = No response

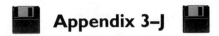 **Appendix 3–J**

TEACHER NOTIFICATION OF SCREENING RESULTS

NAME OF PROGRAM

DATE:_____ SCHOOL: _____

TO: _____ (INSERT TEACHERS' NAMES) _____

FROM: _____ (INSERT AUDIOLOGISTS' NAMES) _____

Based on testing today, the students listed below have a hearing impairment for which they are currently under care of or have been referred to a physician for treatment. Until this condition is resolved, they will benefit from:

1. Being seated close to you or person responsible for instruction.
2. Getting their attention prior to giving instruction.
3. Checking to be sure they have understood directions, etc.
4. Speaking while facing students so they can watch your lips.

Please call me if you feel further intervention is needed or if you have any questions. I can be reached at (INSERT PHONE NUMBER). Thanks for your help with these students.

STUDENTS: _____

_____

_____

_____

_____

_____

_____

_____

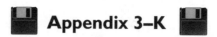

Appendix 3–K

NOTES TO NOTIFY PARENTS OF SCREENING RESULTS

NAME OF PROGRAM

STUDENT:_____ DATE: _____

Dear Parent,

      Hearing is important to your child's ability to learn and to progress satisfactorily at school. For this reason, your child's school recently conducted a hearing screening that included a pure-tone screening (to measure hearing) and an immittance screening (to measure middle-ear function). Your child PASSED all aspects of the screening on the date noted above.

      Please be aware that hearing may change at any time. If you become concerned about your child's hearing in the future, please contact his/her school to request another hearing screening. If you have any questions about the results or about the hearing screening program at your child's school, please contact me at (INSERT PHONE NUMBER).

Sincerely,

Educational Audiologist

NAME OF PROGRAM

STUDENT:_____ DATE: _____

Dear Parent,

      Hearing is important to your child's ability to learn and to progress satisfactorily at school. For this reason, your child's school recently conducted a hearing screening that included a pure-tone screening (to measure hearing) and an immittance screening (to measure middle-ear function). Your child had difficulty with one or both parts of the screening. This result does *NOT* mean that your child has a hearing loss. His/Her difficulty may have been due to distractions or noise in the test room, a lack of understanding of the test, or any of a number of other reasons.

      It is important that your child's hearing be rescreened in the near future. This rescreening will be done at your child's school in three to four weeks. You will be notified of the results of the rescreening at that time. If you have any questions about the results or about the hearing screening program at your child's school, please contact me at (INSERT PHONE NUMBER).

Sincerely,

Educational Audiologist

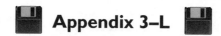 **Appendix 3–L**

PARENT LETTERS TO REFER CHILD
FOR FURTHER EVALUATION

NAME OF PROGRAM

STUDENT: _____ DATE:_____

Dear Parent,

     Hearing is important to your child's ability to learn and to progress satisfactorily at school. Because your child's initial hearing screening at school indicated a concern, he/she was recently rescreened. Your child continued to have difficulty with one or both parts of the hearing screening. This screening test is *NOT* conclusive, but it is recommended that your child be seen in the near future for a complete audiological (hearing) evaluation so we can learn more about his/her hearing.

     Many hearing problems in children are not severe and may not be permanent. It is, however, important that even mild hearing losses be identified so that recommendations can be made to minimize the effects of the loss. A more complete hearing test will help us determine if your child has a hearing loss and, if so, the type and severity of the loss.

     Please call (INSERT PHONE NUMBER) to schedule an appointment for an audiological evaluation as soon as possible. This evaluation is provided for students by the school district at no cost . If you decide to take your child to a private audiologist for evaluation, you may call the same number to obtain the results of the screening to share with the audiologist. If you have any questions, please contact me.

Sincerely,

Educational Audiologist

NAME OF PROGRAM

STUDENT: _____ DATE:_____

Dear Parent,

      Hearing is important to your child's ability to learn and to progress satisfactorily at school. Because the initial hearing screening indicated a concern, your child was recently rescreened. Your child continued to have difficulty with one or both parts of the hearing screening. This screening test is *NOT* conclusive, but it is recommended that:

- Your child be seen by a physician (pediatrician, family physician, or otolaryngologist) to determine if there is a medical problem that is affecting your child's ability to hear. The results of the screening are provided below so you can share them with your physician.

- Your child be seen by an audiologist for a complete audiological evaluation after he/she has seen your physician.

      Many hearing problems in children can be helped with medical attention. It is important that you schedule an appointment for your child as soon as possible. If you have any questions about the screening results or about the hearing screening program at your child's school, please contact me at (INSERT PHONE NUMBER).

Sincerely,

Educational Audiologist

SCREENING RESULTS

STUDENT: _____ DATE:_____

	HEARING (Screened at 20 dB HL)				MIDDLE EAR (Complete Results or Attach Print-out)		
	500 Hz	1000 Hz	2000 Hz	4000 Hz	Stat Acoustic Compliance	Equiv Ear Canal Vol	Tympanometric Width
Right							
Left							

IMPRESSIONS: _____

_____

_____

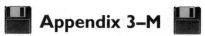 **Appendix 3–M**

REFERRING AGENCY REPORT FORM

NAME OF PROGRAM

STUDENT: _____ DATE:_____

       This student recently participated in a hearing screening at school. The results of the screening and the rescreening indicated that he/she may have some hearing loss. It was therefore recommended that the student be seen by you for further evaluation.

       Your cooperation in completing the information below will help us make appropriate modifications for the student at school. If you have any questions about the hearing screening results, please contact me at (INSERT PHONE NUMBER).

COMPLETE AND RETURN TO:
    Educational Audiologist
    School District
    Street Address
    City, State Zip Code

STUDENT: _____ SCHOOL:_____

PERSON COMPLETING EVALUATION: _____

ADDRESS: _____

RESULTS OF EVALUATION:

RECOMMENDATIONS:

Will the student be returning to you for further care? _____ YES _____ NO

SIGNATURE: _____ DATE:_____

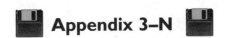 **Appendix 3–N**

DATABASE FOR MONITORING SCREENING FOLLOW-UP

HEARING DATABASE FORMAT

<u>FIELDS FOR DATABASE</u>:

- Last Name
- First Name
- Student ID Number
- School
- Grade

- Date
- Reported By
- Results
- Condition
- Disposition

<u>INSTRUCTIONS FOR FIELDS</u>:

<u>Date</u>:   Use 6-digit code to represent the month, day, and year (e.g., 010697 is the code for January 6, 1997)

<u>Reported By</u>:

SC - Screening	HC - Health clerk
AS - Audiologist at school	RN - Nurse
AU- Audiologist at soundbooth	MD - Physician's notes

<u>Results</u>:   Enter screening results for initial and follow-up screenings (e.g., R+, Labn to mean pass right pure-tone screening and fail left pure-tone screening; RT+, LTabn to mean pass right immittance screening and fail left immittance screening)

Enter actual thresholds obtained (e.g., R5/500, 10/1000, 0/2000, 5/4000; L30/500, 45/1000, 40/2000, 50/4000)

Enter medical or other referral information from physicians and other clarifying data regarding student's hearing status

<u>Condition</u>:   ES - Educationally significant hearing loss
MS - Medically significant hearing loss
ES/MS - Educationally and medically significant hearing loss
O - Other hearing loss that does not meet the ES or MS criteria
NRML - Normal hearing
CAP - Central auditory processing disorder
UNKN - Unknown for students who have failed hearing screening but with whom there has been no follow-up

<u>Disposition</u>:   RK - Recheck at school
RK AU - Recheck in sound booth
MED REF - Medical referral
AUD REF - Audiological referral
MON SCH - Monitor periodically at school
MON ANN - Monitor annually at school
ANN EVAL - Annual evaluation by audiologist in soundbooth
NONE - No further follow-up

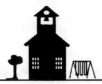

SECTION 4

APPENDIXES

Assessment

CONTENTS

*Appendixes with asterisks (*) are available on an optional computer disk which allows users to customize these forms.

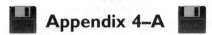 **Appendix 4–A**

PEDIATRIC OBSERVATION, TESTING, AND TALLYING SYSTEM (POTTS)

ARKANSAS DEPARTMENT OF HEALTH
Hearing and Speech Clinics
Pediatric Observation, Testing and Tallying System (POTTS)

Name _____ Age _____ Sex _____ Date _____

Audiometer _____

Procedure: BOA _____ VRA _____ COR _____ Play _____

Mode of Presentation: Soundfield _____ Earphones _____ Inserts _____ Bone _____ Aided _____

dB	SAT	250Hz	500Hz	1kHz	2kHz	4kHz		
0								
5								
10								
15								
20								
25								
30								
35								
40								
45								
50								
55								
60								
65								
70								
75								
80								
90								
95								
100								
105								
110								
115								
120								

Adapted from original by Emily Potts, 1978 - Arkansas Dept. of Health.

Responses

+	definite
✓	possible
–	no response
R	right ear
L	left ear
___	_____
___	_____

COMMENTS:

Reliability _____

**Auditory Behavior Index
(Minimal Response Level Norms)**

Age	F-specific Responses (HL)	Speech Responses (HL)
4–7 mos	50 dB	20 dB
7–9 mos	45 dB	15 dB
9–13 mos	35 dB	5 dB
13–16 mos	30 dB	5 dB
16–21 mos	25 dB	5 dB
21–24 mos	25 dB	0 dB

Adapted from Northern & Downs, 1974

Source: "Pediatric observation, testing, and tallying system (POTTS)" by Arkansas Department of Health, 1978. Reprinted by permission.

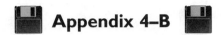

Appendix 4–B

CUMULATIVE RECORD OF THRESHOLDS

NAME: _____   BIRTHDATE: _____

CONDITION: AC = AIR CONDUCTION   BC = BONE CONDUCTION   A = AIDED   S = SOUND FIELD

DATE	COND	Right Ear Thresholds/Aided Results										Left Ear Thresholds/Aided Results									
		SRT	250	500	1K	2K	3K	4K	6K	8K		SRT	250	500	1K	2K	3K	4K	6K	8K	

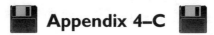 **Appendix 4–C**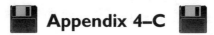

THE FUNCTIONAL LISTENING EVALUATION

Cheryl DeConde Johnson   Peggy Von Almen
Weld County School District 6, Greeley, Co   Utah State University

Purpose of The Functional Listening Evaluation:
The purpose of this evaluation is to determine how a student's listening abilities are affected by noise, distance, and visual input. It is designed to simulate the student's listening ability in a situation that is more representative of his or her actual listening environment than the sound booth. This protocol is based on a listening paradigm suggested by Ying (1990), and by Ross, Bracken, and Maxon (1992).

Materials Needed:	Cassette Tape Recorder
	Sound Level Meter (can be purchased inexpensively from Radio Shack)
	Noise Tape (Multi-Talker Babble-can be purchased from Auditec)
	Tripod or stand to hold sound level meter (optional)
	Sentence/Word Lists for scoring
	Tape measure or yard stick
	Masking tape or marker (optional)

Environment for Testing:
Use the student's classroom during a time when it is empty; if this is not possible choose a room that most closely simulates the size, ambient noise level, and floor and wall surfaces of the student's classroom.

Physical Set-up of Test Environment:
Close: Noise and examiner are 3 feet in front of the student (see Diagram A).
Distant: Noise remains 3 feet in front of the student; examiner moves back to a distance of 15 feet from the student (see Diagram B).

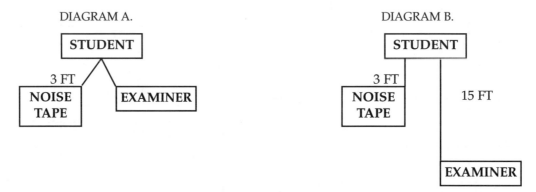

For ease these distances can be marked with masking tape on the floor; be sure that the markers are from the student's ear to the examiner's mouth.

Types of Evaluation Materials:
Whenever possible sentence material should be used since it is more like speech encountered in the classroom. However, due to age and limited language and memory abilities of some students, it may be necessary to use single words. In selecting either sentence or word materials caution should be used to insure that the vocabulary and sentence structure are appropriate for the student's language ability. When the student has poor speech intelligibility, it may be necessary to use materials which allow picture-pointing responses.

Source: "Functional listening evaluation" by C. D. Johnson and P. Von Almen, 1993. Reprinted by permission.

Possible Sentence Materials:	BLAIR Sentences	WIPI Sentences
	SPIN Sentences (older students)	BKB Sentences
	PSI Sentences	
Possible Word Lists:	PB-K	NU-CHIPS
	WIPI	

In most cases there will not be enough lists for the entire protocol (8 lists are needed). When selecting lists to repeat, try to use lists which were more difficult for the student.

Presentation Levels:

Speech: Monitor with sound level meter so that speech averages 75dBA at 1 foot from the examiner's mouth.

Noise: Set with sound level meter so that noise, which is 3 feet from the student, averages 60 dBA at the student's ear.

This will result in a signal-to-noise ratio of +3 dB in the close condition. The signal-to-noise ratio in the distant condition will vary depending upon the acoustics of the room, but it will be approximately –5 dB.

Presentation Protocol:

The evaluation should be conducted in the student's typical hearing mode. If hearing aids are usually worn at school, they should also be worn during the evaluation. This protocol can also be used to demonstrate the improved listening ability with FM amplification.

Eight sentence or word lists should be presented in the following order, as indicated by the numbers on the scoring matrix:

1.	AUDITORY-VISUAL	CLOSE	QUIET
2.	AUDITORY	CLOSE	QUIET
3.	AUDITORY-VISUAL	CLOSE	NOISE
4.	AUDITORY	CLOSE	NOISE
5.	AUDITORY-VISUAL	DISTANT	NOISE
6.	AUDITORY	DISTANT	NOISE
7.	AUDITORY	DISTANT	QUIET
8.	AUDITORY-VISUAL	DISTANT	QUIET

This order was selected to present easier tasks at the beginning and end of the protocol.

The examiner should present the speech materials at a normal, but not slow, rate. The student should repeat the test stimuli or point to the appropriate picture, as dictated by the material used.

It will take approximately 30 minutes to set up and administer the test protocol if sentences are used as the stimulus. If words are used, the protocol will take about 20 minutes.

Scoring:

Scoring should be done using the protocol established for the selected test materials. All scores should be reported in percent correct.

Variations in Protocol:

This protocol is based on the listening situation in a typical classroom. For an individual student, it may be useful to modify this protocol to account for variations in the level and source of noise, classroom size, typical listening distances for the student, or other factors. In order to accommodate these variations, the following modifications should be considered:

1. Placement of noise/tape recorder.
2. Distance of examiner from student for the distant condition.
3. Level of noise.
4. Order of presentation.

Any modifications of the typical protocol should be noted on the test form.

Interpretation:

In order to interpret the effects of noise, distance, and visual input for the individual student, the conditions can be compared on the Interpretation Matrix. These scores can be used to determine educational modifications which would be beneficial for the student. They can also be shared with the student's parents and teachers to help them understand their student's listening abilities and needs.

Scores may be affected by different speakers, rate of speaking, attention of the listener, or status of amplification. As long as variables are kept constant throughout the evaluation, comparisons can be made.

References:

Ross, M., Brackett, D., & Maxon, A. (1991). *Assessment and management of mainstreamed hearing-impaired children.* (Chapter 5: Communication Assessment, pp. 113–127). Austin, TX: Pro-Ed.

Ying, E. (1990). Speech and Language Assessment: Communication Evaluation. In M. Ross (Ed.), *Hearing-impaired children in the mainstream* (pp. 45–60). Parkton, MD: York Press.

FUNCTIONAL LISTENING EVALUATION

NAME: _____ DATE: _____

EXAMINER: _____ AGE/DOB: _____

AUDIOMETRIC RESULTS

HEARING SENSITIVITY: PURE TONE AVE: RIGHT EAR _____ LEFT EAR _____

WORD RECOGNITION: RIGHT EAR _____ % @ _____ dBHL LEFT EAR _____ % @ _____ dBHL

SOUND FIELD: _____ AIDED _____ UNAIDED
QUIET _____ % @ _____ dBHL
NOISE _____ % @ _____ dBHL @ _____ S/N

FUNCTIONAL LISTENING EVALUATION CONDITIONS

AMPLIFICATION: _____ NONE _____ HEARING AIDS _____ FM _____ SOUND FIELD

_____ OTHER

CLASSROOM AMBIENT NOISE LEVEL: _____ dBA

ASSESSMENT MATERIAL: _____ SENTENCES _____ WORDS _____

MODIFICATIONS IN PROTOCOL:

INTERPRETATION MATRIX

	NOISE	
	QUIET	NOISE
CLOSE-AUD	2	4
CLOSE-AUD/VISUAL	1	3
DISTANT-AUD	7	6
DISTANT-AUD/VISUAL	8	5

Average of above scores: _____% QUIET _____% NOISE

	DISTANCE	
	CLOSE	DISTANT
QUIET-AUD	2	7
QUIET-AUD/VISUAL	1	8
NOISE-AUD	4	6
NOISE-AUD/VISUAL	3	5

_____% CLOSE _____% DISTANT

	VISUAL INPUT	
	AUD/VIS	AUD
CLOSE-QUIET	1	2
CLOSE-NOISE	3	4
DISTANT-NOISE	5	6
DISTANT-QUIET	8	7

_____% AUD/VIS _____% AUD

INTERPRETATION AND RECOMMENDATIONS

FUNCTIONAL LISTENING MATRIX

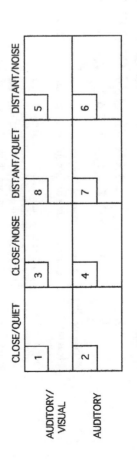

	CLOSE/QUIET	CLOSE/NOISE	DISTANT/QUIET	DISTANT/NOISE
AUDITORY/VISUAL	1	3	8	5
AUDITORY	2	4	7	6

Cheryl Deconde Johnson
Weld County School District 6, Greeley, Co

Peggy Von Almen
Utah State University

Appendix 4–D

RELATIONSHIP OF DEGREE OF LONGTERM HEARING LOSS TO PSYCHOSOCIAL IMPACT AND EDUCATIONAL NEEDS

RELATIONSHIP OF DEGREE OF LONGTERM HEARING LOSS TO PSYCHOSOCIAL IMPACT AND EDUCATIONAL NEEDS

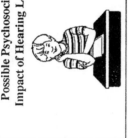

Degree of Hearing Loss Based on modified pure tone average (500-4000 HZ)	Possible Effect of Hearing Loss on the Understanding of Language & Speech	Possible Psychosocial Impact of Hearing Loss	Potential Educational Needs and Programs
NORMAL HEARING -10 - +15 dB HL	Children have better hearing sensitivity than the accepted normal range for adults. A child with hearing sensitivity in the -10 to +15 dB range will detect the complete speech signal even at soft conversation levels. However, good hearing does not guarantee good ability to discriminate speech in the presence of background noise.		
MINIMAL (BORDERLINE) 16-25 dB HL	May have difficulty hearing faint or distant speech. At 15 dB student can miss up to 10% of speech signal when teacher is at a distance greater than 3 feet and when the classroom is noisy, especially in the elementary grades when verbal instruction predominates.	May be unaware of subtle conversational cues which could cause child to be viewed as inappropriate or awkward. May miss portions of fast-paced peer interactions which could begin to have an impact on socialization and self concept. May have immature behavior. Child may be more fatigued than classmates due to listening effort needed.	May benefit from mild gain/low MPO hearing aid or personal FM system dependent on loss configuration. Would benefit from soundfield amplification if classroom is noisy and/or reverberant. Favorable seating. May need attention to vocabulary or speech, especially with recurrent otitis media history. Appropriate medical management necessary for conductive losses. Teacher requires inservice on impact of hearing loss on language development and learning.
MILD 26-40 dB HL	At 30 dB can miss 25-40% of speech signal. The degree of difficulty experienced in school will depend upon the noise level in classroom, distance from teacher and the configuration of the hearing loss. Without amplification the child with 35-40 dB loss may miss at least 50% of class discussions, especially when voices are faint or speaker is not in line of vision. Will miss consonants, especially when a high frequency hearing loss is present.	Barriers beginning to build with negative impact on self esteem as child is accused of "hearing when he or she wants to," "daydreaming," or "not paying attention." Child begins to lose ability for selective hearing, and has increasing difficulty suppressing background noise which makes the learning environment stressful. Child is more fatigued than classmates due to listening effort needed.	Will benefit from a hearing aid and use of a personal FM or soundfield FM system in the classroom. Needs favorable seating and lighting. Refer to special education for language evaluation and educational follow-up. Needs auditory skill building. May need attention to vocabulary and language development, articulation or speechreading and/or special support in reading. May need help with self esteem. Teacher inservice required.
MODERATE 41-55 dB HL	Understands conversational speech at a distance of 3-5 feet (face-to-face) only if structure and vocabulary controlled. Without amplification the amount of speech signal missed can be 50% to 75% with 40 dB loss and 80% to 100% with 50 dB loss. Is likely to have delayed or defective syntax, limited vocabulary, imperfect speech production and an atonal voice quality.	Often with this degree of hearing loss, communication is significantly affected, and socialization with peers with normal hearing becomes increasingly difficult. With full time use of hearing aids/FM systems child may be judged as a less competent learner. There is an increasing impact on self-esteem.	Refer to special education for language evaluation and for educational follow-up. Amplification is essential (hearing aids and FM system). Special education support may be needed, especially for primary children. Attention to oral language development, reading and written language. Auditory skill development and speech therapy usually needed. Teacher inservice required.

Degree of Loss	Possible Impact on Understanding of Language and Speech	Possible Social Impact	Potential Educational Needs and Programs
MODERATE TO SEVERE 56-70 dB HL	Without amplification, conversation must be very loud to be understood. A 55 dB loss can cause child to miss up to 100% of speech information. Will have marked difficulty in school situations requiring verbal communication in both one-to-one and group situations. Delayed language, syntax, reduced speech intelligibility and atonal voice quality likely.	Full time use of hearing aids/FM systems may result in child being judged by both peers and adults as a less competent learner, resulting in poorer self concept, social maturity and contributing to a sense of rejection. Inservice to address these attitudes may be helpful.	Full time use of amplification is essential. Will need resource teacher or special class depending on magnitude of language delay. May require special help in all language skills, language based academic subjects, vocabulary, grammar, pragmatics as well as reading and writing. Probably needs assistance to expand experiential language base. Inservice of mainstream teachers required.
SEVERE 71-90 dB HL	Without amplification may hear loud voices about one foot from ear. When amplified optimally, children with hearing ability of 90 dB or better should be able to identify environmental sounds and detect all the sounds of speech. If loss is of prelingual onset, oral language and speech may not develop spontaneously or will be severely delayed. If hearing loss is of recent onset speech is likely to deteriorate with quality becoming atonal.	Child may prefer other children with hearing impairments as friends and playmates. This may further isolate the child from the mainstream, however, these peer relationships may foster improved self concept and a sense of cultural identity.	May need full-time special aural/oral program for with emphasis on all auditory language skills, speechreading, concept development and speech. As loss approaches 80-90dB, may benefit from a Total Communication approach, especially in the early language learning years. Individual hearing aid/personal FM system essential. Need to monitor effectiveness of communication modality. Participation in regular classes as much as beneficial to student. Inservice of mainstream teachers essential.
PROFOUND 91 dB HL or more	Aware of vibrations more than tonal pattern. Many rely on vision rather than hearing as primary avenue for communication and learning. Detection of speech sounds dependent upon loss configuration and use of amplification. Speech and language will not develop spontaneously and is likely to deteriorate rapidly if hearing loss is of recent onset.	Depending on auditory/oral competence, peer use of sign language, parental attitude, etc., child may or may not increasingly prefer association with the deaf culture.	May need special program for deaf children with emphasis on all language skills and academic areas. Program needs specialized supervision and comprehensive support services. Early use of amplification likely to help if part of an intensive training program. May be cochlear implant or vibrotactile aid candidate. Requires continual appraisal of needs in regard to communication and learning mode. Part-time in regular classes as much as beneficial to student.
UNILATERAL One normal hearing ear and one ear with at least a permanent mild hearing loss	May have difficulty hearing faint or distant speech. Usually has difficulty localizing sounds and voices. Unilateral listener will have greater difficulty understanding speech when environment is noisy and/or reverberant. Difficulty detecting or understanding soft speech from side of bad ear, especially in a group discussion.	Child may be accused of selective hearing due to discrepancies in speech understanding in quiet versus noise. Child will be more fatigued in classroom setting due to greater effort needed to listen. May appear inattentive or frustrated. Behavior problems sometimes evident.	May benefit from personal FM or soundfield FM system in classroom. CROS hearing aid may be of benefit in quiet settings. Needs favorable seating and lighting. Student is at risk for educational difficulties. Educational monitoring warranted with support services provided as soon as difficulties appear. Teacher inservice is beneficial.

NOTE: All children with hearing loss require periodic audiologic evaluation, rigorous monitoring of amplification and regular monitoring of communication skills. All children with hearing loss (especially conductive) need appropriate medical attention in conjuction with educational programming.

REFERENCES

Olsen, W. O., Hawkins, D. B. VanTassell, D. J. (1987). Representatives of the Longterm Spectrum of Speech. Ear & Hearing. Supplement 8, pp. 100-108.

Mueller, H. G. & Killion, M. C. (1990). An easy method for calculating the articulation index. The Hearing Journal. 43, 9, pp. 14-22.

Hasenstab, M. S. (1987). Language Learning and Otitis Media. College Hill Press, Boston, MA.

Adapted from: Bernero, R. J. & Bothwell, H. (1966). Relationship of Hearing Impairment to Educational Needs. Illinois Department of Public Health & Office of Superintendent of Public Instruction. **Peer Review by Members of the Educational Audiology Association, Winter 1991**

Developed by
Karen L. Anderson, Ed.S & Noel D. Matkin, Ph.D (1991)

Source: From "Hearing conservation in the public schools revisited" by K. Anderson, 1991, *Seminars in Hearing, 12*(4), pp. 361–363. Copyright 1991 by Thieme Medical Publishers, Inc. Reprinted by permission.

Appendix 4–E

**COLORADO INDIVIDUAL PERFORMANCE PROFILE
(CIPP) FOR DEAF AND HEARING-IMPAIRED STUDENTS**

Colorado Individual Performance Profile (CIPP) for Deaf and Hearing-Impaired Students

Please send suggestions
for changes to:

Joan Ruberry
Rocky Mountain High School
1300 W. Swallow Rd.
Ft. Collins, CO 80526

© Ruberry and Yoshinaga-Itano, 1993

Colorado Individual Performance Profile (CIPP)
Table of Contents

The following pages can be removed from the back of this packet and copied as needed:

Colorado Individual Performance Profile (CIPP)
Deaf and Hearing-Impaired Students

Purpose

This individual performance profile has been developed for the following purposes:

* to develop a tool to assist staffing teams in determining appropriate services and educational placements for students based on need
* to develop a tool to assist staffing teams in determining progress made by individual students
* to compile ongoing data for the Colorado legislature and the Colorado Department of Education related to the need for improving services for Colorado deaf and hearing impaired youth.

When should the CIPP be used?
Use the CIPP for students age 6 and above whose primary or secondary handicapping condition is hearing (except students in the adaptive skills program). Use the CIPP in the following situations:

* an initial assessment (possible placement),
* a triennial review,
* a possible change a placement,
* a direct transfer,
* advancement to the next age level (e.g., primary to intermediate grades),
* data collection efforts

Directions

1. Briefly **read through this packet** to get an idea of the information that is requested of you. **Copy the necessary number of blank charts and forms** at the end of this packet.

2. **Collect Information** on the most recent standardized test scores (do not use scores older than 12 months), curriculum based-assessments, and/or observation. *When several tests are given for a specific area (e.g., language or math) use average scores of all the tests to plot results.*

3. **Complete the worksheet by listing ratings, student scores, and observations.**

4. **Plot results on the profile chart.** You can plot both standardized scores and curriulum-based scores on the same line by labeling the two different dots. See the sample case for clarification. This can also be done for aided and unaided audiological information.

5. To **Interpret the individual performance profile** for use in the IEP process, use the accompanying guidelines (page 14) and sample cases (pages 2 to 5).

Student Name _____

Summary of Information from Formal and Informal Assessment

Use this worksheet prior to plotting individual results on the student chart.

Area	Performance Rating	Test Names and Scores, Curriculum-Based Assessments, Observations
Audiological Acuity	5 to 6 = 4 to 5 =	*Unaided Responses:* Severe to profound bilateral sensori-neural hearing loss 75db to 110db *Aided Responses:* moderate-severe to severe range 55db to 80db *Use of Residual Hearing -- Comments:* Jane has only been aided since age 4 and has only recently started intense training to use residual hearing.
Communication Skills	5	*Primary Mode of Communication:* speech, listening, speech-reading gestures *Comments:* Speech is often not intelligible, even when familiar with the student's articulation pattern. Some staffing team members have recommended that the parents consider a total communication approach with Jane.
English/Language Skills	6	*Formal and Informal Assessments (Name tests, level of tests and scores):* *Receptive Skills:* Rhode Island Test of Language Structure = Age 5 Peabody Picture Vocabulary Test (PPVT) = Age 4.5 years *Expressive Skills:* Expressive One Word Picture Voc. Test = Age 4 yrs. (EOWPVT) Jane typically expresses herself in 2-3 word phrases.
Reading Comprehension	4	*Formal Assessments (Name tests, level of tests and scores):* Stanford Achievement Test, Primary 1 Word Reading = K.5 grade Word Study = K.8 grade *Curriculum Based Assessments:* The classroom teacher reports that Jane has problems with grade level story concepts, i.e., reading strategies, and in participating in group reading discussions. Primer level book

Student Name _____

Area	Performance Rating	Test Names and Scores, Curriculum-Based Assessments, Observations
Mathematics	3-4 (ST)* 3 (CBA)*	Formal Assessments (Name tests, level of tests and scores): Stanford Achievement Test, Primary 1 = Number Concepts K.5 grade, Math Computation K.6 grade, Math Application K.7 grade. Curriculum Based Assessments: Math Computation = Near grade level skills (less than 1 yr. delay as reported by teacher) Problems reported in story problems.
Content Subject Areas	4	Formal Assessments (Name tests, level of tests and scores): Stanford Achievement Test, Primary 1 = Environment K.4 Curriculum Based Assessments: The teacher (classroom teacher) reports difficulty in assessing knowledge of content subjects because of low language skills.
Social-Emotional	between 2 to 3	Formal Inventory or Test: Meadow-Kendall Inventory. Social Adjustment = 65 %ile, Self Image = 60 %ile, Emotional Adjustment = 70 %ile Observation: Comfortable with classroom situation but Jane is socially isolated from conversations with peers and from problem solving with adults and peers.
Life Skills	2	Observation Only: Close to age-appropriate domestic and general community skills.
Cognitive Status	3	Standardized Test: WISC-R Performance I.Q. = 100 Average Abilities Observation: Informal observations of performance suggests higher cognitive abilities
Special Characteristics	5	Comments: Jane has no formal language as a native tongue. She was not diagnosed as having a hearing loss until age 4. She was adopted by her parents at age 4.

Note: For students in kindergarten through third grade the English language category is the most critical category to assess when using this rating scale to assist with placement decisions.

* CBA = Curriculum Based Assessment
* ST = Standardized Test

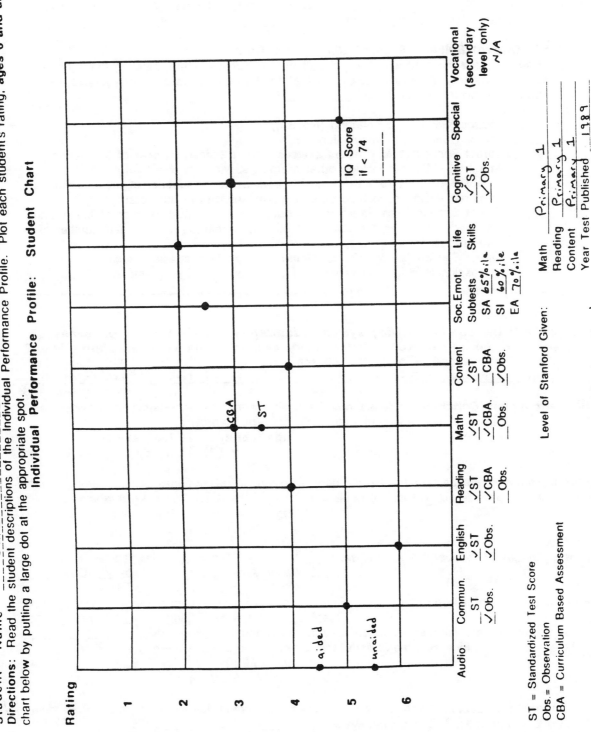

Student Name Jane Doe

Directions: Read the student descriptions of the Individual Performance Profile. Plot each student's rating, **ages 6 and above**, on the chart below by putting a large dot at the appropriate spot.

Individual Performance Profile: **Student Chart**

Rating

	Audio.	Commun.	English	Reading	Math	Content	Soc.Emot.	Life Skills	Cognitive	Special	Vocational (secondary level only)

aided

unaided

CBA

ST

Commun. ST __ / Obs.

English / ST / Obs.

Reading / ST / CBA __ Obs.

Math / ST / CBA __ Obs.

Content / ST __ CBA / Obs.

Soc.Emot. Subtests SA 65%ile SI 60%ile EA 70%ile

Cognitive / ST / Obs.

Special IQ Score if < 74 _____

Vocational N/A

ST = Standardized Test Score
Obs.= Observation
CBA = Curriculum Based Assessment

Level of Stanford Given:

Math Primary 1
Reading Primary 1
Content Primary 1
Year Test Published 1989

Names of Other Tests Administered: PPVT, EOWPVT, Rhode Island

Demographics
For Data Collection Purposes Only

Please complete the following:

Rater's Name ___John Smith___   Administrative Unit Name ___Larimer R-1___
Student Name ___Jane Doe___   DOB _1/5/85_ Grade _1_ Date _1/18/93_
Student's Primary Handicapping Condition ___Hearing___   Other, if any ___—___

Student's **Current Delivery System** *Check One Only.*
Do **not include** the services of an educational **interpreter** when counting these hours to
identify a category of services below. If the student uses an **Interpreter**, record the
number of hours a day here _____

_____ Indirect Service: Monitoring (No IEP)
_____ Indirect Service: Consultation (IEP)
_X_ Direct Service (**1 to 4 hours a week** from a trained teacher of the hearing
impaired -- Do not include other support services in this total.)
_____ Direct Service (**1 to 2 hours daily** from a trained teacher of the hearing
impaired -- Do not include other support services in this total.)
_____ Direct Service (**3 or more hours daily** from a trained teacher of the hearing
impaired. However, the student is still mainstreamed for a limited number of
classes.)
_____ Direct Service (*all academic classes* taken from special education
professionals in hearing services, e.g., self-contained programs and CSDB).
_____ Other: Please explain _____

Do you feel the current delivery system *adequately* **meets the student's needs?**
___ yes _X_ no   IF NOT, what delivery system would be more appropriate ?
Use the list above and write in the choice here:
___Direct Service - 3 or more hours daily from a trained teacher of the
                                                                          hearing impaired

Socio-Economic Condition: Please rate the ability of the student's family to provide the
basic necessities(financial, environmental). *Circle your answer.*

high ability   low ability
1   2   ③   4   5   6

Parent-Family: Please rate the overall degree to which the student's parents/family commit
themselves to provide support for the goals and plans of the IEP. *Circle your answer.*

high support   low support
1   ②   3   4   5   6

Ethnic Origin of Student: *Check One.* ___ Asian ___ Black ___ Hispanic
_X_ Native American ___ White ___ Other

Family Communication Systems: Does the student have deaf parents? ___ yes _X_ no
Deaf/Hearing Impaired Siblings? ___ yes _X_ no
What is the primary language spoken/used in the home? ___English___
If the student uses signs, rate the ability of the family to use signs in the home. N/A

high ability   low ability
1   2   3   4   5   6

Communication System Used at School: Does the student use signs as part of their main N/A
mode of communication? If yes, what system? ___ ASL ___ PSE ___ SEE 2
___ SEE 1 ___ Cued Speech

For students enrolled at CSDB ___ day ___ res   N/A
Reason for CSDB Placement _____

Audiological Acuity

Plot the student's unaided and aided (if available) results on the same vertical line.

Rating	Current Functioning
1	* **avg. pure tone** loss in speech range (500 to 2000 hz) **20-35db** in better ear; or * **avg. high frequency** pure tone loss, **35 -50 db.** in better ear at two or more frequencies of 2,000 ... 3,000 ... 4,000 ... 6,000; or * **permanent unilateral** loss, **35 - 50 db** in speech range *No IEP needed related to hearing.*
2	* **same** audiological criteria as **Rating 1.** However ... *An IEP is needed related to hearing needs.*
3	* **avg. pure tone** loss in speech range (500 to 2,000 hz) **35-50 db** in better ear; or * **avg. high frequency** pure tone loss **50 db. or greater** in better ear at two or more frequencies of 2,000 ... 3,000 ... 4,000 ... 6,000; or * **permanent unilateral** loss of **50 db.** or greater in speech range *An IEP is needed related to hearing needs.*
4	* **avg. pure tone** loss in speech range (500 to 2,000 hz) **50-65 db** in better ear *An IEP is needed related to hearing needs.*
5	* **avg. pure tone** loss in speech range (500 to 2,000 hz) **65-85 db** in better ear *An IEP is needed related to hearing needs.*
6	* **avg. pure tone** loss in speech range (500 to 2,000 hz) **greater than 85 db** in better ear *An IEP is needed related to hearing needs.*

Communication Skills

Primary mode of communication is speech, listening, and speech-reading only.

Rating	Current Functioning
1	* **speech is consistently intelligible** to peers and to the regular classroom teacher. *No IEP is needed related to communication skills.*
2	* **speech is intelligible** to peers and to the regular classroom teacher, even with minor errors. *An IEP is needed to maintain or improve communication skills .*
3	* **speech is intelligible** but may be difficult for the listener to understand. *An IEP is needed to improve communication skills.*
4	* **speech is intelligible** to the listener when familiar with student's articulation pattern *An IEP is needed to improve communication skills.*
5	* **speech is often unintelligible** even when familiar with the student's articulation pattern *An IEP is needed to improve communication skills.*
6	* **speech is unintelligible** to most listeners. *An IEP is needed to improve communication skills.*

Primary mode of communication is sign language or sign language used in combination with speech. Start with rating number 4 for these students.

Rating	Current Functioning
1	Not Applicable
2	Not Applicable
3	Not Applicable
4	* uses sign language and or signs with speech to **effectively communicate** on a consistent basis. *An IEP is needed to maintain or improve communication skills.*
5	* does not use sign language or signs with speech to effectively communicate on a consistent basis -- needs **special training** in the use of sign language and/or simultaneous communication. *An IEP is needed to improve communication skills.*
6	* does not use sign language or signs with speech to effectively communicate on a consistent basis -- needs **intense training** in the use of sign language and/or simultaneous communication. *An IEP is needed to improve communication skills.*

English Language Skills
Reading Comprehension
Mathematics
Content Subjects

All test scores used to rate students in this section should be no older than 12 months. Should you not have recent test scores on these tests, either administer a new test or check the "observation" box or the "curriculum-based assessment" box on the student chart. When using percentile scores for students fully mainstreamed, any appropriate subtest score is acceptable. Such tests may, for example, include the California Achievement Test (CAT) or the Iowa Test of Basic Skills (ITBS).

English Language Skills
Use a combination of the following standardized tests:
   a. Expressive One Word Picture Test (EOWPT),
   b. Stanford Achievement Test -- Reading Vocabulary subtest (hearing grade levels),
   c. Woodcock Johnson Analogies test,
   d. Brown Stages for mean length utterances (for young children),
   e. Peabody Picture Vocabulary Test (PPVT) (for younger children),
   f. Rhode Island Test of Syntactical Structures (for younger children),
   g. Colorado Process Analysis of the Written Language of Hearing-Impaired Children (COPA) -- Yoshinaga-Itano.

Reading Comprehension:
Use **reading comprehension** scores for this section, not word recognition. If reading scores are not available, use curriculum-based materials to assess a delay, if any. For young readers or for multi-handicapped students, curriculum-based assessments may be more useful in determining an appropriate reading level. For non-readers, estimate their readiness to read and the number of years it will require for them to become a reader when comparing them with non-handicapped peers.

For students in grades K- to 3, current functioning in the English language domain may be a better indicator to assist in program placement than would be reading. Reading in the primary grades is too concrete to be a valuable tool. For students in grades 4 to 6, weigh both English and reading scores heavily. For students above the sixth grade, a combination of vocabulary, reading, and writing abilities should be noted.

Mathematics and Content Subjects:
If more than one test score is available for these areas, use an **average of math subtests** (e.g., computation, concepts, applications) and an **average of content areas** (e.g., science and math). The Stanford Achievement Test (Hearing Impaired Edition, 1989 only) is recommended for students ages 8 and older. If no current scores are available or the student is under age 8, assess the student's abilities to handle curriculum offered non-handicapped students their own age.

The above tests should be given to all center-based students and as many fully mainstreamed students as possible. If a student cannot be administered these tests, use curriculum-based assessments or achievement tests administered to all students in the district.

When you record data on the chart, make sure you do the following:

   1. **Check if you rated the student by standardized test, and/or curriculum-based assessment, and/or observation.**
   2. **Write down the name (and level, if needed) of the standardized test by which you rated the student.**

Use the scale below for English, reading, mathematics and content subjects. Use the first scale for students age 12 or below. Use the second scale for students above age 12. When grades and ages don't match in overlap areas (e.g., age 13 - 6th grade), use the student's age.

Ages 6 through 12 (approximately, grades K-6)

Rating	Current Functioning
1	at or above grade level skills *No IEP is needed.* (at or above 60th percentile)
2	at or above grade level skills *IEP is needed to **maintain** skills.* (at or above 60th percentile)
3	**less than a 1 year delay** *IEP is needed to **Improve skills.*** (or 40th to 60th percentile)
4	**1 yr. to less than 2 yr. delay** *IEP is needed to **Improve skills.*** (use tests listed above or curriculum-based assessment only)
5	**2 yr. delay** *IEP is needed to **Improve skills.*** (use tests listed above or curriculum-based assessment only)
6	**3 or more yr. delay** *IEP is needed to **Improve skills.*** (use tests listed above or curriculum-based assessment only)

Ages 13 to 21 (approximately, grades 7 through 12)

Rating	Current Functioning
1	at or above grade level skills *No IEP is needed.* (at or above 60th percentile)
2	**close to age-appropriate skills** (less than 1 yr. delay and/or scores 60th percentile or above on standardized tests) *IEP Is needed to **maintain or Improve** skills.*
3	**1 to 2 yr. delay** *IEP is needed to **Improve** skills.* (or 40th to 60th percentile)
4	**3 yr. delay** *IEP is needed to **Improve** skills.* (use tests listed above or curriculum-based assessments only)
5	**4 yr. delay** *IEP is needed to **Improve** skills.* (use tests listed above or curriculum-based assessments only)
6	**5 or more yr. delay** *IEP is needed to **Improve** skills.* (use tests listed above or curriculum-based assessments only)

Social-Emotional Development

Use an **average** of all three subtests of the Meadow-Kendall Social Emotional Assessment Inventory for deaf and hearing impaired students to rate the student in this area. However, please write in the individual subtests scores on the student chart in addition to graphing the rating.

Rating	Current Functioning
1	Student scores from the 80th to the100th percentile. *No IEP needed related to social-emotional need.*
2	Student scores from the 65th to the 79th percentile. *An IEP may be needed to address specific areas.*
3	Student scores from the 50th to the 64th percentile. *An IEP is needed to address social-emotional needs.*
4	Student scores from the 35th to the 49th percentile. *An IEP is needed to address social-emotional needs.*
5	Student scores from the 20th to the 34th percentile. *An IEP is needed to address social-emotional needs.*
6	Student scores from the zero to the 19th percentile. *An IEP is needed and may address intensive services related to social-emotional needs.*

Life Skills

Rate for all school-age children.

Domestic skills include self-care skills in the home (cooking, laundry, etc. For young children this may include taking care of personal possessions or the ability to assist parents or older siblings with domestic chores).

General community skills include such skills as the ability to handle money, consumer skills, mobility in the community, ability to use the telephone, and the ability to use assistive devices. For young children, this may include the ability to bring notes back and forth to school, ability to handle school bus transportation, visiting friends, etc.

Rating	Current Functioning
1	The student has **age-appropriate** domestic and general community skills. *No IEP is needed.*
2	The student has **close to age-appropriate** domestic and general community skills. Skills may only need "polishing". *An IEP is needed to assist parents and student "fill in minor gaps".*
3	The student **lacks some** domestic and general community skills but they still appear **not significantly different from most students their own age** in their ability to handle their environment. *An IEP is needed. However, such a plan would only require **periodic changes** to the school day. Many of the skills could be taught by parents .*
4	The student **lacks many** of the the domestic and general community skills. They **obviously differ from most students their own age** in their ability to independently function in the home and community environment. *An IEP is needed. Such a plan may require daily changes to the school day, even if only for a limited period of time.*
5	The student is **significantly deficient** in domestic and general community skills. However, such a student would be **expected to function independently** upon graduation from high school. *An IEP is needed. Such a plan should focus on those skills which would enable the student to improve their ability to function independently.*
6	The student is **severely deficient** in ability to handle the environment. They **may never be able to function independently** in the community, but may need domestic and community support indefinitely upon graduation from high school. *An IEP is needed and would focus on adaptive skills.*

Cognitive Status

Use most recent **performance I.Q. results.** Any valid IQ score can be used, regardless of how old the score is. However, the score must represent the student's present abilities. If no valid I.Q. score is available, use **observation of how well the student is able to learn as an indicator.**

Rating	Current Functioning
1	**Superior** Cognitive Abilities (IQ of 120 and above)
2	**Above Average** Cognitive Abilities (IQ of 110-119)
3	**Average** Cognitive Abilities (IQ of 90-110)
4	**Low Average** Cognitive Abilities (IQ of 80 -89)
5	**Borderline** Intellectual Abilities (IQ of 70-79)*
6	**Significantly Limited Intellectual Capacity** (IQ below 70)*

* For students with scores less than 74, please report the exact number on the student chart in addition to graphing the student's rating.

Special Characteristics

Special characteristics may include such things as a second handicapping condition, health condition which interferes with educational progress, and/or a **spoken** language other than English being the primary language of the student. Note: Some hearing handicapped students also have perceptual difficulties (i.e., a learning disability). Please take secondary handicapping conditions into consideration in this section.

Rating	Current Functioning
1	Student has **no special characteristic.**
2	Student has special **characteristic** but it **does not interfere** with educational progress.
3	Student has special **characteristic** which **provides minimal obstacles** to educational progress. Only periodic modifications need to be made .
4	Student has special **characteristic** which **provides significant obstacles** to educational progress such that adaptations need to be made to the daily schedule or the regular education curriculum to accommodate the student's needs.
5	**Same as Rating 4 only more severe.**
6	Same as Rating 4 only more severe. A **short- or long-term extended day program may be necessary** to accommodate student needs.

Pre-Vocational/Vocational Skills
Rate only grades 6 through 12

Grades 6 through 9: Pre-Vocational Skills

As compared to successful hearing students their own age, rate middle and junior high school students on the following: has responsibilities at home, has developed hobbies and interests, does volunteer work, participates in clubs or athletics, or holds part-time or summer employment.

Grades 10 through 12: Vocational Skills

As compared to successful hearing students their own age, rate high school students on the following: identification of a realistic career interest and related plan, skills commensurate with career interest and plan (e.g., experience with part-time employment and/or participation in extra-curricular activities), ability to pursue post-secondary services and post-secondary education to achieve career plans)..

Rating	Current Functioning
1	Student has developed **age-appropriate skills** and plans as listed above *No IEP is needed related to these skills.*
2	Student has developed **age-appropriate** skills and plans as listed above. *An IEP is needed to maintain skills or to assist in planning.*
3	Student has **close to age-appropriate skills** and plans but may need some specific guidance in achieving related goals. *An IEP is needed to improve skills or to assist in the planning. process*
4	Student **lacks many of the pre-vocational or vocational skills** which lead to post-secondary employment or education. Student is **not commensurate with peers** in this area, including experience or lack of experience with part-time employment opportunities, participation in extra-curricular activities, development of leisure time activities etc. *An IEP is needed to improve skills or to assist in the planning process.*
5	Same as rating number four only with **more significant deficits**. However, with appropriate intervention, the student should be able to be competitively employed after graduation or completion of post-secondary training. *An IEP is needed to improve skills and to support the career planning process.*
6	Student is **severely deficient in pre-vocational or vocational skills.** Such a student may never be competitively employed but may need supported employment and assistance from adult agencies throughout part or all of their adult life. *An IEP is needed to support this process.*

...

Guidelines for Interpretation of the Individual Performance Profile

Ratings in the different domains may have varied significance due to the age of the student and the number of high or low ratings a student has in all the areas. The ratings are used to assist in the identification of the *intensity* of services, i.e., the level of weekly or daily service which the student may need to maintain or improve skills. For example, a student may have several ratings of three, at first glance denoting service from a travelling teacher of the hearing impaired. However several ratings of "three" may indicate that a more intense level of service is needed because of the amount of accumulated time involved when addressing needs within each domain. The same may be true for other levels of the rating system.

Care should be exercised when using the year delays to identify the level of service needed. A kindergarten student at the lower end of the age spectrum should not have as severe delays as students at the upper end of the spectrum, i.e., sixth grade. The next level of service may be more appropriate.

Within the array of delivery systems there may be services determined on the IEP, such as speech-language, interpreting, counseling, etc. in addition to the teacher of the hearing impaired. At the resource and self-contained levels, students are pooled in center-based programs, as possible, so that appropriate services and communication practice can be provided.

Indirect Service: Monitoring of Student Progress
The student should have age-appropriate skills in all areas and not need an individual educational plan (IEP). Monitoring of student progress can be implemented through personal and paper follow-up of student.

Indirect Service: Consultation
The student should have age-appropriate skills in all areas but may need an IEP to provide consultation services to help the student maintain skill development.

Direct Service: Travelling Teacher of the Hearing Impaired
1 to 4 hours a week from a trained teacher of the hearing impaired

Student need should not total more than four hours a week from a trained teacher of the hearing impaired. The student should be able to appropriately benefit from all academics within the regular classroom setting with only team-teaching, consultation, and/or "pull-out" services from professionals in the area of hearing service. Therefore, academic delays typically should not exceed one to two years in grades K-6 and not more than two to three years in grades 7-12. Overall, students should have many ratings less than three. If a student has several ratings of three or a language rating higher than three, the student may benefit more appropriately from the next level of service.

Direct Service: Resource Level, Hearing Impaired
1 to 2 hours daily from a trained teacher of the hearing impaired

To maintain or improve educational progress, student need can best be met in a center-based program with other hearing impaired or deaf students for part of the day but yet mainstreamed with hearing students for a majority of the school day. Students typically have no more than a two to three year academic delay at the K-6 level and no more than a three to four year delay in grades 7 -12. Students may need specialized language training not readily accessible in mainstreamed classes. In addition to language related to academics, language training may include skills related to social-emotional development (i.e., problems solving, decision making, understanding feelings, etc). Students needing this level of service may rate high in some areas but have enough cumulative need to warrant more intense services than "travelling" services" can realistically provide.

Students in rural areas needing this level of service, but not near a critical mass of hearing impaired or deaf students, may sometimes benefit from general special education resource room services in addition to services from an itinerant teacher of the hearing impaired. However, caution should be exercised when choosing this option and opportunities should be explored for the student to associate with other hearing impaired or deaf students. Districts may also consider pooling resources with other districts or with CSDB to provide this level of service.

Direct Service: Self-Contained, Hearing Impaired
3 or more hours daily from a trained teacher of the hearing impaired

Student need can best be met in a center-based program with other hearing impaired or deaf students for about half the day and mainstreamed with hearing students for the remainder of the day. Typically, delays should not exceed two to three years at the K-6 level and no more than four to five years at the secondary level. Students at this level of service need considerable modification of the regular curriculum to benefit from instruction. Districts not having a large enough critical mass of students needing this level of service may want to serve both resource level and self-contained level students in the same learning environment and schedule services based on individual need. Districts may also consider pooling resources with other districts or with CSDB to provide appropriate services.

Direct Service: Self-Contained, Hearing Impaired
all academics taken from a trained teacher of the hearing impaired

Students at this level need intense services from trained professionals in deafness, either for short or long-term duration. Typically, students would have a three or more year delay at the K-6 level and a five or more year delay at the 7-12 level. Students usually need specialized curriculum, specific services related to life skills, or those related to the social-emotional domain not readily available in each school district (or administrative unit). Administrative units may want to pool resources and/or work cooperatively with CSDB to provide appropriate services.

Colorado Individual Performance Profile (CIPP)
Deaf and Hearing-Impaired Students (ages 6 through 21)
Overview for Parents

What is this tool?

The Colorado Individual Performance Profile (previously referred to as the Colorado Severity Rating Scale) was originated in 1991 by the Colorado Department of Education, in part (1) to develop a tool to assist staffing teams in determining appropriate services and educational placements for students based on need, and (2) to improve data collection efforts related to improving educational services to Colorado deaf and hearing impaired youth.

How was it developed?

The tool was developed with the assistance of service providers working with deaf and hearing impaired students across Colorado. Special consultation was provided from the University of Colorado, Boulder and from the Poudre R-1 School District, Fort Collins. Information was collected on more than 950 students statewide as part of the process to validate the appropriateness of this tool.

How does the tool work?

Information is collected through formal and informal assessments related to the following areas: audiological acuity, communication, English language skills, reading, mathematics, content areas of social studies and science, social-emotional development, life skills, cognition, and for secondary students, vocational skills. Any special background circumstances related to educational progress is also noted.

The student is then rated on a scale from one to six by using characteristics of the students as noted through the formal and informal information collected. Each rating is charted on an individual student chart to obtain a profile of the student's current functioning.

How is the information used?

Ratings in various domains may have different significance due to the age of the student and the number of high or low ratings a student has in all the areas. The ratings can be used to identify *the intensity of services*, i.e., the level of weekly or daily service which the student needs to improve or maintain skills. The array of possible delivery systems follows:

Indirect Service: Monitoring of Student Progress (no IEP needed)
Indirect Service: Consultation (IEP needed)
Direct Service: Travelling Teacher of the Hearing Impaired -- 1 to 4 hours a week
    from a trained teacher of the hearing impaired
Direct Service Resource Level, Hearing Impaired -- 1 to 2 hours daily from a
    trained teacher of the hearing impaired, some academics taken in the
    mainstream
Direct Service Self-Contained , Hearing Impaired -- 3 hours or more daily from a
    trained teacher of the hearing impaired, but some academics still taken in
    the mainstream
Direct Service: Self-Contained , Hearing Impaired -- all academics taken from a
    trained teacher of the hearing impaired

Within the array of delivery systems noted above, there may be services such as speech-language, counseling, interpreting, etc. in addition to the teacher of the hearing impaired, based on need. At the resource and self-contained levels, students are typically pooled in center-based programs, as possible, so that appropriate services and communication practice can be provided.

Student Name: _____

Summary of Information from Formal and Informal Assessment
Use this worksheet prior to plotting individual results on the student chart.

Area	Performance Rating	Test Names and Scores, Curriculum-Based Assessments, Observations
Audiological Acuity		*Unaided Responses :* *Aided Responses :* *Use of Residual Hearing -- Comments :*
Communication Skills		*Primary Mode of Communication :* *Comments:*
English/Language Skills		*Formal and Informal Assessments (Name tests, level of tests and scores):* *Receptive Skills :.* *Expressive Skills :*
Reading Comprehension		*Formal Assessments (Name tests, level of tests and scores) :* *Curriculum Based Assessments :*

Student Name _____

Area	Performance Rating	Test Names and Scores, Curriculum-Based Assessments, Observations
Mathematics		Formal Assessments (Name tests, level of tests and scores) : Curriculum Based Assessments :
Content Subject Areas		Formal Assessments (Name tests, level of tests and scores) : Curriculum Based Assessments :
Social-Emotional		Formal Inventory or Test : Observation :
Life Skills		Observation Only :
Cognitive Status		Standardized Test : Observation:
Special Characteristics		Comments. :

Note: For students in kindergarten through third grade the English language category is the most critical category to assess when using this rating scale to assist with placement decisions.

Student Name _____

Directions: Read the student descriptions of the Individual Performance Profile. Plot each student's rating, **ages 6 and above**, on the chart below by putting a large dot at the appropriate spot.

Individual Performance Profile:　Student Chart

Rating	Audio.	Commun.	English	Reading	Math	Content	Soc.Emot.	Life Skills	Cognitive	Special	Vocational (secondary level only)
1											
2											
3											
4											
5										IQ Score if < 74	
6											

Sub-column labels:
- Commun.: ST / Obs.
- English: ST / Obs.
- Reading: ST / CBA / Obs.
- Math: ST / CBA / Obs.
- Content: ST / CBA / Obs.
- Soc.Emot. Subtests: SA / SI / EA
- Cognitive: ST / Obs.
- Special: _____

ST = Standardized Test Score
Obs.= Observation
CBA = Curriculum Based Assessment

Level of Stanford Given: _____

Math _____
Reading _____
Content _____
Year Test Published _____

Names of Other Tests Administered: _____

Demographics
For Data Collection Purposes Only

Please complete the following:

Rater's Name _____   Administrative Unit Name _____
Student Name _____   DOB _____ Grade ____ Date _____
Student's Primary Handicapping Condition _____ Other, if any _____

Student's **Current Delivery System** *Check One Only.*
    Do **not include** the services of an educational **interpreter** when counting these hours to identify a category of services below. If the student uses an **Interpreter**, record the **number of hours a day** here _____

    _____ Indirect Service: Monitoring (No IEP)
    _____ Indirect Service: Consultation (IEP)
    _____ Direct Service (**1 to 4 hours a week** from a trained teacher of the hearing impaired -- Do not include other support services in this total.)
    _____ Direct Service (**1 to 2 hours daily** from a trained teacher of the hearing impaired -- Do not include other support services in this total.)
    _____ Direct Service (**3 or more hours daily** from a trained teacher of the hearing impaired. However, the student is still mainstreamed for a limited number of classes.)
    _____ Direct Service (**all academic classes** taken from special education professionals in hearing services, e.g., self-contained programs and CSDB).
    _____ Other: Please explain _____

Do you feel the current delivery system *adequately* meets the student's needs?
___ yes ____no   IF NOT, what delivery system would be more appropriate ?
Use the list above and write in the choice here:

Socio-Economic Condition: Please rate the ability of the student's family to provide the basic necessities(financial, environmental). *Circle your answer.*

                   high ability   **low ability**
                     1 2 3 4 5 6

Parent-Family: Please rate the overall degree to which the student's parents/family commit themselves to provide support for the goals and plans of the IEP. *Circle your answer.*

                   high support   **low support**
                     1 2 3 4 5 6

Ethnic Origin of Student: *Check One.* ___ Asian ___ Black ___ Hispanic
                              ___ Native American ___ White ___ Other

Family Communication Systems: Does the student have deaf parents? ___ yes ___ no
                           Deaf/Hearing Impaired Siblings? ____ yes ___ no
What is the primary language spoken/used in the home? _____
If the student uses signs, rate the ability of the family to use signs in the home.

                   high ability   **low ability**
                     1 2 3 4 5 6

Communication System Used at School: Does the student use signs as part of their main mode of communication? If yes, what system?   ____ ASL _____ PSE ____ SEE 2
                                      ____ SEE 1 _____ Cued Speech

For students enrolled at CSDB ____ day ___ res
Reason for CSDB Placement _____

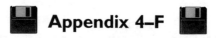

Appendix 4–F

EVALUATION OF CHILDREN WITH SUSPECTED LISTENING DISORDERS

		Ranking Scale		
1	2	3	4	NA
demonstrates all of the time	most of the the time	some of the time	never observed	not applicable

1. *Overall Concerns about Listening*

• Doesn't understand appropriate listening expectations of the classroom	1	2	3	4	NA
• Doesn't seem to listen	1	2	3	4	NA
• Appears to be a good listener but work suggests misunderstandings	1	2	3	4	NA
• Has difficulty following directions	1	2	3	4	NA
• Follows single step commands but has difficulty with multistage commands	1	2	3	4	NA
• Frequently asks for repetition	1	2	3	4	NA
• Tends to quit easily when frustrated	1	2	3	4	NA
• Impulsive—often acts before thinking	1	2	3	4	NA
• Slow at beginning new tasks	1	2	3	4	NA
• Doesn't complete assignments	1	2	3	4	NA
• Has difficulty sustaining attention during oral presentations	1	2	3	4	NA
• Watches the speaker's face for more information	1	2	3	4	NA

2. *Current Strengths and Weaknesses*

• The child shows appropriate listening skills:

In a Large Group Activity:

• When activity is directed	1	2	3	4	NA
• When activity is independent	1	2	3	4	NA
• In the gymnasium	1	2	3	4	NA
• The noise level has impact on the student's performance	Yes _____ No _____				

In a Small Group Activity:

• When activity is directed	1	2	3	4	NA
• When activity is independent	1	2	3	4	NA
• The noise level has impact on the student's performance	Yes _____ No _____				

3. *Child's Level of Awareness of Strengths and Weaknesses*

• Generally unaware of errors in processing information and doesn't attempt to clarify	1	2	3	4	NA
• Recognizes difficult listening situations	1	2	3	4	NA
• Recognizes that it is difficult to understand when people talk too quickly	1	2	3	4	NA
• Has developed preferences for certain speakers	1	2	3	4	NA

4. *Child's Current Strategies*

• Maintains eye contact with speaker	1	2	3	4	NA

• Will choose/request:					
—Seating close to speaker	1	2	3	4	NA
—Seating away from noise sources	1	2	3	4	NA
—use of FM technology	1	2	3	4	NA
• Will ask for repetition:					
—In large group	1	2	3	4	NA
—With classmates	1	2	3	4	NA
—Privately with teacher	1	2	3	4	NA
• Will rehearse information to retain it better	1	2	3	4	NA
• Will clarify by asking questions or paraphrasing	1	2	3	4	NA
• Will close the classroom door	1	2	3	4	NA

• Other strategies:

List _____

_____

Comments _____

_____

5. *Current Modifications by the Teacher*

Environmental Modifications that Improve Listening Performance:

• Use of FM technology	1	2	3	4	NA
• Seating close to teacher	1	2	3	4	NA
• Seating away from constant noise sources (pencil sharpener, hallway, windows, etc.)	1	2	3	4	NA
• Seating in special areas of classroom: _____					
• Use of library/hallways for projects	1	2	3	4	NA
• Use of headphones by the child (for noise reduction during individual work periods)	1	2	3	4	NA

Teaching Strategies that Improve Listening Performance:

• Use of buddy system	1	2	3	4	NA
• Writing instructions on chalkboard	1	2	3	4	NA
• Calling child's name before initiating instructions	1	2	3	4	NA
• Touching child on shoulder to get his/her attention	1	2	3	4	NA
• Simplifying instructions to single steps	1	2	3	4	NA
• Comprehension checks:					
—Ask child to indicate when didn't understand	1	2	3	4	NA
—Ask child to repeat instructions heard	1	2	3	4	NA
—Ask child to summarize instructions before work initiated	1	2	3	4	NA
• Slowing rate of speech	1	2	3	4	NA
• Use of breaks or rest periods from listening	1	2	3	4	NA

6. *Other Factors of Note* (fluid build-up in the middle ear/otitis media, emotional difficulties, attention deficit disorder, etc.) _____

_____

_____

_____

Appendix 4–G

SAMPLE AUDIOGRAMS

Name _____   Referral Source _____

School _____   Grade _____   Date of Birth _____

Date _____   Audiologist _____   Code: ES   MS   O   N   CAP

AUDIOGRAM CODE

	Air	Air Masked	Bone	Bone Masked	Unmasked Bone	AC No Response	BC No Response	
Right (Red)	O	△	<	[		⟲	↙	NR No Response DNT Did Not Test CNT Could Not Test A Sound Field Aided (Personal) FM Sound Field Aided S Sound Field
Left (Blue)	X	□	>	]	⊔	X	↘	

TEST RELIABILITY

Good
Fair
Poor

RIGHT EAR

Low Pitch   FREQUENCY IN HERTZ   High Pitch

LEFT EAR

Low Pitch   FREQUENCY IN HERTZ   High Pitch

↑ Normal

AUDIBILITY INDEX (AI): _____

AUDIBILITY INDEX (AI): _____

Hearing Level in dB (re: ANSI 1969)

AUDIOMETRY

Ear	Pure Tone Average			Speech Reception Threshold	Word Recognition		Most Comfortable Level	
	Air	Bone	High Freq.					
Right	dB	dB	dB	dB	%	dBSL		dBHL
Left	dB	dB	dB	dB	%	dBSL		dBHL

SPECIAL TESTS

Speech Reading: _____ (Test _____)

Ling 5 Sounds : a _____ u _____ i _____ sh _____ s _____

Other: _____

SOUND FIELD

SRT	Word Recognition		
	Stimuli		
	Quiet	%	dBHL
	Noise @	S/N	%
AIDED SRT	Aided Word Recognition		
	Quiet	%	dBHL
	Noise @	S/N	%
AIDED AI	Aud/Vis		%
	Soft	%	dBHL

Uncomfortable Level

| R | dBHL |
| L | dBHL |

R | dDl IL
L | dBHL

HEARING AID

	Right Ear	Left Ear
Brand:		
Ser. #:		
Tone:		
Output:		
Vol:		
Mold:		
Listn ✓:		
Electro:		
Real Ear:		

FM/ALD

System	Right Ear	Left Ear
Coupler:		
Output:		
Tone:		
Gain:		
Vol.:		

ACOUSTIC IMMITANCE

Tympanogram
(Pressure In daPa)

High

Compliance   10 9 8 7 6 5 4 3 2 1 0

Low

-400 -300 -200 -100   0   +100 +200

Physical Vol: R _____ L _____

Gradient: R _____ L _____

STAPEDIUS REFLEX THRESHOLDS

Ear	500	1000	2000	4000	
R					CONTRA
L					CONTRA
R					IPSI
L					IPSI

Otoscopic: R _____ L _____

COMMENTS:

IMPRESSION:

RECOMMENDATIONS:

White Copy - Audiologist   Yellow Copy - _____   Pink Copy - _____   CC _____

Name _____ Referral Source _____

Address _____ Age _____ Date of Birth _____

Date _____ Audiologist _____ Code: ES MS O N CAP

AUDIOGRAM CODE

	Speaker	Unmasked Bone
Right	R	⌐
Left	L	

NR No Response
DNT Did Not Test
CNT Could Not Test
A Sound Field Aided (Personal)
FM Sound Field Aided
S Sound Field

Procedure
____ Behavioral Observation
____ Conditioned Orientation Response

TEST RELIABILITY

Good
Fair
Poor

SOUND FIELD

Low Pitch   FREQUENCY IN HERTZ   High Pitch

AUDIBILITY INDEX (AI): _____   AIDED AI: _____

SOUND FIELD RESULTS

AGE	EXPECTED RESPONSE (dBHL)			OBSERVED RESPONSE
	Startle	Speech	Warble tones	
0 wk - 6 wk	65dB ± 6	40-60dB	78dB	Startle _____dBHL
6 wk - 4 mo	65dB ± 10	47dB ± 2	70dB	Speech _____dBHL
4 mo - 7 mo	65dB ± 9	21dB ± 8	51dB	Warble Tones _____dBHL
7 mo - 9 mo	65dB ± 15	15dB ± 7	45dB	Bone Conduction Speech: _____dBHL
9 mo - 13 mo	65dB ± 8	8dB ± 7	38dB	Speech Localization:
13 mo - 16 mo	65dB ± 10	5dB ± 5	32dB	R_____ L_____
16 mo - 21 mo	65dB ± 10	5dB ± 1	25dB	History of Otitis Media:
21 mo - 24 mo	65dB ± 10	3dB ± 2	26dB	No _____ Yes _____

Frequency per year _____
Tubes _____

Noisemakers:

AUDIOMETRY   HEARING AID   FM/ALD

Ear	Speech Awareness ___ Reception ___ Threshold
Right	
Left	
Sound Field	
Aided S.F.	

	Right Ear	Left Ear
Brand:		
Ser. #:		
Tone:		
Output:		
Vol:		
Mold:		
Listn ✓:		
Electro:		
Real Ear:		

System	Right Ear	Left Ear
Coupler:		
Output:		
Tone:		
Gain:		
Vol.:		

COMMENTS:

ACOUSTIC IMMITANCE
Tympanogram
(Pressure in daPa)

Physical Vol: R _____ L _____
Gradient: R _____ L _____

STAPEDIUS REFLEX THRESHOLDS

Ear Stimulant	500	1000	2000	4000	
R					CONTRA
L					CONTRA
R					IPSI
L					IPSI

Otoscopic: R _____ L _____

IMPRESSION:

RECOMMENDATIONS:

White Copy - Audiologist   Yellow Copy - _____   Pink Copy - _____   CC _____

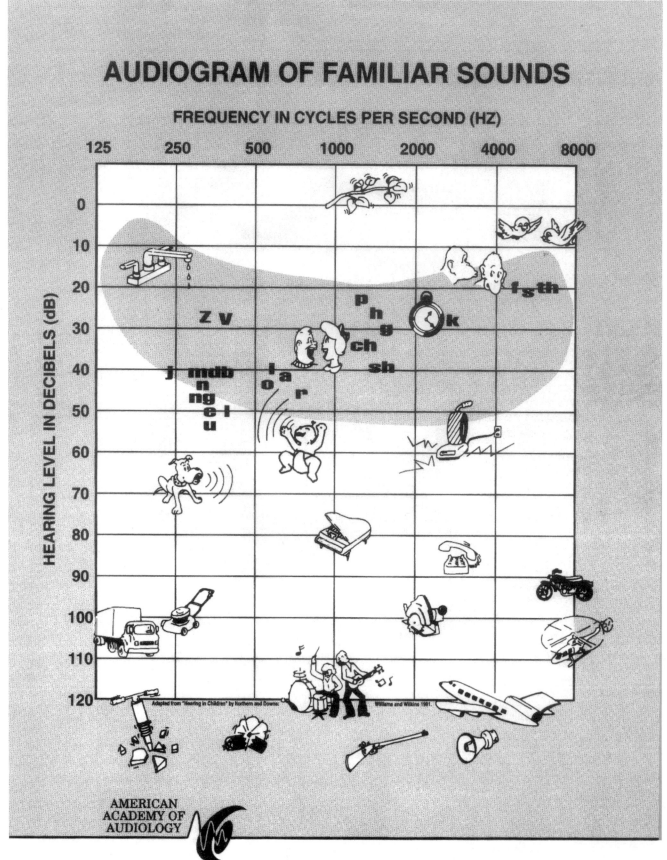

AUDIOGRAM OF FAMILIAR SOUNDS

FREQUENCY IN CYCLES PER SECOND (HZ)

Adapted from "Hearing in Children" by Northern and Downs; Williams and Wilkins 1991.

AMERICAN
ACADEMY OF
AUDIOLOGY

http://www.audiology.com   8201 Greensboro Dr., Ste. 300, McLean VA 22102 • 703-610-9022 • 800-AAA-2336 • Fax: 703-610-9005

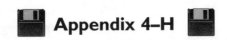

Appendix 4–H

GENERAL TEACHER LETTER

Dear Teacher,

A student in your classroom, _____, has a hearing loss. You can help your student by:

- Promoting acceptance of the student.
- Being sure hearing aids and other amplification devices are used when recommended.
- Providing preferential seating.
- Increasing visual information.
- Minimizing classroom noise.
- Using clear speech and encouraging others to do so.
- Modifying teaching techniques.
- Having realistic expectations.

Specific suggestions to help you accomplish these things are listed in the following material. These guidelines are general and should be adapted as necessary. The items marked with an asterisk (*) are especially important for your student. If you have any questions, please contact me for assistance.

Sincerely,

Educational Audiologist

PROMOTE ACCEPTANCE OF YOUR STUDENT: Your student will benefit from a classroom where he/she feels accepted and where modifications are made without undue attention.

- Welcome the student to your class. Your positive attitude will help other students accept him/her.
- Discuss your student's hearing loss with him/her; let him/her know you are willing to help.
- As appropriate, have your student, the audiologist, or another person explain the student's hearing loss to your entire class.
- Make modifications seem as natural as possible so the student is not singled out.
- Accept your student as an individual; be aware of his/her assets as well as his/her limitations.
- Encourage your student's special abilities or interests.

BE SURE HEARING AIDS AND OTHER AMPLIFICATION DEVICES ARE USED WHEN RECOMMENDED: This will enable your student to use his/her hearing maximally.

- Realize that hearing aids make sounds louder, but not necessarily clearer. Hearing aids don't make hearing normal.
- Be sure your student's hearing aids or other devices are checked daily to see that they are working properly.
- Encourage the student to care for his/her hearing aid(s) by putting it on, telling you when it is not functioning properly, etc.
- Be sure your student always has a spare battery at school.
- Know who to contact if your student's device is not working properly.

PROVIDE PREFERENTIAL SEATING: Appropriate seating will enhance your student's ability to hear and understand what is said in the classroom.

- Seat near where you typically teach. It will be helpful if your student is at one side of the classroom so that he/she can easily turn and follow classroom dialogue.
- Seat where your student can easily watch your face without straining to look straight up. Typically the second or third row is best.
- Seat away from noise sources, including hallways, radiators, pencil sharpeners, etc.
- Seat where light is on your face and not in your student's eyes.
- If there is a better ear, place it toward the classroom.
- Allow your student to move to other seats when necessary for demonstrations, classroom discussions, or other activities.

INCREASE VISUAL INFORMATION: Your student will use lipreading and other visual information to supplement what he/she hears.

- Remember your student needs to see your face in order to lipread!
  - Try to stay in one place while talking to the class so your student does not have to lipread a "moving target."
  - Avoid talking while writing on the chalkboard.
  - Avoid putting your hands, papers, or books in front of your face when talking.
  - Avoid talking with your face turned downward while reading.
  - Keep the light on your face, not at your back. Avoid standing in front of windows where the glare will make it difficult for your student to see your face.
- Use visual aids, such as pictures and diagrams, when possible.
- Demonstrate what you want the student to understand when possible. Use natural gestures, such as pointing to objects being discussed, to help clarify what you say.
- Use the chalkboard—write assignments, new vocabulary words, key words, etc. on it.

MINIMIZE CLASSROOM NOISE: Even a small amount of noise will make it very difficult for your student to hear and understand what is said.

- Seat your student away from noisy parts of your classroom.
- Wait until your class is quiet before talking to them.

USE CLEAR SPEECH AND ENCOURAGE OTHERS TO DO SO ALSO: Clear speech will help your student understand you and others better.

- Speak naturally in a good, clear voice. It is not necessary to shout or exaggerate lip movement.
- Use a moderate rate of speech.
- Pause briefly between phrases to allow time for auditory processing.

MODIFY TEACHING PROCEDURES: Modifications will allow your student to benefit from your instruction and will decrease the need for repetition.

- Be sure your student is watching and listening when you are talking to him/her.
- Be sure your student understands what is said by having him/her repeat information or answer questions.
- Rephrase, rather than repeat, questions and instructions if your student has not understood them.
- Write key words, new words, new topics, etc. on the chalkboard.
- Repeat or rephrase things said by other students during classroom discussions.
- Introduce new vocabulary to the student in advance. The speech-language pathologist or parents may be able to help with this.
- Use a "buddy" to alert your student to listen and to be sure your student has understood all information correctly.

HAVE REALISTIC EXPECTATIONS: This will help your student succeed in your classroom.

- Remember that your student cannot understand everything all of the time, no matter how how hard he/she tries. Encourage him/her to ask for repetition.
- Be patient when student asks for repetition.
- Give breaks from listening when necessary. Your student may fatigue easily because he/she is straining to listen and understand.
- Expect student to follow classroom routine. Do not spoil or pamper your student.

- Expect your student to accept the same responsiblities for considerate behavior, homework, and dependability as you require of other students in your classroom.
- Ask the student to repeat if you can't understand him/her. Your student's speech may be distorted because he/she does not hear sounds clearly. Work with the speech-language pathologist to help your student improve his/her speech as much as possible.

- Be alert for fluctuations of hearing due to middle ear problems.
- Request support from the audiologist, the speech-language pathologist, or others when you feel uncertain about your student and what is best for him/her.

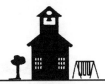

SECTION 5

APPENDIXES

Central Auditory Processing Disorders

CONTENTS

*Appendixes with asterisks (*) are available on an optional computer disk which allows users to customize these forms.

Appendix 5–A

DEFINITIONS OF CENTRAL AUDITORY PROCESSING DISORDERS

Central Auditory Processing Ad Hoc Committee[1]

Central auditory processing disorders are deficits in the formation processing of audible signals not attributed to impaired hearing sensitivity or intellectual impairment. Specifically, CAPD refers to limitations in the ongoing transmission, analysis, organization, transformation, elaboration, storage, retrieval, and use of information contained in audible signals. This processing involves perceptual, cognitive, and linguistic functions which, with appropriate interaction, results in effective receptive communication of passive (e.g., conscious and unconscious, mediated and unmediated) ability to: attend, discriminate, and identify acoustic signals; transform and continuously transmit information through both the peripheral and central nervous systems; filter, sort and combine information at appropriate perceptual and conceptual levels; store and retrieve information efficiently; restore, using phonological, semantic, syntactic, and pragmatic knowledge; and attach meaning to a stream of acoustic signals through utilization of linguistic and non-linguistic contexts.

Task Force on Central Auditory Processing Consensus Development[2]

Central Auditory Processes are the auditory system mechanisms and processes responsible for the following behavioral phenomena:

- ➤ Sound localization and lateralization
- ➤ Auditory discrimination
- ➤ Auditory pattern recognition

- ➤ Temporal aspects of audition, including
  - — temporal resolution
  - — temporal masking
  - — temporal integration
  - — temporal ordering
- ➤ Auditory performance decrements with competing acoustic signals
- ➤ Auditory performance decrements with degraded acoustic signals

These mechanisms and processes are presumed to apply to nonverbal as well as verbal signals and to affect many areas of function, including speech and language. They have neurophysiological as well as behavioral correlates.

Many neurocognitive mechanisms and processes are engaged in recognition and discrimination tasks. Some are specifically dedicated to acoustic signals, whereas others (e.g., attentional processes, long-term language representations) are not. With respect to these nondedicated mechanisms and processes, the term *central auditory processes* refers particularly to their deployment in the service of acoustic signal processing.

A Central Auditory Processing Disorder (CAPD) is an observed deficiency in one or more of the above-listed behaviors. For some persons, CAPD is presumed to result from the dysfunction of processes and mechanisms dedicated to audition; for others, CAPD may stem from some more general dysfunction, such as an attention deficit or neural timing deficit, that affects performance across modalities. It is also possible for CAPD to reflect co-existing dysfunctions of both sorts.

---

[1]*Source:* "Audiological assessment of central auditory processing: An annotated bibliography" by American Speech-Language-Hearing Association, 1990, *Asha, 32*(Suppl. 1), pp. 13–30. Copyright 1990 by American Speech-Language-Heaing Association. Reprinted by permission.

[2]*Source:* "Central auditory processing: Current status of research and implications for clinical practice" by American Speech-Language-Hearing Association, 1996, *American Journal of Audiology, 5*(2), pp. 41–54. Copyright 1996 by American Speech-Language-Hearing Association. Reprinted by permission.

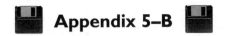 **Appendix 5–B**

CHILDREN'S AUDITORY PROCESSING PERFORMANCE SCALE (CHAPPS)

CHILDREN'S AUDITORY PROCESSING PERFORMANCE SCALE

Child's Name _____ Age (Years _____ Months _____) Date _____

Name of person completing questionnaire _____

Relationship: Parent _____   Teacher _____   Other_____

PLEASE READ INSTRUCTIONS CAREFULLY

Answer all questions by comparing this child to other children of similar age and background. Do not answer the questions based only on the difficulty of the listening condition. For example, all 8-year-old children, to a certain extent, may not hear and understand when listening in a noisy room. That is, this would be a difficult listening condition for all children. However, some children may have more difficulty in this listening condition than others. You must judge whether or not this child has MORE difficulty than other children in each listening condition cited. Please make your judgment using the following response choices: (**CIRCLE** a number for each item.)

RESPONSE CHOICES:

LESS DIFFICULTY ....+1
SAME AMOUNT OF DIFFICULTY...0
SLIGHTLY MORE DIFFICULTY ....–1
MORE DIFFICULTY...–2
CONSIDERABLY MORE DIFFICULTY ....–3
SIGNIFICANTLY MORE DIFFICULTY ....–4
CANNOT FUNCTION AT ALL...–5

Listening Condition—*NOISE:*

If listening in a room where there is background noise such as a TV set, music, others talking, children playing, etc., this child has difficulty hearing and understanding (compared with other children of similar age and background).

1. When paying attention ....+1	0	–1	–2	–3	–4	–5
2. When being asked a question ....+1	0	–1	–2	–3	–4	–5
3. When being given simple instructions . ...+1	0	–1	–2	–3	–4	–5
4. When being given complicated, multiple, instructions .... +1	0	–1	–2	–3	–4	–5
5. When not paying attention ....+1	0	–1	–2	–3	–4	–5
6. When involved with other activities, i.e., coloring, reading, etc...+1	0	–1	–2	–3	–4	–5
7. When listening with a group of children ....+1	0	–1	–2	–3	–4	–5

Listening Condition—*QUIET:*

If listening in a quiet room (others may be present, but are being quiet), this child has difficulty hearing and understanding (compared with other children).

8. When paying attention ....+1	0	–1	–2	–3	–4	–5
9. When being asked a question ....+1	0	–1	–2	–3	–4	–5
10. When being given simple instructions ....+1	0	–1	–2	–3	–4	–5
11. When being given complicated, multiple, instructions ....+1	0	–1	–2	–3	–4	–5
12. When not paying attention ....+1	0	–1	–2	–3	–4	–5

13. When involved with other activities, i.e., coloring,
    reading, etc. ....+1   0   −1   −2   −3   −4   −5

14. When listening with a group of children ....+1   0   −1   −2   −3   −4   −5

Listening Condition—*IDEAL:*

   When listening in a quiet room, no distractions, face-to-face, and with good eye contact, this child has difficulty hearing and understanding (compared with other children).

15. When being asked a question ....+1   0   −1   −2   −3   −4   −5

16. When being given simple instructions . ...+1   0   −1   −2   −3   −4   −5

17. When being given complicated, multiple, instructions .... +1   0   −1   −2   −3   −4   −5

Listening Condition—*MULTIPLE INPUTS:*

   When, in addition to listening, there is also some other form of input (i.e., visual, tactile, etc.), this child has difficulty hearing and understanding (compared with other children).

18. When listening and watching the speaker's face ....+1   0   −1   −2   −3   −4   −5

19. When listening and reading material that is also being
    read out loud by another ....+1   0   −1   −2   −3   −4   −5

20. When listening and watching someone provide an
    illustration such as a model, drawing, information on
    the chalkboard, etc. ....+1   0   −1   −2   −3   −4   −5

Listening condition—*AUDITORY MEMORY/SEQUENCING:*

   If required to recall spoken information, this child has difficulty (compared with other children).

21. Immediately recalling information such as a word,
    word spelling, numbers, etc. . ...+1   0   −1   −2   −3   −4   −5

22. Immediately recalling simple instructions . ...+1   0   −1   −2   −3   −4   −5

23. Immediately recalling multiple instructions ....+1   0   −1   −2   −3   −4   −5

24. Not only recalling information, but also the *order* or
    sequence of the information . ...+1   0   −1   −2   −3   −4   −5

25. When delayed recollection (1 hour or more) of words,
    word spelling, numbers, etc. is required . ...+1   0   −1   −2   −3   −4   −5

26. When delayed recollection (1 hour or more) of simple
    instructions is required ....+1   0   −1   −2   −3   −4   −5

27. When delayed recollection (1 hour or more) of multiple
    instructions is required ....+1   0   −1   −2   −3   −4   −5

28. When delayed recollection (24 hours or more) is
    required ....+1   0   −1   −2   −3   −4   −5

Listening Condition - *AUDITORY ATTENTION SPAN:*

   If extended periods of listening are required, this child has difficulty paying attention, that is being attentive to what is being said (compared with other children).

29. When the listening time is less than 5 minutes ....+1   0   −1   −2   −3   −4   −5

30. When the listening time is 5 to 10 minutes . ...+1   0   −1   −2   −3   −4   −5

31. When the listening time is over 10 minutes ....+1   0   −1   −2   −3   −4   −5

32. When listening in a quiet room ....+1   0   −1   −2   −3   −4   −5

33. When listening in a noisy room . ...+1   0   −1   −2   −3   −4   −5

34. When listening first thing in the morning ....+1   0   −1   −2   −3   −4   −5

35. When listening near the end of the day,
    before supper time . ...+1   0   −1   −2   −3   −4   −5

36. When listening in a room where there are also
    visual distractions . ...+1   0   −1   −2   −3   −4   −5

CHILDREN'S AUDITORY PROCESSING PERFORMANCE SCALE

Performance Analysis (To Be Completed by the Clinic)

_____ ____ Parent ____ Teacher Date _____

Client Last Name   M.I.   First   Informant

_____ Pre Diagnostic _____ Pre Therapy _____ Post Therapy _____ Other: _____

List dates of previous CHAPPS results _____

Client age in months (current years _____ × 12 + current months _____) = _____

INSTRUCTIONS:

1. Enter total raw scores for EACH of the six subsections in the RAW SCORE column. Be careful to take into account the "+" or "−" values when adding.
2. Divide each subsection raw score by the indicated number and enter the result in the AVERAGE SCORE column. Retain the proper sign "+" or "−".
3. Total RAW SCORE and total AVERAGE SCORE are obtained by adding the subsection scores, retaining the proper signs.

SUBSECTION	RAW SCORE	divided by	AVERAGE SCORE (2 decimals)	(comments)
Noise	_____	7	_____	
Quiet	_____	7	_____	
Ideal	_____	3	_____	
Multiple	_____	3	_____	
Memory	_____	8	_____	
Attention	_____	8	_____	
TOTAL	_____	36	_____	

(Raw Score range for: NORMALS (+36 to −11); AT RISK (−12 to −130)

* *

CHAPPS SUBSECTION ANALYSIS

Enter "X" at AVERAGE Score (round to nearest 0.5)

	NOISE	QUIET	IDEAL	MULTIPLE	MEMORY	ATTENTION	TOTAL
+1.0	−	−	−	−	−	−	−
+0.5	−	−	−	−	−	−	−
0.0	−	−	−	−	−	−	−
−0.5	−	−	−	−	−	−	−

(Normal Range)

−1.0 --

(Below Normal Range)

	NOISE	QUIET	IDEAL	MULTIPLE	MEMORY	ATTENTION	TOTAL
−1.5	−	−	−	−	−	−	−
−2.0	−	−	−	−	−	−	−
−2.5	−	−	−	−	−	−	−
−3.0	−	−	−	−	−	−	−
−3.5	−	−	−	−	−	−	−
−4.0	−	−	−	−	−	−	−
−4.5	−	−	−	−	−	−	−
−5.0	−	−	−	−	−	−	−

Appendix 5–C

CENTRAL AUDITORY PROCESSING DISORDERS: A TEAM APPROACH TO SCREENING, ASSESSMENT, AND INTERVENTION PRACTICES

Colorado Department of Education

Central Auditory Processing Disorders: A Team Approach to Screening, Assessment and Intervention Practices

Introduction

These guidelines were developed by the Task Force on Central Auditory Processing (CAP) Disorders, facilitated by the Colorado Department of Education. Task force members represented a variety of viewpoints both in work settings and professions reflecting the multidisciplinary nature of central auditory processing disorders. This Task Force was formed as an outcome of a conference on CAP disorders in Denver, Colorado in May, 1995 to respond to concerns of professionals with the current status of assessment and remediation of CAPD in children. A renewed interest in central auditory processing disorders (CAPD) has been fostered by recent research which has provided a better understanding of the neuroplasticity of brain function and its effect on remediation as well as the increased availability of appropriate instruments for assessing CAP.

Musiek et al. (1990) list the following reasons to conduct CAP assessment: (1) to determine if **"medical aspects"** of the disorder exist which are neurologically based and which may require medical treatment, (2) to increase **"awareness"** of the presence of a disorder which can truly affect a child's ability to learn, (3) to reduce **"shopping around"** by parents for help and understanding of the child's difficulties, (4) to minimize **"psychological factors"** affecting the child and family as a result of not knowing the cause of the child's problem, (5) to enable **"insightful educational planning"** to occur once a problem is confirmed and defined, and, (6) to determine interventions which are helpful to the student's learning process which include **"FM assistive listening devices, auditory training, strategies, and environmental modifications."** The authors further state that **"audiologists have a responsibility to evaluate the entire auditory system, both peripheral and central, and to consider possible disorders involving both areas . . . if such evaluation is not possible, referral and/or appropriate counseling about the possibility of a perceptual problem should be recommended."** Another reason to consider CAPD assessment is to determine the nature of the linguistic and cognitive processing problems to aid in planning language and educational remediation.

The area of CAPD remains controversial and complex. While the interactions among language, audition, and cognitive processing are unclear, it is hoped that this document will provide a working base for all school personnel to make more effective decisions regarding CAP disorders in children.

Definition of CAP

The operational definition used for these guidelines was the definition developed by the ASHA Task Force on Central Auditory Processing Consensus Development (see Appendix A).

CAPD and Special Education Eligibility

Students who are suspected of having CAPD or who are diagnosed with CAPD should be considered for special education services through the same process as any student suspected of having a disability. According to Colorado Department of Education ECEA Rules, CAPD may be considered as a type of perceptual communicative disorder [ECEA 2.02(6) (b) (i)] *"difficulty with cognitive and/or language processing,"* or a type of speech-language disability [ECEA 2.02(7) (a) (ii)] *"auditory processing, including . . . perception (discrimination, sequencing, analysis and synthesis) association, and auditory attention.* To qualify for special education and related services, the disorder must interfere with the student's ability to obtain reasonable benefit from regular education (see Appendix B for the full text of the Rules).

Purpose of Guidelines

These guidelines were developed to provide professionals who work with children with CAP disorders "best practices" to assist with identification and intervention. As with most guidelines, they represent the best of what we know at this time; many questions remain regarding the relationships between screening, assessment, management, and prescriptive intervention therapy as well as the reliability and validity of the instruments used for identification. A very conscious effort was made to insure that the process of identifying and treating children with CAPD is a multi-

Source: "Central auditory processing disorders: A team approach to screening, assessment, and intervention practices" by Colorado Department of Education, 1996. Reprinted by permission.

disciplinary one with participation from the disciplines of audiology, speech/language pathology, learning disabilities, psychology, and health.

How to Use These Guidelines

These guidelines should be used to make decisions regarding the potential evaluation needs of the child. Although it is recommended that observation data (Level I) be obtained, some children may present with such significant concerns, that assessment (Level II) is warranted as the initial point of entry. The success of the intervention procedures should ultimately guide the decision for further assessment; that is, if the management strategies implemented following a screening or preliminary assessment procedure result in an intervention plan which is effective for the child, then further assessment may not be necessary at that time. However, if the intervention strategies are not effective, additional evaluation may be required to develop a more specialized treatment program. Level III assessment should be necessary for only a very small number of students who display unusual symptoms or characteristics of neurological disorders.

The guidelines are set up to consider increasingly more diagnostic procedures as is suggested by the interpretation questions at each level (observation, screening and preliminary assessment, and diagnostic assessment). This approach parallels the school child identification process beginning with the child study review (use of CAP Observation Procedures) to psychoeducational assessment (CAP Assessment Procedures).

Special Considerations

Prior to assessment of CAP, certain factors must be considered to determine the appropriateness of the screening and evaluation. These include:

(1) peripheral hearing—hearing acuity must be normal or child cleared by an audiologist prior to considering CAP testing
(2) age of the child—screening is generally not appropriate until a child is 3 or 4, assessment until 7 or 8 yrs; age criteria recommended with each screening or assessment instrument should be followed; age criteria is important as it reflects the developmental component of the central auditory pathways and resulting developmental abilities of the child [current CAP measures normed on young children (3 and up) are the SCAN (Keith, 1986), SAAT (Cherry, 1980) and the PSI (Jerger & Jerger, 1984); the TAPS may be used for 4 and up].
(3) cognitive ability—performance on central auditory tasks are affected by cognitive ability; therefore any child assessed must have cognitive ability within a normal range.

(4) language competence—children with poor language skills will generally have more difficulty on CAP tasks, particularly those which require more sophisticated language processing (i.e., linguistically loaded); results must be interpreted carefully and extra caution is recommended with bilingual students.
(5) validity and reliability—norms for instruments used must be reviewed and considered; caution must be used in interpretation since some of the measures have limited normative data for children and may require that local norms be developed.
(6) test interpretation and scoring—test manual procedures and interpretation must be adhered to and considered along with the results of the multidisciplinary assessment.
(7) multidisciplinary assessment—the intent of these guidelines is to look holistically at the child; CAP assessment should *not* occur in isolation from other psychoeducational screening or evaluation; consideration must be given to all factors which may affect a child's performance.

Re-evaluation Recommendations

CAP skills should be re-evaluated at a minimum of every three years timed to coincide with triennial assessments if the child receives special education and/or related services. Preschool-age children, children who evidence a change in their classroom performance or auditory behavior, or children who display any other unusual symptoms should be considered for re-evaluation more frequently or as the situation warrants.

Appendices: Handouts, Assessment Materials, and References

Appendix A: ASHA Consensus Statement on CAPD: Definitions
Appendix B: Colorado Department of Education Rules for the Administration of the Exceptional Children's Act (1995): PCD and Speech-Language Disability and Eligibility Criteria
Appendix C: Typical behaviors of children with CAPD
Appendix D: General intervention strategies
Appendix E: Assessment materials/test constructs
Appendix F: CAPD Profiles
Appendix G: Specific Intervention Recommendations (Developmental/compensatory Skills and Essential Learnings)
- classroom management
- instructional modifications
- therapy
- amplification
Appendix H: Parent Information
Appendix I: References

I. Observation Procedures

Purpose: 1. To identify children who may have behaviors associated with CAPD.
2. To identify and implement general intervention strategies which may assist in the child's classroom functioning (Appendix D).
3. To identify children who may need further assessment.

OBSERVATION PROCEDURES

Auditory	Language	Psychological	Educational	Other
• hearing acuity must be normal or candidate cleared by an audiologist prior to considering CAP testing; • auditory behavior checklist (choose one of the following): ▲ Fisher's Auditory Problems Checklist ▲ CHAPPS (Children's Auditory Processing Performance Scale) ▲ Observation Profile of Classroom Communication (Sanger) • optional: parent checklist, student self-checklist	• Observation checklist (Loban's Oral Language Scales) • The Classroom Communication Skills Inventory (Psych Corp)	• behavior checklist (choose one of the following): ▲ Connor's Behavior Rating Scale ▲ BASC (Behavior Assessment for School Age) ▲ ACTeRS	• review classwork, report cards, district assessments	• review of health records for health history & otitis media • review of performance on existing interventions • consideration of social/family/environment factors

Observation Interpretation

1. What behaviors does the child exhibit which may be indicative of or associated with CAPD difficulties?
2. How did the child respond to intervention strategies?
3. Is further assessment needed?
4. What factors need to be considered for further assessment?
   a. age of child
   b. cognitive status
   c. speech/language competence/limited English proficiency
   d. Other factors: attention/distractibility, social emotional/developmental maturity, motivation, motor skills

II. Assessment Procedures

Purpose: 1. To determine the presence of a CAP disorder.

2. To develop and implement an individual therapeutic intervention plan (Appendix G).

Note: Appropriate instruments should be chosen to assess each functional area.

SCREENING AND PRELIMINARY ASSESSMENT PROCEDURES

Auditory	Language	Psychological	Educational	Other
• SCAN/SCAN-A • TAPS (Test of Auditory Perceptual Skills) • ACPT (Auditory Continuous Performance Test • SAAT (Selective Auditory Attention Test) • PSI (Pediatric Sentence Intelligibility)	Choose one • STAL (Screening Test of Adolescent Language) • CELF-screening (elem. students) • Informal speech/language sample	Examination is to rule in/rule out another diagnosis that may look like CAPD • Achenbach Child Behavior Scale • Child Depression Inventory • SNAP IV • Beery Visual-Motor Integration • Beck Depression Inventory • social-emotional & family considerations • Auditory-verbal memory perception	Examination is to determine if CAPD is manifested in the classroom/academic program • nationally normed tests, district standardized assessments	• developmental Health HX • review of previous treatment/management interventions • parent checklist

DIAGNOSTIC ASSESSMENT PROCEDURES

Auditory	Language	Psychological	Educational	Other
Test Battery[1] - to be completed by audiologist; choose at least one from each of the following areas unless otherwise indicated: • Dichotic—(use of one of each): linguistically loaded (SSW, competing sentences, SSI-CCM) and nonlinguistic loaded (dichotic digits, dichotic CV's, dichotic rhyme) • Low redundancy monaural speech (LPFS, time compressed speech, time compressed speech + reverberation) • Temporal processing (frequency patterns and/duration patterns) • Binaural interaction (binaural fusion, masking level diff.) Speech-in-noise (SSI-ICM)	• TOLD-2 • LAC • EOWVT • PPVT-R or ROWVT • WORD-R • Test of Word Knowledge • CELF-R • Detroit II • Woodcock Language Proficiency Battery • Test of Word Finding • TOAL-2 • Fullerton Language Test for Adolescents • Analysis of Language of Learning; Practical Test of Metalinguistics • Language sample	• WISC-III • Woodcock-Johnson-R (cognitive) • Kaufman ABC • Stanford-Binet IV • Boder • MAT (Matrix Analogies Test) • emotional-social considerations (interview/observation) • Detroit III (preschool, school age or adult) • DAS (Differential Abilities Scale, Fisher et al., Psych Corp)	• Woodcock-Johnson Achievement Battery • IRI (Informal Reading Inventory) • GORT (Gray Oral Reading Test III) • WRAT • Bader Reading and Language Inventory	• Incomplete sentences • Interview parents, child, teacher

Assessment Interpretation

1. Based on the multidisciplinary assessment, does the child have a CAP disorder?
2. Does the severity of the disorder qualify this child for special education and/or related services?
3. What are the characteristics or profile of the CAP disorder?
4. What are the possible services that might be considered for this child; i.e., PCD, speech/language, audiology, counseling, health (determination of services must be made by the IEP team).

[1]**Caution:** Some of these measures have limited normative data for children. Therefore local clinical norms may need to be established; see test manuals for each instrument for specific age-normative data and test reliability etc.

Intervention Recommendations

1. What are the specific interventions recommended for this child? Consider each of the following areas when developing the treatment plan.
   - **classroom management:** environmental accommodations to help the student access information more directly; examples include specialized seating, noise reduction.
   - **instructional modifications:** purposeful adaptations made by the teacher to improve the child's opportunity to learn; examples include one-to-one or small group instruction, paraphrasing.
   - **therapy:** direct intervention which is needs driven and is aimed at providing improvement in deficit areas or teaching techniques for learning compensatory strategies; examples include modality specific adaptations, auditory training.
   - **amplification:** improvement of the audibility of the sound source (speaker's voice, audio equipment) using FM sound transmission equipment; examples include personal FM systems, sound field FM systems.

III. Additional Diagnostic Procedures

Additional assessment may be recommended for children with organic-based problems, traumatic brain injury, genetic syndromes (Fragile X, autism, PDD, metabolic) or for children who demonstrate poor progress with a variety of interventions.

ADDITIONAL DIAGNOSTIC PROCEDURES			
Auditory	**Language**	**Psychological**	**Educational**	**Other**
Electrophysiological measures when indicated (ABR, MLR, LEPs, P300, MMN)	• Boston Naming Test • additional measures to supplement as needed	• Neuropsychological Battery	• additional measures to supplement as needed	

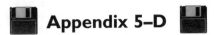

Appendix 5–D

CENTRAL AUDITORY ASSESSMENT PROFILE

SUMMARY OF RESULTS OF CENTRAL AUDITORY ASSESSMENT

NAME: _____ BIRTHDATE: _____ CA: _____

AUDITORY SKILL	BELOW AVER 1 2 3 4 5 6	AVERAGE 7 8 9 10 11 12 13	ABOVE AVER 14 15 16 17 18
CAA SCREENING:			
SCAN:			
Filtered Words			
Aud Figure Ground			
Competing Words			
COMPOSITE			
FISHER'S			
TONI			
SOUND BLENDING:			
LAC			
CAVAT #12			
DISCRIM/FIGURE-GROUND:			
Right (Sent. Noise):			
Left (Sent. Noise):			
Both Ears:			
Words-Quiet:			
Words-Noise:			
Sentences-Quiet:			
Sentences-Noise:			
CLOSURE:			
ITPA Auditory Closure			
SCAN (LP @ 1000 Hz)			
Willeford (LP @ 500 Hz)			
Right Ear			
Left Ear			
MEMORY:			
Related:			
DTLA #2			
CAVAT #10			
Unrelated:			
DTLA #4			
CAVAT #11			
Following Directions:			
DTLA # 3			
ATTENTION:			
LOCALIZATION:			

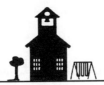

SECTION 6

APPENDIXES

Amplification and Classroom Hearing Technology

CONTENTS

*Appendixes with asterisks (*) are available on an optional computer disk which allows users to customize these forms.

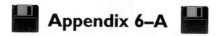 **Appendix 6–A**

CLASSROOM ACOUSTICS DOCUMENTATION FORM

Date_____

Teacher_____   Grade_____

Audiologist_____

FM/SFA System Used_____

CLASSROOM SCHEMATIC DIAGRAM

TEACHER-LISTENER DISTANCE: Nearest_____ feet   Farthest_____ feet

TEACHER VOICE LEVEL IN dBA:

Unamplified	*Amplified*
Location A _____	Location A _____
Location B _____	Location B _____
Location C _____	Location C _____
Location D _____	Location D _____
Location E _____	Location E _____
Location F _____	Location F _____
Location G _____	Location G _____

REVERBERATION TIME

Room Volume (V) = _____ cubic feet

Area Floor	_____ × ABS. Coef. _____ = A Floor	_____
Area Ceiling	_____ × ABS. Coef. _____ = A Ceiling	_____
Area Side Wall 1	_____ × ABS. Coef. _____ = A Wall 1	_____
Area Side Wall 2	_____ × ABS. Coef. _____ = A Wall 2	_____
Area End Wall 1	_____ × ABS. Coef. _____ = A End 1	_____
Area End Wall 2	_____ × ABS. Coef. _____ = A End 2	_____

Total A _____

RT of classroom = .05×_____ (V)/ _____ (A) = _____ seconds

_____

Source: from Acoustic measurements in classrooms by J. Smaldino and C. Crandell, 1995, p. 71. In C.J. Crandell, J. Smaldino, and C. Flexer (Eds.), *Sound-field FM Amplification*. Singular Publishing Group, Inc. Reprinted by permission.

Appendix 6–B

LISTENING INVENTORY FOR EDUCATION (L.I.F.E.)
An Efficacy Tool

L.I.F.E.
Listening Inventory For Education
An Efficacy Tool
Teacher Appraisal of Listening Difficulty
By Karen L. Anderson, Ed.S. & Joseph J. Smaldino, Ph.D.

Name_____ Grade_____ Date_____

School_____ Teacher_____
Hearing Aid User Y / N   Trial Period   Type of Classroom
Trial Period   Y / N   Length____Weeks   Hearing Technology_____

Instructions: Circle the item which best describes the student's listening and learning behaviors.
See reverse for suggestions to aid this student in listening and understanding classroom instruction.

The student's:	AGREE	NO CHANGE	Not Observed	DISAGREE	
1. Focus on instruction has improved (more tuned in to instruction).	(2)	(1)	(0)	(-1)	(-2)
2. Appears to understand class instruction better.	(2)	(1)	(0)	(-1)	(-2)
3. Overall attention span has improved (less fidgety and/or less distracted).	(2)	(1)	(0)	(-1)	(-2)
4. Attention has improved when listening to directions presented to whole class.	(2)	(1)	(0)	(-1)	(-2)
5. Stays on task longer with less need for redirection.	(2)	(1)	(0)	(-1)	(-2)
6. Follows directions more quickly or easily (less hesitation before beginning work).	(2)	(1)	(0)	(-1)	(-2)
7. Answers questions in a more appropriate way or answers appropriately more often.	(2)	(1)	(0)	(-1)	(-2)
8. Improved understanding of instructional videos and/or morning announcements.	(2)	(1)	(0)	(-1)	(-2)
9. More involved in class discussions (volunteers more often, follows better).	(2)	(1)	(0)	(-1)	(-2)
10. Improved understanding of answers or comments by peers during discussions.	(2)	(1)	(0)	(-1)	(-2)
11. Improved attention and understanding when background noise is present (ie., transitions).	(2)	(1)	(0)	(-1)	(-2)
12. Improved ability to discriminate auditorily (understand similar words or sounds).	(2)	(1)	(0)	(-1)	(-2)
13. Attention improved when listening in groups (small group/cooperative learning activities).	(2)	(1)	(0)	(-1)	(-2)
14. Socially involved more with other children or more comfortable in peer conversations.	(2)	(1)	(0)	(-1)	(-2)
15. Rate of learning seems to have improved (quicker to comprehend instruction).	(2)	(1)	(0)	(-1)	(-2)
16. Based on my knowledge and observations I believe that the amplification system is beneficial to the student's overall attention, listening and learning in the classroom.	(5)	(2)	(0)	(-2)	(-5)

Comments: (e.g., absences, equipment use problems)

Total Appraisal Score _____

APPRAISAL SUMMARY (circle one)

Highly Successful   26 - 35

Successful   16 - 25

Minimally Successful   5 - 15

Distributed by the Educational Audiology Association
4319 Ehrlich Rd, Tampa FL 33624 1-800-460-7322

LISTENING INVENTORY FOR EDUCATION
SUGGESTIONS FOR ACCOMMODATING STUDENTS WITH AUDITORY DIFFICULTIES

Students with auditory problems face extra challenges learning in a typical classroom setting. Typically, they can hear the teacher talk, but miss parts of speech or do not hear clearly, especially if noise is present. Students usually do not know what they didn't hear because they didn't hear it. They often may not know that they "misheard" a message unless they have already had experience with the language and topic under discussion. Use of amplification, having fluctuating hearing ability, hearing loss in just one ear, permanent hearing loss of any degree or central auditory processing disorders all compromise a student's ability to focus on verbal instruction and comprehend the fragments of speech information that are heard. The following items are suggestions for accomodating these student's special auditory needs and helping them learn their best in your classroom.

1. **Seat the student close to where you customarily teach.**
Sound weakens as it crosses distance. If a student has any auditory difficulties, how close you are to him/her will make a big difference on how well the student can hear and understand you.
    - Can the student be moved to the front of the room?
    - Can the student be allowed flexible seating so they can move to a better vantage point as classroom activities change? (e.g. move close to TV during movies)
    - If your teaching style causes you to move around the room when you talk, is it possible to stay in close proximity to the student with auditory problems?
    - When giving test directions, can you see the student's face clearly? Are you standing near the student's desk? Is the lighting on your face and not from a window behind you? Be sure the student is watching you.
    - Develop a signal the student can use if he or she does not understand or has missed critical information.

2. **Be aware of the benefits and limitations of lipreading.**
    - Only about 30-40% of speech sounds are visible on the lips. Lipreading supplements a student's hearing but is most helpful when the topic of conversation and vocabulary are known. New concepts and new vocabulary words have little meaning using lipreading.
    - Is the student seated so they can see your face clearly? Too close and they view your face from a skewed angle, too far and the quick, tiny mouth movements are imperceptible.
    - Lipreading is only possible if you are facing the student. If you use the chalkboard, do not provide verbal instruction while writing or be prepared to summarize or repeat that information for the student.
    - Reading aloud to the class with your face downward makes lipreading very difficult. Hold the book below your chin so your face is easily visualized.
    - Students cannot lipread and take notes at the same time. Classroom notetakers can use carbonized (NCR) paper and share notes easily. The student can use these notes from other students to fill in gaps in understanding.
    - The extra demands of trying to understand using only speech fragments and of constantly trying to lipread can be very fatiguing. Listening breaks are natural, especially after rapid class discussions, lectures or new information.

3. **Noise is a barrier to learning.**
    - Adults and children with normal hearing usually can tolerate a small amount of background noise without having their speech understanding compromised. Students with auditory problems are already missing fragments of what is said, especially if a message is spoken farther than from 3-6 feet away. Noise covers up word endings and brief words, reverberation smears the word fragments that are perceived.
    - Can the student be allowed flexible seating so they can move away from noise sources? (e.g. lawn mower)
    - Overhead projectors allow the student to clearly view the teacher's face, however, their fan noise interferes with understanding. If the student has a poorer hearing ear, face that one toward the overhead projector (or noisy ventilator, etc.) and seat close, but not next to the projector.
    - If possible, eliminate or dampen unnecessary noise sources. Sometimes apsorbtive material, such as styrofoam or a thick bathtowel placed under an aquarium heater or animal cage will absorb some noise. Seat the student away from animal distractions.
    - Keep your classroom door closed, especially when classes pass in the hall, gym or lunchroom activities are audible.
    - One of the main causes of noise in the classroom is due to the activity of students. Seat away from peers who are very active or habitually noisy. Allow student's time to search their desks so that the noise generated will not occur during verbal instruction. Inform the custodian of especially squeaky desks.

4. **Control or allow for distance.**
    - During group discussion, students with auditory problems typically can understand the students seated next to them but cannot understand students who are answering from more distant seats.
    - Use a student's name when calling on them to answer a question. This will allow the student with hearing needs a chance to turn to face the answering student and to lipread if at all possible.
    - Summarize key points given by classmates, especially brief messages like numeric answers, yes/no, etc.
    - Allow or assign a student buddy that the student with auditory problems can ask for clarification or cueing.

L.I.F.E.

Listening Inventory For Education
An Efficacy Tool
Student Appraisal of Listening Difficulty
By Karen L. Anderson, Ed.S. & Joseph J. Smaldino, Ph.D.

Name _____ Grade _____ Date_____

School _____ Teacher _____

Hearing Aid User Y / N   Trial Period   Type of Classroom

Trial Period Y / N   Length____Weeks   Hearing Technology_____

Instructions: Circle the item which best describes the student's difficulty listening in the situations shown on picture card items 1-10. Optional items 11-16 can be scored if these situations are encountered in the listening environment. See reverse for intervention suggestions to improve listening and understanding.

Classroom Listening Situations	ALWAYS		SOMETIMES		NEVER
1. Teacher talking in front of room Comments:	(0)	(2)	(5)	(7)	(10)
2. Teacher talking during transition time Comments:	(0)	(2)	(5)	(7)	(10)
3. Teacher talking with back turned Comments:	(0)	(2)	(5)	(7)	(10)
4. Listening with hallway noise present Comments:	(0)	(2)	(5)	(7)	(10)
5. Other students making noise Comments:	(0)	(2)	(5)	(7)	(10)
6. Student answering during discussion Comments:	(0)	(2)	(5)	(7)	(10)
7. Listening with overhead projector fan on Comments:	(0)	(2)	(5)	(7)	(10)
8. Teacher talking while moving Comments:	(0)	(2)	(5)	(7)	(10)
9. Word recognition during a test or directions Comments:	(0)	(2)	(5)	(7)	(10)
10. Watching a video movie in classroom Comments:	(0)	(2)	(5)	(7)	(10)

Additional Listening Situations					
11. Cooperative small group learning	(0)	(5)	(10)	(15)	(20)
12. Listening in gym (inside & outside)	(0)	(5)	(10)	(15)	(20)
13. Listening in school assembly	(0)	(5)	(10)	(15)	(20)
14. Listening to students during lunch	(0)	(5)	(10)	(15)	(20)
15. Students talking while coats are hung up	(0)	(5)	(10)	(15)	(20)

Scoring

		PRE-TEST		POST-TEST
Sum of Items 1 - 10	(100 possible)	_____	CLASSROOM LISTENING SCORE	_____
Sum of Items 11-16	(100 possible)	_____	ADDITIONAL SITUATIONS SCORE	_____
Total Score of Items	(200 possible)			

The LIFE Student Appraisal was inspired by the Hearing Performance Inventory for Children. The authors recognize T. Giolas, A. Brancia Maxon & A. Riordan Kessler for their work in developing the HPIC.

LISTENING INVENTORY FOR EDUCATION
SUGGESTIONS FOR IMPROVING CLASSROOM LISTENING

Mark an X next to each statement that corresponds with the situations indicated on the reverse side in which the student is experiencing any difficulty.

Classroom Difficult Listening Situations

_X_ 1. Let the teacher know that you cannot understand. Develop a signal system with your teacher.

_X_ 1. Be sure that you are seated near the teacher. Ask to move if needed.

_____ 2. Ask a student buddy to explain the directions ("Did she say page 191?).

_____ 2. Before the teacher hands out a test to the class, ask what kind of test it is and how you take it (fill in all blanks, true/false, multiple choice).

_____ 3. Have another student or two in your class that will share their class notes with you; the teacher can help to arrange this and provide carbonized paper. It is still your job to listen very carefully as your teacher talks. Notes can help you fill in gaps you may have missed as you study later.

_____ 3. Be sure that the teacher is aware of how important it is for you to see his/her face. Ask your parent to send a note to the teacher. Ask for the teacher to repeat information, ask a neighbor, use your signal.

_____ 4. If there is noise in the hall, ask for door to be closed. Arrange with your teacher ahead of time to have permission to get up and close the door whenever it's noisy.

_____ 5. Let your teacher know that noise from classmates is interfering with your understanding; use your signal system to alert your teacher that it's too noisy.

_____ 6. Ask your teacher to say student's names when calling on them to answer questions. Watch her face and listen carefully for names so you can quickly turn to face the talking student.

_____ 6. If you miss information from student answers or discussion: 1) ask answering student to repeat the information, 2) ask the teacher to repeat, 3) ask a neighbor

_____ 7. If you did not hear all of the announcements, ask the teacher or a neighbor what they were about.

_____ 8. If you cannot understand what the teacher is saying as he or she talks when the class is getting out books or papers it is important to be sure you are ready and watching the teacher during these times. If you miss a page number or other information be sure to raise your hand and ask - you are probably not the only one who didn't hear the teacher clearly in all the noise of changing activities.

_____ 9. Spelling tests are easiest if you really know the word list and can tell the difference between similar words (e.g., champion and trampoline have similar sounds but have different endings). Sit close and watch the teacher's face carefully. If you are not sure you clearly heard a word, let the teacher know immediately (you could use your signal).

_____ 10. Hearing speech clearly in a movie can be hard because of the background music on some videos. Sit close to the TV even if it means sitting in a different seat. If used, ask the teacher to put the FM microphone next to the TV. Have a note taker. Request closed captioned videos be used.

Additional Difficult Listening Situations

_____ 11. In small group work, be sure to sit close to other students and try to be able to see all of their faces. If used, pass the FM microphone from student to student. Ask students to repeat what you missed. It helps if your group could meet in a quieter spot of the class or in the hall while you work.

_____ 12. While in the gym, stand close to the teacher for directions and ask other children for directions you may have missed. Ask the teacher to repeat what you missed. Use a signal system to let your teacher know you didn't understand.

_____ 13. To hear in an assembly it is important to be near the front. If you have a personal FM the person speaking should wear the transmitter.

_____ 14. Ask your friends to repeat or clarify when something is missed (Did you say tomorrow night?"). Sit where you can easily see their faces and try to sit away from noisier children or noisy areas of your classroom. Remind your friends they may need to tap you to get your attention when it's really noisy and if you are not watching their faces.

_____ 15. You need to depend on your friends to catch your eye, tap you or for them to wait until they see you looking at them before they talk to you. Ask them to repeat what you have missed (Practice is at what time? You called Suzy when?).

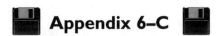

Appendix 6–C

EVALUATION OF CLASSROOM LISTENING BEHAVIOR

STUDENT_____ SCHOOL _____ GRADE _____

COMPLETED BY _____ DATE _____

TYPE OF AMPLIFICATION_____

PRE_____ POST_____ LENGTH OF TRIAL _____

Please evaluate this student for the behaviors described below using a 1–5 rating scale:

1	**3**	**5**
SELDOM	**SOMETIMES**	**USUALLY**

_____ 1.   Responds when name is called at close distance (3–6 ft).

_____ 2.   Responds when name is called at a far distance (6–20 ft).

_____ 3.   Attends to a single oral direction.

_____ 4.   Attends to a series of oral directions.

_____ 5.   Attends to oral instruction.

_____ 6.   Comprehends oral instruction in a one to one situation.

_____ 7.   Comprehends oral instruction in a group situation.

_____ 8.   Comprehends oral instruction in a quiet environment.

_____ 9.   Comprehends oral instruction in a noisy environment.

_____ 10.   Comprehends oral instruction without visual cues.

____/50   TOTAL SCORE

Source: From "Evaluation of classroom listening behavior" by L. VanDyke, 1985, *Rocky Mountain Journal of Communication Disorders, (1).* Adapted by permission.

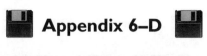

Appendix 6–D

FM FITTING PROTOCOL

1. Preselection Considerations

<u>Dates</u>

I. Present Levels of Receptive Auditory Functioning

_____ Audiological evaluations (attached)

_____ Observations in appropriate settings (attached)

_____ Consultations with students and teacher(s)

_____ Questionnaires/scales (attached)

II. Other Factors Related to Device Use

_____ Style of devices available (See Feature Matching, attached)

_____ Compatibility with personal hearing aids (see Feature Matching)

_____ User's ability to use, adjust, and manage device: _____

_____ Environment checked for external source interference (computers, pagers, etc.)

_____ **III. Identification of team members who will support use of FM system (helping with management and monitoring of equipment), <u>including parent</u>:**

A)

B)

C)

D)

Source: From Kristina M. English. 1996.

FM FITTING PROTOCOL

2. Teacher Pre-Evaluation

Student's Name _____ Date _____

Teacher's Name_____

	Not a concern	A concern
AUDITORY CONCERNS:		
Consistently responds to voice	_____	_____
Attends to voice from a distance	_____	_____
Understands stereotypical phrases (e.g., "Close the door," "Turn off the lights") presented orally	_____	_____
Follows simple directions in small groups	_____	_____
Follows simple directions in large groups	_____	_____
Follows directions after repetition	_____	_____
Follows directions after rephrasing	_____	_____
Overall academic functioning	_____	_____
BEHAVIOR CONCERNS:		
Attention span	_____	_____
Volunteers answers/comments	_____	_____
Strained behavior while attending to speaker	_____	_____
Frustration	_____	_____
Peer interactions	_____	_____

COMMENTS:

FM FITTING PROTOCOL

3. Student Questionnaire

1. It is hard for me to understand the teacher.

      YES   SOMETIMES   NO

2. It is hard for me to understand my classmates.

      YES   SOMETIMES   NO

3. It is hard for me to understand people when there is noise around.

      YES   SOMETIMES   NO

4. It is hard for me to understand people when they are far way.

      YES   SOMETIMES   NO

5. It is hard for me to understand people when they turn away.

      YES   SOMETIMES   NO

FM FITTING PROTOCOL

4. Feature Matching

Team Members:

       Student   Date

       Audiologist   School

       Teacher

       Others

	Student's Preferences	Audiologist's Recommendations	Teachers'/Others' Suggestions
RECEIVER OPTIONS 1 2 3 4 5 6			
TRANSMITTER OPTIONS 1 2 3 4 5 6			
COUPLING OPTIONS 1 2 3 4 5 6			

FM FITTING PROTOCOL

5. Selection and Comparison of Devices

From Feature Matching matrix:

Features preferred by student:

Features recommended by audiologist:

Features suggested by teachers and others:

Select use, and evaluate FM system with most appropriate features:

Device #1	Device #2	Device #3
Model #s Serial #s	Model #s Serial #s	Model #s Serial #s
Frequency of Use:	Frequency of Use:	Frequency of Use:
Advantages:	Advantages:	Advantages:
Limitations:	Limitations:	Limitations:
Comments:	Comments:	Comments:

Electroacoustic anaylses, probe mic measurements, behavioral measurements attached.

FM FITTING PROTOCOL

6. Evaluation Process

Device # _____

Checklist for evaluation process:

_____ Functional gain measurements obtained (report attached)

_____ Probe mic measurements obtained (report attached)

_____ 2cm^3 coupler measurements obtained (report attached)

_____ Orientation/Training conducted (see "Management & Monitoring")

_____ Timeline for trial period established (from _____ to _____)

_____ Observations of FM use conducted in normal-use settings (see attached)

_____ Student interview conducted to measure level of acceptance of device

_____ Student questionnaire completed (attached)

_____ Teacher questionnaire completed (attached)

_____ Decision made to continue use of this device or continue evaluation of other devices

When decision is made to continue use of an FM system:

_____ Document on IEP, under Present Level of Performance, student's use of FM system. (Example: Student uses FM system approximately 80% of school day, 5 days a week.)

_____ Document on IEP, under Accommodations, Modifications and/or Assistive Technology, a descriptive statement of the important features of the FM system. (Example: An FM system is used to provide an appropriate signal-to-noise ratio necessary for learning with hearing impairment.)

Evaluation as an ongoing process will continuously reconsider student preferences and changes in educational environment and programs.

FM FITTING PROTOCOL

7. Management & Monitoring

Date:

_____ I.   **Orientation: Hands-on Demonstration**

   _____ Student

   _____ Teacher

   _____ Aide

   _____ Classroom Peers

   _____ Other(s): _____

_____ II. **Training for Troubleshooting Minor Problems**

   _____ Student

   _____ Teacher

   _____ Aide

   _____ Other(s): _____

_____ III. **Schedule of FM Use Developed and Agreed Upon**

   _____ Student

   _____ Teacher

   _____ Other(s): _____

_____ IV. **Daily Checklists Provided**

FM FITTING PROTOCOL

8. Teacher Post-Evaluation

Student's Name _____ Date_____

Teacher's Name _____

	Identified as a concern	Improvement noted	No change noted
AUDITORY CONCERNS:			
Consistently responds to voice	_____	_____	_____
Attends to voice from a distance	_____	_____	_____
Understands stereotypical phrases (e.g., "Close the door," "Turn off the lights") presented orally	_____	_____	_____
Follows simple directions in small groups	_____	_____	_____
Follows simple directions in large groups	_____	_____	_____
Follows directions after repetition	_____	_____	_____
Follows directions after rephrasing	_____	_____	_____
Overall academic functioning	_____	_____	_____
BEHAVIOR CONCERNS:			
Attention span	_____	_____	_____
Volunteers answers/comments	_____	_____	_____
Strained behavior while attending to speaker	_____	_____	_____
Frustration	_____	_____	_____
Peer interactions	_____	_____	_____

ADJUSTMENT CONCERNS:

Has child accepted use of FM?

Have peers accepted use of FM?

FM FITTING PROTOCOL

9. Student Questionnaire

1. The FM makes it easier for me to understand the teacher.

      YES   SOMETIMES   NO

2. The FM makes it easier for me to understand my classmates.

      YES   SOMETIMES   NO

3. The FM makes it easier for me to understand people when there is noise around.

      YES   SOMETIMES   NO

4. The FM makes it easier for me to understand people when they are far way.

      YES   SOMETIMES   NO

5. The FM makes it easier for me to understand people when they turn away.

      YES   SOMETIMES   NO

Teacher's Last Name_____

Student's First Name_____

STUDENT'S OPINIONS ABOUT
USING AN FM SYSTEM

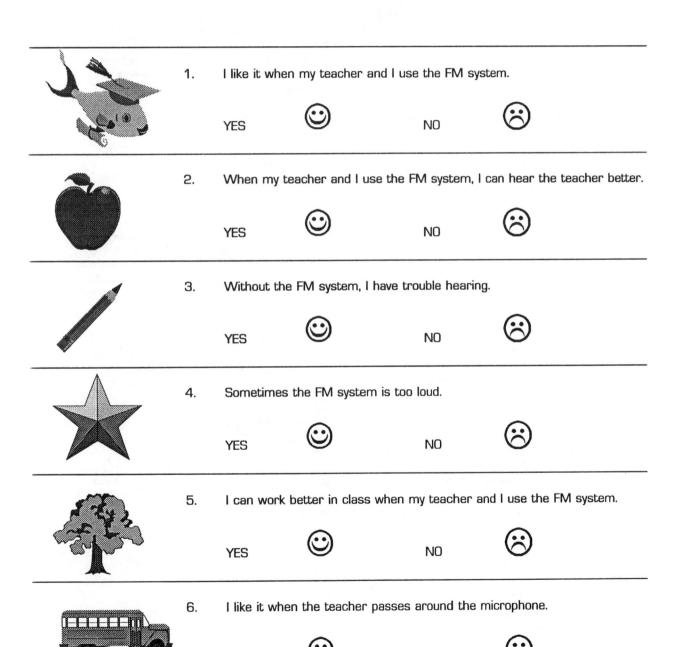

1. I like it when my teacher and I use the FM system.

   YES ☺   NO ☹

2. When my teacher and I use the FM system, I can hear the teacher better.

   YES ☺   NO ☹

3. Without the FM system, I have trouble hearing.

   YES ☺   NO ☹

4. Sometimes the FM system is too loud.

   YES ☺   NO ☹

5. I can work better in class when my teacher and I use the FM system.

   YES ☺   NO ☹

6. I like it when the teacher passes around the microphone.

   YES ☺   NO ☹

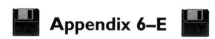

Appendix 6–E

HEARING AID ADJUSTMENT PROGRAM

HEARING AID(S) FOR CHILDREN

TO PARENTS:

Your child has been fitted with the best hearing aid(s) available. However, the use of hearing aids is just one part of the treatment program for your child. Although children hear more sounds when they put on hearing aids, it takes a long time for most children to receive maximum hearing benefit from them. Of course, the length of time depends on many things. If your child is an infant, the adjustment period is often very short because infants usually accept their hearing aids easily. If your child is a toddler, it may be more difficult to establish regular daily use of the aids. Children with mild or moderate losses tend to adjust and show benefit from their hearing aids sooner than those with severe and profound hearing losses. For other children, it may take as long as six months to a year with training before the sound received from the aid(s) becomes meaningful. Some children may show no benefit at all; your audiologist will explore other options if this situation occurs.

Any child who is beginning to hear for the first time has a very difficult challenge. Everyday your child will be hearing more and more sounds without always understanding them. It may seem like "noise". If you have normal hearing, you learn to recognize all the different sounds and to disregard the ones you do not want to hear. To understand your child's problem, listen now to all the background noises—you will be surprised how many there are! No wonder your child finds "sounds" very tiring at first. Your child has been living in a very quiet world, and now must adjust to a very noisy one. **It is worth the adjustment**—don't ever forget that!

When adults or other children show interest in the aid(s), make a point of explaining that some people cannot see very well and wear glasses which help them to see more clearly; your child cannot hear well, and must wear hearing aid(s). If your child cannot talk, explain that now that sounds may be heard more clearly, talking should soon begin to develop. Parents have noticed that other children like to hold the hearing aid to their ears and listen—they may call it a little "radio" and say how neat it is and wish they could have one.

You should also be clear about what you should expect from the hearing aid(s). Even at best, it will take some time before the sounds that are heard through the aid(s) become meaningful. It takes a newborn baby a full year of just **listening** to speech before beginning to speak. Your child may be like a newborn baby in relation to learning what sounds mean. Therefore, it may take more than a year to develop the understanding of what speech means. Hopefully, it will take less time.

This packet includes some basic rules for developing listening skills and learning to talk and a hearing aid adjustment program. Your child's audiologist and therapist will help guide you and provide more specific information as you work towards the goal of full-time use of the hearing aids.

Note: The Hearing Aid Adjustment Program was designed for use with toddlers and preschool-age children with the goal that full-time use be established in a one-month period of time. This program may not be appropriate for infants who usually adjust to their aids in a much shorter time period.

Source: "Hearing aid orientation" by University Hospital, Division of Audiology, University of Colorado Health Sciences Center, Denver, CO. Adapted by permission.

BASIC RULES TO DEVELOP LISTENING SKILLS

1. Select sounds and call them to your child's attention.
2. Respond to these sounds by pointing to your ear with a wide-eyed expression saying, "I hear it, do you?
3. Always associate sounds and their sources.
4. Always praise your child when he/she reacts to sounds.
5. Construct listening and responding games that are fun for your child.

BASIC RULES FOR TALKING

1. How do you get and maintain your child's attention?

   ➤ Get down on the child's level and face him/her so he/she can watch your lip movements and facial expressions.
   ➤ Talk in a normal voice. You don't need to shout or exaggerate lip movements.
   ➤ Let your face and your voice tell your child that what you are doing is interesting and fun.
   ➤ Let your child actively participate whenever possible; language is best learned while doing.

2. How do you make your talking meaningful?

   ➤ Talk about the here and now.
   ➤ Tune into your child; talk about what interests him/her.
   ➤ Use short simple sentences.
   ➤ Say the obvious.
   ➤ At times, talk for your child.
   ➤ Everything has a name—use the name.
   ➤ Put your child's feelings into words.
   ➤ Give your child a chance to respond.
   ➤ Say things over and over.
   ➤ When using a single word, put it back into a sentence.

3. How do you respond when your child talks?

   ➤ Encourage and give your child a chance to talk; be a listener as well as a talker.
   ➤ Respond when your child tries to talk.
   ➤ Reward your child when he/she attempts to say a word.
   ➤ Repeat the child's word and put it back into a sentence.
   ➤ Build on your child's present vocabulary by adding new words.
   ➤ When a child uses incorrect language, repeat it correctly.
   ➤ When your child expresses an idea, expand his/her thoughts by adding more information.

HEARING AID ADJUSTMENT

Home Program for_____

THE FIRST WEEK:

1. Wear the aid(s) in a quiet place at home for at least 2 to 3 periods a day, (insert time) minutes per time.
2. There should not be too many people in the room or too much noise. For the first week, it is very important to be with your child the entire time the hearing aids are worn.
3. Have an activity ready to do so these periods are enjoyable. You may also want to prepare a snack during this time, as eating usually is a pleasant experience and, you can also talk about the food your child is eating. Activities will be suggested for you as the program moves along.
4. After the (insert time) minute period, turn off and remove the hearing aid(s). You may feel your child wants to wear them longer, but to keep the experience positive and to insure supervision, short periods are recommended at the beginning of the orientation program. Many times children will want to wear the aid(s) longer because like a new toy, they are fun at first. But when the newness wears off, they may no longer want to wear them. By following this program, we hope to avoid any negativeness which could develop toward the hearing aid(s). It also takes a while for children to get used to having something in their ear. If your child wears their aid(s) too long at first, the ear canal could become irritated and then pain might be associated with wearing the aid(s).

REMEMBER:

1. YOU decide when _____ can take the aid(s) on and off; if your child wants the aid(s) off, say "no", wait a few minutes, and then take them out.
2. TALK to your child as much as possible using the Basic Rules for Talking. Until _____"hears" a lot of talking, speaking will not develop. Children with hearing impairments must hear information on the average of 10 times as much as children with normal hearing to obtain some meaningful benefit; deaf children need even more repetition and experience.
3. Give _____ time to talk and encourage talking even if it is unintelligible. If necessary, don't give your child something that is wanted until an effort is made to ask for it.
4. Let your child play with friends as much as possible. It is amazing how well young children can get along. It is good for them to talk to each other.
5. If you get frustrated, don't let _____ know. If your child wants the aid(s) off, say "no", wait a few minutes, and then remove the aid(s).
6. Don't panic! It's not easy to put the aid(s) in at first; it takes practice to learn. In the end, it will be worth the trouble and better for you and _____. Don't expect drastic changes in your child's speech—that takes time too.

SOME FIRST WEEK ACTIVITIES:

1. Read stories, talk about the pictures.
2. Together pick out simple, interesting pictures from old magazines. Cut them out and paste them on construction paper. Starting with two pictures at a time, say the word and have _____ repeat it, or at least attempt to say something. As these pictures are learned, add on new ones. Stop the activity before either one of you gets frustrated. As time goes on, you can set out pictures, say one of the words, and see if _____ can pick out the right picture.
3. Model clay or play dough. Talk about color, shape, and how it feels.
4. Draw or color, talking about what the child is making and colors the child in using.
5. Bake or cook.
6. Look out the window; talk about what your see.
7. Play simple games.

THE SECOND WEEK:

1. If your child has successfully worn the aid(s) for the 1st week as recommended, it is time to increase each period to (insert time) hours. If your child has not been able to wear them without pulling them out, continue with (insert time) minute periods until _____ can do this.
2. Have an activity prepared to do with your child during the period the aid(s) are on. If your child can wear them for an hour, do an activity for half of the time and let _____ play on his/her own during the remainder of the time, watching closely to be sure that the aid(s) are not removed.
3. Remember that **YOU** remove the hearing aid(s) when the time is finished.

ACTIVITIES:

➤ Let _____ listen to the radio or records and watch TV.
➤ Add sounds around the house: listen to the telephone ring, the vacuum cleaner, water running, the clock ticking, the doorbell. Show your reaction to these sounds with a wide eyed expression and point to your ear saying "oh, I hear it, do you?"
➤ Go outdoors and take a walk. Listen carefully and identify all of the sounds you hear: voices, dogs barking, cars. Be sure to let your child know who or what made the sounds.

THE THIRD WEEK:

1. If _____ has successfully worn the aid(s) as prescribed for the first two weeks, increase time to what ever is manageable to allow for activities and adequate supervision.
2. Continue with activities that you have chosen or that have been prepared for you.
3. When the hearing aid time is over, remove the aid(s) and put them away!

THE FOURTH WEEK:

By now your child should realize that enjoyable sounds are being missed without the hearing aid(s) and should be wearing them with little difficulty. Now is the time to teach that wearing the aid(s) is as necessary as wearing shoes or brushing teeth. Put the aid(s) on as part of dressing every morning and leave them on for as along as possible (most of the day unless napping or bathing). However, it is best if you can provide some quiet times during the day since the constant strain of listening can be tiring. Let your child's behavior be your guide. Continue with this schedule, trying to keep the time while the aid(s) are worn enjoyable. The aid(s) can be worn wherever your child goes (except water play activities).

➤ Remember to check the aid(s) daily to be sure they are working properly (check batteries and make sure earmolds are clean).
➤ Play games in which your child has to depend on hearing. Using toys that make noise, see if _____ can tell which sound is made. For example, ring a bell, beat a drum, ring a play phone, or bang blocks together when your child is not watching you. Children with hearing impairments also have difficulty locating the direction of sound. Have _____ close his/her eyes and point to the corner of the room from where your child's name is called or from where noise is made. If your child is beginning to understand words, ask him/her to find or bring to you common objects such as shoes, or favorite toys.
➤ Begin requiring that _____ try to talk when he/she wants something. When your child wants a cookie, you can show it to him/her, say "cookie" and tell _____ to say "cookie". At first, if any attempt is made to speak, even if unintelligible, reward the child with the cookie. Gradually, try to get your child to say the word more clearly.

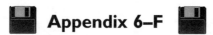 **Appendix 6–F**

PEDIATRIC COCHLEAR IMPLANT FACT SHEET

 Colorado

Cochlear Implant

Consortium

PEDIATRIC COCHLEAR IMPLANT FACT SHEET

The following introductory facts are designed to give a brief overview to cochlear implants. Contact a member of the Colorado Cochlear Implant Consortium for more specific information. Additional materials (also in Spanish and other languages) are available.

<u>Device Description:</u> A cochlear implant is an electronic device designed to provide useful sound information to individuals who are deaf. The device consists of internal and external components. The internal component is surgically implanted completely under the skin. The external equipment consists of a body-worn speech processor connected to an ear-level microphone/transmitter assembly. The transmitter is held in place using internal and external magnets.

<u>Demographic Data:</u> Research on cochlear implants has been conducted for over thirty years. The Nucleus 22 Channel Cochlear Implant System is the only cochlear implant commercially available for children with profound sensorineural hearing loss (aged 2 years and older), and for postlinguistically deafened adults with severe to profound hearing loss who gain minimal benefit from amplification and for pre-/perilinguistically deafened adults with profound hearing loss.

The Nucleus 22 Channel Cochlear Implant System continues to improve. Recently, a new external speech processor, the Spectra 22, was released, and based on clinical trial data, patients showed significant improvements in speech perception, especially in noisy environments.

Research and clinical trials through the United States Food and Drug Administration (FDA) are ongoing with other cochlear implant systems. The Clarion Multi-Strategy Cochlear Implant System is currently under investigational evaluation for both adults and children and the All-Hear Cochlear Implant is under investigation for adults.

More than 14,000 people worldwide have received cochlear implants. Over 5,000 children have received the Nucleus 22 Channel Cochlear Implant worldwide; 3,000 of those children live in North and South America. Over half of the children in North and South America received their implants between the ages of two to five years. Cochlear implants are available in over 40 countries and at 550 centers in the world. There are over 225 recognized cochlear implant centers in the United States.

<u>Pediatric Cochlear Implant Procedure:</u> After a child is referred to a cochlear implant center, the candidacy process begins. This is child specific and usually involves evaluations by an audiologist, speech-language pathologist, psychologist, surgeon, and perhaps an occupational therapist. During the candidacy process, coordination with local service providers is crucial. If a child is a candidate for the cochlear implant, the surgery is followed four to six weeks later by the programming of the external equipment and initial stimulation of the child with the device. The most important component of the cochlear implant procedure is ongoing habilitation, with close coordination between parents, educators, therapists, and the implant center.

<u>Pediatric Criteria for Candidacy:</u> The following are general criteria for cochlear implants in children:
- Profound sensorineural hearing loss in both ears
- Children must be at least 2 years of age
- Little or no useful benefit from hearing aids
- No medical contraindications
- High motivation and appropriate expectations of family and child (when appropriate)
- Placement in an educational program that emphasizes development of auditory skills after the implant has been fitted

The candidacy process is individualized for each child, and centers often consider more specific criteria, such as: amount of residual hearing, age of the child, length of deafness, availability of appropriate educational options, communication methodology, and parent commitment to success.

Source: From Colorado Cochlear Implant Consortium, April 1996. Reprinted by permission.

A controversy exists within the Deaf Community regarding the use of cochlear implants in children. Parents should thoroughly investigate and understand the implications of this controversy so that they may make an informed choice about the options available to their child. The cochlear implant is a widely recognized medical treatment for childhood deafness and is just one of many choices available for parents of children who are deaf.

<u>Results:</u> It is important for parents and professionals to know that the amount of benefit varies greatly between children. A child's ability to use the cochlear implant for communication appears to be dependent upon a variety of factors, such as:

- the amount of time the device is used each day
- the extent to which sound is integrated meaningfully into the child's daily life
- the habilitation services the child receives
- parental involvement and appropriate expectations
- auditory nerve survival
- duration of deafness
- age at implantation

Numerous research studies have investigated the results seen in children using cochlear implants. Some of these results include the following:

- significant increases in speech intelligibility and speech perception
- significant, continued increases in receptive and expressive language
- a trend for better performance with those children implanted before the age of five to seven years
- children who lost their hearing before or during the time that they were learning spoken language (pre- or perilinguistically deafened) may have as much success when implanted early as children who lost their hearing after acquiring spoken language

<u>Risks and post-surgical precautions:</u> Few significant problems have been reported. The risks of implant surgery are the same basic risks associated with any inner ear surgery which requires general anesthesia. Potential damage to the internal device can be minimized by protecting the implant site from knocks or blows to the head and static electricity discharge, which can be generated, for example, when playing on plastic playground equipment. Certain medical procedures are contraindicated (e.g., MRI). Sports and other physical activities may continue after the implant with advise from the surgeon.

<u>Cost:</u> Like any sophisticated medical device, the cochlear implant is expensive, but full or partial costs are reimbursed by most private insurances or Medicaid. The implant team can help families determine the amount of coverage in advance.

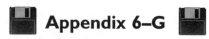

Appendix 6–G

INSTRUCTIONS FOR HEARING AID CHECK

Materials needed (should be assembled in kit such as a zipper pencil case):

Stethoscope
Battery Tester
Batteries
Brush, wire loop
Instructions
Picture of hearing aid with parts labeled
Information regarding how to contact the audiologist

Instructions for conducting a hearing aid check:

• Check the Battery
    1. Open the battery door.
    2. Remove the battery, place in the appropriate slot of a battery tester, and check according to tester instructions.
    3. Obtain new battery if indicator on tester says battery is dead.
    4. Replace battery into the hearing aid - the battery usually only fits one way; DO NOT FORCE THE DOOR CLOSED.

• Listen to the Hearing Aid
    1. Snap the tube onto the listening piece of the stethoscope and place stethoscope in your ears.
    2. Place the end of the tube over the opening of the earmold.
    3. Adjust the volume of the hearing aid to number "2" and turn the hearing aid on (for most hearing aids "M" stands for microphone which means the hearing aid is turned on).
    4. Rotate the volume wheel up and down. Listen for any crackling sound, cutting in or out, or no sound at all. If any of these problems exist, contact the audiologist.
    5. While listening through the aid, say the sounds "OO, EE, AH, S, SH, MM." They should be clear and the hearing aid should not cut off and on. No buzzing or hissing sound should be present.
    6. Shake and squeeze the hearing aid to see if the aid cuts off.
    7. Check for cracks in the case of the hearing aid and the earmold and tubing.
    8. If the hearing aid whistles in the ear, feedback is occurring. Check to see if the earmold is inserted into the ear properly. If not, reinsert. Check for gaps around the earmold. If gaps are present, the earmold might need to be replaced.

• Check the Earmold
    1. Examine the earmold to check for any build-up of wax in the canal end of the mold.
    2. If there is wax build-up, insert the wax loop to remove the wax. The loop will collect wax from the earmold. Wipe off the loop and insert again until all the wax is removed.
    3. Wipe off any foreign materials from the earmold. The earmold may be washed in warm soapy water. Do not use any alcohol to clean the earmold or hearing aid case.
    4. If the earmolds or hearing aid case still looks dirty after the above cleaning, send a note home to notify parents of the problem or contact the audiologist.

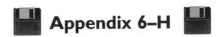

Appendix 6–H

HEARING AID/FM MONITORING CHART

STUDENT_____   SCHOOL_____

KEY: + = OK   − = PROBLEM (explain under comments)

DATE	RT HA	LT HA	FM	SOUND TEST						COMMENTS	ACTION
				oo	ee	ah	s	sh	mm		

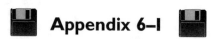

Appendix 6–I

HEARING AID SERVICE - PARENT NOTIFICATION

NAME: _____ DATE: _____ NOTICE # _____

EXAMINER'S NAME: _____ POSITION: _____ AUD. INIT. _____

A problem with your child's hearing aid(s) was brought to our attention by:

_____ routine check   _____ annual evaluation
_____ teacher/specialist   _____ parent
_____ your child   _____ other _____
Problem reported: _____

Problem Found:

_____ dead battery   _____ damage to outside of hearing aid
_____ no battery   _____ malfunctioning hearing aid(s)
_____ clogged earmold   _____ hearing aid(s) are not being worn consistently
_____ poor fitting earmold   _____ tubing/earhook problem
_____ no problem found   _____ other _____

School Action Taken:

_____ a battery had to be replaced. Your child has _____ batteries left.
_____ your child has no batteries left; a batter was loaned to your child.
_____ your child's earmolds needed to be cleaned in order for the hearing aid(s) to work properly.
_____ the tubing/earhook was replaced in order for the hearing aid(s) to work properly.
_____ a listening check or computer analysis was performed on the hearing aid(s).
_____ a school owned hearing aid was loaned to your child (ser# _____).
_____ other _____

Parent Action Needed:

_____ send _____ package(s) of batteries to school for your child.
_____ send _____ batteries to the school audiologist to replace loaned batteries.
_____ wash earmolds frequently with warm water and soap; remember to remove them from the hearing aids first and dry completely before reattaching to the hearing aid(s).
_____ write on the bottom of this form where you will be obtaining new earmolds (private clinic or school).
_____ contact your private clinic to repair hearing aid(s) and to provide a loaner hearing aid.
       right aid serial # _____ left aid serial # _____
_____ please contact the school audiologist at _____
_____ other _____

Please sign and return the bottom of this form to school

-enter your school name here-

STUDENT'S NAME: _____ DATE OF NOTICE: _____

PARENT COMMENTS:

PARENT SIGNATURE _____ DATE _____

        white copy - parents   yellow copy - audiologist   pink copy _____

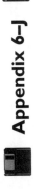 **Appendix 6–J**

HEARING AID/FM MONITOR RECORD

Name _____

AMPLIFICATION: _____ School _____

Hearing Aids: Right Ear _____ Left Ear _____

Assistive Listening System _____

DIRECTIONS: If aids/FM are functioning properly, check appropriate boxes below for each ear. If not functioning properly, identify problem(s) by inserting an R-for right aid or L-for left aid in the box(es) which correspond to the problem(s). For FM, either check satisfactory box, or, if not working properly, identify problem (indicate R for receiver, T for transmitter).

DATE	SATISFACTORY HA FUNCTION		AID NOT WORN (check reason)							PROBLEM OR DEFECTIVE AID (check cause)														BATTERY		EARMOLD (check problem)					FM: REC/ TRANSMITTER					
	Right	Left	Sensitive ear	Refuses	In pocket	Left home	Lost	No battery	In for repair	Turned off	Dirty	Mic	Distortion	Volume control	No output	Battery compartment	Loose hook	Cracked case	Wet	Intermittent	Low gain	Internal feedback	Unknown problem	Weak/dead	Missing	Lost	Poor fit	Dirty	Plugged	Damaged	Poor tubing	Satisfactory	Defective	battery dead	interference	no FM	other

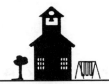

SECTION 7

APPENDIXES

Case Management and Aural (Re)habilitation

CONTENTS

*Appendixes marked with asterisks (*) are available on an optional computer disk which allows users to customize these forms.

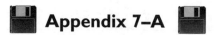 **Appendix 7–A**

STUDENT SERVICES AND SERVICE PROVIDER INFORMATION

STUDENT NAME: _____ DATE: _____

SCHOOL: _____

Services Needed	No	Yes (describe briefly)	Person Responsible
Audiological			
Medical			
Amplification			
Educational			
Communication			
Visual Technology			
Transportation			
Interpreting			
Notetaking			
Tutoring			
Counseling			
Recreation			
Vocational			

Other (list, if needed):

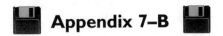

Appendix 7–B

FORM TO FACILITATE WRITTEN COLLABORATION
[BETWEEN TEACHER/ SCHOOL PROVIDER AND PHYSICIAN]

The student identified below is in my class, and it would be helpful if you would provide information on your assessment and recommendations. I have also included my primary concerns/questions concerning this student. Thank you.

STUDENT NAME: DATE OF BIRTH:

SCHOOL PLACEMENT:

MY 3 PRIMARY CONCERNS ABOUT THIS STUDENT ARE:

     1.

     2.

     3.

SIGNATURE & TITLE OF PERSON REQUESTING INFORMATION:

_____

- -

Please complete the following information and send back to school with _____
                                                                 (Student's name)

RESULTS OF EXAMINATION COMPLETED BY   _____
                                                    (Physician's name)

DATE OF EXAM: _____

MY 3 PRIMARY RECOMMENDATIONS FOR THIS STUDENT ARE:

     1.

     2.

     3.

SIGNATURE: _____

ADDRESS & PHONE:

THE BEST TIME TO CONTACT ME IS: _____

[When completed form is returned to school, <u>please cc all service providers</u>.]

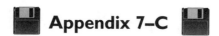

Appendix 7–C

LISTENING DEVELOPMENT PROFILE

Listening Development Profile

Name_____ DOB_____ Age@ID_____

Age@beginning intervention_____ Age@initial amplification_____ Type/Model_____

Amplification:

Date													
Unaided AI													
Aided AI													
Hrs/day of HA use													
ALD used/ freq of use													

Rating: 1=skill introduced   Mode: AVQ = auditory-visual/quiet
         2=skill emerging   AQ = auditory/quiet
         3=skill in progress   AVN = auditory-visual/noise
         4=skill established   AN = auditory/noise

Stage 1: Beginning Listener

STUDENT OUTCOMES	PERFORMANCE INDICATORS	RATING: MODE/DATE			
		1	2	3	4
• increases auditory detection/awareness	• can differentiate the presence or absence of sound				
	• responds to sounds around the home e.g. doorbell, telephone (response may be voluntary or involuntary)				
	• reponds to people's voices				
	• increases time on listening task				
• directs attention to sound) (auditory localization	• turns head in response to sound				
	• turns directly to sound source				
• increases linguistic interaction	• parents use appropriate communication strategies (turntaking, eye contact, child initiated conversation)				
	• child begins to demonstrate age appropriate conversation behavior				
• increases auditory attention	• child indicates desire to wear hearing aids, amplification device & demonstrates a listening attitude				

Stage 2 - Intermediate Listener

• identifies when amplification is not working	• child reports that equipment is not working without prompting				
• demonstrates benefit of listening	• student enjoys listening tasks, initiates desire to hear				
• responds to loud/quiet sounds	• startle response (loud sounds)				
	• says "huh" or looks puzzled (quiet sounds)				
	• demonstrates use of appropriate loud vs quiet sound				
• responds to fast/slow sounds	• moves appropriately to speed of sound				
	• demonstrates fast & slow through vocalizations				
• responds to high/low sounds	• matches pitch of voice				
	• demonstrates high & low through vocalizations				
• understands rhythm of songs	• follows rhythmic patterns of songs				

Source: From "The Development of Listening Function" by Z. R. Razack, 1994, *Toward Excellence in Listening*, pp. 26–30. Copyright May 1994, by The Waterloo County Board of Education, Kitchener, Ontario, Canada. Adapted by permission.

Stage 2 - Intermediate Listener-continued

STUDENT OUTCOMES	PERFORMANCE INDICATORS	RATING: MODE/DATE			
		1	2	3	4
• understands words in songs	• performs action i.e. demonstrates understanding of words				
• increases linguistic interaction	• uses of more complex sentence forms and vocabulary				
	• discriminates words with similar speech sounds (bat vs pat)				
	• uses language for a variety of purposes				
	• uses appropriate intonation patterns				

Stage 3: Advanced Listener

STUDENT OUTCOMES	PERFORMANCE INDICATORS	1	2	3	4
• participates in groups -listens in groups -uses appropriate language & conversation rules	• takes turns				
	• uses appropriate clarification strategies for misunderstood messages				
	• uses discussion to complete assignments				
	• uses phrases appropriately for content				
• increases awareness of pronunciation of words, phrases, sound & symbol connections	• asks for auditory representation or repetition of words so that he/she can internalize auditory images (modeling)				
• increases use of words/concepts in various contexts	• discriminates/self corrects between correct & incorrect productions				
• increases responsibility for understanding oral messages	• follows multi-step instructions				
	• more frequent interactions with teachers, peers				
	• reduce frequency of conversation repair ("huh", "what", "I didn't understand')				
• begins to troubleshoot amplification systems	• reports dead battery or static sounds, intermittency, spill over of signal, clogged mold				
• advocates for services	• asks teacher to check transmitter using appropriate language				

Stage 4: Sophisticated Listener/Communicator

STUDENT OUTCOMES	PERFORMANCE INDICATORS	1	2	3	4
• demonstrates knowledge of audiograms	• explains audiograms in terms of degree and configuration (shape)				
• knowledge of various types of amplification & assistive devices (HA, ALD, TDD, captioner, phone)	• discuss characteristics of various hearing aids, cochlear implants & assistive devices				
	• demonstrates appropriate use of ALD, TDD, captioner, phone				
• uses amplification equipment appropriately	• reports malfunctioning equipment & conducts basic troubleshooting				
• increases awareness of communication/listening environment & appropriate accommodations	• requests appropriate physical accommodations (seating, sound system, etc.)				
	• requests appropriate support services (interpreter, captioning, written materials, notetaker)				
• utilizes professionals & agencies appropriately (audiology, ENT, SLP, interpreter, relay systems, vocational rehabilitation, etc.)	• identifies roles of professionals & community agencies				
	• uses professionals & community services appropriately				
• able to educate others about hearing loss & its implications	• selects target audience for presentation on hearing & communication				
	• does presentation to peers, other schools				
	• explains listening needs in work situations				

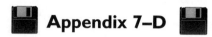

Appendix 7–D

PARENT LETTER ON SPEECHREADING

Dear Parents:

Lipreading is the term commonly used to describe when a listener focuses on the speaker's lips to interpret a message. Through lipreading alone, a person can distinguish between the words *man* and *fan*, but not between *man* and *pan*. More information is needed. *Speechreading* is the more accurate term that accounts for how facial expressions, gestures, other body language, and context contribute to overall understanding.

Speechreading is not used only by people with hearing loss. Everyone, especially people in difficult listening situations, benefits from the additional information received from visual cues. The following activities can be used to improve the natural speechreading skills of *all* children. Remember, speak using natural speech/lip movements. Exaggerated movements or slowed speech makes speechreading more difficult.

- **Develop vocabulary lists, phrases, or sentences that are related to a specific topic.** For example, practice speechreading the vocabulary of school subjects and activities, common classroom instructions, predictable situations, or the names of family members, classmates, and school personnel.

- **Use familiar speech found in nursery rhymes, commercial jingles, commonly used phrases, or sayings. Ask the listener to identify the title or product.**

- **Tell a short story or riddle with everyone watching and listening. Periodically drop your voice while saying certain words or phrases that must be speechread.**

- **Play word games, such as hangman or Scrabble. Write spelling words or key vocabulary words with some missing letters to practice the skill of visualizing a whole word by seeing only part of it.**

- **Point out commonly understood gestures, such as those used for, "Come here," "Wait a minute," and "Stop."** Identifying gestures and the related phrases without gestures can be an entertaining form of family charades.

Remember: understanding usually does not come from visual cues alone. Use some voice, but don't make it too loud or have competing noise in the background. Simply mouthing words may result in exaggerated movements that are difficult to understand.

Sincerely,

Source: From the American Speech-Language-Hearing Association. Adapted by permission.

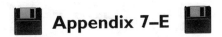

Appendix 7–E

STUDENT SELF-ADVOCACY LETTER

Dear _____:

My name is _____, and because I have a hearing loss, it is sometimes difficult for me to understand what goes on in a busy classroom. This letter lists some suggestions
that can help me to do my best work in your class.

Every person who is hearing impaired has a different kind of loss, and you may have already
read some information about mine. If you do not have this information, please contact

_____.
(audiologist's name & phone no.)

In your classroom, it will help if I:

_____ have special seating (describe or draw diagram on back):
_____ can see your face when you talk to the class. It also helps me to see the other students
during a class discussion.
_____ can change my seat for different activities, if it would help me to see better.
_____ wear 1 hearing aid.
_____ wear 2 hearing aids.
_____ wear an FM unit that includes a microphone for you. This can be very helpful to me
if the room is even a little bit noisy.
_____ I don't need to use any special equipment.

It will also help me if you:

_____ show videos, films, and filmstrips *with captions,* if at all possible, since it is very hard
for me to understand when the room is dark. If captions aren't included, it would
help me to have a written script to study.
_____ will write homework assignments on the chalkboard, so I won't miss these requirements.
_____ would help me choose a "buddy" who can take notes for me and help me find my
place if I get lost (it's really hard to watch you and take notes at the same time).

The other members of my support team would be happy to meet with you to talk about other
ways we can work together in your class. They include:

Name _____ Title _____ Phone Number

I hope we will have a good year together. Please let me know if I'm not keeping up with the
class or if you have trouble understanding my speech.

Sincerely,

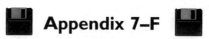

Appendix 7–F

CLASSROOM OBSERVATION CHECKLIST

Student: Age: Grade:

School: Teacher:

Date of Observation: Observer:

I. Physical Characteristics

1. Type of School:
a. Open space_____
b. Modified open space_____
c. Traditional_____
d. Other_____

2. Room Size:
a. Large_____
b. medium_____
c. small_____

3. Number of Students in Class_____

4. Number of Teacher Aides:
a. Full-time_____
b. Part-time_____

5. Type of Seating Used:
a. Desks_____
b. Tables & chairs_____
c. Chairs with writing arms_____
d. Combination of tables & desks_____
e. Other (Identify)_____

6. Lighting:
a. Adequate_____
b. Not adequate_____

7. Windows:
a. Complete wall_____
b. Individual windows_____
c. Covered (describe)_____
d. None_____

8. Floor Surface:
a. Rubber tile_____
b. Hardwood_____
c. Carpeting_____

9. Wall Surface:
a. Wood_____
b. Brick_____
c. Acoustic tile_____
d. Other_____

10. Blackboards:
a. Visible to child_____
b. Teacher usage:
1) Good_____
2) Fair_____
3) Poor_____
c. Glare_____

11. Room Location:
a. Next to disturbing space_____
Describe:

12. General Room Noise Level:
a. High_____
b. Medium_____
c. Low_____
d. SPL_____

II. Teacher-Student Characteristics

13. **Child's Seating is:**
    a. Appropriate_____
    b. Inappropriate_____

14. **Teacher's Speech/Voice:**
    a. Loud_____
    b. Soft_____
    c. Well modulated_____
    d. Good articulation_____
    e. Poor articulation_____
    f. Good voice quality_____
    g. Poor voice quality_____
    h. Readability of lips:
       1) Good_____
       2) Fair_____
       3) Poor_____

15. **Teacher Mobility:**
    a. Faces children when speaking_____
    b. Moves while speaking_____
    c. Uses hand gestures while speaking_____
    d. Talks with back to class_____

16. **Child's Attention:**
    a. Always attends to speaker_____
    b. Usually attends to speaker_____
    c. Sometimes attends to speaker_____
    d. Rarely attends to speaker_____
    e. Difference between attending to teacher and classmates (describe):_____

17. **Child's Speech in the Classroom:**
    a. Very intelligible_____
    b. Usually intelligible_____
    c. Unintelligible_____
    d. Teacher shows adequate comprehension of child's speech_____

18. **Child's Speechreading Skills:**
    a. Speechreading utilized_____
    b. Speechreading not utilized_____
    c. Speechreading skills are successful:
       1) Large group_____
       2) Small group_____
       3) Not at all_____

19. **Child's Participation in Class:**
    a. Volunteers information_____
    b. Answers questions when they are directed to him/her
       1) Accurately most of the time
       2) Inaccurately most of the time
    c. Does not participate in class discussion_____
    d. Asks questions when he/she does not understand_____
    e. Pretends to understand when he/she doesn't_____

20. **Child's Social Interactions:**
    a. Tries to interact with other children_____
    b. Other children try to interact with child_____
    c. Joins group activities on playground_____
    d. Plays alone_____

21. **Friends of Student:**
    a. No friends_____
    b. Some friends_____
    c. Many friends_____

22. **Child's Attendance Is:**
    a. Regular_____
    b. Irregular_____
    c. No. days missed this year_____

23. **Amplification:**
    a. Hearing aid_____
       1) Monaural_____
       2) Binaural_____
    b. FM (Personal, SF)_____
       1) Set up is correct_____
       2) Set up is incorrect_____
    c. Used inconsistently_____
    d. Not used at present_____

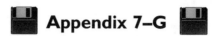

Appendix 7–G

COMMUNICATION OPTIONS MOST COMMONLY USED TO COMMUNICATE WITH AND EDUCATE DEAF AND HARD OF HEARING CHILDREN

COMMUNICA-TION OPTIONS → ATTRIBUTES ↓	American Sign Language/English as a Second Language (ASL/ESL) *Bilingual/Bicultural*	Auditory-Verbal Unisensory Acoupedics	Cued Speech
Definition	A philosophy of education which employs a visual language used by Deaf people in the United States and Canada. English is taught as a second language.	The development of listening, speech and language skills through the maximized use of residual (usable) hearing or other current technology.	A visual representation of spoken language, which uses hand cues in combination with the natural mouth movements of speech, to make all sounds of spoken language look different.
Primary Goals	Goals are development of ASL as the primary language and English as a second language with assimilation into the deaf community, if desired.	Goals are development of spoken language, primarily through the use of current hearing technology, and assimilation into the hearing community.	Goals are development of spoken language through a combination of listening and visual cues, and assimilation into the hearing community.
Language Development (Receptive)	Language is developed through the use of American Sign Language. English is taught as a second language after ASL has been established.	Spoken language is developed through the use of current hearing technology.	Spoken language is developed primarily through speech reading and hand cues which represent consonant and vowel sounds as well as use of current hearing technology.
Expressive Language	ASL is primary language with written English given equal significance.	Spoken and written English.	Spoken English, sometimes with use of cues and written English.
Audition	Use of personal amplification (hearing aids, cochlear implant, FM system) is not required.	Aggressive amplification (hearing aids, cochlear implant, FM system) to maximize residual (usable) hearing is critical to this approach. Early auditory stimulation is required to determine auditory ability.	Use of amplification (hearing aids, cochlear implant, FM system) is encouraged to maximize residual (usable) hearing. Clear visual communication provided by Cued Speech.
Family Responsibility	Deaf and/or hearing adults fluent in ASL are considered to be the primary language facilitators. Deaf and hearing peers are also used as language models.	Family is primary language facilitator. The family must create an auditory learning environment in which sound becomes a meaningful part of daily experience and communication.	Family is primary language facilitator. At least one parent must cue fluently and consistently for age-appropriate language to develop.
Parent Training	Intensive ASL training and education about deaf culture for the family is desired in order for the family to become proficient in the language.	Parents participate in ongoing training with child's teacher or therapist in creating an auditory learning environment.	Cued Speech can be learned through classes offered by trained Cued Speech therapists teachers. To become proficient in the language, many hours of practice are necessary.

Source: From BEGINNINGS FOR PARENTS OF HEARING IMPAIRED CHILDREN, INC., 1996.

COMMUNICATION OPTIONS → ATTRIBUTES ↓	Oral *Auditory/Oral*	Total Communication
Definition	The development of speech and language through the maximized use of residua (usable) hearing and speech reading.	A philosophy of education/communication which employs a combination of oral and manual teaching modes using a sign system, speechreading, finger-spelling, use of residual (usable) hearing, speech, and sometimes Cued Speech.
Primary Goals	Goals are development of spoken language, through a combination of listening and speech reading and assimilation into the hearing community.	Goals are development of language through a combination of manual sign systems, speechreading, listening, and the ability to participate in either the hearing or deaf community.
Language Development (Receptive)	Spoken language is developed through speech reading, and/or use of current hearing technology.	Language is developed through the use of manual sign systems, speech reading, and/or use of current hearing technology.
Expressive Language	Spoken and written English.	Signing and finger-spelling accompanied by spoken and written English.
Audition	Aggressive amplification (hearing aids, cochlear implant, FM system) to maximize residual (usable) hearing is critical to this approach.	Use of personal amplification (hearing aids, cochlear implant, FM system) is encouraged.
Family Responsibility	Family is the primary language facilitator. The family is expected to integrate audition and speech reading throughout the day and in structured play activities.	Family is primary language facilitator. At least one parent must learn the sign system fluently and use it consistently for age-appropriate language to develop.
Parent Training	Parents participate in ongoing training with child's teacher or therapist to learn how to create an oral learning environment.	Signing can be learned through classes available in the community with the supplement of video tapes and books. To become fluent, many hours of practice are necessary

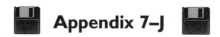 **Appendix 7–J**

AUDITORY LEARNING PROGRAM

Parent/School/Student Contract

The use of audition for children who are deaf and hard of hearing requires patience, perseverance, and commitment. Auditory learning must be integrated into all of a child's daily activities if the use of hearing is to be maximally developed. Success with audition is based on appropriate expectations, cooperation between the family and the school and/or habilitation program, and hard work.

Auditory learning is based on the following principles:

- early diagnosis of hearing loss and early appropriate intervention
- consistent use of appropriate amplification
- good listening conditions (acoustic environment)
- implementation of auditory learning principles
- informed, sustained and systematic efforts by staff, student, parent, and community to collaborate

PREREQUISITES FOR AUDITORY LEARNING

Parent Expectations:
1. Recognition of importance of audition and its implications for the development of hearing and speech.
2. Commitment to providing a learning environment which enhances the use of audition.
3. Assume responsibility for the child's amplification
   (a) fitting of hearing aids and/or assistive listening device
   (b) maintenance of amplification including daily monitoring for proper functioning, providing batteries and proper fitting earmolds, timely repairs, and regular contact with an audiologist
4. Work with school or habilitation program to optimize coordination and consistency of program.
5. Maintain record, such as a journal, regarding child's auditory learning to assist with monitoring child's progress and to determine appropriate goals.

School/Habilitation Program Expectations:
1. Provide information regarding importance of audition and its implications for the development of hearing and speech.
2. Provide opportunities and support for parents to learn about amplification, auditory development, and auditory learning principles including appropriate activities to support auditory learning.
3. Provide a learning environment which optimizes the use of audition.
4. Provide a positive, supportive, and non-judgmental atmosphere for communication which encourages parents to participate as a team member to promote their child's development.
5. Provide assessment to monitor child's progress and determine appropriate goals.

Child Expectations:
1. Child wears hearing aids or amplification device during all waking hours.

STATEMENT OF COMMITMENT

We agree with the expectations outlined above and will work together to promote auditory learning for:

_____ Date _____

Parent/Guardian _____   _____

Student _____   _____

Deaf/HOH Program Representative
_____   _____

Appendix 7–I

EARLY AUDITORY SKILL DEVELOPMENT FOR SPECIAL POPULATIONS

Stage 1. Sound awareness and early attending; beginning to relate to sound as meaningful event.
- Overt response to intense sound (startle, diminished activity, vocalization, eye widening or eye blinking).
- Overt response to softer sounds (see #1).
- Overt response to caregiver's voice.
- Eye contact with soundmaker or caregiver.

Note: Child may habituate if sound stimuli occur frequently, or if the environment contains competing noise. Reinforce any potential response with touch by the soundmaker or caregiver, unless child exhibits tactile defensiveness.

Stage 2. Beginning localization; early sound recognition; beginning deliberate vocalization.
- Attempts to maintain eye contact with moving soundmaker or caregiver.
- Begins to search for sound by looking or reaching.
- Smiling to caregiver's voice.
- Increased vocalizations during dressing, being held, or with diaper change.
- Different body responses to varying emotional tone of voice (happy, sad, angry).
- Beginning vocal play (vocalization increases to caregiver's voice).
- Vocalizes to objects.
- Vocalizes to singing or music.

Note: This stage requires some awareness of cause and effect. Reinforce responses immediately, whenever possible.

Stage 3. Accurate localization and tracking; meaningful sound recognition; deliberate vocalization.
- Manipulates sound maker purposefully to make sound.
- Attends to and follows voice for longer periods of time.
- Vocalizes to persuade caregiver to continue play time or pleasurable attention.
- Searching behavior for any change in sound within immediate environment.
- Different vocalizations to indicate pleasure and displeasure.
- "Calls" to caregiver to indicate basic needs (wet, hungry, desire for physical contact).
- Unfamiliar sounds are unsettling.
- Beginning to initiate and maintain repetitive sound activities (clapping, hand-waving, banging toys, primitive vocal play).
- Begins to anticipate daily activities and familiar persons from auditory cues (different response to sounds of cooking, water running, voices, animal sounds, repetitive songs used in the classroom, door slam, car keys).
- Begins to respond to routine words plus gestures (bye-bye, all gone, pat-a-cake).

Note: Child's cognitive, motor, and visual development is critical in this stage, as well as hearing acuity and whether or not the child uses amplification. Accurate localization requires good head control; students who are motorically involved or delayed will require firm support to develop this skill. If vision is severely impaired, multi-sensory stimulation and reinforcement will be required. Beginning use of co-active gestures should be considered for these students. Knowledge of hearing status is critical to select appropriate loudness and distance for auditory signals. Always check for auditory awareness before working on localization or auditory tracking activities.

Stage 4. Increased sound/speech comprehension; improved control of vocalizations as communication.
- Understands familiar phrases, such as no-no, bye-bye, all gone.
- Responds to name by turning, smiling, reaching, vocalizing, in different fashion than to any other name.
- Initiates and participates in imitative vocal play (attempts to change vocalization when stimulated by different vocal pattern).
- Vocalizations are beginning to sound like words or meaningful units.
- More consistent use of appropriate inflectional patterns (pitch, loudness, and duration) for questions, demands, comments, confusion, scolding toys, etc.
- Uses consistent vocal approximations of names for caregivers or other meaningful individuals (ma-ma, da-da, na-na).
- Purposeful play with more complex sound-making toys (pushes button, squeezes toys).
- Shakes head for no.
- Increasingly attentive to speakers for longer periods of time.
- "Dances" to music.

Note: Child's fine and gross motor skills affect responses during this stage. If mobility is impaired, adult should attempt to substitute an appropriate response, such as pushing a button to make a doll dance whenever the music begins. Use of switches for motorically involved students may assist in assessment and teaching of auditory comprehension tasks. Oral-motor difficulties can interfere with performance of imitative speech tasks, and alternative or augmentative communication systems may need to be considered at this stage. Participation in turn-taking activities should be mastered during this stage.

Stage 5. Early auditory comprehension; meaningful use of oral language; ability to initiate and maintain conversations.
- Follows simple one-step directions without gestures.
- Expressive vocabulary increases.
- Uses clusters of speech that sound like sentences, accompanied by gestures, interspersed with intelligible words.
- Lets speaker know when message is not understood (primitive requests for clarification)
- Talks about objects that are not in sight by name.
- Recognizes names of family members, classmates, and a few body parts.
- Child can attend to primary signals (teacher, peers) when other noise is in the background.

Note: The child's progress during this stage will depend on cognitive development and oral-motor function. Beyond this stage, progress in auditory comprehension can be measured using appropriate receptive language scales

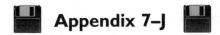 Appendix 7–J

AUDITORY RESPONSE DATE SHEET

AUDITORY RESPONSE DATA SHEET

Student Name: School: Class:

Teacher(s): Observer(s):

Observed Behavior	Stimulus	Distance/ conditions (quiet vs noise)	Amplification (yes/no)	Date
No Response				
Cessation of Activity				
Quieting				
Jerk/startle (extension)				
Jerk/startle (flexion)				
Increased activity				
Vocalization				
Cry				
Laugh				
Smile				
Frown				
Eye blink				
Eye widening				
Eye localization				
Head turning				
Body localization				
Reaching				

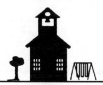

SECTION 8

APPENDIXES
Hearing Conservation

CONTENTS

*Appendixes marked with asterisks (*) are available on an optional computer disk which allows users to customize these forms.

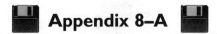 **Appendix 8–A**

HEARING CONSERVATION PARENT LETTER (PRESCHOOL)

Dear Parent:

We have been learning about our ears at school. We have learned that loud noises can hurt our ears, but there are ways that we can take special care that this doesn't happen. Listed below are a few activities that you can do at home to help your child,_____, remember the things we have talked about at school.

- Identify and count all the ears in your household. Include dolls, pets, and all the friends and relatives present. Send the total with your child to school, and we'll see which child found the most ears.

- Close your eyes and listen for about a minute. Then name all the things you hear.

- Help your child draw a picture of something you hear.

- Identify loud and soft sounds in each room in your home. Put stickers or tape on the things that make loud sounds.

- Talk about how fireworks can hurt your ears (we discussed this at school). Remind your child that it is important never to play with fireworks alone.

- Activities that could damage your hearing include the following:
  *Auto racing
  *Riding on a tractor
  *Motorcycle riding
  *Snowmobiling
  *Recreational shooting

If your family participates in any of these activities, discuss with your child ways to protect your ears during these activities.

Please let us know if you have any questions, or if you and your child came up with another activity to share.

Sincerely,

HEARING CONSERVATION PARENT LETTER (ELEMENTARY)

Dear Parents:

Noise fills your child's day, beginning with the alarm clock in the morning and continuing through the school bus ride, band practice, lunch in the cafeteria, and "studying" with personal headsets.

Too much noise can cause a hearing loss. Sometimes the loss comes from a one-time exposure to an extremely loud noise. Other times the loss comes from repeated exposure to moderately loud noise.

Please read and discuss with your child the following suggestions for protecting hearing.

- Turn down the volume on stereos and headsets. If a friend can hear the music from 3 feet away, the volume is too high. Also keep the volume turned down for both the television and stereo speakers at home.

- Wear special hearing protectors during activities that involve loud noise, such as hunting, going to rock concerts, watching auto races, or riding vehicles with noisy motors like motor bikes, jet skis, or snowmobiles. *Cotton does not work and neither do earplugs made for swimming.* Special earplugs for noise can be purchased at your local drug or sporting goods store.

- Sit at a safe distance from the front of loudspeakers at home and at concerts.

- Avoid noisy toys like cap guns. Check all the labels on toys to make sure they do not carry a warning about possible hearing damage from noise. If there is a warning, avoid buying the toy, if at all possible, unless you can control its noise level.

Remind your child of the good things that might not be heard if you have a hearing loss. Ask your child to tell you about ways we discussed at school to protect your ears from loud noises and how we can tell if noise may be hurting our ears.

Please contact me if you have any concerns or want further information on how to protect your family's hearing.

Sincerely,

Educational Audiologist

Source: From the American Speech-Language-Hearing Association. Adapted by permission.

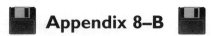

Appendix 8–B

HEARING CONSERVATION HANDOUT FOR MIDDLE/HIGH SCHOOL STUDENTS

DO YOU HAVE A NOISY LIFESTYLE?

Pete Townshend, lead guitarist for The Who, has tinnitus and noise-induced hearing loss from his years of exposure to loud music.

Recent studies have shown that aerobic exercise can increase the danger of temporary hearing loss from loud music through a headset.

Orlando Brown, an offensive tackle with the Cleveland Browns, uses a hearing protective device to tone down crowd noise and help him distinguish audible signals from the quarterback.

Bobby Unser and other drivers on the national racecar circuit have reported experiencing significant hearing difficulties as a result of failing to use ear protection.

Firearms (including rifles, pistols, shotguns and revolvers) have been measured to produce an average of 134 to 164.5 dB SPL when fired. All of these levels put the shooter at risk of immediate, permanent hearing loss.

HOW'S YOUR HEARING LIFESTYLE?

Have you been exposed to noise from the following sources?

> Farm machinery
> Power tools
> Hunting
> Firecrackers
> Snowmobiles
> Lawnmowers
> Aircraft
> Stereo loudspeakers
> Stereo earphones
> Motorcycles
> Live music
> Boom cars
> Go-carts
> Video arcade

HOW CAN I TELL IF MY EARS ARE HURTING?

Am I shouting to be heard?
Does speech sound muffled?
Are my ears ringing?

IF YES, WHAT CAN I DO?

Turn down the stereo.
Wear professional ear protection.
Move away from the speakers.
Take a break from the music.
Open the windows in your car.
Use headphones that have output measured below 115 dB.
Get a hearing test.

Appendix 8–C

HEARING CONSERVATION PERIODICAL REFERENCES FOR HIGH SCHOOL STUDENTS

Cohen, P. (1990). Drumming: How risky is it to your hearing? *Modern Drummer, October,* 24-29, 95-99.

Emmett, R. (1991). Hear today, gone tomorrow. *Guitar Player, June,* 108.

Emmett, R. (1991). Ear damage control. *Guitar Player, July,* 101.

Jaret, P. (1990). The rock and roll syndrome. *Health, July/August,* 51-57.

Lanpher, K., & K. Keller (1991). Turn down that noise. *Redbook, April,* 58-64.

Murphy, E. (1989). Townshend, tinnitus and rock and roll. *Rolling Stone, July,* 101.

Saunders, A. (1990). Motorcycles and hearing. *Rider, January,* 56-57.

Silverman, L. (1989). Earning a deaf ear: Loud music and hearing loss. *Audio, January,* 76-82.

Tennis, C. (1990). Crank it down. *EQ, Sept/Oct,* 22-33

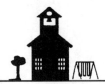

SECTION 9

APPENDIXES

Community Collaboration

CONTENTS

*Appendixes marked with asterisks (*) are available on an optional computer disk which allows users to customize the forms

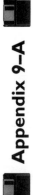 **Appendix 9–A**

COMMUNITY NEEDS ASSESSMENT FORM

PART I - PROGRAMS/AGENCIES/HOSPITALS/CLINICS

Program Name Address, Phone	Services (describe)	Fees	Schedule	Contact (Name, phone)	Comments (Personnel, funding constraints)

PART II - LOCAL PHYSICIANS

Name Address, Phone	Satellite Office(s)	Schedule	Audiologist(s)	Comments (Reimbursement)

PART III - COMMUNITY AUDIOLOGISTS

Name Address, Phone	Services	Schedule	Comments (Special equipment, Communication and/or pediatric skills)

PART IV - SERVICE CLUBS

Club Name/Contact Address. Phone	Meeting Time	Fiscal Year	Program Chair Phone	Special Projects(describe)

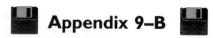

Appendix 9–B

LETTER TO COMMUNITY RESOURCES

Dear

This letter is to follow up our conversation last week when we discussed the _____ Educational Audiology Program. We provide the following services for children birth–21 who live in the _____ School District:

Hearing Screenings
Comprehensive Audiologic Evaluations
Hearing Aid Orientation and Management
Loaner Hearing Aids
Provision of Individual and Classroom Amplification Systems
Habilitation Services for Educational Needs related to hearing loss
Parent-Infant Home Program

We are continuing to work with other local professionals and agencies to insure that all children who have hearing loss are identified as early as possible and to help families obtain the necessary equipment and services once a hearing loss is identified. This year we have been able to add testing equipment that is appropriate for very young children who cannot be tested by traditional methods. As I mentioned last week, _____ has joined our audiology staff to concentrate on hearing evaluations and rehabilitation for preschool children and other students who are difficult to test, because these services have not been available anywhere else in our region.

The _____ Educational Audiology Services are provided at no direct charge to families and children who are residents of _____ County. I have enclosed a brochure and several referral forms. Please call us at _____, if you need more forms or additional information.

Thank you again for your time last week.

Sincerely,

Educational Audiologist

Appendix 9–C

SUGGESTED TOPICS FOR COMMUNITY PRESENTATIONS

Overview of Hearing Loss

What Is an Audiologist?

Local School Audiology and Hearing Impaired Program

Prevention of Hearing Loss

Technological Advances in Hearing Aids

Assistive Devices

Infant Hearing Loss Identification

Treatment and Effects of Ear Infections (joint program with MD)

The ADA

Deaf Culture

Sign Language

Hearing Ear Dogs

Noise/Hearing Conservation

Recreational Audiology

Communication Methodologies

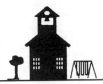

SECTION 10

APPENDIXES

Relationships With Families

CONTENTS

*Appendixes marked with asterisks (*) are available on an optional computer disk which allows users to customize the forms.

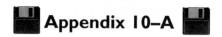 **Appendix 10–A**

WELCOME TO HOLLAND!
by Emily Perl Kingsley

I am often asked to describe the experience of raising a child with a disability—to try to help people who have not shared that unique experience to understand it, to imagine how it would feel. It's like this . . .

When you're going to have a baby, it's like you're planning a fabulous vacation trip—to Italy. You buy a bunch of guide books and make your wonderful plans. The Coliseum. The Michelangelo David. The gondolas in Venice. You may learn some handy phrases in Italian. It's all very exciting.

After months of eager anticipation, the day finally arrives. You pack your bags and off you go. Several hours later, the plane lands. The stewardess comes in and says, "Welcome to Holland."

"**Holland**?!?" you say. "What do you mean Holland?? I signed up for Italy! I'm supposed to be in Italy. All my life I've dreamed of going to Italy."

But there's been a change in the flight plan. They've landed in Holland and there you must stay.

The important thing is that they haven't taken you to a horrible, disgusting, filthy place, full of pestilence, famine and disease. It's just a different place.

So you must go out and buy new guide books. And you must learn a whole new language. And you will meet a whole new group of people you would never have met.

It's just a **different** place. It's slower-paced than Italy, less flashy than Italy. But after you've been there for a while and you catch your breath, you look around . . . and you begin to notice that Holland has windmills . . . and Holland has tulips. Holland even has Rembrandts.

But everyone you know is busy coming and going from Italy . . . and they're all bragging about what a wonderful time they had there. And for the rest of your life, you will say, "Yes, that's where I was supposed to go. That's what I had planned."

And the pain of that will never, ever, ever go away . . . because the loss of that dream is a very significant loss.

But . . . if you spend your life mourning the fact that you didn't get to Italy, you may never be free to enjoy the very special, the very lovely things . . . about Holland.

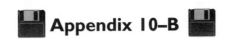

Appendix 10–B

FAMILY NEEDS SURVEY

(Adapted for Families of Children Who Are Deaf or Hard of Hearing)

Child's Name:______________________ Date Completed:__________

Person Completing Survey:______________________ Relationship to Child:________

Dear Parent:

Many families of young children who are deaf or hard of hearing have needs for information or support. Listed below are some of the needs frequently identified by families. It would be helpful if you would check the topics below for which you would like more information or to discuss with a staff person from our program. At the end there is a place for you to add other areas not included on this list.

If you choose to complete this form, the information you provide will be kept confidential. If you would prefer not to complete the survey at this time, you may keep it for future reference.

Would you like more **Information** or to **discuss** this topic with a staff person from our program?

TOPICS	NO	NOT SURE	YES - DISCUSS	YES - INFO
General Information:				
1. How children grow and develop				
2. How to play or talk with my child				
3. How to teach my child				
4. How to handle by child's behavior				
Information - Hearing & Hearing Loss:				
1. How the normal ear hears & how the ear works				
2. How my child hears, cause of hearing loss				
3. About hearing aids				
4. How hearing aids will help my child				
5. About other types of hearing devices				
6. How to keep the hearing aid(s) on				
Communication:				
1. How to teach my child to listen				
2. How will the hearing loss affect my child's ability to learn to talk				
3. How language develops				
4. About sign language				
5. How my child will communicate				
6. How I can communicate with my child				
Services & Educational Resources				
1. Information about special services available for my child				
2. Information about special services my child may need in the future				

Source: From "The Family Needs Survey" by D. Baily and R. Simeonsson, 1990. Adapted by permission.

TOPICS	NO	NOT SURE	YES - DISCUSS	YES - INFO
3. More time to talk with to my child's teacher or therapist				
4. Information about other conditions my child may have				
5. Reading materials, videos, local, state & national organizations & resources about hearing loss				
Family & Social Support				
1. Talk with someone in my family, or a friend, about my concerns				
2. Opportunities to meet with other parents of children who are deaf or hard of hearing				
3. Opportunities to meet deaf and hard of hearing adults				
4. Information about parent support groups				
5. More time for myself				
6. Help our family to accept the hearing loss				
7. Meet with a counselor who specializes in hearing loss issues				
8. Explaining my child's hearing problem to others				
Child Care & Community Services				
1. Help locating good baby-sitters for my child				
2. Help locating a day care program for my child				
3. Help locating a doctor, dentist, etc.				
4. Help with transportation				
Financial				
1. Paying for hearing aids				
2. Paying for therapy				
3. Paying for child care/respite care				
4. Paying for other special equipment my child needs				
5. Paying for food, housing, medical care, clothing, or transportation				

Please list other topics or information that you feel would be helpful to receive or discuss:

_____

_____

Is there a particular person with whom you would prefer to meet?

_____

Thank you for your time.
We hope this form will be helpful to you in identifying the services that you feel are important.

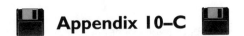

Appendix 10–C

PARENT CHECKLIST
PLACEMENT OF A HEARING-IMPAIRED CHILD IN THE CLASSROOM

This checklist's aim is to help you find the most appropriate placement for your hearing-impaired child in a mainstreamed classroom setting.

The authors recommend that each of the following items be evaluated through classroom observation(s). Note your observations even though you may not have a lot of objective data and may find yourself reacting to gut level feelings. Trust your instincts. Ask other parents of children in the classroom (or parents of other students in the school) what their experiences have been.

No placement decision is final. You should have the opportunity to observe and interact with the teacher and other school personnel, especially if you have concerns or other negative feelings about the classroom or school situation. Your review of these issues should be an ongoing process of reassessment. Good luck to you in this exciting but potentially anxiety-provoking time.

I.   Physical Environment
    Structure:
    °   Is the room size conducive to learning? (A large room/high ceiling can distort sound; a small room may be noisier.)
    °   What is the number of and size of the windows? (Large number may increase noise levels and distractions.)
    °   Is the school set up as an open school (open classrooms) or is it more traditional?
    °   Is the room adequately lit? (Lighting and shadows may affect speech reading.)
    Acoustic Treatment for Noise Reduction:
    °   Is the entire classroom carpeted?
    °   Is the hallway carpeted?
    °   Are there acoustical tiles on the ceiling?
    °   Are there shades, blinds, curtains, drapes, etc., on the windows? (These reduce noise and/or distractions.)
    °   Are there cork boards/bulletin boards on the walls? (These boards decrease noise levels.)
    Noise Levels:
    What is the noise level:
    °   In the classroom? (Note: Students, heater, fish tank, fan, etc.)
    °   In the hallway? (Note: Students, lockers, etc.)
    °   Outside the building? (Note: Traffic, playground, etc.)
    Other Considerations:
    °   Are assorted visual aids used (blackboard, pictures, teaching aids, etc.)?
    °   How many students are in the class?
    °   What is the adult/student ratio?
    °   What is the average distance between the teacher and the students?
    °   Does the school rely on the public address system for announcements? (If so, is a signal given before the message?)
    Observations/Comments: _____

II. Teacher
    Teaching Style:
    °   Does the teacher provide a good language model for the students?
    °   How does the teacher present information? (Does the teacher typically face the students?)
    °   What are the teacher's speaking skills (enunciation, clarity of speech, rate of speech, loudness of voice, intonation/rhythm, facial expression, etc.)?
    °   Are the instructions clear to the students? (Does the teacher repeat himself/herself?)
    Other Features to Note:
    °   What is the teacher's attitude towards having a hearing-impaired student in the classroom?
    °   Is the teacher willing and able to spend time with the parent(s)?
    °   Has the teacher ever taught a hearing-impaired student?
    °   Has the teacher received any formal training regarding hearing impairment?

    °   What does the teacher know about personal hearing aids/group amplification systems (FM auditory trainers)?

    °   What is the teacher's attitude regarding child management and discipline?

    °   Consider evaluating other personnel regarding the above issues (for example, teacher aides, interpreters, tutors, notetakers, etc.)

Observations/Comments: _____

_____

III. Attitude of School

    °   Have there been other special-needs children in the school?

    °   Do the teacher, principal, and other personnel seem agreeable to having a hearing-impaired student in the school?

Observations/Comments: _____

_____

IV. Information Regarding the Student

Student's Management of Hearing Loss:

    °   What does your child do when he/she does not hear? (Tells speaker he/she did not hear, requests repetition, etc.)

    °   What is your child's attitude towards his/her hearing loss?

Hearing Aid Maintenance/Monitoring Skills:

    °   Does your child take responsibility for his/her hearing aids? (Inserts own earmolds, hearing aids; tells adult if the battery is not working, etc.)

Child Characteristics:

Compare your child's performance with the other students in the classroom in the following areas:

    °   Attending behavior   °   Listening behavior in quiet

    °   Listening behavior in noise   °   Social/emotional maturity

    °   Communication skills in speech, reading, writing, understanding, and verbal expression (spoken language)

Other Important Issues to Consider:

    °   Child's physical size/development   °   Academic/intelligence level

    °   Play skills   °   Peer acceptance

    °   Independence (for example, in completing tasks, in resolving conflicts and confrontations, etc.)

    °   Sibling relationships

Observations/Comments: _____

_____

V. Special Services

Are qualified personnel available to provide evaluation and/or intervention in the following areas:

    °   Speech-language pathology   °   Educational audiology   °   Hearing impaired resources

    °   Occupational therapy   °   Physical therapy   °   Resource room

    °   Guidance/counseling   °   Psychology   °   Gifted program

    °   Educational interpreters (manual or oral)   °   Notetakers

Observations/Comments: _____

_____

VI. Miscellaneous:

    °   Transportation to/from school   °   Cost (if any)   °   Family concerns

The above information may lead to questions, concerns and/or requests to be discussed at the Child Study Team or Individual Education Plan/Program (IEP) meeting. Some of the above issues must be acted upon as objectives/special needs in the IEP.

Be your child's best advocate!

Source: From Goldberg, Niehl, Metropoulos, 1989, *The Volta Review 91* (7). Reprinted with permission.
Copyright © 1989 by the Alexander Graham Bell Association for the Deaf, 3417 Volta Place N.W., Washington, D.C. 20007, Reprinted with permission from the *The Volta Review*.

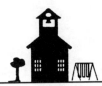

SECTION 11

APPENDIXES

Individual Planning

CONTENTS

*Appendixes with asterisks (*) are available on an optional computer disk which allows users to customize these forms.

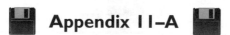 **Appendix 11–A**

IEP CHECKLIST: RECOMMENDED ACCOMMODATIONS
AND MODIFICATIONS FOR STUDENTS
WITH HEARING IMPAIRMENT

Name: _____   Date: _____

Amplification Options
___ Personal hearing device (hearing aid, cochlear implant, tactile device)
___ Personal FM system (hearing aid + FM)
___ FM system/auditory trainer (without personal hearing aid)
___ Walkman-style FM system
___ Sound-field FM system

Assistive Devices
___ TDD
___ TV captioner
___ Other _____

Communication Accommodations
___ Specialized seating arrangements:
    _____
___ Obtain student's attention prior to speaking
___ Reduce auditory distractions (background noise)
___ Reduce visual distractions
___ Enhance speechreading conditions (avoid hands in front of face, mustaches well-trimmed, no gum chewing)
___ Present information in simple, structured, sequential manner
___ Clearly enunciate speech
___ Allow extra time for processing information
___ Repeat or rephrase information when necessary
___ Frequently check for understanding
___ Educational interpreter (ASL, signed English, cued speech, oral)

Physical Environment Accommodations
___ Noise reduction (carpet & other sound absorption materials)
___ Specialized lighting
___ Room design modifications
___ Flashing fire alarm

Instructional Accommodations
___ Use of visual supplements (overheads, chalkboard, charts, vocabulary lists, lecture outlines)
___ Captioning or scripts for television, videos, movies, filmstrips
___ Buddy system for notes, extra explanations/directions
___ Check for understanding of information
___ Down time/break from listening
___ Extra time to complete assignments
___ Step-by-step directions
___ Tutor
___ Notetaker

Curricular Modifications
___ Modify reading assignments (shorten length, adapt or eliminate phonics assignments)
___ Modify written assignments (shorten length, adjust evaluation criteria)
___ Pre-tutor vocabulary
___ Provide supplemental materials to reinforce concepts
___ Provide extra practice
___ Alternative curriculum

Evaluation Modifications
___ Reduce quantity of tests
___ Use alternative tests
___ Provide reading assistance with tests
___ Allow extra time
___ Other modifications:_____

Other Needs/Considerations
___ Supplemental instruction (speech, language, pragmatic skills, auditory, speechreading skills)
___ Counseling
___ Sign language instruction
___ Vocational services
___ Family supports
___ Deaf/hard of hearing role models
___ Recreational/social opportunities
___ Financial assistance
___ Transition services

Appendix 11–B

SUGGESTED ANNUAL GOALS AND SHORT TERM OBJECTIVES RELATING TO AUDIOLOGY NEEDS

The following goals and their accompanying objectives were developed to be used with students with hearing impairment when developing IEP's. The goals represent developmentally-based skills which students should acquire to maximize their residual hearing. These goals and objectives should be used as basic guidelines and be expanded as needed for each student. Every student with hearing impairment should have audiology goals on their IEP until competency or maximal potential has been reached.

ANNUAL GOALS

INDEPENDENT USE OF AMPLIFICATION.

DEVELOP AND IMPROVE AUDITORY SKILLS.

DEMONSTRATE APPROPRIATE COMPENSATORY STRATEGIES RELATED TO HEARING IMPAIRMENT.

KNOWLEDGE OF HEARING LOSS AND ITS IMPLICATIONS.

ADVOCATE APPROPRIATELY FOR HEARING-RELATED NEEDS.

ANNUAL GOALS AND SHORT TERM OBJECTIVES

Goal 1:
The student will demonstrate independent use of amplification (hearing aids, cochlear implants, FM device, or other system).

Objectives:

1. The student will arrive at school wearing properly functioning amplification _____ out of _____ times as measured by daily checks.
2. The student will be able to correctly insert and remove amplification _____ out of _____ times as measured by observation.
3. The student will monitor his/her own amplification function (batteries, volume settings, cleaning of earmolds) _____ out of _____ times as measured by observation or checklist.
4. The student will notify appropriate personnel when amplification is not functioning properly _____ out of _____ times as measured by observation.
5. The student will demonstrate basic knowledge, use and/or care of assistive listening device utilized in his/her academic settings, _____ out of _____ times as measured by demonstration or observation.
6. The student will be responsible for the use of his/her FM system in all appropriate education situations _____ out of _____ times as measured by observation.

Goal 2:

The student will develop or improve his/her auditory skills.

Objectives:

1. The student will develop/improve sound awareness skills _____ out of _____ times across a variety of settings (quiet, noise, close, distant, with and without visual clues, familiar, unfamiliar,) as measured by an auditory curriculum.[1]

2. The student will develop/improve suprasegmental listening skills (pitch, duration, intensity, rate etc.) _____ out of _____ times across a variety of settings as measured by an auditory curriculum.

3. The student will develop/improve vowel discrimination and identification across a variety of settings as measured by an auditory curriculum.

4. The student will auditorially discriminate his/her name _____ out of _____ times across a variety of settings as measured by observation or a teacher made test.

5. The student will develop/improve consonant discrimination and identification _____ out of _____ times across a variety of settings as measured by an auditory curriculum.

6. The student will develop/improve auditory comprehension skills by following _____ out of _____ step directions across a variety of settings as measured by an auditory curriculum.

7. The student will discriminate common phrases _____ out of _____ times across a variety of settings as measured by an auditory curriculum.

8. The student will identify familiar language patterns _____ out of _____ times across a variety of settings.

9. The student will increase his/her ability to answer questions following auditorially presented information _____ out of _____ times as measured by observation or teacher made test.

Goal 3:

The student will demonstrate appropriate compensatory strategies (accommodations and modifications).

Objectives:

1. The student will explain his/her need for preferential seating _____ out of _____ times as measured by informal evaluation.

2. The student will independently choose or request to sit in an appropriate seat _____ out of _____ times as measure by observation and teacher feedback.

3. The student will ask for repetition/clarifications _____ out of _____ times as measured by observation and teacher feedback.

4. The student will utilize available clues (visual, contextual, lipreading, etc.) to aid in comprehension _____ out of _____ times as measured by observation and teacher feedback.

Goal 4:

The student will demonstrate knowledge of his/her hearing loss and resulting needs.

Objectives:

1. The student will describe the type, amount and cause of his/her hearing loss _____ out of _____ times as measured by informal evaluation.

2. The student will demonstrate an understanding of the benefits/limitations of amplification as they relate to his/her own hearing loss _____ out of _____ times as measured by informal evaluation.

Goal 5:

The student will advocate appropriately for his/her needs.

Objectives:

1. The student will inform teachers of his/her hearing loss and resulting needs _____ out of _____ times as measured by teacher feedback and observation.

---

[1]The *Developmental Approach to Successful Listening* (DASL) or the *Auditory Skills Curriculum* are examples of curriculums which include a variety of subskills for each of these objective areas that are measurable in a variety of settings.

2. The student will request appropriate visual and or supplementary materials as needed (copy of notes, film script, captioning, lecture outline...) _____ out of _____ times as measured by teacher feedback and observations.

3. The student will demonstrate and make use of appropriate assistive technology (TTY, captioner, Relay COLORADO, etc.) _____ out of _____ times as measured by teacher feedback, observations, and/or informal evaluations.

Source: From "Effectiveness Indicators for Audiological Services," Appendix F, The Colorado Department of Education, Special Education Unit, January 1993. Reprinted by permission.

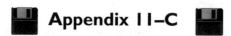

Appendix 11–C

SECTION 504 INDIVIDUALIZED PLAN

Student: _____   Date: _____

Date of Birth: _____   School: _____

Date of Meeting: _____   Grade Level: _____

      As a result of a special education evaluation and staffing procedure, it was determined that this student does not qualify for special education services as defined by The Individuals With Disabilities Education Act (IDEA).

      Nevertheless, the school recognizes that _____ is or may experience challenges in school. Therefore, the school has agreed to modify or adapt the classroom and/or other school environments to accommodate _____ individual needs as follows by:

_____ Providing a structured learning environment by allowing the student to keep his/her desk removed from other students and providing a daily written schedule to follow the class

_____ Supplementing verbal instructions with visual instructions

_____ Using behavioral management techniques, such as _____

_____ Adjusting class schedule

_____ Modifying test delivery by _____

_____ Giving the student additional time to complete assignments

_____ Using tape recorders, computer-aided instruction, or other audiovisual equipment

_____ Selecting modified textbooks or workbooks

_____ Tailoring homework assignments

_____ Use of one-to-one peer tutors, aides, and/or note takers

_____ Involvement of a "services coordinator" to oversee implementation of these accommodations

_____ Modification of nonacademic times such as lunchroom, recess, and physical education by:

_____

_____ Use of assistive listening device

_____ Specialized seating arrangement to enhance ability to hear in the classroom

_____ Special communication strategies such as getting student's attention, facing student, speaking clearly, and speaking in close proximity to student, minimizing background noise

_____ Other: _____

           _____

           _____

           _____

           _____

Participating Team Members:

_____   _____
Signature   Signature

_____   _____
Signature   Signature

_____   _____
Signature   Signature

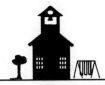

SECTION 12

APPENDIXES

Inservice

CONTENTS

*Appendixes with asterisks (*) are available on an optional computer disk which allows users to customize these forms.

Appendix 12–A

SUGGESTED INSERVICE TOPICS

Introduction to Hearing Loss
Overview of District Audiology and Hearing Impaired Program
Effects of Hearing Loss on Learning
Strategies to Support Students Who are Deaf or Hard of Hearing
Integrating Auditory Skill Practice into the Classroom
Inclusion of Students With Hearing Loss
Hearing Aid Management
Use of FM in the Classroom
Assistive Devices
Communication Metholodologies
Deaf Culture
Use of Tutor/Interpreter/Notetaker
New Techniques in Hearing Loss Assessment
Infant Identification Programs
Prevention of Hearing Loss/Hearing Conservation
Minimal Hearing Loss
Classroom Management for Central Auditory Processing Disorders
Hearing Screening
Classroom Acoustics

Appendix 12–B

INSERVICE OUTLINES

TIPS FOR USING OUTLINES:

- Copy on 5×8 index cards.
- Start a new index card for each segment.
- Write down stopping points for each video or audio segment. Set at next beginning point immediately after playing segment.
- Color code supplementary materials (handouts, transparencies, video, equipment) and insert in sequence of use.
- Write out important points to emphasize for each segment.

TITLE: INTRODUCTION TO HEARING LOSS (3 hours)

TARGET AUDIENCE: TEACHERS/OTHER SCHOOL PERSONNEL

OBJECTIVES:

- Participants will acquire basic information related to the identification of hearing loss in the school-age population.
- Participants will gain knowledge about the impact of hearing loss on learning and the importance of early identification of hearing loss.
- Participants will be exposed to communication methods used by individuals who are deaf and hard-of-hearing, parent opinions concerning the selection of educational options, and equipment used in the assessment and management of hearing loss.

Initial Activity (3 minutes): Write one "burning question" on index cards

I. **Introduction** (20 minutes): Discussion of definitions, labels, perceptions that can limit expectations; IDEA language (person with disability); $ rationale for labels

    Supplementary Materials: *Access for All* video (from Gallaudet)
                                              Overhead of can labeled "Beans"
                                            Handout of current state definitions

    Activity: Discuss knowledge about can contents

II. **Anatomy of the Ear and Conductive Hearing Loss** (20 minutes): Briefly discuss how we hear and resources to teach topic in classrooms; high incidence of SOM in preschool/elementary population and effects on learning; importance of medical follow-up and current medical guidelines for Rx; other etiologies and Rx

    Supplementary Materials: *Access for all* video
                                              Handout: Diagram of ear
                                            Transparency: Same as handout
                                            Mock ossicles
                                            PE tube

    Activity: Identify audience members who have had children of their own or in class with otitis media and have them participate in discussion of treatment options.

III. **Sensorineural Hearing Loss** (20 minutes): Describe; incidence in local hearing impaired program; etiologies; treatment options/misperceptions—hearing aids, cochlear implants, acupuncture, chiropractic; importance of genetics in identification of etiology; noise and prevention; time of onset affects language learning (prelinguistic vs. postlinguistic)

    Supplementary Materials: *Access for all* video
                                              Earplugs
                                            Brochures on commercial hearing conservation programs

IV. Interpreting the Audiogram (20 minutes): Describe testing procedures and professionals' roles; screening vs. diagnostic testing and documentation on audiogram; amount and configuration of hearing loss; unilateral vs. bilateral; implications of hearing loss; percentage not accurate descriptor of what heard.

> Supplementary Materials: *Access for all* video
> Audiometer; tympanometer; otoscope
> Transparency: Audiologist; otologist, etc.
> Handouts/transparencies: Blank audiogram;
> *Audiogram of familiar sounds* (from AAA)

> Activity: Screen hearing and/or middle ear function during break.

V. Referral Procedures (10 minutes): Briefly review symptoms of hearing loss and how to refer for testing; describe need for early ID and recommendations for universal screening

> Supplementary Materials: Handouts: Signs of possible hearing loss;
> Referral steps for local program(s); *Your child's
> speech and hearing* (checklist from ASHA)

****BREAK****

VI. Impact of Hearing Loss (30 minutes): Overview of effect on communication, language, classroom learning; impact of noise and distance; discuss how state/system assesses eligibility for support services; importance of assessing individual needs and individualizing programs

> Supplementary Materials: *Access for all* video
> *Say what...?* audiotape
> Transparency: Eligibility components
> Handout: Psychosocial/Educational Impact (Anderson & Matkin)
> Sound field amplification system

> Activity: Audience pairs converse while turning backs to each other
> Activity: Identify reverberant surfaces in current classroom

Note: Sound field amplification system should be used during total inservice and turned off during discussion of the impact of noise, distance, and reverberation

VII. Support Strategies (30 minutes): Overview of support personnel and technology; communication methodologies

> Supplementary Materials: Samples of amplification equipment (hearing aid,
> personal FM system)
> Brochures on cochlear implants and assistive devices
> *State resource guide for hearing impaired*
> Transparencies: Support people and technology;
> Communication methodologies
> Handouts: *Do's and dont's for teachers;*
> *Communication options* (from Beginnings)

> Activity: Pass around amplification attached to stethoscope during this section; use mike for FM system while receiver being passed around

VIII. Summary (5 minutes or less): Hearing loss significantly affects communication, language, and learning, but many individual differences. Importance of early identification and individualized programming.

Final activity: Leave 5 minutes at a minimum to address any unanswered "burning questions."

TITLE: CLASSROOM AMPLIFICATION (45 minutes)

TARGET AUDIENCE: ADMINISTRATORS

OBJECTIVES:
- Participants will gain knowledge about sound-field FM amplification.
- Participants will experience sound-field amplification.
- Participants will receive information concerning benefits of using sound-field amplification in the classroom.

Initial activity (3–5 minutes): Participants and instructor introduce themselves while an audiotape of classroom noise is being played; show transparency and turn off tape. Reactions??

Materials needed:	Audiotape made in local classroom
	Transparency IV-1 from *Improving classroom acoustics*
	(ICA), "Classroom Acoustics and Listener Distress"

I. System Overview (15 minutes): Turn on sound-field FM system and identify microphone and speakers being used; explain equipment, advantages, and other system options (alternate microphone styles and speaker arrangements) following *ICA* transparencies

Materials needed:	Working sound-field FM
	Transparency IV-2, "Premise for Using FM Soundfield Amplification in Classrooms"
	Transparency IV-4, "Basis of FM Soundfield Amplification"
	Transparency IV-5, "Classroom Amplification System"
	Transparency IV-6, "Primary Advantages of FM Soundfield Amplification"

II. Benefits (15 minutes): Summarize research demonstrating benefit from soundfield amplification (MARRS study); identify at-risk populations with local statistics for each category.

Materials needed:	ICA Transparency IV-8, "Summary of FM Soundfield Benefits Based on Research Findings"
	Handout—annotated research studies on soundfield FM
	Transparency IV-9, "Other Pediatric Populations That May Benefit from FM Soundfield Classroom Amplification"
	Handout of transparency with local info for each category

III. Summary (10 minutes): Present classroom info for initial audiotape using classroom grid from ICA manual; proposal for trial period in local classrooms; questions and answers

Materials needed:	Classroom audiotape
	Transparency of classroom noise measurements
	Commercial packets

Activity:	Replay classroom tape while using soundfield FM and explaining grid
	Pass out commercial package on equipment proposed for trial, which includes estimated costs if purchased
	Schedule follow up appointments to select classrooms and develop plan for training and data collection

TITLE: HEARING AID MONITORING (1 hour)

TARGET AUDIENCE: SUPPORT PERSONNEL

OBJECTIVES:
- Participants will accurately identify parts of behind-the-ear (BTE) and in-the-ear (ITE) hearing aids.
- Participants will demonstrate competency in routine visual and listening checks for BTE and ITE hearing aids.
- Participants will demonstrate knowledge of solutions for typical hearing aid malfunctions.

Initial activity: Pre-test (5 minutes): Fill in the blank illustration of BTE and ITE hearing aids

I. Review parts of aids, using loaner BTE and ITE hearing aids (10 minutes): battery, on-off switch, volume control, microphone, tone/output controls, amplifier, tone hook, tubing, earmold. Identify make, model and serial number for each aid used. Distribute battery warning and demonstrate child-proof battery compartment. Group asked to ID parts on transparency.

> Materials needed: BTE and ITE hearing aids—no less than 1 for every 2 participants
> Handout/Transparency of Pre-test

II. Visual inspection and possible problems (20 minutes): Case, battery compartment, OTM switch, tone control, tubing, earmold; basic cleaning instructions; moisture problems and solutions

> Materials needed: Handout listing visual inspection components.
> Hearing aids with hole in tubing, scratched/dirty case, cerumen in earmold, loose/broken
> tone hook, missing battery door/tone control cover
> Cleaning "supplies," air blower
> Dri-aid kit and instructions

III. Listen check and possible problems (20 minutes): feedback; Ling sound check using stethoscope.
> Materials needed: Handout listing problems and trouble-shooting techniques
> Hearing aid stethoscopes
> Battery testers
> Hearing aids with battery upside down/dead; dead aid;
> aids with internal feedback, distortion, static

IV. Summary (5 minutes): Procedure for reporting problems that can't be solved during daily check; post-test (connect problems and trouble-shooting technique); questions and answers.

Note: Schedule follow-up classroom visit ASAP for any support personnel who are responsible for daily monitoring of hearing aids.

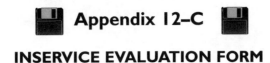

Appendix 12–C

INSERVICE EVALUATION FORM

INSERVICE TITLE:

DATE:

Please mark 1–5, with 1 = Strongly Agree to 5 = Strongly Disagree

1. Inservice content was appropriate for my needs   1 2 3 4 5

2. Inservice information was targeted for my level of knowledge   1 2 3 4 5

3. Presentations were interesting   1 2 3 4 5

4. Presentations were informative   1 2 3 4 5

5. Presenter was knowledgable about topic   1 2 3 4 5

6. I acquired relevant information during this inservice   1 2 3 4 5

7. I obtained materials/resources that I can apply in my work situation.   1 2 3 4 5

8. I would recommend that my colleagues attend this inservice if it were presented again.   1 2 3 4 5

9. What I liked best about this inservice:

10. What I liked least about this inservice:

11. Suggestions for improving this inservice in the future:

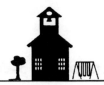

SECTION 13

APPENDIXES

Marketing

CONTENTS

*Appendixes marked with asterisks (*) are available on an optional computer disk which allows users to customize these forms.

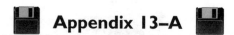

Appendix 13–A

18 REASONS WHY YOUR SCHOOL NEEDS AN EDUCATIONAL AUDIOLOGIST

- Provide community leadership to ensure that all infants, toddlers, and youth with impaired hearing are promptly identified, evaluated, and provided with appropriate intervention services

- Collaborate with community resources to develop a high-risk registry, newborn screening, and follow-up

- Coordinate hearing screening programs for preschool and school-aged children

- Train audiometric technicians or other appropriate personnel to screen for hearing loss

- Perform comprehensive, educationally relevant, hearing evaluations

- Assess central auditory function

- Make appropriate medical, educational, and community referrals

- Interpret audiological assessment results to other school personnel

- Assist in program placement as a member of the educational team to make specific recommendations for auditory and communication needs

- Provide inservice training on hearing and hearing impairments and their implications to school personnel, children, and parents

- Educate about noise exposure and hearing loss prevention

- Make recommendations about the use of hearing aids, cochlear implants, assistive listening devices, group and classroom amplification

- Ensure the proper fit and functioning of hearing aids and other auditory devices

- Analyze classroom noise and acoustics and make recommendations for improving the listening environment

- Manage the use and calibration of audiometric equipment

- Collaborate with school, parents, teachers, special support personnel, and relevant community agencies and professionals to ensure delivery of appropriate services

- Make recommendations for assistive devices (radio/television, telephone, alerting, convenience) for students with hearing impairments

- Provide services, including home programming if appropriate, in the areas of speechreading, listening, communication strategies, use and care of amplification, including cochlear implants, and self-management of hearing needs

Source: From the American Speech-Language-Hearing Association (1993). *Guidelines for audiology services in the schools.* Adapted by permission.

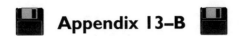

Appendix 13–B

MARKETING LETTER TO PARENTS AND TEACHERS

Dear Parents and Teachers:

Are you worried about your child's or student's hearing? Does he or she often ask you to repeat what you've said, miss instructions, turn up the volume of radio or TV? Has your child experienced frequent ear infections, or does he or she misunderstand what is said when it's noisy?

If you are concerned, an educational audiologist is available at your child's school.

WHAT DOES AN EDUCATIONAL AUDIOLOGIST DO?

• **TESTS HEARING**

The educational audiologist uses special equipment to determine if a child has a hearing loss and, if so, how much of a loss is present. Students with a hearing loss need to be seen by the educational audiologist on a regular basis. If you think your child may have a hearing loss or needs his/her hearing retested, contact your school's audiologist at the address or phone number above about scheduling an appointment.

• **PROVIDES EDUCATIONALLY-RELATED MANAGEMENT FOR HEARING LOSS**

Educational audiologists select, recommend, and work with hearing aids and other listening devices that benefit children with temporary or permanent hearing loss. They also provide information to children, teachers, and parents about hearing loss and how it affects learning.

Educational audiologists can offer suggestions to help a child with a hearing loss in school, such as which seat might be the best for listening and watching, as well as what equipment might be helpful to the student in the classroom. They also help students and teachers with ways to keep this equipment working well.

Educational audiologists can also help students learn ways to function better in the classroom, including help with lipreading (or speechreading), listening skills, and ways to cope with hearing loss at school and at home.

• **HELPS PREVENT HEARING LOSS**

Educational audiologists help all children by assisting with hearing conservation programs and increasing awareness about the dangers of noise on hearing. As your school's educational audiologist, I have information about ways to protect hearing which I would be happy to share with you.

Please contact me if you would like additional information.

Sincerely,

Educational Audiologist

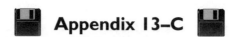

Appendix 13–C

MARKETING LETTER TO STUDENTS

Dear

       My name is _____, and I am your EDUCATIONAL AUDI-OLOGIST. Even though we have talked before, I thought it might help for you to know what I do in my job.

—I test students' hearing and help them learn about their ears.

—I often recommend hearing aids or other equipment that can help students hear better in school.

—I help students who use hearing aids learn how to take care of them and what to do when they break.

—For students who use other equipment (like personal FM or speaker systems), I can help with the care of this equipment, too.

—Sometimes I see students once or twice a week to help with learning to listen and understand teachers and other students.

—I also help students learn about their ears, their hearing, and ways to prevent hearing loss.

—I can help students explain their hearing loss to teachers and other students.

—Sometimes I help students learn new ways to understand other people when they are in situations where it is hard to hear.

—I also teach teachers, parents, and other people in the school about hearing and hearing loss.

I have checked the things you and I have already decided we should do. If you would like me to help with anything else, just let me know the next time I see you, or you can contact me at

_____.

                                    Sincerely,

                                    Educational Audiologist

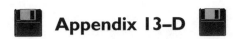

Appendix 13–D

INDEX CARD INFORMATION FOR MARKETING

DID YOU KNOW . . .

⇒   that _____ school system serves ____ students with hearing impairment?

⇒   that we have _____ teachers of the hearing impaired and _____ interpreters in our district?

⇒   that our students in _____ grade are learning sign language and each one has a sign for his or her name?

⇒   that _____ students have had their hearing screened so far this year?

⇒   that one of our students who is hearing impaired received a "75 Stars" award from Miss America last year?

⇒   that one of our high school students who is deaf plays on the soccer team and is teaching the coach to sign to him on the field?

⇒   that you can contact you school's audiologist, _____, by calling _____?

EQUIPMENT AVAILABLE FOR STUDENTS
AND TEACHERS IN _____ DISTRICT

The following equipment is available for short- or long-term loan for use in your classroom:

⇒   Sound Field Amplification System
⇒   Personal FM Units
⇒   TDD (Telephone Device for the Deaf)
⇒   TV Caption Adaptor
⇒   Amplified Telephone Training Unit
⇒   Sound Level Meter
⇒   3-D Model of the Ear
⇒   Sample Earplugs

Contact _____, Educational Audiologist, at
_____ for details.

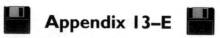 **Appendix 13–E**

CONSUMER SURVEY OF AUDIOLOGY SERVICES

School District _____ Date _____

Name of Individual Completing Survey_____

Agency or Clinic Name _____

Directions: Please rate the indicated service according to the following scale:

1 = In place and working well
2 = In place but needs modification
3 = Developing
4 = Not present at this time
5 = Not applicable

- School-based audiology services are coordinated with community-based services to increase family access to services.   1 2 3 4 5

- School-based audiology services support community resources in the development and delivery of the following:

	1	2	3	4	5
High-risk registry	1	2	3	4	5
Newborn screening	1	2	3	4	5
Follow-up services to identify and manage infants, toddlers, and children with hearing loss	1	2	3	4	5
Information for families regarding service and equipment options for children with hearing loss	1	2	3	4	5

- School-based audiology services have ongoing communication with community resources.   1 2 3 4 5

Please identify the major strengths of the educational audiology service program:

Please identify your major concerns about the educational audiology service program:

How did you first learn of the_____ educational audiology services?

Thank you for assisting us in improving our educational audiology program. Write your address below if you would like current information on our services.

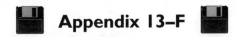

Appendix 13–F

MARKETING EFFECTIVENESS LOG

Marketing Strategy	Date	Target Audience	Response	Date

Key to responses: 1 = Referral or request for specific service   2 = Request for information   3 = Request for repeat presentation   4 = Financial or other program support   5 = Other (describe)

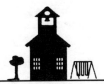

SECTION 14

APPENDIXES

Program Development, Evaluation, and Management

CONTENTS

*Appendixes marked with asterisks (*) are available on an optional computer disk which allows users to customize these forms.

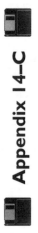

Appendix 14–C

SELF-ASSESSMENT: EFFECTIVENESS INDICATORS FOR AUDIOLOGY SERVICES IN THE SCHOOLS

Educational Audiologist _____ Date _____ School District _____

EFFECTIVENESS INDICATORS	STATUS[1]				ACTION PLAN/COMMENTS
	A	E	G	NA	
I. Community/Family Collaboration:					
a. Audiologist conducts on-going awareness activities regarding hearing loss.					
b. Audiologist networks with local ENTs, hearing aid dispensers, children's disability programs, and other audiologists.					
c. Audiologist collaborates with other community agencies dealing with hearing loss.					
d. Audiologist seeks input from Deaf/hard-of-hearing community members/groups.					
e. Audiologist recognizes and respects the ethnic, cultural and language backgrounds of families.					
f. All notices and conference notes are provided to parents in their native language.					
g. Audiologist provides a network which enables "experienced" parents of HI child to support parents of children newly diagnosed.					
h. Audiologist provides support to parents on coping with hearing loss and helping them to understand the importance of accepting their child with a HI.					
i. Audiologist maintains regular and frequent, formal and informal, home-school communication to ensure coordination and consistency of services.					
j. Audiologist helps families understand the nature and implications of hearing loss and the importance of consistent communication with their child.					
k. Audiologist informs family of community resources and financial aid and how to access them, of available assistive devices such as TDDs, and closed captioning devices, of functions and publications for HI.					

individuals, and of opportunities for interaction with HI role models when appropriate.

II. Prevention

a. Yearly awareness efforts include information about normal auditory, speech and language development, establishment of at-risk registers, the value of early identification, and where and how to obtain screening and audiologic evaluation.

b. Hearing loss prevention is part of school health curricula.

III. Identification

a. A community interagency process for the identification of hearing loss is in place which includes local ENTs, pediatricians, family physicians, county health departments, and local audiologists.

b. Hearing screening opportunities are available year round.

c. Hearing screening is provided annually for all state mandated ages and grade levels (including children in private schools) or in accordance with accepted professional guidelines.

d. Screening includes tympanometry for all young children and other children at risk for OM.

e. Hearing screening is conducted in accordance with professionally acceptable procedures and referral criteria.

f. Audiometers used for screening are calibrated to ANSI S3.6, 1996 specifications and are checked at least annually and recalibrated when necessary.

g. Screening facilities are checked for ambient noise so as not exceed acceptable levels.

h. Hearing screening information is recorded and parents and teachers are informed of results.

---

[1]A = Accomplished   E = Emerging   G = Goal   NA = Not Applicable at this time.
When determining program status, consider the following characteristics of the service: comprehensiveness, accessibility, coordination, consistency, accountability, efficiency, and collaboration.

EFFECTIVENESS INDICATORS	STATUS[1]				ACTION PLAN/COMMENTS
	A	E	G	NA	
i. All screening failures are referred for either audiologic assessment by an audiologist at no expense to the parents, or for medical examination.					
j. Follow-up procedures exist to ensure that individuals who are referred for audiologic assessment or medical treatment or who need annual monitoring of their hearing status receive the recommended service.					
k. All children who meet the state's criteria for educationally significant hearing loss (ESHL) are referred to either a building level conferences or to a full special education assessment and staffing.					
l. Audiologist attends pre-referral conference to represent unique needs of HI students.					
IV. Assessment					
a. Assessment is multidisciplinary and multifaceted and includes at least one specialist in the area of hearing.					
b. Audiology assessment is comprehensive with additional tests (e.g., ABR, OAEs) recommended when necessary. Audiology assessment minimally includes: case history, otoscopic inspection, acoustic immittance, pure tone audiometry, speech reception or detection threshold, word recognition/speech discrimination; speech in noise, quiet, and visual only conditions are included for students with ESHL.					
c. For individuals with hearing aids and FM or other devices, assessment includes aided speech testing, electroacoustical analysis of amplification, and real ear verification procedures.					
V. Amplification					
a. Audiologist evaluates and determines need for assistive amplification device (all students					

with educationally significant hearing loss should be considered candidates for amplification until ruled out).				
b. Amplification equipment is provided to support all needs identified on the IEPs.				
c. Hearing aids worn by Deaf/HH children are checked daily for proper functioning.				
VI. Management and Habilitation/Rehabilitation				
a. Audiologist provides specific, on-going training relating to the development of communication skills including auditory training, expansion of speech and language, use of hearing aid(s) and assistive listening devices(ALDs), and hearing aid/ALD maintenance.				
b. Audiologist is a regular team member in IEP development.				
c. IEPs are developed jointly by staff, specialists trained in hearing, and the family.				
d. IEP goals and objectives are written and implemented for hearing needs across a variety of environments and situations.				
e. Audiologist provides consultation services to teachers such as inservice on appropriate accommodations and technical assistance regarding equipment.				
f. Audiologist provides specific information and training to student on accommodations, hearing aid maintenance, and community resources related to hearing needs.				
VII. Program Management and Development				
a. Audiologist has a sufficient budget to carry out effective identification and services to HI students.				
b. District minimally employs audiologist at 1:12,000 (average daily membership).				
c. Facilities are adequate for all instructional and related services to students with HI				

[1]A = Accomplished   E = Emerging   G = Goal   NA = Not Applicable at this time.
When determining program status, consider the following characteristics of the service: comprehensiveness, accessibility, coordination, consistency, accountability, efficiency, and collaboration.

STATUS[1]

EFFECTIVENESS INDICATORS	A	E	G	NA	ACTION PLAN/COMMENTS
including accommodations where appropriate for noise, lighting, and special seating.					
d. A needs assessment, program evaluation, and planning process is conducted.					
e. Promising practices in audiology are known and utilized.					
f. Audiologist is provided with opportunities to attend workshops and inservice training.					
g. Audiologist is evaluated regularly by a special education supervisor who understands issues in hearing or a combination of a selected peer audiologist and a program administrator.					

[1]A = Accomplished　E = Emerging　G = Goal　NA = Not Applicable at this time.
When determining program status, consider the following characteristics of the service: comprehensiveness, accessibility, coordination, consistency, accountability, efficiency, and collaborative.

Source: From "Administrative Unit On-site Checklist," the Colorado Department of Education Special Education Unit. Adapted by permission.

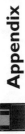 Appendix 14–B

GOAL PRIORITIZATION WORKSHEET

In the boxes across the top, write the goals or objectives that are under consideration. Rate them using the listed criteria. The higher the total score, the more likely that the objective is appropriate.

Goals/objectives 1 2 3 4 5 Little Great						
Importance What is the urgency or impact?						
Control To what extent do you have control?						
Difficulty What is the relative difficulty of achieving it?						
Time Required How much time is required to achieve it?						
Return on Investment What is the expected payoff?						
Resource Requirement What skills, space, etc. are needed?						
Total Points						

Appendix 14–C

LONG-RANGE PLANNING FORM[1]

PROGRAM COMPONENT	GOALS	1ST YEAR		2ND YEAR	
		ACTIVITIES	BUDGET/RESOURCES	ACTIVITIES	BUDGET/RESOURCES

[1]Activities, budget, and resources may be added for subsequent years to attain desired length of long-range plan.

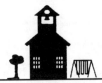

SECTION 15

APPENDIXES

Sentence and Phrase Lists

CONTENTS

*Appendixes with asterisks (*) are available on an optional computer disk which allows users to customize these forms.

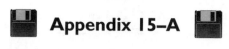

Appendix 15–A

WIPI SENTENCES

<u>List 1</u>

PRACTICE: The boy swung his <u>bat</u> in the baseball game.

1. We go to <u>school</u> to play and learn.
2. We throw the <u>ball</u> and play catch.
3. The fire sends <u>smoke</u> up the chimney.
4. We walk on the <u>floor</u> and then we sweep it.
5. The sharp teeth of a <u>fox</u> can bite you.
6. Daddy wears a <u>hat</u> when it is raining.
7. We cook eggs in the <u>pan</u> for breakfast.
8. We like sandwiches made with <u>bread</u> and butter.
9. Your <u>neck</u> helps you move your head.
10. We walk up and down the <u>stair</u> in the house.
11. We must open each <u>eye</u> to see.
12. I fell on my <u>knee</u> and hurt it.
13. The cars on the <u>street</u> were driving to the park.
14. The bird uses its <u>wing</u> to fly.
15. The cheese in the trap scared the <u>mouse</u> in the house.
16. Daddy wears a <u>shirt</u> with his uniform.
17. The cowboy used his <u>gun</u> to shoot wild animals.
18. We ride on the <u>bus</u> to go to school.
19. We ride on the <u>train</u> when we go on a trip.
20. The muscles in your <u>arm</u> help you move your hand.
21. The baby <u>chick</u> came out of the egg.
22. The baby in the <u>crib</u> was sleeping.
23. The car's <u>wheel</u> turned very fast.
24. We use a <u>straw</u> to drink soda.
25. We put water in the <u>pail</u> at the beach.

<u>List 2</u>

PRACTICE: The furry grey <u>cat</u> played with a string.

1. We use the <u>broom</u> to sweep the floor.
2. We eat cereal from a <u>bowl</u> at breakfast.
3. We wear a <u>coat</u> when it is cold and windy.
4. Open the <u>door</u> and go in the house.
5. We wear <u>socks</u> to keep our feet warm.
6. The American <u>flag</u> was blowing on the pole.
7. When it is warm, the <u>fan</u> blows cool air.
8. Where is that <u>red</u> apple?
9. Sit at the <u>desk</u> and do your homework.
10. In the forest the <u>bear</u> was eating honey.
11. I like to eat <u>pie</u> for dessert.
12. I drink hot <u>tea</u> when I have a cold.
13. We eat <u>meat</u> for dinner.
14. We need a <u>string</u> to fly the kite.
15. We laughed at the funny <u>clown</u> at the circus.
16. We go to <u>church</u> to pray.
17. I can wiggle my <u>thumb</u> and fingers.
18. We walked on the <u>rug</u> on the floor.
19. I like to eat chocolate <u>cake</u> on my birthday.
20. The animals in the <u>barn</u> were cows and horses.
21. I played with a <u>stick</u> in the sand.
22. The pirates sailed the <u>ship</u> in the water.
23. In the water was a slippery <u>seal</u> playing ball.
24. When I pet the <u>dog</u>, he stops barking.
25. Daddy hammered the <u>nail</u> into the wood.

List 3

PRACTICE: We sat on the <u>grass</u> and ate our lunch.

1. At night, the <u>moon</u> shines in the sky.
2. In the morning, the school <u>bell</u> will ring.
3. I want to drink <u>coke</u> with my lunch.
4. We eat <u>corn</u> on the cob in summer time.
5. Mother put some toys in the <u>box</u> to surprise us.
6. We filled the grocery <u>bag</u> with food from the market.
7. The cook opened a <u>can</u> of food to eat for lunch.
8. The tailor uses <u>thread</u> to sew the clothing.
9. The mother bird in the <u>nest</u> sat on the eggs.
10. Dad was sitting in the <u>chair</u> reading the newspaper.
11. There was a <u>fly</u> buzzing around the room.
12. We turned the <u>key</u> to unlock the door.
13. We use our two <u>feet</u> to walk and run.
14. The rocking horse <u>spring</u> jumps up and down.
15. The queen wears a <u>crown</u> on her head.
16. We played in the <u>dirt</u> and got very messy.
17. On a warm day, the <u>sun</u> shines brightly.
18. Father drinks coffee from his <u>cup</u> after dinner.
19. The poisonous <u>snake</u> in the grass can bite you.
20. Mother drove the <u>car</u> to the store.
21. We use a <u>dish</u> when we eat our cereal.
22. The baby wears a <u>bib</u> to keep his clothes from getting dirty.
23. The king and <u>queen</u> live in the castle.
24. Dad used the <u>saw</u> to cut the wood.
25. The bad people in the <u>jail</u> wanted to go home.

List 4

PRACTICE: We drink juice from a <u>glass</u> for breakfast.

1. We use a <u>spoon</u> to eat our soup.
2. The little girl wore a <u>bow</u> in her hair.
3. At the farm, the <u>goat</u> was eating grass.
4. The clown blew the <u>horn</u> and made a loud noise.
5. We can play with the <u>blocks</u> and build a house.
6. At night, the color of the sky is <u>black</u> and very dark.
7. My father is a <u>man</u> who is very strong.
8. I sleep in my <u>bed</u> with my head on the pillow.
9. The girl was wearing a <u>dress</u> made of cotton.
10. We picked a <u>pear</u> from the tree to eat.
11. The man wore a <u>tie</u> around his neck.
12. If you take his honey, the <u>bee</u> might sting you.
13. Inside his mouth are <u>teeth</u> that can bite.
14. The bride wore a <u>ring</u> on her finger.
15. We use our <u>mouth</u> to smile.
16. The plaid <u>skirt</u> was worn with a belt.
17. I like to chew <u>gum</u> and eat candy.
18. I see a <u>bug</u> crawling in the garden.
19. The pilot will fly a jet <u>plane</u> to England.
20. It is night when a <u>star</u> shines in the sky.
21. We tried to catch a <u>fish</u> swimming in the water.
22. Mother kissed my <u>lip</u> and smiled.
23. The grass is <u>green</u> on the hillside.
24. The green <u>frog</u> jumped and said, "Ribbet!"
25. The horse's <u>tail</u> was long and brown.

Source: "A sentence test for measuring speech discrimination in children" by S. Weber and R.C. Reddell, 1976, *Audiology and Hearing Education, 2,* pp. 25–31. Copyright 1976 by Audiology & Hearing Education. Reprinted by permission.

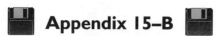

Appendix 15–B

PEDIATRIC SPEECH INTELLIGIBILITY (PSI) SENTENCES, LEVEL I

Card A:

1. Show me a rabbit painting an egg.

2. Show me a bear brushing his teeth.

3. Show me a horse eating an apple.

4. Show me a rabbit putting on his shoes.

5. Show me a bear combing his hair.

Card B:

6. Show me a bear drinking milk.

7. Show me a fox roller skating.

8. Show me a rabbit kicking a football.

9. Show me a bear eating a sandwich.

10. Show me a rabbit reading a book.

Source: "Pediatric speech intelligibility test: Manual for administration" by S. Jerger and J. Jerger, 1984, St. Louis, MO: Auditec of St. Louis. Reprinted by permission.

Appendix 15–C

BLAIR SENTENCES

Group 1

1. The <u>bean</u> is in the <u>jar</u>.
2. A <u>goose</u> is a large <u>bird</u>.
3. That yellow <u>jug</u> costs a <u>dime</u>.
4. This <u>hat</u> is made from <u>wool</u>.
5. Please <u>lock</u> the <u>van</u> doors.
6. The man <u>dug</u> a long <u>ditch</u>.
7. I left my <u>knife</u> at <u>home</u>.
8. I <u>wish</u> we had a <u>kite</u>.
9. Sew the <u>patch</u> on my <u>shirt</u>.
10. Go <u>pick</u> a big, <u>ripe</u> apple.
11. The <u>wheel</u> will <u>fit</u> the cart.
12. The young <u>king</u> was very <u>mad</u>.
13. The <u>tooth</u> is <u>thin</u> and white.
14. His <u>name</u> is <u>tough</u> to spell.
15. A <u>rose</u> died in the <u>fall</u>.
16. The <u>sun</u> warmed the lake <u>shore</u>.
17. Freddy <u>sees</u> a <u>toad</u> beside him.
18. I <u>hope</u> you have a <u>robe</u>.
19. <u>Make</u> a <u>loop</u> in your rope.
20. The chicken soup will <u>boil</u> <u>soon</u>.
21. Try to <u>guess</u> the correct <u>route</u>.
22. <u>Sell</u> me <u>that</u> little, brown dog.
23. <u>Leave</u> your <u>cape</u> on the bed.
24. Your <u>mail</u> is on the <u>chair</u>.
25. The teacher will <u>check</u> each <u>page</u>.

Group 2

1. Jim will <u>beg</u> for a <u>car</u>.
2. The big zooming <u>jet</u> is <u>late</u>.
3. Father will <u>choose</u> a car <u>tire</u>.
4. Put your <u>coat</u> on that <u>rail</u>.
5. I saw mother <u>burn</u> the <u>beef</u>.
6. Fix the <u>leak</u> in the <u>dam</u>.
7. <u>Dodge</u> the big, round, <u>red</u> ball.
8. Girls <u>love</u> to <u>suck</u> yellow candy.
9. I <u>met</u> Susan at the <u>gate</u>.
10. <u>Tall</u> trees are full of <u>sap</u>.
11. The <u>cub</u> made a lot of <u>noise</u>.
12. The big <u>nurse</u> killed every <u>germ</u>.
13. Tell me <u>which</u> <u>goal</u> is ours.
14. I ate <u>four</u> pieces of <u>ham</u>.
15. That green <u>ring</u> is a <u>fake</u>.
16. <u>Dive</u> under the water to <u>hide</u>.
17. <u>Wash</u> your dishes in a <u>pail</u>.
18. <u>Lead</u> me to your new <u>house</u>.
19. The <u>moon</u> <u>should</u> come up tonight.
20. The big <u>pan</u> is too <u>large</u>.
21. The <u>pup</u> will <u>wag</u> his tail.
22. Your <u>chin</u> moves when you <u>talk</u>.
23. That <u>vine</u> has a long <u>root</u>.
24. <u>This</u> little <u>seal</u> loves to swim.
25. The <u>ship</u> sailed <u>south</u> last night.

Group 3

1. You <u>did</u> get my little <u>note</u>.
2. The <u>dog</u> <u>caught</u> the blue ball.
3. I <u>have</u> a <u>lame</u> foot today.
4. I like a big <u>cool</u> <u>coke</u>.
5. <u>Shoot</u> one <u>young</u> rabbit for dinner.
6. <u>Save</u> the <u>bun</u> for the hamburger.
7. Please <u>pass</u> me more good <u>fish</u>.
8. <u>Join</u> me for a long <u>nap</u>.
9. That <u>sure</u> was a <u>dumb</u> letter.
10. Paint a <u>mouth</u> on that <u>face</u>.
11. I can almost <u>reach</u> that <u>far</u>.
12. The <u>hill</u> was a <u>mile</u> high.
13. <u>Geese</u> are <u>such</u> pretty big birds.
14. Stick the <u>gun</u> in his <u>rib</u>.
15. I <u>bet</u> you feel very <u>sad</u>.
16. That man has a <u>big</u> <u>laugh</u>.
17. That tall <u>pine</u> tree is <u>mine</u>.
18. I <u>lose</u> money on that <u>ride</u>.
19. Get the <u>third</u> can of <u>tar</u>.
20. He <u>led</u> me to <u>big</u> John.
21. The water <u>hole</u> <u>was</u> very deep.
22. <u>Jim</u> went to <u>vote</u> last night.
23. <u>Tap</u> one <u>cheek</u> with your finger.
24. You got my new <u>tape</u> <u>wet</u>.
25. Put the <u>pearl</u> in a <u>sack</u>.

Group 4
1. That is a <u>nice</u> <u>birch</u> tree.
2. Your <u>foot</u> has a broken <u>bone</u>.
3. The <u>bug</u> fell in his <u>lap</u>.
4. <u>Shake</u> the <u>can</u> before you pour.
5. We will <u>give</u> mother a <u>wig</u>.
6. <u>Take</u> the <u>date</u> off the calendar.
7. The <u>chief</u> will <u>hire</u> three men.
8. The man <u>said</u> it would <u>hail</u>.
9. You can <u>read</u> by the <u>pool</u>.
10. The <u>path</u> led to a <u>mill</u>.
11. <u>Keep</u> working on that hard <u>job</u>.
12. The <u>lone</u> ranger <u>shut</u> the door.
13. The new <u>towel</u> was very <u>long</u>.

14. Put the <u>phone</u> in my <u>room</u>.
15. <u>Pack</u> the <u>mop</u> in the car.
16. Catch a <u>moth</u> with a <u>net</u>.
17. The <u>bus</u> stopped for some <u>gas</u>.
18. Spell the <u>word</u> "<u>tool</u>" for me.
19. Please <u>serve</u> the boys some <u>rice</u>.
20. My <u>cough</u> has lasted five <u>days</u>.
21. Take your <u>thumb</u> off that <u>dish</u>.
22. That is <u>your</u> dirty, black <u>sock</u>.
23. Your <u>voice</u> sounds <u>loud</u> to me.
24. Please <u>write</u> <u>when</u> you get home.
25. Go try to <u>cheer</u> <u>him</u> up.

Group 5
1. Go <u>bathe</u> that dirty, old <u>doll</u>.
2. Lie on your <u>back</u> and <u>sing</u>.
3. Put the <u>peg</u> in the <u>cup</u>.
4. I will <u>sail</u> by the <u>beach</u>.
5. <u>Tell</u> me when the <u>cab</u> comes.
6. An egg <u>yolk</u> can be <u>food</u>.
7. The <u>man</u> fell off the <u>limb.</u>
8. Take <u>care</u> of my new <u>purse</u>.
9. Get me <u>five</u> pieces of <u>chalk</u>.
10. <u>Dip</u> you doughnut in <u>hot</u> chocolate.
11. A <u>town</u> needs <u>coal</u> for heat.
12. Put the <u>wire</u> on the <u>dock</u>.
13. He <u>let</u> me wear one <u>boot</u>.

14. The <u>judge</u> wore a <u>knit</u> sweater.
15. The paper <u>match</u> is <u>half</u> burned.
16. Be careful <u>with</u> your <u>sore</u> foot.
17. With <u>luck</u> I'll get some <u>gum</u>.
18. <u>Run</u> and get me a <u>rock</u>.
19. That green <u>vase</u> really looks <u>good</u>.
20. It is really <u>mean</u> to <u>tease</u>.
21. <u>Hush</u> or the <u>worm</u> will move.
22. I <u>need</u> a long, thin <u>nail</u>.
23. He <u>shot</u> at the lion's <u>paws</u>.
24. That <u>light</u> yellow flower is <u>real</u>.
25. It rained, <u>then</u> the <u>roof</u> leaked.

Group 6
1. Go <u>sit</u> down you <u>bad</u> boy!
2. I watched the <u>birth</u> of a <u>calf</u>.
3. <u>Move</u> that small <u>tube</u> of water.
4. I go to <u>bed</u> at <u>night</u>.
5. <u>Get</u> a <u>cage</u> for the rabbit.
6. <u>Turn</u> around and <u>hit</u> the ball.
7. The blue <u>cheese</u> is all <u>gone</u>.
8. Put the <u>chain</u> on the <u>door</u>.
9. Jack <u>paid</u> me for the <u>whip</u>.
10. My <u>niece</u> played in the <u>rain</u>.
11. Go <u>fan</u> the <u>fire</u> a little.
12. Take your <u>map</u> on the <u>hike</u>.
13. Some TV <u>shows</u> are very <u>dull</u>.

14. <u>Search</u> under the <u>rug</u> for money.
15. Tell me one <u>more</u> funny <u>joke</u>.
16. You can <u>hop</u> on my <u>lawn</u>.
17. <u>Look</u> at that pretty flower <u>bud</u>.
18. <u>Knock</u> the long, blue <u>pole</u> down.
19. The <u>cat</u> bit the bird's <u>wing</u>.
20. All the <u>team</u> wore red <u>shoes</u>.
21. The <u>vowel</u> ee is in <u>piece</u>.
22. <u>Dig</u> a <u>well</u> to find water.
23. <u>Rush</u> home and <u>call</u> your father.
24. I <u>live</u> with my pretty <u>wife</u>.
25. This <u>jam</u> tastes <u>sour</u> to me.

Source: "The contributing influences of amplification, speechreading, and classroom environments on the ability of hard of hearing children to discriminate sentences" by J.C. Blair, 1976, Unpublished doctoral dissertation, Northwestern University, Evanston, IL. Reprinted by permission.

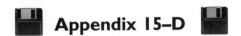

Appendix 15–D

BAMFORD-KOVAL-BENCH/STANDARD AMERICAN ENGLISH (BKB/SAE) SENTENCES

Sentence List 1

1. The clown had a funny face.
2. The car engine's running.
3. She cut with her knife.
4. Children like strawberries.
5. The house had nine rooms.
6. They're buying some bread.
7. The green tomatoes are small.
8. He played with his train.
9. The mailman shut the gate.
10. They're looking at the clock.
11. The bag sits on the ground.
12. The boy did a handstand.
13. A cat sits on the bed.
14. The truck carried fruit.
15. The rain came down.
16. The ice cream was pink.

Sentence List 2

1. The ladder's near the door.
2. They had a lovely day.
3. The ball went into the basket.
4. The old gloves are dirty.
5. He cut his finger.
6. The thin dog was hungry.
7. The boy knew the game.
8. Snow falls at Christmas.
9. She's taking her coat.
10. The police chased the car.
11. A mouse ran down the hole.
12. The lady's making a toy.
13. Some sticks were under the tree.
14. The little baby sleeps.
15. They're watching the train.
16. The movie finished early.

Sentence List 3

1. The glass bowl broke.
2. The dog played with a stick.
3. The kettle's quite hot.
4. The farmer feeds a bull.
5. They say some silly things.
6. The lady wore a coat.
7. The children are walking home.
8. He needed his vacation.
9. The milk came in a bottle.
10. The man cleaned his shoes.
11. They ate the lemon jelly.
12. The boy's running away.
13. Father looked at the book.
14. She drinks from her cup.
15. The room's getting cold.
16. A girl kicked the table.

Sentence List 4

1. The wife helped her husband.
2. The machine was quite noisy.
3. The old man worries.
4. A boy ran down the path.
5. The house had a nice garden.
6. She spoke to her son.
7. They're crossing the street.
8. Lemons grow on trees.
9. He found his brother.
10. Some animals sleep on straw.
11. The jam jar was full.
12. They're kneeling down.
13. The girl lost her doll.
14. The cook's making a cake.
15. The child grabs the toy.
16. The mud stuck on his shoe.

Sentence List 5

1. The bath towel was wet.
2. The matches are on the shelf.
3. They're running past the house.
4. The train had a bad crash.
5. The kitchen sink's empty.
6. A boy fell from the window.
7. She used her spoon.
8. The park's near the road.
9. The cook cut some onions.
10. The dog made an angry noise.
11. He's washing his face.
12. Somebody took the money.
13. The light went out.
14. They wanted some potatoes.
15. The naughty girl's shouting.
16. The cold milk's in a jug.

Sentence List 6

1. The paint dripped on the ground.
2. The mother stirs the tea.
3. They laughed at his story.
4. Men wear long pants.
5. The small boy was asleep.
6. The lady goes to the shop.
7. The sun melted the snow.
8. The father's coming home.
9. She had her pocket money.
10. The truck drove up the road.
11. He's bringing his raincoat.
12. A sharp knife's dangerous.
13. They took some food.
14. The clever girls are reading.
15. The broom stood in the corner.
16. The woman cleaned her house.

Sentence List 7

1. The children dropped the bag.
2. The dog came back.
3. The floor looked clean.
4. She found her purse.
5. The fruit lies on the ground.
6. Mother gets a saucepan.
7. They washed in cold water.
8. The young people are dancing.
9. The bus went early.
10. They had two empty bottles.
11. A ball's bouncing along.
12. The father forgot the bread.
13. The girl has a picture book.
14. The orange was quite sweet.
15. He's holding his nose.
16. The new road's on the map.

Sentence List 8

1. The boy forgot his book.
2. A friend came for lunch.
3. The match boxes are empty.
4. He climbed his ladder.
5. The family bought a house.
6. The jug stood on the shelf.
7. The ball broke the window.
8. They're shopping for cheese.
9. The pond water's dirty.
10. They heard a funny noise.
11. The police are clearing the road.
12. The bus stopped suddenly.
13. She writes to her brother.
14. The teacher lost a boot.
15. The three girls are listening.
16. The coat lies on a chair.

Source: "BKB Sentence Lists" by J. Bamford, A. Koval, and J. Bench in *Speech-hearing tests and the spoken language of partially-hearing children* by J. Bench and J. Bamford, 1979, New York: Academic Press. Copyright 1979 by Academic Press. Adapted by permission. "BKB/SAE Sentence Lists" by O.T. Kenworthy, T. Klee, and A. Tharpe, 1990. Reprinted by permission.

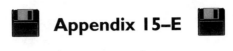

Appendix 15–E

SPIN SENTENCES

The H or L at the left of each sentence indicates whether the key word has high or low predictability.

Sentence List 1

H 1. The watchdog gave a warning <u>growl</u>.
H 2. She made the bed with clean <u>sheets</u>.
L 3. The old man discussed the <u>dive</u>.
L 4. Bob heard Paul called about the <u>strips</u>.
L 5. I should have considered the <u>map</u>.
H 6. The old train was powered by <u>steam</u>.
H 7. He caught the fish in his <u>net</u>.
L 8. Miss Brown shouldn't discuss the <u>sand</u>.
H 9. Close the window to stop the <u>draft</u>.
H 10. My T.V. has a twelve-inch <u>screen</u>.
L 11. They might have considered the <u>hive</u>.
L 12. David has discussed the <u>dent</u>.
H 13. The sandal has a broken <u>strap</u>.
H 14. The boat sailed along the <u>coast</u>.
H 15. Crocodiles live in muddy <u>swamps</u>.
L 16. He can't consider the <u>crib</u>.
H 17. The farmer harvested his <u>crop</u>.
H 18. All the flowers were in <u>bloom</u>.
L 19. I am thinking about his <u>knife</u>.
L 20. David does not discuss the <u>hug</u>.
H 21. She wore a feather in her <u>cap</u>.
L 22. We've been discussing the <u>crates</u>.
L 23. Miss Black knew about the <u>doll</u>.
H 24. The admiral commands the <u>fleet</u>.
L 25. She couldn't discuss the <u>pine</u>.
L 26. Miss Black thought about the <u>lap</u>.
H 27. The beer drinkers raised their <u>mugs</u>.

H 28. He was hit by a poisoned <u>dart</u>.
H 29. The bread was made from whole <u>wheat</u>.
L 30. Mr. Black knew about the <u>pad</u>.
L 31. You heard Jane called about the <u>van</u>.
H 32. I made the phone call from the <u>booth</u>.
L 33. Tom wants to know about the <u>cake</u>.
L 34. She's spoken about the <u>bomb</u>.
H 35. The cut on his knee formed a <u>scab</u>.
L 36. We hear you called about the <u>lock</u>.
L 37. The old man discussed the <u>yell</u>.
H 38. His boss made him work like a <u>slave</u>.
H 39. The farmer baled the <u>hay</u>.
L 40. They're glad we heard about the <u>track</u>.
H 41. A termite looks like an <u>ant</u>.
H 42. Air mail requires a special <u>stamp</u>.
H 43. Football is a dangerous <u>sport</u>.
L 44. Sue was interested in the <u>bruise</u>.
L 45. Ruth will consider the <u>herd</u>.
H 46. We saw a flock of wild <u>geese</u>.
L 47. The girl talked about the <u>gin</u>.
L 48. Paul can't discuss the <u>wax</u>.
H 49. Drop the coin through the <u>slot</u>.
L 50. I hope Paul asked about the <u>mate</u>.

Sentence List 2

L 1. You're glad they heard about the <u>slave</u>.
L 2. The girl knows about the <u>swamps</u>.
H 3. Hold the baby on your <u>lap</u>.
H 4. For your birthday I baked a <u>cake</u>.
H 5. The railroad train ran off the <u>track</u>.
L 6. They did not discuss the <u>screen</u>.
L 7. They were interested in the <u>strap</u>.
H 8. Tear off some paper from the <u>pad</u>.
L 9. I had a problem with the <u>bloom</u>.
L 10. Peter should speak about the <u>mugs</u>.
H 11. The fruit was shipped in wooden <u>crates</u>.
H 12. The rancher rounded up his <u>herd</u>.
L 13. She wants to speak about the <u>ant</u>.

L 14. We're discussing the <u>sheets</u>.
L 15. The boy would discuss the <u>scab</u>.
H 16. The lonely bird searched for its <u>mate</u>.
L 17. Tom could have thought about the <u>lock</u>.
L 18. You'd been considering the <u>geese</u>.
H 19. They drank a whole bottle of <u>gin</u>.
H 20. On the beach we play in the <u>sand</u>.
L 21. Mr. Black considered the <u>fleet</u>.
H 22. The airplane went into a <u>dive</u>.
H 23. We're lost so let's look at the <u>map</u>.
L 24. I want to know about the <u>crop</u>.
H 25. Household goods are moved in a <u>van</u>.
H 26. The honey bees swarmed round the <u>hive</u>.
L 27. Betty has talked about the <u>draft</u>.

L 28.   Tom discussed the <u>hay</u>.
L 29.   Jane was interested in the <u>stamp</u>.
H 30.   The airplane dropped a <u>bomb</u>.
H 31.   Cut the bacon into <u>strips</u>.
L 32.   I had not thought about the <u>growl</u>.
H 33.   The drowning man let out a <u>yell</u>.
H 34.   I gave her a kiss and a <u>hug</u>.
L 35.   Paul should know about the <u>net</u>.
H 36.   I cut my finger with a <u>knife</u>.
H 37.   The candle flame melted the <u>wax</u>.
L 38.   Tom heard Jane called about the <u>booth</u>.

Sentence List 3

H   1.   A rose bush has prickly <u>thorns</u>.
L   2.   We should have considered the <u>juice</u>.
H   3.   The shipwrecked sailors built a <u>raft</u>.
L   4.   Bob could have known about the <u>spoon</u>.
H   5.   Ruth poured the water down the <u>drain</u>.
H   6.   The boy gave the football a <u>kick</u>.
L   7.   Bill might discuss the <u>foam</u>.
H   8.   The cop wore a bullet-proof <u>vest</u>.
L   9.   Tom could not discuss the <u>barn</u>.
L 10.   You were considering the <u>gang</u>.
H 11.   After his bath he wore a <u>robe</u>.
L 12.   Nancy should consider the <u>fist</u>.
H 13.   I can't guess so give me a <u>hint</u>.
H 14.   The soup was served in a <u>bowl</u>.
L 15.   I've spoken about the <u>pile</u>.
L 16.   Jane has a problem with the <u>coin</u>.
H 17.   The bomb exploded with a <u>blast</u>.
L 18.   Mary could not discuss the <u>tack</u>.
L 19.   They have a problem with the <u>limb</u>.
L 20.   Nancy had considered the <u>sleeves</u>.
H 21.   Lubricate the car with <u>grease</u>.
H 22.   The workers are digging a <u>ditch</u>.
L 23.   Bill heard Tom called about the <u>coach</u>.
H 24.   They marched to the beat of the <u>drum</u>.
H 25.   No one was injured in the <u>crash</u>.
L 26.   The old man thinks about the <u>mast</u>.
H 27.   The sailor swabbed the <u>deck</u>.

Sentence List 4

L   1.   Miss White would consider the <u>mold</u>.
L   2.   Ruth has a problem with the <u>joints</u>.
L   3.   The boy might consider the <u>trap</u>.
H   4.   To store his wood he built a <u>shed</u>.
H   5.   The lion gave an angry <u>roar</u>.
L   6.   He is considering the <u>throat</u>.
L   7.   They hope he heard about the <u>rent</u>.
H   8.   The car was parked at the <u>curb</u>.
L   9.   Peter should consider the <u>bow</u>.
L 10.   The old woman discussed the <u>thief</u>.
H 11.   A round hole won't take a square <u>peg</u>.
L 12.   You're discussing the <u>plot</u>.

L 39.   We can't consider the <u>wheat</u>.
H 40.   This key won't fit in the <u>lock</u>.
L 41.   We have not discussed the <u>steam</u>.
L 42.   Miss Brown might consider the <u>coast</u>.
L 43.   Mr. Brown can't discuss the <u>slot</u>.
H 44.   The little girl cuddled her <u>doll</u>.
H 45.   Tom fell down and got a bad <u>bruise</u>.
L 46.   He hasn't considered the <u>dart</u>.
H 47.   The furniture was made of <u>pine</u>.
H 48.   How did your car get that <u>dent</u>?
L 49.   Mr. Smith thinks about the <u>cap</u>.
H 50.   The baby slept in his <u>crib</u>.

L 28.   Tom will discuss the <u>swan</u>.
L 29.   Ann was interested in the <u>breath</u>.
H 30.   This nozzle sprays a fine <u>mist</u>.
L 31.   Ruth hopes he heard about the <u>hips</u>.
L 32.   Tom is talking about the <u>fee</u>.
L 33.   Miss Smith considered the <u>scare</u>.
H 34.   The ship's captain summoned his <u>crew</u>.
H 35.   They fished in the babbling <u>brook</u>.
H 36.   The hockey player scored a <u>goal</u>.
L 37.   David should consider the <u>blame</u>.
H 38.   They played a game of cat and <u>mouse</u>.
L 39.   He's glad you called about the <u>jar</u>.
L 40.   Tom will discuss the <u>cot</u>.
H 41.   The steamship left on a <u>cruise</u>.
H 42.   She faced them with a foolish <u>grin</u>.
L 43.   He hopes Tom asked about the <u>bar</u>.
L 44.   Miss Black could have discussed the <u>rope</u>.
H 45.   A chimpanzee is an <u>ape</u>.
H 46.   He wiped the sink with a <u>sponge</u>.
H 47.   We shipped the furniture by <u>truck</u>.
L 48.   Ruth's grandmother discussed the <u>broom</u>.
L 49.   I've been considering the <u>crown</u>.
H 50.   A bear has a thick coat of <u>fur</u>.

L 13.   The woman knew about the <u>lid</u>.
H 14.   Peter dropped in for a brief <u>chat</u>.
L 15.   You were interested in the <u>scream</u>.
H 16.   The gambler lost the <u>bet</u>.
H 17.   The burglar escaped with the <u>loot</u>.
L 18.   He could discuss the <u>bread</u>.
H 19.   He was scared out of his <u>wits</u>.
L 20.   He doesn't discuss the <u>mop</u>.
H 21.   Eve was made from Adam's <u>rib</u>.
L   .   <u>row</u>.
H 22.   Get the bread and cut me a <u>slice</u>.
L 23.   Bill won't consider the <u>brat</u>.

H 24. We heard the ticking of the <u>clock</u>.
H 25. Greet the heroes with loud <u>cheers</u>.
H 26. This camera is out of <u>film</u>.
L 27. Ruth wants to speak about the <u>sling</u>.
H 28. My jaw aches when I chew <u>gum</u>.
L 29. The man could consider the <u>spool</u>.
H 30. The bloodhound followed the <u>trail</u>.
H 31. The doctor prescribed the <u>drug</u>.
H 32. He rode off in a cloud of <u>dust</u>.
L 33. He was interested in the <u>hedge</u>.
L 34. Ruth hopes he called about the <u>junk</u>.
H 35. Playing checkers can be <u>fun</u>.
L 36. We're glad Ann asked about the <u>fudge</u>.
H 37. The super highway has six <u>lanes</u>.

H 38. Unlock the door and turn the <u>knob</u>.
L 39. Ruth is speaking about the <u>meal</u>.
H 40. Maple syrup is made from <u>sap</u>.
L 41. Bill cannot consider the <u>den</u>.
L 42. We are speaking about the <u>prize</u>.
H 43. The car drove off the steep <u>cliff</u>.
L 44. Miss Smith couldn't discuss the <u>row</u>.
H 45. The glass had a chip on the <u>rim</u>.
H 46. Old metal cans were made with <u>tin</u>.
L 47. Miss White thinks about the <u>tea</u>.
L 48. Miss White doesn't discuss the <u>cramp</u>.
H 49. That job was an easy <u>task</u>.
L 50. Mr. White spoke about the <u>firm</u>.

Source: "Development of a test of speech intelligibility in noise using sentence materials with controlled word predictability" by D. N. Kalikow, K.N. Stevens, and L.L. Elliott, 1977, *Journal of Acoustical Society of America, 61,* pp. 1337–1351. Copyright 1977 by Acoustical Society of America. Reprinted by permission.

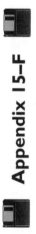

Appendix 15–F

COMMON CHILDREN'S PHRASES[1]

LIST 1

1. He fell down.
2. Clean this up.
3. It's not for you.
4. Can you see me?
5. Can I play now?
6. Look over there.
7. It's lunch time.
8. Can you help me?
9. Close your eyes.
10. Give it to me.
11. Clean up the mess.
12. Hold this toy.
13. Bring it here.
14. Who is missing?
15. Take my hand.
16. Ring the bell.
17. Let me have it.
18. You can't make me.
19. Can I have some?
20. Go right now.
Score (@ 5% each) _____

LIST 2

1. Can I go play?
2. Who is that?
3. Can we go?
4. Have a nice day.
5. What's the matter?
6. What's going on?
7. How are you?
8. Can you play?
9. I don't want to.
10. It's snowing outside.
11. That is neat.
12. No way man.
13. Leave me alone.
14. Do I have to?
15. Where's the crayons?
16. Why can't I go?
17. I want that.
18. That's cool.
19. When can I?
20. No way.
Score (@ 5% each) _____

LIST 3

1. See you later.
2. Got to go now.
3. Let me have it.
4. I'm tired.
5. That's awesome.
6. Way to go.
7. That's tough.
8. Turn the light off.
9. Stop that now.
10. Guess what?
11. Do you want to play?
12. Give it over.
13. Can we be friends?
14. She did it.
15. Do you know what?
16. You can't do that.
17. Watch this.
18. Tie my shoe.
19. What's up?
20. I can't find it.
Score (@ 5% each) _____

LIST 4

1. Can I watch TV?
2. Where is it?
3. Let's go play.
4. I don't feel good.
5. Can we draw?
6. I want to.
7. Like my picture?
8. Can I go too?
9. Can we play that?
10. I want that toy.
11. Where are we going?
12. Where's my shoe?
13. Leave me alone.
14. Can we stop?
15. I want some.
16. That one is mine.
17. I get the front.
18. It was my turn.
19. Did you see mine?
20. Let's stop there.
Score (@ 5% each) _____

LIST 5

1. Why can't I?
2. Do we have to?
3. Soccer is cool.
4. Can I open it?
5. Pick a team.
6. Where's my shoe?
7. How come?
8. I get to go.
9. Stop it now.
10. School was fun.
11. We played outside.
12. I know a song.
13. Can you do that?
14. Come in my house.
15. I don't know.
16. It's time for art.
17. Make my day.
18. I am hungry.
19. Go for it.
20. Why not?

Score (@ 5% each) _____

LIST 6

1. Know what Mom?
2. I'm sick.
3. Where's my present?
4. Give me that.
5. I didn't do it.
6. Put your shoes on.
7. That's so cool.
8. Who is it?
9. He threw it.
10. What time is it?
11. He tripped me.
12. Let's play Nintendo.
13. It's time for lunch.
14. Want to ride bikes?
15. This is dumb.
16. It's my turn.
17. I wrecked my bike.
18. Watch out.
19. My tooth is loose.
20. I want money.

Score (@ 5% each) _____

LIST 7

1. I broke my arm.
2. My lunch is gone.
3. Is it recess?
4. Do I have to?
5. Stay off the hill.
6. Don't worry.
7. That's my sweater.
8. My dog is gone.
9. I want an A.
10. Buy me that book.
11. I hate spinach.
12. I don't feel good.
13. You can't make me.
14. That's my phone.
15. Get that off.
16. Change the channel.
17. What a ride.
18. It's mine now.
19. Finders keepers.
20. Get off my bed.

Score (@ 5% each) _____

LIST 8

1. I bit the dust.
2. He kept it.
3. That song is sad.
4. He poked my eye.
5. I like candy.
6. Get the ball.
7. He kicked me.
8. Why can't I?
9. No thank you.
10. Where's the ball?
11. I don't know.
12. You know what?
13. My homework is late.
14. I hate that.
15. I don't get it.
16. Don't mess with me.
17. Keep your hands off.
18. That's my steak.
19. Let's get pizza.
20. I skinned my knee.

Score (@ 5% each) _____

[1]Phrase lists have been matched for length and for comprehension difficulty using the Flesch Reading Ease Index; they have not yet been field tested.

Source: C. DeConde Johnson & L. Owens, 1996.

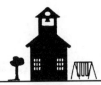

SECTION 16

APPENDIXES

Resources and Ordering Information

CONTENTS

*Appendixes marked with asterisks (*) are available on an optional computer disk which allows users to customize these forms.

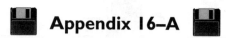 **Appendix 16–A**

RESOURCES FOR PARENTS OF CHILDREN
WHO ARE DEAF AND HARD-OF-HEARING

I.   Organizations and Programs

Alexander Graham Bell Association for the Deaf
3417 Volta Place NW
Washington, DC 20007-2778
(202) 337-5220 (Voice/TTY)

Organization for parents, individuals with hearing losses, and professionals committed to support for auditory-oral option. Excellent publications; free first-year membership for parents.

American Academy of Audiology
8201 Greensboro Drive, Suite 300
McLean, VA 22102
1-800-222-2336

Professional organization which provides information about hearing, listening devices, and audiology services.

American Society for Deaf Children
2848 Arden Way, Suite 210
Sacramento, CA 95825-1373
1-800-942-2732 (Voice/TTY)

Organization which advocates for use of American Sign Language. Will provide referrals to support groups for parents.

American Speech-Language-Hearing
     Association(ASHA)
10801 Rockville Pike
Rockville, MD 20852
1-800-638-8255 (Voice/TTY)

Professional organization which offers brochures on hearing and speech and language-related topics.

Aspen Camp School for the Deaf
P.O. Box 272
Snowmass, CO 81654
(970) 923-2511 (Voice/TDY)

Summer camp emphasizing self-esteem independence, fun.

Auditory-Verbal International
2121 Eisenhower Avenue, Suite 402
Alexandria, VA 22314
(703) 739-1049 (Voice)
(703) 739-0874 (TTY)

Organization which advocates for use of amplified residual hearing to develop listening and speaking skills.

Beginnings for Parents of
   Hearing-Impaired Children, Inc.
3900 Barrett Drive, Suite 100
Raleigh, NC 27609
1-800-541-4327 (Voice/TTY)

Group which provides emotional support and information for parents.

Better Hearing Institute
P.O. Box 1840
Washington, DC 20013
(703) 642-0580 (Voice/TTY)

Organization which provides information and resources on all aspects of hearing impairment from medical to hearing instruments.

Central Institute for the Deaf
818 S. Euclid Avenue
St. Louis, MO 63110
(314) 652-3200 (Voice/TTY)

School which publishes tests and classroom materials for professionals in deaf education.

Cochlear Corporation
61 Inverness Drive East, Suite 200
Englewood, CO 80112
1-800-458-4999

Manufacturer which produces and disseminates information packets and materials useful for children who have or are considering a cochlear implant. Maintains regional list of implant centers. Many materials are free of charge and some are available in Spanish as well as English.

Cochlear Implant Club International (CICI)
P.O. Box 464
Buffalo, NY 14223-0464
(716) 838-4662 (Voice/TTY)

Organization to support users of cochlear implants and their families. Publishes a quarterly newsjournal, <u>Contact</u>.

Deaf Life Magazine
MSM Productions, Ltd.
85 Farrugut St.
Rochester, NY 14611

Magazine that covers Deaf news and related issues.

DEAFPRIDE
1350 Potomac Ave., SE
Washington, DC 20003
(202) 675-6700 (Voice/TDY)

Organization which provides advocacy for the rights of Deaf people and their families.

Educational Audiology Association
4319 Ehrlich Road
Tampa, FL 33624
1-800-460-7322

Professional organization that supports educational services to students with hearing losses and auditory processing disorders.

The Geoffrey Foundation
P.O. Box 1112
Ocean Avenue
Kennebunkport, ME 04046

Foundation which provides financial aid to parents for auditory-verbal services.

HEAR NOW
9745 E. Hampton Avenue, Suite 300
Denver, CO 80231-4923
1-800-648-HEAR

Foundation which provides free hearing aids and cochlear implants to children whose families do not qualify for public assistance and cannot afford them.

House Ear Institute
2100 W. Third St, 5th Floor
Los Angeles, CA 90057
1-800-352-3888,
213-484-2642 (TTY), 213-483-4431 (Voice)

Toll-free hotline for parenting information and information on early childhood deafness.

International Hearing Dog, Inc.
5909 E. 89th Ave.
Henderson, CO
(303) 287-3277 (Voice/TDY)

Provides hearing dog training and placement.

John Tracy Clinic
806 West Adams Boulevard
Los Angeles, CA 90007
1-800-522-4582

Clinic which has a free correspondence course for families of preschool children. Lessons cover the development of oral language skills and are also available in Spanish.

Miracle-Ear Children's Foundation
1-800-234-5422 (Voice)
1-800-234-5422, Ext. 751 (TTY)

Foundation which provides free hearing aids to children whose families do not qualify for public assistance and cannot afford to purchase hearing aids.

National Association for the Deaf (NAD)
814 Thayer Avenue
Silver Spring, MD 20910-4500
(301) 587-1788 (Voice)
(301) 587-1789 (TTY)

Organization of Deaf individuals, parents, and professionals committed to support sign language option.

National Captioning Institute
5203 Leesburg Pike, Suite 1500
Falls Church, VA 22041
(703) 998-2400 (Voice/TTY)

This group provides closed captioning of television programs.

National Cued Speech Association
c/o Dr. Katheine Quenin
Speech-Language Pathology Department
Nazareth College of Rochester
4245 East Avenue
Rochester, NY 14168

Organization which supports the use of cued speech and provides a list of local instructors.

National Information Center on Deafness,
    Gallaudet University
NICD, Dept. P-94
800 Florida Avenue, NE
Washington, DC 20002
(202) 651-5000 (Voice/TTY)

Center which provides information on all topics dealing with deafness and hearing loss, including hearing aids, cochlear implants, assistive listening devices, communication, and educational methodologies.

National Institute on Deafness &
    Other Communication Disorders
    Hereditary Hearing Impairment Resource
    Registry (NIDCD-HHIRR)
555 N. 30th St
Omaha, NE 68131-9909

Provides a registry of hereditary hearing loss, support and resources for parents, and information on a variety of genetic hearing disorders for professionals.

Network of Educators of Children with
    Cochlear Implants (NECCI)
Cochlear Implant Center
Manhattan Eye, Ear & Throat Hospital
210 East 64th Street, 4th Floor
New York, NY 10021
(212) 605-3793 (Voice/TTY)

Organization of professionals which publishes a practical newsletter and an annual directory of professionals who have experience with children using cochlear implants.

Oticon 4 Kids
Oticon, Inc.
29 Schoolhouse Road
Somerset, NJ 08875
1-800-526-3921

Manufacturer's program that provides a club for children with hearing losses and support material for teachers and parents.

Self Help for Hard of Hearing People, Inc.
    (SHHH)
7910 Woodmont Ave., Suite 1200
Bethesda, MD 20814
(301) 657-2248 (Voice)
(301) 657-2249 (TTY)

Organization of individuals with hearing impairments and professionals who promote awareness of and information about hearing loss and options for hearing impaired. Publishes a bimonthly journal.

Signing Exact English Center for Advancement of
    Deaf Children
P.O. Box 1181
Los Alamitos, CA 90720
310-430-1467 (Voice/TTY).

Information for parents and professionals on Signing Exact English (SEE II).

Tripod
2901 N. Keystone St.
Burbank, CA 91504
818-972-2080 (Voice/TDY)

Support and information services on
any aspect of deaf education and advice
for parents of children with hearing losses.

II. Articles, Books, Videotapes, Electronic Media

Articles and Books

Altman, E. (1988). *Talk with me: Giving the gift of language and emotional health to the hearing-impaired child.* Washington DC: A. G. Bell Association for the Deaf.

Bradford, T. (1991). *Say that again, please.* Dallas, TX: Thomas H. Bradford.

Fletcher, L. (1987). *Ben's story: A deaf child's right to sign.* Washington DC: Gallaudet University Press.

Forecki, M. (1985). *Speak to me!* Washington DC: Gallaudet University Press.

Freeman, R., Carbin, C., & Boese, R. (1981). *Can't your child hear? A guide for those who care about deaf children.* Baltimore: University Park Press.

Greene, J. Craig. (1993). *BEGINNINGS: A parent manual for parents of deaf and hard of hearing children.* North Carolina: BEGINNINGS for Parents of Hearing Impaired Children, Inc.

House Ear Institute. *Parent to parent: Parents of deaf children sharing and caring–Resource catalog.* Los Angeles, CA: House Ear Institute.

Kisor, H. (1990). *What's that pig outdoors? A memoir of deafness.* New York: Penguin Books.

Lane, Harlan. (1984). *What the mind hears: A history of the Deaf.* New York: Random House Press.

Luterman, D. (1987). *Deafness in the family.* Boston: Little, Brown.

Luterman, D. (1991). *When your child is deaf.* Parkton, MD: York Press.

McArthur, S. (1982). *Raising your hearing impaired child: A guide for parents.* Washington, DC: A.G. Bell Association for the Deaf.

Mindel, E.D., & Vernon, M. (1987). *They grow in silence: Understanding deaf children and adults* (2nd ed.). San Diego: College-Hill Press.

Moore, C. (Ed.) (1990). *A resource guide for parents of children with mental, physical, or emotional disabilities.* Rockville, MD: Woodbine House.

Moores, D. (1987). *Educating the deaf: Psychology, principles, and practices* (3rd ed.). Boston: Houghton Mifflin.

National Center for Law and Deafness. (1992). *Legal Rights: The guide for deaf and hard of hearing people.* Washington, DC: Gallaudet University Press.

Ogden, P. (1996). *The silent garden: Raising your deaf child.* Washington DC: Gallaudet University Press

Padden, C., & Humphries, T. (1988). *Deaf in America: Voices from a culture.* Cambridge, MA: Harvard University Press.

Sacks, O. (1989). *Seeing voices.* Berkeley/Los Angeles: University of California Press.

Schwartz, S. (Ed.) (1987). *Choices in deafness: A parents' guide.* Rockville, MD: Woodbine House.

Tucker, B. (1995). *The feel of silence.* Washington, DC: A.G. Bell Association for the Deaf.

Walker, L. (1986). *A loss for words: The story of deafness in a family.* New York: Harper & Row.

Other sources for books (call for a catalogue):

Gallaudet University Press	Dawn Sign Press	Harris Communicatons
800 Florida Ave, NE	6130 Nancy Ridge Drive	15159 Technology Drive
Washington, DC 20002	San Diego, CA 92121	Eden Prarie, MN 55344
1-800-672-6720	1-800-549-5350	1-800-825-9187

A.G. Bell Association for the Deaf
3417 Volta Place NW
Washington, D.C. 20007-2778
202-337-5220 (Voice/TTY)

Videotapes

A.G. Bell Association, 3417 Volta Place, NW, Washington, DC 20007   202-337-5220 (Voice/TDY)
   Do you Hear That?
   Auditory-Verbal Therapy for Parents & Professionals
   Show & Tell
   I Can Hear!

Boys Town Press, 13603 Flanagan Blvd. Boys Town, NE 68010   1-800-282-6657 (Voice/TDY)
   Read with Me (a 3-set series of stories available in MCE or ASL)
   Sign with Me (3 volumes availabe in MCE or ASL)
   Families with Deaf Children: Discovering Your Needs, Exploring Your Choices
   Families with Hard-of-Hearing Children: What if Your Child Has a Hearing Loss?

HOPE, Inc., 809 North 800 East, Logan, UT 84321   801-752-9533
   Home Total Communication Videotapes (signed English)
   Signed Cartoons (signed English)

Maryland State Department of Education and Maryland Instructional Television (Prod.)(1985). *Beginnings: Handicapped Children Birth to Age 5.* Communication: Disorders, Language & Development. PBS; 919-733-5920 Voice/TDY.

Modern Signs Press, P.O. Box 1181, Los Alamitos, CA 90720
   A Mother's Look at Total Communication

National Cued Speech Association, Dr. Katherine Quenin, Speech-Language Pathology Department, Nazareth College of Rochester, 4245 East Avenue, Rochester, NY 14168
   I See What You Say

Sign Enhancers   1-800-76-SIGN-1
   Sign Enhancers (ASL)

Tranchin, R. (Prod.),
   For a deaf son. Alexandria, VA: PBS Video.

T.J. Publishers, Inc.   301-585-4440
   Sign Me a Story (ASL)

Electronic Media

Websites:

These addresses change frequently; the authors apologize in advance if any addresses are not active or current.

A.G. Bell Association for the Deaf: www.agbell.org

American Academy of Audiology: www.audiology.org

American Speech-Language-Hearing Association: www.asha.org

Auditory-Verbal International: www.digitalnation.com/avi

Boys Town National Research Hospital: www.boystown.org

Central Institute for the Deaf: www.cidmac.wust.edu

Deaf/Hard of Hearing: www.familyvillage.wisc.edu/lib_deaf.htm

Deaf World Web, Cyberkids: www.deafworldweb.org/dww/kids

Ear infections and ear tube surgery: http://kidshealth.org/parent/healthy/ent/ear_infection.html

Educational Audiology Association: www.ehhs.cmich.edu/eaa

Gaullaudet University: www.gallaudet.edu

Where Do We Go From Hear?   www.gohear.org

HIP Magazine (for hearing impaired children):   ww.hipmag.org

Self Help for Hard of Hearing People   www.ourworld.compuserve.com/homepages/shhh

TRIPOD   TRIPOD@sure.net

Chat Rooms:

PC Pals Deaf Teen Chat (second & last Sunday of each month, 7:00 pm EST), sponsored by A.G. Bell;
       Facilitator: Kbuehl
       Room: Equal Access Cafe
       Keyword: PEN or deaf

Deaf Community (8 pm)
       Room: Equal access Cafe
       Keyword: PEN or deaf

Appendix 16–B

ORGANIZATIONS AND AGENCIES WITH AUDITORY DEVELOPMENT CHECKLISTS

American Academy of Audiology: "Your Baby's Hearing"
    8201 Greensboro Drive, Suite 300
    McLean, VA 22102
    (703) 610-9022; (800) 222-2336

American Speech-Language-Hearing Association: "How Does Your Child Hear and Talk"
    10801 Rockville Pike
    Rockville, MD 20852
    (301) 897-5700; (800) 638-6868

New York League for the Hard of Hearing: "Does Your Baby Hear?"
    71 West 23rd Street
    New York, NY 10010
    (212) 741-7650

NIDCD Information Clearinghouse: "Silence Isn't Always Golden"
    1 Communication Avenue
    Bethesda, MD 20852-3456
    (800) 241-1044 (Voice); (800) 241-1055 (TDD/TT)

Appendix 16–C

COMPANIES PROVIDING PRODUCTS USEFUL IN INFECTION CONTROL

Oaktree Products, Inc.
2134 Heather Glen Drive
Chesterfield, MO 63017
(800) 347-1960
(314) 530-1664

Manufacturer of Audiologist's Choice products and supplier of a full line of infection control products including disinfectants, sterilants, and gloves.

Hal-Hen Company, Inc.
35-53 24th Street
Long Island City, NY 11106
(800) 242-5436
(718) 392-6020

Distributer of ultrasonic cleaners and other supplies for cleaning hearing instruments.

Appendix 16–D

ORDERING INFORMATION FOR SELECTED ASSESSMENT PRODUCTS

Audiogram of Familiar Sounds

American Academy of Audiology
8201 Greensboro Dr., Suite 300
McLean, VA 22102
(800) 222-2336

Auditory Perception of Alphabet Letters
(APAL)

Auditec of St. Louis
2515 S. Big Bend Blvd.
St. Louis, MO 63143
(314) 781-8890

Developmental Approach to Successful
Listening (DASL) II
(Placement Test)

Resource Point
61 Inverness Drive East, Suite 200
Englewood, CO 80112-9726
(800) 688-8788

Early Speech Perception Test
(ESP)

Central Institute for the Deaf
818 South Euclid Avenue
St. Louis, MO 63110
(314) 977-0000

Fisher's Auditory Problems Checklist

Educational Audiology Association
4319 Ehrlich Road
Tampa, FL 33624
(800) 460-7322

Minimal Auditory Capabilities Battery
(MAC Battery)

Auditec of St. Louis
(See Auditory Perception of
Alphabet Letters above)

Northwestern University Children's
Perception of Speech
(NU-CHIPS)

Auditec of St. Louis
(See Auditory Perception of
Alphabet Letters above)

Pediatric Speech Intelligibility
(PSI)

Auditec of St. Louis
(See Auditory Perception of
Alphabet Letters above)

Screening Instrument for Targeting
Educational Risk
(S.I.F.T.E.R.)

Educational Audiology Association
(See Fisher's Auditory Problems
Checklist above)

Screening Instrument for Targeting
Educational Risk in Preschool Children
(Preschool S.I.F.T.E.R.)

Educational Audiology Association
(See Fisher's Auditory Problems
Checklist above)

Sound Effects Recognition Task
(SERT)

Auditec of St. Louis
(See Auditory Perception of
Alphabet Letters above)

Test of Auditory Comprehension
    (TAC)

Word Intelligibility by Picture Identification
    (WIPI)

Foreworks Publications
Box 82289
Portland, OR 97282
(503) 653-2614

Auditec of St. Louis
(See Auditory Perception of
Alphabet Letters above)

Appendix 16–E

ORDERING INFORMATION FOR SELECTED CENTRAL AUDITORY PROCESSING TESTS

Auditory Continuous Performance Test

The Psychological Corporation
Harcourt, Brace, Jovanovich
555 Academic Court
San Antonio, TX 78204-2498
(800) 228-0752

Auditory Fusion Test, Revised

Auditec of St. Louis
2515 S. Big Bend Blvd.
St. Louis, MO 63143
(314) 781-8890

Auditory Sequential Memory Test

Western Psychological Services
12031 Wilshire Boulevard
Los Angeles, CA 90025
(800) 648-8857

Binaural Fusion Tests

Auditec of St. Louis
2515 S. Big Bend Blvd.
St. Louis, MO 63143
(314) 781-8890

Clinical Evaluation of Language
Fundamentals-Revised

The Psychological Corporation
(See Auditory Continuous
Performance Test)

Compressed WIPI

Auditec of St. Louis
(See Binaural Fusion Tests)

Detroit Test of Learning Aptitude-2

American Guidance Service
4201 Woodland Road
P. O. Box 99
Circle Pines, MN 55014-1796
(800) 328-2560

Dichotic C-V Test

Auditec of St. Louis
(See Binaural Fusion Tests)

Dichotic Digits Test

Auditec of St. Louis
(See Binaural Fusion Tests)

Dichotic Sentence Identification Test

Auditec of St. Louis
(See Binaural Fusion Tests)

Expressive One-Word Picture Vocabulary
Test-Revised

Academic Communication
Associates
Publications Division, Dept. 195
4149 Avenida de la Plata
Oceanside, CA 92058-6249
(619) 758-9593

Fisher's Auditory Problems Checklist

Educational Audiology Association
4319 Ehrlich Road
Tampa, FL 33624
(800) 460-7322

Goldman-Fristoe-Woodcock Auditory
Skills Test Battery

American Guidance Service
(See Detroit Test of Learning
Aptitude-2)

Goldman-Fristoe-Woodcock Test of
Auditory Discrimination

American Guidance Service
(See Detroit Test of Learning
Aptitude-2)

Lindamood Auditory Conceptualization Test

Pro-Ed
8700 Shoal Creek Blvd.
Austin, TX 78757-9965
(512) 451-3246

Peabody Picture Vocabulary Test-Revised

American Guidance Service
(See Detroit Test of Learning
Aptitude-2)

Pediatric Speech Intelligibility Test

Auditec of St. Louis
(See Binaural Fusion Tests)

Pitch Pattern Sequence Tests

Auditec of St. Louis
(See Binaural Fusion Tests)

SCAN: A Screening Test for Auditory
Processing Disorders

The Psychological Corporation
(See Auditory Continuous
Performance Test)

SCAN-A: A Test for Auditory Processing
Disorders in Adolescents and Adults

The Psychological Corporation
(See Auditory Continuous
Performance Test)

Selective Auditory Attention Test

Auditec of St. Louis
(See Binaural Fusion Tests)

Speech Perception in Noise Test

Robert C. Bilger, Ph.D.
Department of Speech and
    Hearing Science
901 South Sixth Street
Champaign, IL 61820
(217) 244-4140

Staggered Spondaic Words Test

Precision Acoustics
411 NE 87th Street, Suite B
Vancouver, WA 98664
(360) 892-9367

Synthetic Sentence Identification

Auditec of St. Louis
(See Binaural Fusion Tests)

Test of Auditory Comprehension of Language

Pro-Ed
(See Lindamood Auditoy
Conceptualization Test)

Test of Auditory-Perceptual Skills

Psychological and Educational
Publications, Inc.
1477 Rollins Road
Burlingame, CA 94010
(800) 523-5775

Test of Language Competence-
Expanded Edition

The Psychological Corporation
(See Auditory Continuous
Performance Test)

Test of Word Knowledge

The Psychological Corporation
(See Auditory Continuous
Performance Test)

Tests of Language Development

Pro-Ed
(See Lindamood Auditoy
Conceptualization Test)

Time Compressed Tests

Auditec of St. Louis
(See Binaural Fusion Tests)

Token Test for Children

Pro-Ed
(See Lindamood Auditory
Conceptualization Test)

Tonal and Speech Materials for Central
Auditory Assessment (CD)

Richard Wilson
Department of Audiology & Speech
Services
126 VA Medical Center
Johnson City, Mtn Home, TN 37684

Wepman Auditory Discrimination Test

Western Psychological Services
(See Auditory Sequential Memory Test)

Willeford Central Auditory Test Battery

Jack A. Willeford, Ph.D.
Colorado State University
Department of Communication
Disorders
Fort Collins, CO 80523

Appendix 16–F

ORDERING INFORMATION FOR AMPLIFICATION

Advanced Bionics Corp
12740 San Fernando Rd.
Sylmar, CA 91342
818-362-7588

Cochlear Implants (Clarion)

American Loop Systems
29 Silver Hill Rd, Suite 100
Milford, MA 01757-1311
800-438-5667

3-D Loop FM System

All Hear Systems
20833 67th Ave. West, Suite 107
Lynnwood, WA 98036
800-355-7525

Sound Field FM Amplification

Audio Enhancement
12613 S. Redwood Rd.
Riverton, UT 84065
800-383-9362

Personal & Sound Field FM
Amplification

Audiologic Engineering Corp.
35 Medford St.
Sommerville, MA 02143
800-283-4601

Vibrotactile aids (Tactaid), personal FM
(Chorus)

AVR/Sonovation Inc.
1450 Park Court
Chanhassesn, MN 55317
800-462-8336

Frequency transposition hearing aids
(Transonic), personal FM (Extend Ear),
vibrotactile aids (Trill)

Cochlear Corp.
61 Inverness Dr. E., Suite 200
Englewood, CO 80112
800-523-5798

Cochlear Implants (Nucleus 22)

Lifeline Amplification Systems
55 South 4th St.
Platteville, WI 53818
800-236-4327

Sound Field FM Amplification

LightSpeed Technologies, Inc.
15812 SW Upper Boones Ferry Rd.
Lake Oswego, OR 97035
800-732-8999

Personal & Sound Field FM systems,
Infrared systems

Oval Window Audio
33 Wildflower Ct.
Nederland, CO 80466
303-447-3607

Induction Loops, Sound Lab,
vibrotactile aids, miscellaneous
amplification

Phonak
P.O. Box 3017
Naperville, IL 60566-7017
800-777-7333

Personal FM (Microlink, Microvox)

Phonic Ear, Inc.
3880 Cypress Dr.
Petaluma, CA 94954-7600
800-227-0735

Personal FM (Free Ear, Easy Listener),
auditory trainers, Sound Field FM
(StarSound), & Infrared systems

Radio Shack

All purpose amplifiers, Sound Field
amplification components

Telex Communications, Inc.
9600 Aldrich Ave. South
Minneapolis, MN 55420
800-328-3102

Personal & Sound Field FM, group
auditory trainers

Williams Sound Corp.
10399 W. 70th St.
Eden Prarie, MN 55344-3446
800-328-6190

Personal & Sound Field FM systems

Appendix 16–G

ORDERING INFORMATION FOR AUDITORY AND TACTILE CURRICULA

Auditory enhancement guide (1992). Developed by B. David Shea and Clarke School for the Deaf. Published by Alexander Graham Bell Association for the Deaf, 3417 Volta Place, Washington, DC 20007-2778.

Auditory skills curriculum (1976). Developed at Los Angeles County School District. Published by Foreworks, Box 82289, Portland, OR 97282, 503-653-2614.

Auditory skills curriculum preschool supplement (1986). Developed by the Lexington School for the Deaf. Published by Foreworks (see above).

CHATS: The Miami cochlear implant, auditory and tactile skills curriculum (1994). Edited by Kathleen C. Vergara & Lynn W. Miskiel. Published by Intelligent Hearing Systems, 10689 North Kendall Drive, Miami, FL 33176. Also distributed by Alexander Graham Bell Association for the Deaf (see above).

DASL II (1992). Developed by Gayle Stout, Jill Windle, and the Houston School for Deaf Children. Published by Resource Point, Inc., 61 Inverness Drive East, Suite 200, Englewood, CO 80112-5128.

Five steps to improving your child's use of a cochlear implant (1993). Developed by Danielle Kelsay, Nancy Tye-Murray, Karen Iler Kirk, & Lorianne Schum. Published by University of Iowa Hospitals and Clinics, Department of Otolaryngology, Iowa City, IA 52242. Accompanying workbook, *Stepping out: Specific activities to do at home.*

Foundations in speech perception (1993). Software package including manual, CD, supplementary user materials, and blank diskettes. Distributed by Cochlear Corporation, 61 Inverness Drive East, Suite 200, Englewood, CO 80112.

SPICE: Speech perception instructional curriculum and evaluation (1996). Developed by Jean Moog, Jill Biedenstein, & Lisa Davidson at Central Institute for the Deaf, 818 S. Euclid Avenue, St. Louis, MO 63110.

TARGO: Tactaid reference guide and orientation (1993). Developed by Amy Robbins, Linda Hesketh, & Cindy Bivins in cooperation with the Indiana University School of Medicine. Published by Audiological Engineering Corporation, 35 Medford Street, Somerville, MA 02143.

Appendix 16–H

SPEECHREADING RESOURCES FOR CHILDREN

Craig lipreading inventory (1964). Distributed by Cochlear Corporation, Suite 200, 61 Inverness Drive East, Englewood, CO 80112.
Four-choice picture test using single word stimuli, developed for 6 years and older.

Deyo, D. *Speechreading in context.* Washington, DC: Gallaudet University, Pre-College Programs. Order from Gallaudet University Bookstore, 800 Florida Avenue NE, Washington, DC 20002-3695.
Teacher guide including speechreading activities for elementary and middle school.

DeFilippo, C., & Scott, B. (1978). A method for training and evaluating the reception of ongoing speech. *Journal of the Acoustical Society of America, 63,* 1186–1192.
Article which describes connected discourse tracking, an approach used to develop speechreading skills in both children and adults.

Haspiel, G. (1987). *Lipreading for children.* Washington, DC: A.G. Bell Association.
Lesson plans to develop speechreading skills for elementary-aged children.

NTID Speechreading Videotapes (1987). Washington, DC: A.G. Bell Association.
Series of 11 videotapes of daily living situations, plus workbooks, teacher's manual, and speechreading strategies developed for young adults.

Pluznik, N., & Sobel, R. (1986). *Messy monsters, jungle joggers, and bubble baths.* Washington DC: A.G. Bell Association. Also available from Gallaudet University Bookstore.
Children's workbook which lends itself to speechreading activities for elementary children.

Yoshinaga-Itano, C. (1988). Speechreading instruction for children. *Volta Review, 90,* 241–259.
Chapter in monograph on speechreading which briefly describes a wholistic approach for use with children. Includes annotated bibliography.

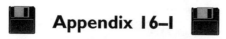

Appendix 16–1

RESOURCES/MATERIALS FOR MAINSTREAM TEACHERS
AND STUDENTS WHO ARE DEAF/HARD-OF-HEARING

A.G. Bell Association for the Deaf, Inc.
3417 Volta Place, NW
Washington, DC 20007-2778

Information on PC Pals, a computer network for students who are deaf/HOH; catalog includes mainstream publications.

HiP Magazine
1563 Solano Avenue, #137
Berkeley, CA 94707

Bi-monthly periodical for students, 8–14 years of age, who are deaf/HOH; comes with companion teaching guide, *HiP TiPs.*

KIP - Knowledge Is Power
Audiological & Education
HI Services Department
Attn: KIP
Mississippi Bend Area Education Agency
729-21st Street
Bettendoft, IA 52722-5096

Program designed to help students learn about their hearing losses.

The Mainstream Center
Clarke School
Round Hill Road
Northampton, MA 01060-2199

Publishes *The Mainstream News,* monthly school-year periodical for school personnel; publishes *The note-writer,* a system for student notetakers.

Oticon 4 Kids
29 Schoolhouse Road
Somerset, NJ 08875-6724
1-800-227-3951, or -0735, ext. 258

Support program sponsored jointly with Phonic Ear; publishes *Teacher guide* pamphlet and quarterly teacher newsletter; teacher-to-teacher computer network directory.

Pre-College Outreach
Gallaudet University
KDES PAS-6
800 Florida Avenue NE
Washington, DC 20078-0603

Publishes *Perspectives in Education and Deafness,* 5 times/year for educators; publishes *World Around You,* 5 times/year for teens who are deaf/HOH; manages Educational Resource Centers on Deafness; catalog includes current mainstream modules, videos, publications.

Self-Advocacy for Students who are
    Deaf and Hard of Hearing
Kristina M. English
Pro-Ed
8700 Shoal Creek Blvd.
Austin, TX 78757-9965
512-451-3246

Fourteen lesson curriculum designed for high school students.

Unitron Kids Club
333 West Fort Street
Suite 2010
Detroit, MI 48226

Publishes booklets on hearing aids and their use for teachers, parents, elementary and middle school students in English and Spanish.

Appendix 16–J

ORDERING INFORMATION FOR COMMERCIAL HEARING CONSERVATION MATERIALS

Preschool Level

Cartoon Poster on Healthy Hearing. Order from ASHA Fulfillment Operations, 10801 Rockville Pike, Rockville, MD 20852-3279. Minimal cost for classroom packet & shipping.

Elementary Level

Quiet pleases III, listen up for the sounds of your life. Order through local Sertoma Club or from Sertoma Foundation, 1912 East Meyer Boulevard, Kansas City, MO 64132. Charge for module.

Operation Shhh. Order from Self Help for Hard of Hearing People, Inc., 7910 Woodmont Avenue, Suite 1200, Bethesda, MD 20814. Charge for classroom package. Teacher kits can be purchased separately for minimal fee.

Know noise. Order from Sight & Hearing Association, 674 Transfer Road, St. Paul, MN 55114-1402. Charge for program, plus shipping fee. Free 30-day trial (money refunded if not satisfied).

Good vibes. Submit requests through local Sertoma Club to Sertoma Sponsorships Department-NIE, 1912 E. Meyer Boulevard, Kansas City, MO 64132-1174.

I love what I hear! Order from NIDCD Clearinghouse, P.O. Box 37777, Washington, DC 20013-7777. Materials are free and can be duplicated.

Have you ever wondered about . . . the ear and hearing? Order from National Information Center on Deafness, Gallaudet University, 800 Florida Avenue NE, Washington, DC 20002-3695. Materials are free.

Middle School Level

Hip talk. Order from House Ear Institute, 2100 W. Third Street, 5th Floor, Los Angeles, CA 90057. Charge for full program (8-minute demo video available free of charge.)

Say what . . . ? Order from American Academy of Audiology, 8201 Greensboro Dr., Suite 300, McLean, VA 22102. Minimal charge for AAA members; cost slightly higher for non-members.

Stop that noise. Request from New York League for the Hard of Hearing, 71 West 23rd Street, New York, NY 10010. Free to audiologists and elementary and secondary school teachers.

High School Level

Hip talk—See Middle School Level.

People vs. noise. Order from Better Hearing Institute, 5021-B Backlick Road, Annandale, VA 22003. Cost depends on length of video requested.

Can't hear you knocking. Produced by H.E.A.R. (Hearing Education and Awareness for Rockers), P.O. Box 460847, San Francisco, CA 94146. Minimal cost for program if ordered through Sertoma Club.

Additional H.E.A.R. materials (buttons, bumper stickers, posters, etc.). See address above. Contact producer for specific item prices.

An earful of sound advice about hearing protection. Free on request from EAR, 7911 Zionsville Road, Indianapolis, IN 46268

National Hearing Conservation Association materials (slides and posters). Order from NHCA, 611 East Wells Street, Milwaukee, WI 53202-3892. Charges based on quantities ordered, plus minimal postage fee.

Appendix 16–K

SERVICE CLUBS THAT SUPPORT PROGRAMS FOR PERSONS WITH DISABILITIES
(*Organizations Whose Focus is Speech and Hearing)

Business and Professional Women's Clubs, National
   Federation
2012 Massachusetts Avenue NW
Washington, DC 20036
(202) 293-1100

Civitan International
1 Civitan Place
Birmingham, AL 35213-1983
(205) 591-8910
(800) CIVITAN

Lions Clubs International*
300 22nd Street
Oak Brook, IL 60521
(708) 571-5466

Quota International*
1420 21st Street NW
Washington, DC 20036
(202) 331-9694

Sertoma International*
1912 East Myer Boulevard
Kansas City, MO 64132
(816) 333-8300

Kiwanis, International*
3636 Woodview Trace
Indianapolis, IN 46268-3196
(317) 875-8755
(800) 549-2647

Pilot International
244 College Street
PO Box 4844
Macon, GA 31213-0599
(912) 743-7403

Rotary International
1 Rotary Center
1560 Sherman Avenue
Evanston, IL 60201
(708) 866-3000

Telephone Pioneers*—Contact through your local telephone company.

In general, these organizations may be listed in the phone book, or you can contact your local Chamber of Commerce to obtain the phone number of local chapters of civic organizations. Also, many of these organizations list their meetings and contact persons in your local newspaper.

Appendix 16–L

RESOURCES FOR COMMUNITY EDUCATION PRESENTATIONS

American Academy of Audiology (AAA)
8201 Greensboro Dr., Suite 300
McLean, VA 22102
(703) 610-9022 Voice/TDY:
Audiotape demonstrating hearing loss; brochures and written materials on audiology, hearing loss, prevention, infant hearing loss

American Speech-Language-Hearing Association (ASHA)
10801 Rockville Pike
Rockville, MD 20852
(301) 897-5700 Voice/TDY; (800) 638-8255
Brochures on audiology, school audiology, hearing loss, prevention, ADA; video modules on assistive technology, audiology, and ADA.

Better Hearing Institute (BHI)
P.O. Box 1840
Washington, DC 20013
(703) 642-0580 Voice; (800) EAR-WELL TDY
Videos on hearing loss, noise-induced loss, and amplification; brochures and written materials on most hearing related topics

International Hearing Dogs, Inc.
5909 E. 89th Avenue
Henderson, CO
(303) 287-2277
Information on obtaining and training hearing dogs.

National Association for the Deaf (NAD)
814 Thayer Avenue
Silver Spring, MD 20910-4500
(301) 587-1788 Voice
(301) 587-1789 (TDY)
Information on deafness, Deaf culture, and sign language.

National Information Center on Deafness (NIDCD)
Gallaudet University
800 Florida Avenue, NE
Washington, DC 20002
(202) 651-5051 Voice; (202) 651-5052 TDY
Brochures and written information on hearing and hearing loss, infant assessment, universal hearing screening, otitis media, prevention, and most other hearing related topics.

Self-Help for Hard of Hearing People, Inc. (SHHH)
7910 Woodmont Avenue, Suite 1200
Bethesda, MD 20814
(301) 657-2248 Voice
(301) 657-2249 TDY
Brochures and written materials on hearing impairment, amplification, assistive devices, the ADA.

ADDITIONAL RESOURCES/MATERIALS

Getting the most out of your hearing aids. Video featuring former Surgeon General, C. Everett Koop. Distributed by CDR Communications, Inc., 9310-B Old Keene Mill Road, Burke, VA 22015-4204. (703) 569-3400; (800) 729-2237

Local distributors and/or equipment manufacturers will frequently provide brochures, written information, and demo models for new equipment and assistive devices.

Additional resources for noise and hearing conservation listed in Appendix 16–J.

Appendix 16–M

COMMERCIAL MATERIALS FOR INSERVICE PRESENTATIONS

Deaf and hard of hearing students: Educational service guidelines. Manual compiled by the Deaf Education Initiative Project that details best practice guidelines and contains excellent glossary and appendixes. Order from National Association of State Directors of Special Education, Inc., King Street Station, I, 1800 Diagonal Road, Suite 320, Alexandria, VA 22314 (nominal charge).

Access for all. Video and manual includes information on hearing loss and deafness, communication options, and interagency collaboration at the preschool level. Order through Gallaudet University Bookstore, Pre-College Outreach Program, 800 Florida Avenue, NE, Washington, DC 20002-3695.

There's a hearing impaired child in my class. Book, plus audiotape that simulates effects of hearing loss. Order from Gallaudet University Bookstore (see above).

How to have a winning year teaching the student who is deaf or hard of hearing. Brochure for teachers that provides an overview of the effects of hearing loss with suggestions for strategies to use in the classroom. Order from A.G. Bell Association for the Deaf, 3417 Volta Place NW, Washington, DC 20007-2778 (first copy free).

Beginnings: Communication options. Video of parents discussing and demonstrating the various methodologies they have chosen for their children who are deaf or hard-of-hearing. Order from Beginnings for Parents of Hearing Impaired Children, Inc., 3900 Barrett Drive, Raleigh, NC 27609.

Aural-oral and sign options for hearing families in early home programming. Video discussion and demonstration of auditory-verbal, oral, and total communication, as well as manually coded English, American Sign Language, and bilingualism. Order from Hope, Inc., 55 East 100 North, Logan, UT 84321.

Technology in the classroom: Listening and hearing. Manual and accompanying video demonstrates assistive technology use by children. Order from American Speech-Language-Hearing Association, 10801 Rockville Pike, Rockville, MD 10852.

Improving classroom acoustics (1995). Inservice training manual developed by the Sarasota, FL, County Schools covering classroom need for and use of sound field FM systems. Includes teacher guide and accompanying manual with transparency masters. Order from Clearinghouse/Information Center, Bureau of Student Services and Exceptional Education, Division of Public Schools, Florida Department of Education, Florida Education Center, Suite 614, Tallahassee, FL 32399-0400 (nominal fee for printing, shipping, and handling).

Amplification handbook. Loose-leaf notebook compiled by Phonic Ear that includes information related to the use of FM technology and the Americans with Disabilities Act. Material for handouts, transparencies, and related published articles are included. Request from Phonic Ear, Inc., 3880 Cypress Drive, Petaluma, CA 94954-7600 (no charge).

Issues in infant hearing screening and follow-up. Building blocks module compiled by ASHA that addresses early identification programs and family counseling. Includes extensive bibliography and related ASHA Guidelines. Request from American Speech-Language-Hearing Association, 10801 Rockville Pike, Rockville, MD 20852.

Early identification. Video promoting universal newborn hearing screening that also describes and demonstrates evoked otoacoustic emissions testing. Order from National Center for Hearing Assessment and Management, Parent Education, Department of Psychology, Utah State University, Logan, UT 84322-2810 (nominal charge).

Between you and me. Training module for parents, teachers, and support personnel to facilitate the development of conversational skills in preschool children. Includes video, viewer's guide, and facilitator's guide. (Additional modules on language skills available for teachers and parents working with children from birth–8 years.) Order from Educational Productions Inc., 7412 SW Beaverton Hillsdale Highway, Suite 210, Portland, OR (free preview copies).

Additional listed in Appendix 16–I (Resources/Materials for Mainstream Teachers and Students Who are Deaf/Hard-of-Hearing), Appendix 16–J (Ordering Information for Commercial Hearing Conservation Material), and Appendix 16–L (Resources for Community Education Presentations).

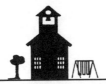

REFERENCES

American Academy of Audiology. (1993). *Audiogram of familiar sounds.* Arlington, VA: Author.

American National Standards Institute. (1987). *Specification of hearing aid characteristics.* (ANSI Section 3.22). New York: Author.

American Speech-Language-Hearing Association. (1985). Guidelines for identification audiometry. *Asha, 27,* 49–52.

American Speech-Language-Hearing Association. (1989). Audiologic screening of newborn infants who are at risk for hearing impairment. *Asha, 31,* 89–92.

American Speech-Language-Hearing Association. (1990a). Audiological assessment of central auditory processing: An annotated bibliography. *Asha, 32*(Suppl. 1), 13–30.

American Speech-Language-Hearing Association. (1990b). Guidelines for screening for hearing impairment and middle-ear disorders. *Asha, 32*(Suppl. 2), 17–24.

American Speech-Language-Hearing Association. (1991a). Amplification as a remediation technique for children with normal peripheral hearing. *Asha, 33*(Suppl. 3), 22–24.

American Speech-Language-Hearing Association. (1991b). Guidelines for the audiologic assessment of children from birth through 36 months of age. *Asha, 33*(Suppl. 5), 37–43.

American Speech-Language-Hearing Association. (1991c). The use of FM amplification instruments for infants and preschool children with hearing impairment. *Asha, 33* (Suppl. 5), 1–2.

American Speech-Language-Hearing Association. (1993). Guidelines for audiology services in the schools. *Asha, 35*(Suppl. 10), 24–32.

American Speech-Language-Hearing Association. (1994a). Clinical practice by certificate holders in the profession in which they are not certified. *Asha, 36*(Suppl. 13), 11.

American Speech-Language-Hearing Association. (1994b). Guidelines for fitting and monitoring FM systems. *Asha, 36*(Suppl. 12), 1–9.

American Speech-Language-Hearing Association. (1995). *ASHA desk reference for audiology and speech-language pathology,* II. Rockville, MD: Author.

American Speech-Language-Hearing Association. (1996). Central auditory processing: Current status of research and implications for clinical practice. *American Journal of Audiology, 5*(2), 41–54.

American Speech-Language-Hearing Association Task Force on Treatment Outcomes and Cost Effectiveness. (1994). *Functional communication measures and codes.* Rockville, MD: Author.

Americans with Disabilities Act of 1990, Public Law 101–336, 42, U.S.C. 12101 *et seq.: U.S. Statutes at Large, 104,* 327–378 (1991).

Anderson, K. (1989). *Screening instrument for targeting educational risk (S.I.F.T.E.R.).* Tampa, FL: Educational Audiology Association.

Anderson, K. (1991). Hearing conservation in the public schools revisited. *Seminars in Hearing, 12*(4), 340–364.

Anderson, K., & Matkin, N. (1996). *Screening instrument for targeting educational risk in preschool children (age 3–kindergarten) (Preschool S.I.F.T.E.R.).* Tampa, FL: Educational Audiology Association.

Anderson, K., & Smaldino, J. (1996). *Listening inventory for education (L.I.F.E.): An efficacy tool.* Tampa, FL: Educational Audiology Association.

Anderson, K., & Whalen, M. J. (1996). Qualifying as hard of hearing in the U.S. *Educational Audiology Monograph, 4,* 35–37.

Arkansas Department of Health. (1978). *Pediatric observation, testing and tallying system.* Little Rock, AR: Author.

Babbidge, H. (1965). *Education of the deaf: A report to the Secretary of Health, Education, and Welfare by his Advisory Committee of the Education of the Deaf.* Washington, DC: U.S. Department of Health, Education, and Welfare.

Bailey, D., & Simeonsson, R. (1988). *Family assessment in early intervention.* Columbus, OH: Merrill.

Baran, J., Musiek, F., & Gollegly, K. (1987, November). *Auditory duration pattern sequences in the assessment of CANS pathology.* Paper presented at the American Speech-Language-Hearing Association annual meeting, New Orleans, LA.

Beasley, D., Maki, J., & Orchik, D. (1976). Children's perception of time-compressed speech using two measures of speech discrimination. *Journal of Speech and Hearing Disorders, 41,* 216–225.

Bellis, T. (1995, May). *Central auditory processing disorders: Current perspectives.* Workshop presented in Denver, CO.

Benafield, N. (1990). *The effects of sound field amplification on the attending behaviors of speech and language-delayed preschool children.* Unpublished master's thesis, University of Arkansas at Little Rock.

Bench, J., & Bamford, J. (1979). *Speech-hearing tests and the spoken language of partially-hearing children.* New York: Academic Press.

Bench, J., Koval, A., & Bamford, J. (1979). The BKB (Bamford-Koval-Bench) sentence lists for partially-hearing children. *British Journal of Audiology, 13,* 108–112.

Berg, F. (1970). Educational audiology. In F. Berg & S. Fletcher (Eds.), *The hard of hearing child* (pp. 275–318). New York: Grune & Stratton.

Berg, F. (1976). The hard of hearing child and educational audiology. In F. Berg (Ed.), *Educational audiology: Hearing and speech management* (pp. 1–37). New York: Grune & Stratton.

Berlin, C. (1973). *Dichotic C-V test.* St. Louis: Auditec of St. Louis.

Berry, V. S. (1988). Classroom intervention strategies and resource materials for the auditorily handicapped child. In R. J. Roeser & M. P. Downs (Eds.), *Auditory disorders in school children* (pp. 325–349). New York: Thieme Medical Publishers.

Bess, F. H. (1985). The minimally hearing–impaired child. *Ear and Hearing, 6,* 43–47.

Bess, F. H., Klee, T., & Culbertson, J. L. (1986). Identification, assessment and management of children with unilateral sensorineural hearing loss. *Ear and Hearing, 7,* 43–51.

Blair, J. C. (1976). *The contributing influences of amplification, speechreading, and classroom environments on the ability of hard of hearing children to discriminate sentences.* Unpublished doctoral dissertation, Northwestern University, Evanston, IL.

Blair, J. C. (1986). Assessing the hearing impaired. In F. S. Berg, J. C. Blair, S. H. Viehweg, & A. Wilson-Vlotman (Eds.), *Educational audiology for the hard of hearing child* (pp. 37–80). Orlando, FL: Grune & Stratton.

Blair, J. (1991). Educational audiology and methods for bringing about change in schools. *Seminars in Hearing, 12*(4), 318–328.

Blair, J., EuDaly, M., & Von Almen, P. (1993, November). *The effectiveness of communication used by audiologists with classroom teachers.* Paper presented at the meeting of the American Speech-Language-Hearing Association, Anaheim, CA.

Blair, J. C., Wilson-Vlotman, A., & Von Almen, P. (1989). Educational audiologists: Practices, problems, directions, recommendations. *Educational Audiology Monograph, 1,* 1–14.

Blake, P. E., & Hall, J. W. (1990). The status of state-wide policies for neonatal hearing screening. *Journal of the American Academy of Audiology, 1,* 67–74.

Bluestone, C. D., Fria, T. J., Arjona, S. K., Casselbrant, M. L., Schwartz, D. M., Ruben, R. J., Gates, G. A., Downs, M. P., Northern, J. L., Jerger, J. F., Paradise, J. L., Bess, F. H., Kenworthy, O. T., & Rogers, K.D. (1986). Controversies in screening for middle ear disease and hearing loss in children. *Pediatrics, 77,* 57–70.

Bollela-Sample, K. A. (1994). Practicing "seat-of-the-pants" audiology in New York City. *Advance for Speech–Language Pathologists and Audiologists, 4,* 18.

Boothroyd, A. (1987). CASPER: Computer assisted speech perception evaluation and training. In *Proceedings of the 10th Annual Conference on Rehabilitative Technology* (pp. 734–736). Washington, DC: Association for Advancement of Rehabilitative Technology.

Boothroyd, A. (1992). The FM wireless link. In M. Ross (Ed.), *FM auditory training systems: Characteristics, selection, and use* (pp. 1–19). Timonium, MD: York Press.

Brundage, D., Keane, R., & Makneson, R. (1993). Implications of learning theory to the instruction of adults. In T. Barer-Stein & J. A. Draper (Eds.), *The craft of teaching adults* (pp. 131–145). Toronto, Canada: Culture Concepts.

Carrow-Woolfolk, E. (1985). *Test of auditory comprehension of language—revised.* Chicago: Riverside Publishing Company.

Chermak, G. D. (1992, July). *Beyond diagnosis: Strategies and techniques for management of central auditory processing disorders across the lifespan.* Presentation given at Institute for Management of the Communicatively Handicapped, Logan, UT.

Chermak, G. D., & Musiek, F. E. (1992). Managing central auditory processing disorders in children and youth. *American Journal of Audiology, 1*(3), 61–65.

Cherry, R. (1980). *Selective auditory attention test (SAAT).* St. Louis, MO: Auditec of St. Louis.

Colorado Department of Education. (1995). *RESOURCES for families of children with hearing loss in Colorado.* Denver, CO: Author.

Colorado Department of Education. (1996a). *Central auditory processing disorders: A team approach to screening, assessment, and intervention practices.* Denver, CO: Author.

Colorado Department of Education. (1996b). *Planning and preparing quality individual education programs.* Denver, CO: Author.

Commission on Education of the Deaf. (1988). *Toward equality: Education of the deaf.* Washington, DC: U.S. Government Printing Office.

Consensus Panel on Support Personnel in Audiology. (1997). *Position statement and guidelines of the consensus panel on support personnel in audiology.* Unpublished manuscript.

Council of Organizational Representatives. (1992). *COR bill of rights for children who are deaf and hard-of-hearing.* Unpublished manuscript.

Crandell, C. (1991). Classroom acoustics for normal-hearing children: Implications for rehabilitation. *Educational Audiology Monograph, 2,* 18–38.

Crandell, C. (1996). The effects of sound-field FM amplification on the speech perception of ESL children. *Educational Audiology Monograph, 4,* 1–5.

Diefendorf, A. (1988). Pediatric audiology. In J. Lass, L. McReynolds, J. Northern, & D. Yoder (Eds.), *Handbook of speech-language pathology and audiology* (pp. 1315–1338). Toronto, Canada: B. C. Decker.

DiSimoni, F. (1978). *The token test for children.* Boston: Teaching Resources Corporation.

Downs, M. P. (1988). Contribution of mild hearing loss to auditory learning problems. In R. J. Roeser & M. P. Downs (Eds.), *Auditory disorders in school children* (2nd ed., pp. 186–199). New York: Thieme Medical Publishers.

Dunn, L., & Dunn, L. (1981). *Peabody picture vocabulary test—revised.* Circle Pines, MN: American Guidance Service.

Education for All Handicapped Children Act of 1975, Public Law 94–142, 20, U.S.C. 1401–1461: *U.S. Statutes at Large, 89,* 773–779 (1975).

Education of the Handicapped Amendments of 1974, Public Law 93–380.

Education of the Handicapped Act Amendments of 1986, Public Law 99–457, 20, U.S.C. 1400 *et seq.: U.S. Statutes at Large, 100,* 1145–1177 (1986).

Educational Audiology Association. (1994). Minimum competencies for educational audiologists. *Educational Audiology Association Newsletter, 11*(4), 7.

Edwards, C. (1991). Assessment and management of listening skills in school–aged children. *Seminars in Hearing, 12*(4), 389–401.

Elfenbein, J. (1992). Coping with communication breakdown: A program of strategy development for children who have hearing losses. *American Journal of Audiology, 1,* 25–29.

Elfenbein, J. (1993). *Developing communication strategies.* Iowa City, IA: University of Iowa.

Elliot, L., & Katz, D. (1980). *Development of a new children's test of speech discrimination.* St. Louis, MO: Auditec of St. Louis.

English, K. M. (1995). *Educational audiology across the life-span.* Baltimore: Paul H. Brookes.

English, K. M. (1996). Marketing tips: When you provide a HC program, tell someone! *Educational Audiology Association Newsletter, 13,* 7.

Erber, N. (1980). Use of the auditory numbers test to evaluate speech perception abilities of children who are hearing impaired. *Journal of Speech and Hearing Disorders, 45*(4), 527–532.

Erber, N. (1982). *Auditory training.* Washington, DC: Alexander Graham Bell Association for the Deaf.

Erber, N., & Alencewicz, A. (1976). Audiologic evaluation of deaf children. *Journal of Speech and Hearing Disorders, 41*(2), 256–267.

Ferre, J., & Wilber, L. (1986). Normal and learning disabled children's central auditory processing skills: An experimental test battery. *Ear and Hearing, 7,* 336–343.

Fifer, R., Jerger, J., Berlin, C., Tobey, E., & Campbell, J. (1983). Development of a dichotic sentence identification test for hearing impaired adults. *Ear and Hearing, 4,* 300–305.

Finitzo–Hieber, T., Matkin, N., Cherow-Skalka, E., & Gerling, I. (1977). *Sound effects recognition test.* St. Louis, MO: Auditec of St. Louis.

Firszt, J., & Reeder, R. (1996). *Classroom goals: Guide for optimizing auditory learning skills.* Washington, DC: Alexander Graham Bell Association for the Deaf.

Fisher, L. I. (1985). Learning disabilities and auditory processing. In R. J. Van Hattam (Ed.), *Administration of speech language services in schools: A manual* (pp. 231–290). San Diego, CA: College-Hill Press.

Flexer, C., Millin, J., & Brown, L. (1990). Children with developmental disabilities: The effects of sound field amplification on word identification. *Language, Speech, and Hearing Services in Schools, 21,* 177–182.

Flowers, A., & Costello, R. (1970). *Flowers-Costello test of central auditory abilities.* Dearborn, MI: Perceptual Learning Systems.

Fuchs, D., & Fuchs, L. (1994). Inclusive schools movement and the radicalization of special education reform. *Exceptional Children, 60*(4), 294–309.

Gantz, B., Tyler, R., Woodworth, G., Tye-Murray, N., & Fryauf-Bertschy, H. (1994). Results of multichannel cochlear implants in congenital and acquired prelingual deafness in children: Five-year follow-up. *The American Journal of Otology, 15*(Suppl. 2), 1–8.

Gardner, M. F. (1985). *Test of auditory-perceptual skills.* Burlingame, CA: Psychological and Educational Publications, Inc.

Gardner, M. F. (1990). *Expressive one-word picture vocabulary test—revised.* Oceanside, CA: Academic Communication Associates.

Geers, A., & Moog, J. (Eds.) (1994). The effectiveness of cochlear implants and tactile aids for deaf children: A report of the CID sensory aids study. *Volta Review Monograph, 96*(5). Washington, DC: Alexander Graham Bell Association for the Deaf.

Gillet, P. (1993). *Auditory processes.* Novato, CA: Academic Therapy Publications.

Gitlin, R. (1995). Custom device "intercepts" crowd noise. *Hearing Instruments, 46,* 16–18.

Goldman, R., Fristoe, M., & Woodcock, R. (1974a). *Goldman-Fristoe-Woodcock auditory skills test battery.* Circle Pines, MN: American Guidance Service.

Goldman, R., Fristoe, M., & Woodcock, R. (1974b). *Goldman-Fristoe-Woodcock test of auditory discrimination.* Circle Pines, MN: American Guidance Service.

Greenblatt, H., & Daar, L. (1994). A support program: Audiological counseling. *Language, Speech, and Hearing Services in Schools, 25,* 112–114.

Haley, J. (1976). *Problem solving therapy.* New York: Harper Colomon Books.

Hall, J. W., Baer, J. E., Byrn, A., Wurm, F. C., Henry, M. M., Wilson, D. S., & Prentice, C. H. (1993). Audiologic assessment and management of central auditory processing disorder (CAPD). *Seminars in Hearing, 14*(3), 254–264.

Hall, J., & Santucci, M. (1995). Protecting the professional ear: Conservation strategies and devices. *The Hearing Journal, 48,* 37–45.

Hammill, D. (1985). *Detroit tests of learning aptitude* (2nd ed.). Austin, TX: Pro–Ed.

Hammill, D., & Newcomer, P. (1988). *Tests of language development—2.* San Antonio, TX: The Psychological Corporation.

Hampton, D. (1992). Internal marketing for the established audiology practice. *American Journal of Audiology, 1,* 57–60.

Hanin, L., & Adams, S. (1996, April). *Use of soundfield FM amplification with cochlear implants.* Paper presented at the annual convention of the American Academy of Audiology, Salt Lake City, UT.

Haskins, H. A. (1949). *A phonetically balanced test of speech discrimination for children.* Unpublished master's thesis, Northwestern University, Evanston, IL.

Hawkins, D. (1984). Comparisons of speech recognition in noise by mildly to moderately hearing impaired children using hearing aids and FM systems. *Journal of Speech and Hearing Disorders, 49*(4), 409–418.

Hendrich Hudson School District Board of Education v. Rowley (1982). 102 S. Ct. 3034.

Hirsh, I. J., Davis, H., Silverman, S. R., Reynolds, E. G., Eldert, E., & Bensen, R. W. (1952). Development of materials for speech audiometry. *Journal of Speech and Hearing Disorders, 17,* 321–337.

Individuals with Disabilities Education Act of 1990 (IDEA), Public Law 101–476, 20, U.S.C. 1400 *et seq.: U.S. Statutes at Large, 104,* 1103–1151 (1990).

Jerger, J., & Jerger, S. (1974). Auditory findings in brainstem disorders. *Archives of Otolaryngology, 99,* 342–349.

Jerger, S. (1987). Validation of the pediatric speech intelligibility test in children with central auditory system lesions. *Audiology, 26,* 298–311.

Jerger, S., & Jerger, J. (1984). *Pediatric speech intelligibility test: Manual for administration.* St. Louis, MO: Auditec of St. Louis.

Johnson, C. D. (1991). The "state" of educational audiology: Survey results and goals for the future. *Educational Audiology Monograph, 2,* 71–80.

Johnson, C. D., & Rees, K. (1995). Amplification options for infants and toddlers. *Seminars in Hearing, 16*(2), 140–150.

Johnson, C. D., & Von Almen, P. (1993, April). *Assessing speech recognition using a functional listening paradigm.* Paper presented at the meeting of the American Academy of Audiology, Phoenix, AZ.

Johnson, C. D., & Von Almen, P. (1993, November). *Beyond the soundbooth: Using a functional listening paradigm.* Paper presented at the annual convention of the American Speech-Language-Hearing Association, Anaheim, CA.

Johnson, R., & Cohen, O. (Eds.). (1994). *Implications and complications for deaf students of the full inclusion movement.* Washington, DC: Gallaudet Research Institute.

Joint Committee on Infant Hearing. (1994). Joint Committee on Infant Hearing 1994 position statement. *Audiology Today, 6*(6), 6–9.

Kalikow, D. N., Stevens, K. N., & Elliott, L. L. (1977). Development of a test of speech intelligibility in noise using sentence materials with controlled word predictability. *Journal of Acoustical Society of America, 61,* 1337–1351.

Katz, J. (1962). The use of staggered spondaic words for assessing the integrity of the central auditory system. *Journal of Auditory Research, 2,* 327–337.

Katz, J. (1983). Phonemic synthesis. In E. Lasky & J. Katz (Eds.), *Central auditory processing disorders: Problems of speech, language, and learning* (pp. 269–295). Baltimore: University Park Press.

Katz, J., Kushner, D., & Pack, G. (1975, November). *The use of competing speech (SSW) and environmental sounds (CES) tests for localizing brain lesions.* Poster presented at the American Speech-Language-Hearing Association annual meeting, Washington, DC.

Keith, R. (1986). *SCAN: A screening test for auditory processing disorders.* San Diego, CA: The Psychological Corporation.

Keith, R. (1988). Tests of central auditory function. In R. J. Roeser & M. P. Downs (Eds.), *Auditory disorders in school children* (2nd ed., pp. 83–97). New York: Thieme Medical Publishers, Inc.

Keith, R. (1993). *SCAN-A: A test for auditory processing disorders in adolescents and adults.* San Diego, CA: The Psychological Corporation.

Keith, R. (1994). *Auditory continuous performance test.* San Diego, CA: The Psychological Corporation.

Kemp, R. J., Roeser, R. J., Pearson, D., & Ballachanda, B. (1995). *Infection control for the professions of audiology and speech–language pathology.* San Diego, CA: Singular Publishing Group.

Kenworthy, O. T., Klee, T., & Tharpe, A. (1990). Speech recognition ability of children with unilateral sensorineural hearing loss as a function of amplification, speech stimuli and listening condition. *Ear and Hearing, 11*(4), 264–270.

Kirk, S., McCarthy, J., & Kirk, W. (1968). *Illinois test of psycholinguistic abilities* (rev. ed.). Urbana: University of Illinois Press.

Koppitz, E. M. (1975). Bender gestalt test, visual aural digit span test and reading achievement. *Journal of Learning Disabilities, 8*(3), 32–35.

Lankford, J., & West, D. (1993). A study of noise exposure and hearing sensitivity in a high school woodworking class. *Language, Speech, and Hearing Services in Schools, 24,* 167–173.

Lewis, D. (1994). Assistive devices for classroom listening. *American Journal of Audiology, 3*(1), 58–69.

Lindamood, C. H., & Lindamood, P. C. (1975). *Lindamood auditory conceptualization (LAC) test.* Allen, TX: Developmental Learning Materials.

Ling, D., & Ling, A. (1978). *Aural habilitation: The foundations of verbal learning in hearing–impaired children.* Washington, DC: The Alexander Graham Bell Association for the Deaf.

Lipscomb, M., Von Almen, P., & Blair, J. (1992). Students as active participants in hearing aid maintenance. *Language, Speech, and Hearing Services in Schools, 23,* 208–213.

Madell, J. R. (1992). FM systems as primary amplification for children with profound hearing loss. *Ear and Hearing, 13*(2), 102–107.

Marttila, J. (1994). For your students' information. *EAA Newsletter, 11,* 14.

Marttila, J., & Mills, M. (1993). *Knowledge is power.* Bettendorf, IA: Mississippi Bend Area Educational Agency.

Matkin, N. (1994). *Key considerations in the provision of family centered services.* Paper presented at the Colorado State Symposium on Deafness, Colorado Springs, CO.

Mauk, G. W., White, K. R., Mortensen, L. B., & Behrens, T. R. (1991). The effectiveness of screening programs based on high–risk characteristics in early identification of hearing impairment. *Ear and Hearing, 12,* 312–319.

Maxon, A. B., & Smaldino, J. (1991). Hearing aid management in children. *Seminars in Hearing, 12*(4), 365–379.

McCroskey, R. (1984a). *Wichita auditory fusion test.* Tulsa, OK: Modern Education Corp.

McCroskey, R. (1984b). *Wichita auditory processing test.* Tulsa, OK: Modern Education Corp.

Medwetsky, L. (1994). Educational audiology. In J. Katz (Ed.), *Handbook of clinical audiology* (4th ed., pp. 503–518). Baltimore: Williams & Wilkins.

Meyen, E. (1978). An introductory perspective. In E. Meyen (Ed.), *Exceptional children and youth: An introduction* (pp. 2–84). Denver, CO: Love Publishing Co.

Moog, J., & Geers, A. (1990). *Early speech perception test (ESP).* St. Louis, MO: Central Institute for the Deaf.

Moore, J. R. (1988). Guidelines concerning adult learning. *Journal of Staff Development, 9,* 1–4.

Moore, J., Wilson, W., & Thompson, G. (1977). Visual reinforcement of head-turn responses in infants under twelve months of age. *Journal of Speech and Hearing Disorders, 42,* 328–334.

Morlock, G. (1995). Calling all teachers . . . and calling all students! *Volta Voices, 2,* 26–27.

Mueller, G., & Killion, M. (1990). The count–the–dot audiogram for calculation of the articulation index. *The Hearing Journal, 43*(9), 15.

Musiek, F. (1983). Assessment of central auditory dysfunction: The dichotic digits test revisited. *Ear and Hearing, 4,* 79–83.

National Association of State Directors of Special Education (NASDSE). (1991). Section 504 of the Rehabilitation Act of 1973; Old problems and emerging issues for public schools. *LIAISON Bulletin, 17,* 8.

National Commission on Excellence in Education. (1983). *A nation at risk: The imperative for educational reform.* Washington, DC: U.S. Government Printing Office.

National Institutes of Health. (1993). Early identification of hearing impairment in infants and young children. *NIH Consensus Statement, 11*(1), 1–24.

National Institutes of Health. (1995). Cochlear implants in adults and children. *NIH Consensus Statement, 13*(2), 1–30.

Nobelpharma. (1993). Bone anchored applications. *Nobelpharma International Updates 2*(1).

Occupational Safety and Health Administration. (March 8, 1983). Rules and regulations, Department of Labor, Occupational Safety and Health Administration, 29 CFR 1910.95, Occupational noise exposure; Hearing conservation amendment; Final rule. *Federal Register, 48,* 46.

Office of Los Angeles County Superintendent of Schools. (1976). *Test of auditory comprehension.* North Hollywood, CA: Foreworks.

Olsen, W., Hawkins, D., & Van Tassell, D. (1987). Representation of long-term spectra of speech. *Ear and Hearing, 8*(5 Suppl.), 100S–108S.

Owens, E., Kessler, D., Raggio, M., & Schubert, E. (1985). *The minimal auditory capabilities battery.* St. Louis, MO: Auditec of St. Louis.

Oyler, R. F., Oyler, A. L., & Matkin, N. D. (1988). Unilateral hearing loss: Demographics and educational impact. *Language, Speech, and Hearing Services in Schools, 19,* 201–210.

The Pediatric Working Group of the Conference on Amplification for Children with Auditory Deficits. (1996). Amplification for infants and children with hearing loss. *American Journal of Audiology, 5*(1), 53–68.

Phonic Ear, Inc. (1993). *Phonic Ear frequency reference chart.* Petaluma, CA: Phonic Ear, Inc.

Pinheiro, M. (1978). Central auditory test profile in children with learning disabilities. In L. Bradford (Ed.), *Communication disorders: An audio journal for continuing education* (Vol. 3). New York: Grune & Stratton.

Regional Research Institute for Human Services, Research and Training Center. (1988). *Focal Point, 2*(2). Portland, OR: Portland State University.

Rehabilitation Act of 1973, Section 504, 29, U.S.C. 794 *U.S. Statutes at Large, 87,* 335– 394 (1973).

Robbins, A., Svirsky, M., & Kirk, K. (1996, February). *Implanted children can speak, but can they communicate?* Paper presented at the Sixth Annual Symposium on Cochlear Implants in Children, Miami, FL.

Rose, D. E. (1994). Cochlear implants in children with prelingual deafness: Another side of the coin. *American Journal of Audiology, 3*(1), 6.

Rosenberg, G., & Blake-Rahter, P. (1995). Sound-field amplification: A review of the literature. In C. Crandell, J. Smaldino, & C. Flexer (Eds.), *Sound-field FM amplification: Theory and practical applications* (pp. 107–123). San Diego, CA; Singular Publishing Group.

Ross, M., Brackett, D., & Maxon, A. B. (1991). Communication assessment. In *Assessment and management of mainstreamed hearing-impaired children* (pp. 113–139). Austin, TX: Pro–Ed.

Ross, M., & Lerman, J. (1970). A picture identification test for hearing impaired children. *Journal of Speech and Hearing Research, 5,* 44–72.

Ross, M., & Randolph, K. (1988). *The auditory perception of alphabet letters.* St. Louis, MO: Auditec of St. Louis.

Roush, J. (1992). Screening school-age children. In F. H. Bess & J. W. Hall (Eds.), *Screening children for auditory function* (pp. 297–313). Nashville, TN: Bill Wilkerson Center Press.

Ruberry, J., & Yoshinaga-Itano, C. (1993). *Colorado individual performance profile (CIPP) for deaf and hearing-impaired students.* Denver, CO: Colorado Department of Education.

Schum, R., & Gfeller, K. (1994). Requisites for conversation: Engendering social skills. In N. Tye-Murray (Ed.), *Let's converse* (pp. 147–176). Washington, DC: Alexander Graham Bell Association for the Deaf.

Seaton, J. B. (1991). Educational audiology: Integrating community-based and school-based audiology services. *Audiology Today, 3,* 21–23.

Seaton, J., Von Almen, P., & Blair, J. C. (1994). Autonomy of audiologists in educational settings. *Journal of the American Academy of Audiology, 5,* 412–416.

Seewald, R., Ramji, K., Sinclair, S., Moodoe, K., & Jamieson, D. (1993). *Computer-assisted implementation of the desired sensation level method for electroacoustic selection and fitting in children: User's manual.* London, Canada: University of Western Ontario.

Semel, E., Wiig, E., & Secord, W. (1987). *Clinical evaluation of language fundamentals—revised.* San Antonio, TX: The Psychological Corporation.

Smaldino, J., & Crandell, C. (1995). Acoustic measurements in classroom. In C. Crandell, J. Smaldino, & C. Flexer (Eds.), *Sound-field FM amplification: Theory and practical applications* (pp. 69–81). San Diego, CA: Singular Publishing Group.

Smoski, W. (1990). Use of CHAPPS in a children's audiology clinic. *Ear and Hearing, 11*(5 Suppl.), 53S–56S.

Stone, P. (1988). *Blueprint for developing communication competence: A planning instructional model with detailed scenarios.* Washington, DC: Alexander Graham Bell Association for the Deaf.

Stout, G., & Windle, J. V. (1992). *Developmental approach to successful listening II.* Englewood, CO: Resource Point.

Sweetow, R., & Reddell, R. (1978). The use of masking level differences in the identification of children with perceptual problems. *The Journal of the American Audiology Society, 4,* 52–56.

Thompson, G., & Folsom, R. (1984). A comparison of two conditioning procedures in the use of visual reinforcement audiometry (VRA). *Journal of Speech and Hearing Disorders, 49,* 241–245.

Tillman T. W., & Carhart, R. (1966). *An expanded test for speech discrimination utilizing CNC monosyllabic words.* (Northwestern University Auditory Test No. 6, Technical Report No. SAM–TR–66–55). Brooks Air Force Base, TX: USAF School of Aerospace Medicine.

Tsantis, L., & Keefe, D. (1996). Reinventing education. *Asha, 38,* 38–41.

Tye-Murray, N. (Ed.). (1994). *Let's converse: A how-to guide to develop and expand conversational skills of children and teenagers who are hearing impaired.* Washington, DC: Alexander Graham Bell Association for the Deaf.

Tye-Murray, N., & Woodworth, G. (1995). Acquisition of speech by children who have prolonged cochlear implant experience. *Journal of Speech and Hearing Research, 38*(1), 1–11.

U.S. Congress. Technology-related assistance for individuals with disabilities act of 1988. PL 100-407.

U.S. Department of Education. (September 29, 1992). Assistance to states for the education of children with disabilities program and preschool grants for children with disabilities; Final rule (34 CFR Parts 300 and 301). *Federal Register, 57,* 189.

U.S. Department of Education. (October 30, 1992). Deaf students education services; Policy guidance; Notices. *Federal Register (Part VI), 57,* 211.

U.S. Department of Education. (July 30, 1993). Early intervention program for infants and toddlers with disabilities; Final rule (34 CFR Part 303). *Federal Register, 58,* 145.

U. S. Department of Education. (1994a). *Goals 2000: Educate America Act.* Washington, DC: Author.

U.S. Department of Education. (1994b). *Sixteenth annual report to Congress on the implementation of the individuals with disabilities education act.* Washington, DC: U.S. Government Printing Office.

U.S. Department of Education. (1995). *Seventeenth annual report to Congress on the implementation of the individuals with disabilities education act.* Washington, DC: U.S. Government Printing Office.

U.S. Department of Health, Education, and Welfare. (August 23, 1977). Rules and regulations for the administration of the education for all handicapped children act. *Federal Register (Part IV), 42,* 163.

VanDyke, L. (1985). Evaluation of classroom listening behavior. *Rocky Mountain Journal of Communication Disorders, 1.*

Ventry, I. (Ed.). (1965). *Audiology and education of the deaf.* Washington, DC: Joint Committee on Audiology and Education of the Deaf.

Von Almen, P., Blair, J., & Spriet, S. (1990). Central auditory assessment. *Educational Audiology Newsletter, 7*(2), 10–11.

Waltzman, S., Cohen, N., Gomolin, R., Shapiro, W., Ozdamar, S., & Hoffman, R. (1994). Long-term results of early cochlear implantation in congenitally and prelingually deafened children. *The American Journal of Otology, 15*(Suppl. 2), 9–14.

Watkins, S. (Ed.). (1993). *Graphics to accompany the SKI*HI resource manual.* Logan, UT: H.O.P.E., Inc.

Weber, S., & Reddell, R. C. (1976). A sentence test for measuring speech discrimination in children. *Audiology and Hearing Education, 2*(30), 25–31.

Weintraub, F., Abeson, A., Ballard, J., & LaVor, M. (Eds.). (1976). *Public policy and the education of exceptional children* (p. 103). Reston, VA: The Council for Exceptional Children.

Wepman, J. (1973). *Wepman auditory discrimination test.* Los Angeles: Western Psychological Services.

Wepman, J., & Morency, A. (1973). *The auditory sequential memory test.* Los Angeles: Western Psychological Services.

Wiig, E., & Secord, W. (1989). *Test of language competence—expanded edition.* San Antonio, TX: The Psychological Corporation.

Wiig, E., & Secord, W. (1992). *Test of word knowledge.* San Antonio, TX: The Psychological Corporation.

Willeford, J. (1977). Assessing central auditory behavior in children: A test battery approach. In R. Keith (Ed.), *Central auditory dysfunction* (pp. 43–72). New York: Grune & Stratton.

Wilson-Vlotman, A., & Blair, J. C. (1986). A survey of audiologists working full-time in school systems. *Asha, 28*(11), 33–38.

Ying, E. (1990). Speech and language assessment: Communication evaluation. In M. Ross (Ed.), *Hearing-impaired children in the mainstream* (pp. 45–60). Parkton, MD: York Press.

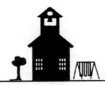

INDEX